Interdisciplinary Approaches to Game Design in Healthcare and Education

David Bonilla Carranza
https://orcid.org/0000-0002-8690-4865
Universidad de Guadalajara, Mexico

Adriana Peña Pérez Negrón
https://orcid.org/0000-0001-6823-2367
Universidad de Guadalajara, Mexico

Marco Pérez-Cisneros
https://orcid.org/0000-0001-6493-0408
Universidad de Guadalajara, Mexico

IGI Global
Scientific Publishing
Publishing Tomorrow's Research Today

Vice President of Editorial Melissa Wagner
Director of Acquisitions Mikaela Felty
Director of Book Development Jocelynn Hessler
Production Manager Mike Brehm
Cover Design Jose Rosado

Published in the United States of America by
IGI Global Scientific Publishing
701 East Chocolate Avenue
Hershey, PA, 17033, USA
Tel: 717-533-8845 | Fax: 717-533-7115
Website: https://www.igi-global.com E-mail: cust@igi-global.com

Library of Congress Cataloging-in-Publication Data

Names: Bonilla Carranza, David editor | Peña Pérez Negrón, Adriana, 1961- editor | Pérez-Cisneros, Marco editor

Title: Interdisciplinary approaches to game design in healthcare and education / edited by David Bonilla Carranza, Adriana Peña Pérez Negrón, Marco Pérez-Cisneros.

Description: Hershey, PA : IGI Global Scientific Publishing, 2026. | Includes bibliographical references and index. | Summary: "This book aims to establish a comprehensive framework for understanding how game design bridges education and healthcare"-- Provided by publisher.

Identifiers: LCCN 2025042007 (print) | LCCN 2025042008 (ebook) | ISBN 9798337346571 hardcover | ISBN 9798337346588 paperback | ISBN 9798337346595 ebook

Subjects: LCSH: Video games in education--Case studies | Video games--Psychological aspects--Case studies | Video games--Physiological aspects--Case studies

Classification: LCC LB1028.75 .I583 (print) | LCC LB1028.75 (ebook) | DDC 794.8--dc23/eng/20260122

LC record available at https://lccn.loc.gov/2025042007

LC ebook record available at https://lccn.loc.gov/2025042008

British Cataloguing in Publication Data

A Cataloguing in Publication record for this book is available from the British Library.

Table of Contents

Detailed Table of Contents

The high school Regional of Ixtlahuacan de los Membrillos belongs to the Higher Middle Education System of the University of Guadalajara, it is located in a suburban town, specifically Capilla-Atequiza road, close to the Metropolitan Area of Guadalajara, approximately 40 km away. It is worth mentioning that in Mexico, Guadalajara acquires great importance in educational, economic, political, social issues, among others. Interested in contributing to the excellent academic training of young people at a national and international level, the University of Guadalajara contributes with human capital, infrastructure and other essential processes in education. For this purpose, the Higher Secondary Education System was created in 1984, which of course carries out teaching, research and dissemination functions at this level. Its schools are distributed throughout the state of Jalisco.

The rapid digital transformation of higher education demands innovative strategies to address the growing challenges of cybersecurity. Universities must prepare students not only with technical skills but also with the ability to act responsibly in interconnected digital environments. Gamification has emerged as a powerful pedagogical approach to engage learners, foster motivation, and translate complex concepts into meaningful experiences. This chapter introduces a gamified learning platform designed to raise cybersecurity awareness and promote digital responsibility among university students. The platform integrates interactive scenarios, self-assessment tools, and educational games to develop essential skills such as critical thinking, decision-making, and ethical digital behavior. Early results suggest its potential to strengthen students' understanding of digital risks and encourage safer online practices. Future iterations envision adaptive content, AI-driven personalization, and advanced analytics to enhance impact.

This chapter explores the intersection of gamification, culturally responsive pedagogy, and professional Spanish instruction within a Doctor of Occupational Therapy program at a U.S.–Mexico border university. Focusing on instructors' perspectives, it examines how interdisciplinary collaboration between language educators and occupational therapy faculty can enhance students' linguistic, cultural, and clinical competencies. Observations reveal how these approaches fostered student engagement, rapid thinking, peer support, and confidence in using Spanish in professional contexts. By integrating cultural responsiveness and authentic language practice, the courses modeled a replicable framework for preparing healthcare professionals to deliver equitable, high-quality care to Spanish-speaking populations. Findings suggest that gamification and interdisciplinary course design can serve as effective strategies for bridging language learning, cultural competence, and clinical readiness in health education.

This work proposes a methodology based on STEM, game-based learning, and gamification to develop a game that strengthens the teaching of programming at the university level. This game considers the programming languages C, C++, and Python, each with levels of difficulty, feedback, and global report generation. In this project, quality tests were applied to the use of the game, based on the ISO/IEC 25022 standard. The tests consisted of completing a task (effectiveness), measuring the task time (efficiency), and determining the proportion of users with complaints (satisfaction). The results show that out of ten participants, eight rated the user experience positively and others rated it as attractive, fun, and interesting. On average, it took 45 seconds to complete a basic level for C++. An interview was conducted to identify opportunities for improvement in this game, particularly in terms of the graphical interface, and to ensure that it meets the requirements for sharing this game on the GameMaker platform.

This chapter presents a conceptual proposal for an educational video game, Macromolecules in Play, designed to connect polymer structures and their material properties. Instead of learning through static formulas, players apply polymer properties—such as adhesion, thermal resistance, and elasticity—to navigate challenges. Each gameplay choice is directly linked to molecular principles; for example, players learn that increasing crosslinking enhances thermal stability but reduces flexibility. The game's design emphasizes the critical concept of "trade-offs," compelling players to balance competing properties for optimal solutions. By embedding these concepts into interactive mechanics, abstract chemical knowledge becomes a tangible experience. Grounded in research on gamification, this work illustrates how interactive tools can enrich teaching in chemistry, materials science, and engineering.

Gamification uses elements like stars, shields, and avatars to boost motivation, engagement, and active learning in primary education. It proved vital during the pandemic for remote learning and aligns with Sustainable Development Goals by helping reduce the educational gap. Its key benefits include fostering motivation through immediate feedback, strengthening emotional development and self-esteem

and dissolution—essential for ensuring drug efficacy, quality and safety. To address this challenge, BioSimuLab was developed as a pedagogical simulator that reproduces dissolution processes in accordance with NOM-177-SSA1, generating simulated data for reference and test drugs. This tool enables the analysis of dissolution profiles, application of statistical reasoning, and evaluation of bioequivalence through parameters such as the similarity factor (f_2) and linear regression. By promoting discovery-based learning and evidence-driven decision-making, BioSimuLab enhances analytical, technical, and interpretive skills, strengthens understanding of pharmacokinetic principles, and bridges the gap between theory and professional practice in pharmaceutical sciences, aligning educational outcomes with professional competencies.

Immersive maze-based memory tasks in virtual reality represent a novel intersection between game design and neuroscience, providing controlled yet ecologically valid environments for investigating spatial memory, navigation strategies, and executive functions. This chapter explores how VR-based adaptations of classical paradigms (radial arm, Morris water, and floor mazes) enable dynamic manipulation of environmental complexity, multisensory cues, and cognitive load. By integrating principles of serious game design, these immersive tasks enhance engagement and motivation while preserving experimental rigor, allowing researchers to evaluate hippocampal-dependent learning and memory consolidation. Evidence from experimental and clinical studies demonstrates VR's potential for early detection of cognitive decline, rehabilitation of spatial deficits, and personalized cognitive training. Bridging interactive game mechanics with neuroscientific inquiry, this work highlights VR as a transformative platform for translational research and next-generation neurorehabilitation.

This chapter presents a longitudinal case study on the integration of generative artificial intelligence (AI), specifically Large Language Models (LLMs), into the teaching of cryptography at the undergraduate level. Conducted over eight academic terms at the Universidad de Guadalajara, the study analyzes how LLM-driven activities—such as personalized explanations, automated problem generation, and cryptanalysis simulations—impacted student learning. The implementation of a standardized final examination beginning in 2024B enabled consistent cross-cohort comparisons. Results show an initial performance dip during the transition phase, followed by stabilization and improved consistency. The findings suggest that LLMs can serve as adaptive scaffolding tools, supporting diverse learners in mastering abstract technical content. The chapter also explores the ethical, legal, and pedagogical considerations of using AI in education, offering a replicable model for integrating generative AI into STEM curricula.

Molecules and Missions is a point-and-click strategy game that makes nanoscale science accessible through gamified learning. Set in a steampunk lab, players use virtual tools to explore cells, conduct experiments, and progress through campaigns. The chapter presents a citizen science proposal in which researchers can design downloadable content used so that players' results can be indicative of real

Preface

In recent years, game design has established itself as a powerful catalyst for innovation across multiple sectors, particularly in healthcare and education. As digital technologies advance and pedagogical approaches evolve, interactive systems—from gamified environments and serious games to mixed-reality simulations—are transforming how learners engage with complex concepts, develop practical skills, and sustain intrinsic motivation.

This edited volume emerges from this dynamic landscape, bringing together interdisciplinary perspectives that highlight the transformative potential of game-based methodologies. Its relevance extends beyond novelty or entertainment; it addresses urgent educational and societal needs. Healthcare professionals must navigate demanding clinical environments, students need to develop socio-emotional competencies, and educators must adapt to learners whose expectations are shaped by constant technological change. In this context, interdisciplinary thinking is no longer optional. Effective learning and professional development require collaboration among educators, engineers, clinicians, designers, cognitive scientists, and technologists. The chapters in this collection illustrate how these intersections generate creative, robust, and meaningful learning experiences.

We have prepared this book with the conviction that academic rigor can coexist with accessible, exploratory design. Each contribution demonstrates not only the theoretical foundations of gamification and game-based learning but also offers pragmatic strategies, empirical findings, and innovations applicable in real educational and healthcare contexts. Our goal is to provide researchers, practitioners, and students with a resource that bridges theory and practice while fostering a deeper understanding of the interdisciplinary nature of contemporary game design.

CHAPTER OVERVIEW

The book opens by exploring the role of gamification in emotional and psychological well-being. **Chapter 1** presents a teaching intervention model designed to support students experiencing stress, anxiety, or a lack of academic motivation. **Chapter 2** extends this focus to the high school level, examining how a gamified life-planning course fosters psycho-emotional development and academic engagement.

Chapters 3 and 4 examine the use of gamification in professional and disciplinary training. The former presents a university platform aimed at enhancing cybersecurity awareness and digital responsibility; the latter analyzes culturally responsive language teaching within a healthcare program, demonstrating how interdisciplinary collaboration strengthens clinical and cultural readiness.

A group of chapters focuses on game design for STEM fields. **Chapter 5** discusses the creation of an educational video game to support introductory programming instruction. **Chapter 6** proposes a conceptual game that helps students understand polymer structures and material properties through interactive challenges. Together, these chapters reflect how game mechanics can make abstract scientific principles accessible and intuitive.

Chapters 7 and 8 shift attention to early childhood and primary education. The seventh highlights how stars, shields, and avatars foster motivation and emotional development in young learners, while the eighth presents a participatory design case study for a literacy-focused serious game co-developed with teachers and children in Mexico.

The cognitive and neuroscientific dimensions of gameplay are addressed in **Chapter 9**, which examines how analog and digital games influence executive functioning, motivation, and neural processes. This exploration is extended in **Chapter 12**, which introduces Virtual Reality (VR) maze paradigms for researching spatial memory and cognitive performance.

The volume also showcases simulation and VR applications in clinical and professional training. **Chapter 10** explores a collaborative VR-based surgical training system for medical residents.

Finally, **Chapters 11, 13, and 14** highlight advanced technological integrations. Chapter 11 introduces a simulator aligned with national pharmaceutical standards for dissolution profile analysis. Chapter 12 examines a multi-term implementation of generative Artificial Intelligence for personalized learning in cryptography. **Chapter 14** concludes the volume with a gamified citizen-science platform that enables learners to explore nanoscale science and contribute to collaborative pharmaceutical innovation.

CONCLUSION

The works collected in this volume demonstrate that game design is far more than an instructional add-on; it is an emerging framework for cultivating agency, deepening understanding, and transforming educational and healthcare environments. Whether addressing emotional well-being, scientific reasoning, clinical decision-making, or early literacy, these chapters illustrate how interactive systems can support both the cognitive and affective dimensions of learning. This interdisciplinary field continues to grow as new tools, pedagogies, and collaborative models redefine how we teach and learn.

As editors, we are encouraged by the diversity of innovations represented here—from VR-based memory research and complex engineering simulations to culturally responsive language instruction and gamified emotional support systems. These contributions reaffirm that impactful game design requires the convergence of diverse perspectives—educational, clinical, technological, design, and research—demonstrating that interdisciplinarity is not merely beneficial but essential for addressing contemporary challenges in education and health.

We hope this volume serves as a valuable resource for scholars, practitioners, and students seeking to advance their understanding of game-based methodologies. Furthermore, we trust it will inspire readers to explore new collaborations, adopt creative strategies, and continue pushing the boundaries of what games and interactive systems can offer. The future of learning resides not in isolated disciplines, but in the rich intersections this book explores.

Chapter 1

Gamification for Student Mental Well-Being: A Teaching Intervention Model in the National Technology

Carmen Leticia Salcedo-Quevedo
https://orcid.org/0009-0008-8601-0969
Instituto Tecnológico Superior de Jalisco en Chapala, Mexico

Jesus Cabral-Araiza
https://orcid.org/0009-0006-9078-6044
Universidad de Guadalajara, Mexico

Madeleine Gabriela Contreras Davito
Universidad de Guadalajara, Mexico

Francisco Javier González Siordia
https://orcid.org/0009-0006-4883-986X
Instituto Tecnológico Superior de Jalisco en Chapala, Mexico

ABSTRACT

This chapter presents the development of a gamification proposal, whose methodological design aims to address one of the identified needs among students at the Tecnológico Superior de Jalisco, Chapala campus. This need is closely linked to the personal and academic consequences experienced by students when indicators of emotional health issues—such as anxiety, depression, and behaviors associated with procrastination—are identified or manifested. A key actor in fostering interest and engagement in the gamification process is the teacher, who guides students to approach this space as one that, among other core areas, seeks to provide orienta-

DOI: 10.4018/979-8-3373-4657-1.ch001

tion, emotional support, facilitate communication and trust, and, given its integral nature, incorporate functions such as biofeedback and practical tools to promote emotional well-being.

BACKGROUND AND CONTEXT

Mental health in higher education has become a critical challenge for the academic and personal development of students globally, a situation that has reached worrying dimensions in Mexico. Recent national studies confirm this crisis; the National Health and Nutrition Survey (ENSANUT) 2024 reveals that, in the population aged 10 to 19, the prevalence of depressive symptoms is 15.6%, while anxiety symptoms reach 30.1%. This problem is intensified in the university population, where academic pressure, the transition to adult life and socioeconomic factors act as significant triggers. The situation was exacerbated by the COVID-19 pandemic, after which there was an alarming increase of at least 200% in the demand for psychological and mental care in university centers such as the University of Guadalajara (UdeG-2023. June 27).

In the state of Jalisco, headquarters of the institution where this project is proposed to be piloted, the figures are especially serious. The prevalence of mental disorders affects 23.9% of the population, with anxiety (16%) and depression (4.4%) as the most common conditions. The Ciénega region, where the Chapala campus is located, has an even higher prevalence of 30%. Added to this situation is an alarming suicide rate that positions Jalisco in second place nationally, with cases registered in the municipality of Chapala during 2024, underscoring the urgent need for effective interventions. University students in the region are not oblivious to this reality, as it has been observed that 60% suffer from academic stress and there is a direct correlation between high levels of anxiety and poor school performance.

In addition to this, we must consider that the population of Upper Secondary Education will be five million 508 thousand 572 students for this cycle according to official figures (SEP-Bulletin 113, 2025). It is even worth noting the proximity to the number of secondary education students that in the state of Jalisco maintains similar figures according to the same SEP.

This mental health crisis faces two crucial systemic barriers. First, an insufficient traditional mental health infrastructure, particularly in rural and semi-urban areas, where access to professionals is limited and often stigmatized. Second, a persistent digital divide in access to the internet in homes; in Chapala, for example, only 39.6% of homes had this service in 2018. However, this gap coexists with a high penetration of mobile telephony. According to the Federal Telecommunications Institute (IFT-2024), in 2023, 90% of the rural population and 97% of the urban population in

Mexico are mobile phone users, and the smartphone is the main internet connection device for the vast majority of young people (IFT, 2024).

In addition to this statistical context, in the daily life of the Tecnológico Superior de Jalisco, Chapala Academic Unit, the academic body and the areas of psychopedagogical support have identified a growing concern about manifestations of stress, academic exhaustion (burnout) and anxiety among the student population, as well as the need to attend to isolated cases of depression and risk of suicidal behavior. Although there is no formal statistical diagnosis at the campus level, which reinforces the relevance of this project, these qualitative observations, recognized by the teaching and management community, are the driving force behind this proposal. The absence of a standardized method for early detection and referral underscores the urgency of implementing the technological intervention described here.

This panorama defines the problem to be solved: there is a critical need for mental health care for students of the Tecnológico Superior de Jalisco that can impact the entire community of the Tecnológico Nacional de México (TecNM), who face a high prevalence of anxiety and depression, but lack access to scalable support tools. and adapted to their digital context. The community of the Tecnológico Superior de Jalisco, Chapala campus, has explicitly recognized the urgency of having defined strategies and roles to mitigate this psycho-emotional deterioration. Therefore, the development of a gamified digital platform such as "Soul-Mind Hackers" directly addresses this problem, taking advantage of the high penetration of mobile devices to offer a preventive, training and channeling intervention that overcomes geographical and infrastructure barriers, being a first step towards a model applicable to the entire TecNM network.

Adolescence has been a concept that has been strongly hit by society by providing a conception with dark overtones, mainly sustained by rebellious and apathetic behaviors, which have helped to encourage the creation of repressive sanctioning measures, and even to limit access to certain rights. This results in the creation of conflictive relationships between adults and young people, a victim of social prejudice, and in turn, these stigmas work as a prophecy, causing the young people themselves to adopt these transgressive behaviors as a way of living their adolescence (Gutierrez, et. al., 2024).

The same study carried out by Gutierrez, et. al. (2024) in a group of adolescents highlighted the importance of mental health care and promotion in adolescents, since in the course of their intervention it was found that, thanks to the lack of knowledge of the symptoms of psychological distress, and the lack of tools acquired to cope with them, they react with fear and uncertainty and some even resort to self-injurious techniques as a means of relieving the feelings of anxiety and stress that exist in their daily lives.

Thus, this stigma highly shared by today's society about adolescence has helped the development of symptoms of stress, anxiety and any sign of psychological discomfort thanks to the pressure that exists on adolescents in the face of the alleged appearance of behaviors strongly condemned by adults. This discomfort caused has a negative impact on the meaning that adolescents give to life, since according to the results of the 2023 National Health and Nutrition Survey, (GOB June 27) 4.4% of the adolescent population has carried out self-injurious behaviors in order to end their lives, it also highlights a higher prevalence in adolescent women with 7.7% compared to the male population who only 1.2% have tried, of this population group, 50.2% tried to do so in the last 12 months prior to the survey (Ministry of Health & National Institute of Public Health, 2024).

Background

Today, increasing enrollment in Mexico by up to 60% is possible, however, not with the same traditional policies that only reached an average rate of (43.8%). The profile of the average student has changed and this change requires an adaptation of institutions (technological and labor disruption). The financing of public institutions and adherence to the new policies in private institutions must be equally adapted.

It also implies a greater capacity for innovation in university systems and public policies, to experiment with new educational models that focus on student success and well-being. (Moreno, A. 2025. pp.39-40).

> *In the last school year (2023-2024) enrollment at the undergraduate level was 4.9 million students and graduate enrollment was 466.9 thousand students, compared to 2009, the growth was 66.7% and 86% respectively. [...] Between 2009 and 2012, undergraduate enrollment grew at a rate of 4.8%, then decreased to 3.9% in the 2013-2018 period and to 2% between 2019 and 2023. If the growth rate had been maintained, undergraduate enrollment would have been higher than 5.1 million students in the 2023-2024 cycle (Moreno. A., 2025. p. 23).*

On the other hand, from 1995 to 2002 enrollment in higher education increased from 23% to 32%, and a growth of private schools of 72% in this period. Private institutions usually do not have watchdog, control, regulation, evaluation or oversight bodies to verify the quality of the vocational training services they offer, such as degrees and degrees, in record time and tailored to all pockets (Guzmán. 2025. p. 72. Cited in Perfiles Educativos, 2002).

The use of technology for mental health, or *e-mental health*, has grown exponentially, giving rise to a wide range of digital interventions. These range from general wellness applications to structured therapeutic platforms. In the current market, applications such as Calm and Headspace stand out, which focus mainly on guided meditation, mindfulness and sleep hygiene to reduce stress and anxiety (Team

2021) Although they are very popular and have proven to be effective for general well-being, their approach is not primarily therapeutic nor is it designed with game dynamics (gamification) as the central axis. but rather as a repository of resources.

A second category of applications uses principles of Cognitive Behavioral Therapy (CBT) and positive psychology to offer a more active approach. Happify, for example, employs science-based games and activities to help users overcome negative thoughts and build emotional resilience (Happify, Inc., n.d.). While these platforms incorporate gamification elements, they often focus on task completion and habit tracking rather than an immersive narrative experience, which is a key differentiator of the proposed project.

The field most directly related to this project is that of *Serious Games* for health, which are video games designed with a purpose that goes beyond mere entertainment, such as education or therapy. In this area, the scientific literature reports very relevant antecedents that validate the approach of this proposal. A pioneering and successful example is SPARX, a fantasy video game designed to deliver CBT sessions to young people with depression (Merry et al., 2012). In a controlled clinical trial, SPARX proved to be non-inferior to conventional treatment and even obtained significantly higher remission rates, validating the use of immersive storytelling to teach therapeutic skills (Merry et al., 2012).

Another important precedent is Reach Out Central (ROC), a serious narrative game developed to improve the mental health of young people between 16 and 25 years old (Shandley et al., 2010). ROC uses real-life scenarios and role-playing to teach practical coping skills, improve the ability to challenge negative thoughts, and reduce psychological distress (Shandley et al., 2010). Both SPARX and ROC demonstrate that a unified story and a virtual companion that evolves with the user's progress are crucial elements in increasing immersion and intervention effectiveness.

In the context of the "Soul-MindHackers" project, the proposal draws on this background by combining a solid psychoeducational foundation, based on Beck's inventories for depression and anxiety, with validated game mechanics. It seeks to integrate daily lessons and "streaks" to promote consistency; a system of points, badges and levels to reinforce achievement; and interactive exercises such as puzzles and role-playing scenarios. Unlike general wellness apps, "Soul-MindHackers" is conceived as an early warning system that can guide the user towards professional care when needed. Finally, its model is designed to be a support resource that any teacher at the Tecnológico Superior de Jalisco Chapala campus can use to create a bridge of trust with students, positioning itself as a relevant and necessary innovation in the current panorama.

It is worth noting how attractive it is for a pubescent or adolescent to be close to an electronic device and to interact with it. Adolescence is an important stage for the growth and consolidation of the subject. Electronic devices have become the most chosen medium by adolescents for one of the most important activities of this stage: socializing. (UN-UNICEF-Uruguay, 2020)

In this sense, it is an area of opportunity to broaden the focus for this population, that taking care of health and seeking emotional well-being is part of the tools that can be used on a daily basis from the individual level to their interactions.

There are also studies that investigate how students have changed their perception of health based on crucial situations such as the consequences of having lived through a pandemic and analyze healthy lifestyle habits, behaviors, beliefs, knowledge, habits, and actions of people. (Cárdenas, A., et al., 2023) based on the pandemic, this proposal seeks to focus not only on the sphere of physical health but also on how it is an integrated whole to conceptualize their personal identities.

Something that the authors cited in the previous paragraph revealed is how topics such as physical activity were paused, bringing, for example, the repercussion of an increase in weight, if it is revealed with this parallelism, what happened then with emotional health and psychological well-being? Surely there will be important issues on which young people could stop and reflect.

Addressing student mental health is a major concern on college campuses. In 2023, the American College Health Association found that 45.9% of undergraduate students reported a history of at least one mental disorder diagnosis (Taylor, et. al., 2024. p.683. Cited by Department of Psychological Sciences, University of California).

In this work, Taylor points out the importance of the updated study of the new advances in the application of video games as coping strategies towards specific aspects of mental health, an aspect that is very important worldwide, not only post-pandemic, but other aspects were already affecting the health of people in the world, with specific particularities that could be from economic aspects, to those of social security as a result of regular crime or natural disasters of various kinds.

On the other hand, Tin Ting, et.al (2024) week some interesting aspects in his work on the impact of video games on mental health, as he points out, for example, that in Malaysia it is a key sector in the consumer industry, which has also taken economic relevance and that the psychological significance has not been sufficiently evaluated to know precisely the consequences in this regard.

> *The projected revenue in the video game market in Malaysia is expected to reach US$649.30 million by 2024. Forecasts suggest that the market is poised for a steady annual expansion, with a projected compound annual growth rate (CAGR 2024-2027) of 7.55%. This trajectory is expected to culminate in a market volume that reaches US$ 807.80 million by 2027. (p. 23915).*

However, in the same work, Tin Tin (2024) points out that a study found that video games contribute to improving cognitive skills and decision-making: High school and undergraduate students who played video games exhibit better results when assigned tasks related to cognitive skills compared to students who do not play video games. (pp. 23915-23916). In other words, there is an attitude and data that support significant support for the use of video games and activities with devices, which favor other cognitive skills, such as visual-spatial comprehension, problem solving, language, among others.

It is no secret to anyone that large polling models on various aspects of human actions are in full swing. The same is the case of research and comparative studies on gamification and the use of video games or electronic devices, whether for entertainment or educational purposes.

One of these examples is found with Tianjie Ju and Zhenyu Shao. et. al. (2025), these authors analyze with their comparative studies from aspects of language to other aspects concerning the personality of the subjects.

According to the data stated by Zamani, (2025) more than 280 million people around the world are being affected by depression, which is equivalent, if we want to see it differently, to several countries together. This, in addition to implying a deterioration in the quality of life of people, results in a deterioration in the economy of individuals, families and society itself. But beyond these losses, there is an ethical and moral obligation to understand and attack the problem with concrete strategies and according to each context and culture.

Zamani (2025) and his collaborators reach important conclusions about the use of AI and gamification strategies in the aforementioned work, some of them are:

> *This study presents an AI-powered gamified system for monitoring and managing depression, integrating therapeutic micro-games, adaptive momentary ecological assessments, detection of environmental context, and machine learning analytics. Evaluated using synthetic data, the platform was rigorously tested for classification accuracy, adaptability, and research potential without immediate real-world data collection. (p. 25).*

Important studies such as Zamani's opened the door for more detailed work with increasingly powerful intelligences and processors. Even this same author states about the work to come, "The next phase will involve real-world pilot implementations to evaluate system performance with live data, assess long-term user engagement, and improve model generability. Integration with passive sensing through wearable devices and smartphones, including objective monitoring of sleep, activity, and physiological signals, will improve multimodal data collection." (p. 25).

The importance of the study and approach to mental disorders in youth takes on a nuance of high relevance today. Not only because it is a highly relevant topic in itself, but also because many of the disorders or the degree of affectation are the reason for various studies associated with video games and electronic devices that are often used in a way that is often poorly regulated by parents or guardians or even by the educational institutions themselves in various countries and school levels.

Some countries have begun to limit the use of time or a total ban on bringing such devices into educational institutions. In this sense, and according to a study carried out by Wanniarachchi (2025. p.20), on the impact of personalization on user participation and adherence in digital mental health interventions (DMHI) where he analyzes 67 articles, he highlights the following findings:

A. Therapeutic content is the most common object of personalization, and interventions favor the user's choice as a personalization mechanism.
B. While incorporating personalization elements into DMHIs has the potential to improve them, there is not enough research on their impact on user experience and adherence among teens and young adults.
C. Additionally, while machine learning techniques have frequently been employed to personalize the user experience, the limited use of generative AI and LLM is noteworthy.
D. Future studies could address these research gaps to improve the experience of young people in DMHI, ultimately contributing to more effective mental health interventions and policies.

As in other cases, we can observe that even when we cannot make conclusive conclusions, we are on the right track when research shares common objectives of evaluation on the effects of the use of video games or other applications without minimum regulation time on their use.

So it is precisely to start from promoting, on the one hand, a culture of prevention, of self-awareness and why not start from previous experiences, which already involved personal and family issues, in terms of what we have learned even as humanity.

This stage where young people learn through technology, where social networks favor access to a large amount of information, is also an area that allows transforming concepts such as access to health issues is only the competence of professionals.

THE WAY FORWARD

Recapitulating the previous context, the development of scalable technological intervention models has been considered, such as considering gamification postulates for the creation of this platform that has been named "Soul-Mind Hackers", which is aligned with international recommendations to train teachers to identify mental health problems and guide students to the appropriate resources. Thus generating a "domino effect" of support throughout the national network, especially supported by data that outstandingly position anxiety and depression as the most widespread and debilitating conditions among students, since they are the ones who in the symptomatology process see their functionality affected in different areas, including, of course, school. (Angulo et al., 2018).

Thus, technology emerges as a promising way to transform mental health care. The field of *e-mental health* is taking advantage of the ubiquity of mobile devices to offer interventions that are scalable, accessible, and able to overcome the stigma associated with traditional therapy. In Mexico, this approach is particularly relevant, as a high penetration of mobile telephony (97% in urban areas and 90% in rural areas) coexists with a persistent digital divide in household internet access (IFT, 2024). This makes the *smartphone* the main, and sometimes only, digital hotspot for most young people.

The "Soul-Mind Hackers" proposal represents a strategic opportunity. This type of tool can work as an early warning system, identifying risk patterns through user interaction and, if necessary, channeling it towards professional care. By integrating these resources into the university ecosystem, a bridge of trust can be created between teachers and students, offering an accessible, private and destigmatized first line of support.

Considering the specific context of Chapala, with its digital divide and the mental health needs of university students, a concrete gamified intervention is proposed, designed to generate a significant impact on the community.

It is essential to recognize the significant digital divide in Chapala, where only 39.6% of households have access to the internet (Government of the State of Jalisco, 2021). Therefore, any proposed intervention must adopt a hybrid approach. This involves designing solutions that can work effectively without an internet connection for the core gameplay, or be easily accessible through university computer labs and designated community centers, in addition to any online components. This strategy ensures equitable access and maximizes reach.

METHODOLOGY AND METHODS

The issue of emotional well-being is something that still requires special attention to focus on a range of responses based, among other variables, on contextual ones that also involve reciprocity between participants and put the teacher-student binomial at the center. In other words, a methodological approach must be chosen that starts from openness that thus guarantees the proper development of the project.

Returning to what Creeswell (2014) provides, a mixed methodology has been chosen, since, as this author mentions, it is an approach in which the researcher collects, analyzes and integrates both quantitative and qualitative data in the same study or in a series of studies, to better understand a research phenomenon.

The proposed methodology is mixed and sequential exploratory (Creeswell 2014), where the researcher begins with the qualitative phase, exploring the opinions of the participants, data are analyzed and this information will be useful for the quantitative phase that is the basis for the construction of the product "Soul-MindHackers" that has already been explained that it is a comprehensive technological system designed for the promotion of mental health.

Thus, on the one hand, integrating the qualitative perspective and thus validating data as unique, which reflect the subjectivity of the study subjects, allow for a contextualized characterization, and on the other hand, the quantitative perspective will provide concrete, measurable data that will allow us to have parameters to continue, as explained in previous paragraphs, with the action research, based on what a pilot study implies.

> *The methods to be used, qualitative made up of the realization of focus groups, individual interviews and analysis of user testimonies to understand their subjective experiences, the challenges encountered and the perceived value of the intervention. In this case, a detection of the teacher's needs is first contemplated, since they are the ones who will position themselves as activators of the essence of the integral system.*

However, regarding the quantitative methods, they will include engagement metrics (time in the application, frequency of use, mission completion rates), user retention rates and performance data in mini-games or challenges.

> *The integration of both methods is key for the phase of both the development and evaluation processes that are being considered, since, as has been defined, it is a pilot study.*

Delving into aspects of the integral system, where not only emphasis is placed on gamification, but as explained above, the teacher-student binomial is the essence of it, and it is intended to enhance a "domino effect" where a trained teacher can impact a large number of students. This strategy aligns with UNESCO IESALC's recommendation to train faculty and staff to identify mental health issues and guide students to appropriate resources (UNESCO IESALC, 2024).

In this methodological framework, it is essential to specify not only the approach and the data collection instruments, but also the measurement criteria that will guide the evaluation of the pilot. The combination of qualitative and quantitative techniques makes it possible not only to collect perceptions and testimonies, but to translate them into concrete and comparable indicators. These indicators, or evaluation metrics, operate as success parameters that make it easier to judge the relevance of the technological system and its impact on student well-being. In this way, the definition of metrics is not an isolated addition, but a structural piece that articulates action research, offering an objective framework for interpreting the results and making decisions about the continuity or scaling of the project.

Assessment metrics include 7- and 30-day retention indicators, number of missions completed per week, improvements in identifying cognitive distortions, as well as reductions in anxiety (BAI) and depression (BDI-II) scores. Initial goals are set for 70% retention in the first week and 60% per month, the completion of at least four weekly missions and an average three-point decrease in anxiety and depression

THE PROPOSAL

The Soul-MindHackers project arises as an educational and technological innovation initiative within the framework of the Tecnológico Nacional de México (TecNM), particularly at the Tecnológico Superior de Jalisco (TSJ) in the Chapala Academic Unit, with the aim of comprehensively addressing mental health in academic environments through interactive digital tools. This proposal is not conceived only as an application or a device, but as an ecosystem of psychoeducational intervention that combines gamification, psychometrics and biometrics to strengthen the emotional well-being of students.

The system is inspired by the Beck Inventories for Anxiety (BAI) and Depression (BDI), instruments recognized for their validity and reliability in clinical assessment (Beck, et al., 1996; Beck et al., 1988). However, Soul-MindHackers proposes a gamified reinterpretation of these inventories, replacing traditional questions with interactive mini-games that behaviorally represent the Beck's items. In this way, instead of answering self-administered questionnaires, the user participates in digital experiences that identify or associate their emotional and cognitive responses.

The purpose of this innovation is to transform psychological assessment into a meaningful and playful experience, integrating the collection of physiological data through a bracelet. This device records in real time variables such as heart rate, blood pressure, temperature, blood oxygenation, physical activity, galvanic skin response, respiratory rate, among others, which correlate with the user's reactions within the minigames. By merging behavioral performance data with biometric data, the system can offer contextualized data, making it possible to distinguish between symptoms of physical or mental origin.

From a pedagogical perspective, Soul-MindHackers seeks to destigmatize psychological care and promote a culture of emotional self-care in the university environment. In the TSJ-Chapala community, where students face high levels of academic stress, anxiety, and demotivation, this tool is proposed as an accessible and empathetic means to detect, prevent, and accompany symptoms of anxiety and depression before they translate into major crises or school dropouts.

The system also works as a support model for the specialist, as it allows the user's data to be visualized in interpretive panels that show behavioral trends, physiological changes, and emotional variations (stress and anxiety) over time. Thus, a specialist can access a more complete representation of the student's status.

In methodological terms, Soul-MindHackers is built under an applied research approach, in which psychologists, engineers, designers, and education specialists collaborate in an iterative process of design, testing, and improvement. This approach makes it possible to integrate scientific validity with user experience, ensuring that the final product is not only functional, but ethically responsible and clinically useful.

Finally, the project is conceived as a scalable model. The initial implementation in Chapala will serve as a pilot for its subsequent expansion to other campuses of the Tecnológico Nacional de México. This replicable character is based on its hybrid architecture, its inclusive design and its potential to adapt to different cultural and socioeconomic contexts within the national education system.

ELEMENTS OF GAMIFICATION

The essence of Soul-MindHackers lies in its ability to transform psychological and pedagogical processes into interactive experiences that promote motivation, curiosity and emotional self-regulation. Gamification is not a superficial add-on, but the engine that structures the user experience and makes it emotionally meaningful. Inspired by the principles of Self-Determination Theory (Ryan & Deci, 2000) and meaningful learning models, the proposal seeks to generate an environment where students actively participate in their own process of well-being, experiencing autonomy, competence and social connection.

Gamified design is based on three essential principles: association, feedback, and progression. Through them, an environment of identification - association is created that promotes constant practice, self-observation and emotional identification. The dynamics of play allow emotional learning to be internalized in a natural way, without the rigidity or stigmatizing weight that usually accompanies traditional psychological treatments.

The first element, association, is built through an immersive narrative that places the user as the protagonist of their own emotional process. Instead of a linear "role-playing" story, the system is organized as a panel of levels, where each session represents a mini-game or emotional challenge. The user can freely choose when and how many times to play each challenge; however, upon completing them, your progress level increases and new activities are unlocked.

This approach offers a more flexible and personalized experience: each participant progresses at their own pace, but with a constant sense of accomplishment and growth. In addition, minimum levels can be set as a requirement to access certain mini-games, which stimulates engagement without imposing a rigid sequence.

In this way, the environment maintains its symbolic component, the "inner sanctuary" that evolves visually, reflecting the player's progress and strengthening their perception of emotional advancement and self-knowledge (Kapp, 2012).

The second principle, feedback, is present in every interaction. Instead of penalizing mistakes, the system offers an immediate, empathetic, and constructive response that reinforces positive learning. This approach is inspired by the theories of experiential learning (Kolb, 1984) cited in Romero et. al (2010) and by educational gamification practices that prioritize intrinsic reinforcement. Each mini-game provides small visual, sound, or tactile rewards such as lights, sounds, or vibrations that convey a sense of accomplishment and keep the user focused and emotionally connected to the activity. Finally, progression manifests itself on multiple levels. The user earns points, unlocks badges, advances in their "Emotional Skill Tree" and watches their inner sanctum blossom with each completed module. These mechanics of tangible advancement function as visual markers of psychological growth, reinforcing constancy and generating a clear perception of personal evolution. In addition, the Wellness Points and achievements earned can be used to unlock additional content or avatar customizations, reinforcing the sense of autonomy.

Together, these elements not only guarantee adherence to the system, but also turn the process of evaluation and emotional training into an act of self-discovery, reinforcing the idea that taking care of the mind is as valuable and everyday an experience as training the body. Gamification, in this sense, becomes a digital emotional literacy strategy, an accompaniment tool that helps TecNM students develop resilience, self-awareness and well-being habits from an accessible and attractive approach.

Gamification in Soul-MindHackers is not limited to including rewards or points, but is conceived as a language that connects emotions with action. Each interaction is designed to generate a meaningful experience, in which the user feels that they are progressing, learning and getting to know themselves better. Game mechanics such as immediate feedback, progressive challenges, freedom of choice, and symbolic reinforcement function as scaffolds that sustain emotional learning and active participation.

In this system, feedback takes on a central role. Instead of punishing mistakes, the environment offers immediate and empathetic responses that invite reflection and improvement. Every action has a visible or perceptible consequence: a color that changes, a subtle vibration, an animation that recognizes effort. These small symbolic gestures strengthen the user's relationship with the tool and encourage persistence in practice.

Another key element is visual progression, which replaces traditional scorecards with personal growth indicators. Progress is shown by colors, medals, or badges that reflect levels of mastery, but without promoting competition between users. The goal is not to "win," but to recognize one's own emotional progress and maintain intrinsic motivation. This logic is inspired by the principles of the Self-Determination Theory (Ryan & Deci, 2000), which states that the most lasting motivation arises when the person feels autonomous, competent, and connected to a meaningful goal.

Likewise, the mechanics incorporate moments of pause or self-regulation, where the user can stop, observe their breathing or simply reflect on the experience lived. These spaces are not interruptions of play, but essential components of the social-emotional learning process. In this way, the environment combines the cognitive stimulation of play with the calm necessary for introspection.

Together, these mechanics create a balance between action and reflection, challenge and well-being, reinforcing the idea that gamification can also be a form of emotional accompaniment. Unlike the competitive dynamics of digital entertainment, Soul-MindHackers proposes an empathetic gamification, oriented towards awareness and self-care.

In line with these principles, the design of the system evolves towards a more flexible structure focused on personal exploration: the Soul-MindHackers emotional circuit. This model replaces the linear narrative with a modular path that translates the psychometric dimensions of the Beck Inventory into interactive experiences of self-knowledge and emotional practice.

SOUL-MINDHACKERS EMOTIONAL CIRCUIT

Narrative and logical integration of design.

In line with the idea of transforming emotional assessment into a meaningful experience, Soul-MindHackers adopts a new structure called Emotional Circuit, which replaces the linear narrative of "missions" with a modular and progressive format. This change responds to the intention of offering a more flexible, intuitive environment focused on the user's personal exploration.

The emotional circuit is composed of ten mini-games or modules that represent emotional and cognitive dimensions taken directly from Beck's Inventories. Each one addresses a particular aspect of the human experience such as attention, stress regulation or self-perception and translates these psychological constructs into simple, understandable and measurable playful dynamics.

The circuit structure avoids rigid hierarchies or sequences: the user can freely choose where to start, repeat activities or advance in the order he wants. This freedom encourages more genuine participation, motivated by curiosity and self-interest. Unlike conventional games, the purpose is not to win, compete or accumulate points, but to get to know each other, observe each other and understand how one reacts to different emotional situations.

The approach combines three axes: emotional self-exploration, immediate feedback, and constant practice. Playing thus becomes a form of emotional learning. Each game session acts as a micro-experience of self-awareness: the user observes their performance, their physical sensations and the way they respond to controlled stimuli.

Modular design and self-exploration principles.

Each mini-game within the emotional circuit is designed to activate a specific cognitive or physiological response and translate it into observable data. These indicators are not used for clinical diagnostic purposes, but as guideline references that help identify emotional tendencies and patterns of self-regulation.

In technical terms, each module collects basic data (such as response time, accuracy, or heart rate) and combines it with narrative and visual elements that reinforce motivation. However, from the user's perspective, the experience is perceived as a friendly and personalized journey, where each challenge offers the opportunity to improve in a specific aspect of emotional well-being.

1. Mental pulse (Attention and concentration)

This module tests the ability to maintain attention in repetitive tasks and mental resistance to increasing stimuli. The player must play visual or sound sequences that become progressively more complex, a process that reveals their level of concentration and tolerance for fatigue. Assesses: difficulty concentrating, mental fatigue (BDI-19 / BAI-17). Indicators: response time, heart rate, and error rate.

2. Internal balance (Emotional regulation)

In this exercise, the user synchronizes their breathing and heart rate with visual stimuli, such as light waves that change color or intensity. The activity invites you to regulate the body and mind, reinforcing the connection between the two. Assesses: emotional control, calmness and stress management (BDI-2 / BAI-5). Indicators: heart rate variability (HRV) and galvanic skin response.

3. Decide on time (Decision making under pressure)

This module simulates quick decisions in ambiguous or changing situations. Through a set of options that change over time, the player learns to react with agility without losing coherence. Assesses: indecision, anticipatory anxiety (BDI-15 / BAI-11). Indicators: blood pressure, reaction time, and consistency in choices.

4. Emotional Memory (Affective Retention)

Here, the user must remember and associate stimuli, faces, sounds or colors, with certain emotions. This process helps to recognize how memory relates to affectivity and emotional bonding. Assesses: loss of interest, affective disconnection (BDI-13 / BAI-10). Indicators: number of correct answers, physiological stability and sustained attention.

5. Tolerance to failure (Frustration and resilience)

This mini-game exposes the player to tasks that are impossible to complete or with inevitable errors. The goal is not perfection, but to observe the reaction to frustration and the ability to persist without giving up. Assesses: irritability, frustration, loss of control (BDI-9 / BAI-4). Indicators: persistence, micro variations of the pulse and dropout rate.

6. Rhythm and calmness (Physiological anxiety)

In this exercise, a constant rhythm must be maintained, either breathing or following a movement pattern, while distracting stimuli appear. Assesses: body tension, difficulty relaxing (BAI-17). Indicators: heart rate and physiological rhythm stability.

7. Perspective (Self-esteem and self-concept)

This module introduces a visual metaphor: the player constructs or balances figures that represent different "parts of the self." As the figure is completed, the environment brightens or changes color, symbolizing personal balance. Assesses: self-criticism, feelings of failure (BDI-7 / BDI-14). Indicators: consistency of progress and continuity of interaction.

8. Trail of Light (Motivation and Pleasure)

The user follows light paths that respond to their level of participation. The greater the constancy, the brighter the environment becomes. Assesses: loss of interest or pleasure (BDI-12 / BAI-8). Indicators: emotional reactivity and physiological constancy.

9. Mental Clarity (Automatic Thought Control)

The player clears a screen of negative phrases or words that appear at different rates. The activity symbolizes the effort to clear the mind of intrusive thoughts. Assesses: ruminative thoughts, negativity (BDI-3 / BAI-9). Indicators: response time, heart rate, and voluntary return to the task.

10. Daily Balance (Self-Observation and Closure)

It works as a visual emotional log. The user sorts icons or cards based on how they felt during the day. This exercise reinforces emotional awareness and the ability to reflect on oneself. Assesses: self-perception and emotional stability (cross-sectional dimension). Indicators: coherence of records, physiological stability and affective tendency.

Progression and visual accompaniment

Each mini-game has mastery levels represented by colors (blue - green - gold), symbolic badges or medals and a visible progress number. These levels do not seek to hierarchize, but to show the personal growth of the user, helping them to visualize their emotional progress in a simple way.

Progression is based on three criteria:

1. Frequency of practice, which reflects the user's consistency.
2. Improved performance, seen in accuracy and reaction time.
3. Physiological stability, measured by the coherence between heart rate, breathing, and attention.

As the user reaches new levels, narrative resources, backgrounds or sounds that represent balance and well-being are unlocked. This sensory-visual, auditory and tactile feedback maintains motivation without resorting to external or competitive rewards.

System scalability and projection

The design of the emotional circuit is designed to grow over time. New modules may be added progressively, retaining the same structure and correspondence with the items in the Beck Inventory. This allows the system to remain scalable and adaptable to different populations or educational contexts within the Tecnológico Nacional de México.

In addition, this modularity facilitates integration with other research projects or complementary applications. For example, relaxation modules, mindfulness dynamics or brief cognitive exercises could be incorporated. Thus, Soul-MindHackers can evolve as a comprehensive platform for digital emotional accompaniment.

CONCEPTUAL SYNTHESIS

Together, the Soul-MindHackers Emotional Circuit translates Beck's psychological constructs into a visual and participatory language. Each mini-game functions as a window into emotional experience: an opportunity to observe, understand, and learn about oneself through play.

The system does not seek to replace the traditional psychometric assessment, but to expand it, incorporating the experiential and physiological dimension of emotion. Thanks to its modular structure, Soul-MindHackers offers a more human, close and educational experience, where diagnosis becomes dialogue and measurement becomes self-discovery.

ADAPTATION OF THE KIRKPATRICK MODEL

Evaluating the effectiveness of Soul-MindHackers requires a framework that considers both the emotional and cognitive aspects of the gamified experience and its educational and social impact within the university environment. To this end, the assessment model of Donald Kirkpatrick (1994) Smidt A. et. al., (2009), widely used in training environments, but here reinterpreted under the logic of educational gamification and emotional assessment, is taken up and adapted.

Kirkpatrick's model proposes four levels of assessment: reaction, learning, behavior, and outcomes, which can be applied holistically to the processes of interaction and emotional learning within Soul-MindHackers.

At the first level, reaction, the user's subjective experience of the gamified environment is measured. In gamification, this dimension is directly related to motivation and commitment. Here we look at how students perceive the system: whether they find it useful, attractive, and relevant to their well-being. Metrics include degree of satisfaction, time of use, perception of difficulty, and empathy with the "Keeper of Balance" narrative. This level seeks to ensure that the experience is emotionally positive, a key element to maintain adherence and engagement (Deterding et al., 2011).

The second level, learning, assesses the knowledge, skills, and attitudes acquired through interaction. At Soul-MindHackers, this translates into emotional awareness: the ability to identify, understand, and self-regulate one's emotions. Minigames, being designed from the principles of cognitive and emotional psychology, generate learning that goes beyond entertainment: the player recognizes thought patterns, develops coping strategies and strengthens their self-knowledge. According to Gee, J. (2007), well-designed games promote deep learning by allowing users to experiment, reflect, and adjust their actions in simulated contexts in meaningful ways.

The third level, behavior, examines the transfer of what has been learned to real contexts. In gamification, this level is linked to behavioral transformation: whether students apply the skills developed in the virtual environment in their daily lives. In the case of the TSJ-Chapala, it is expected to observe improvements in emotional self-regulation, reduction of impulsive behaviors, increase in academic concentration and greater use of psychological support services. This level reflects the effectiveness of the system not only as a diagnostic tool, but as a means of emotional training.

Finally, the fourth level, the results, analyzes the overall impact of the program on the educational community. In this context, we seek to measure the institutional effects of the use of Soul-MindHackers: decrease in reported anxiety and depression rates, reduction in school dropout associated with emotional factors and strengthening of the culture of mental well-being in the TSJ Chapala. At the macro level, this level connects with the project's vision of becoming a replicable model for the entire system of the Tecnológico Nacional de México.

This adaptation of the Kirkpatrick model demonstrates that gamification can not only be used as a pedagogical tool, but also as an evaluative framework of emotional impact. By combining gamification theory with Kirkpatrick levels, Soul-MindHackers offers a comprehensive approach to understanding how playful interaction can lead to measurable cognitive, emotional, and social changes. In this way, the model ensures that the intervention is not limited to an engaging experience, but contributes in a tangible way to the psychological and educational well-being of students.

COMPLEMENTS TO THE PROPOSAL

The Soul-MindHackers proposal is not limited to a technological application or a set of mini-games; it constitutes a comprehensive ecosystem of emotional accompaniment and socio-affective learning that is based on conceptual, pedagogical and ethical pillars. This system recognizes that mental health is a complex phenomenon that requires a multidimensional intervention, in which technology, psychology, education and digital ethics converge. Consequently, the complements of the proposal are structured around three main axes: the psychoeducational model, the ethical and persuasive design and the functional interaction between the components of the system.

The psychoeducational model is based on the conception of emotional well-being as a competence that can be developed through meaningful and sustainable learning experiences. Soul-MindHackers operates under the premise that self-knowledge, emotional regulation, and empathy are skills that are strengthened through practice and reflection (Fernández-Abascal, 2018). In this sense, the system acts as a mediator between psychological self-assessment and emotional training, promoting affective literacy through playful interaction. Every mini-game, every feedback, and every physiological metric are not ends in themselves, but means to foster self-reflection and emotional awareness.

From the point of view of ethical design, Soul-MindHackers assumes the responsibility of building digital experiences that respect the autonomy, privacy and dignity of the user. The system is based on the principles of ethical persuasive design, understood not as manipulation, but as facilitators of positive changes in behavior (Fogg, 2003). In this context, gamification is used as an empathetic language that motivates without coercing, that invites without imposing. The rewards and game mechanics are not oriented towards addiction or excessive competition, but towards the construction of healthy, resilient and sustainable habits. In addition, sensitive data protection measures and intervention protocols are integrated in case of detecting signs of emotional risk, guaranteeing confidentiality and adequate support.

In functional terms, Soul-MindHackers articulates a synergistic interaction between hardware, software, and human specialist. The biometric bracelet acts as a physiological state sensor; gamified software interprets, contextualizes and translates that data into interactive experiences; and the specialist (psychologist or tutor) analyzes the information to accompany the emotional processes of the users. This triangulation ensures that technology does not replace the human relationship, but rather enhances it. The tool thus becomes a bridge between the subjectivity of the student and the professional interpretation of the specialist.

The system also incorporates an analytical panel to support specialists, in which real-time indicators and trends over time are visualized. This component, developed under an emotional educational analytics approach, allows identifying patterns of improvement or regression, as well as critical areas of attention. In turn, the user module offers understandable visual reports that reflect their emotional progress in a symbolic and motivating way, encouraging self-management of well-being.

A fundamental aspect of the complements of the proposal is their alignment with the institutional values of the Tecnológico Nacional de México, especially with the axis of integral training. Soul-MindHackers is integrated into the TecNM's human development and emotional health strategy, functioning as an accompaniment tool that complements the work of tutors, psychologists and teachers. In this framework, technology acts as a catalyst for institutional change towards a culture of digital emotional well-being.

Finally, the conceptual and functional complements of the project are articulated with a vision of digital ethics and emotional citizenship (Berson & Berson, 2019), where the use of technology is aimed at strengthening empathy, a sense of community, and social responsibility. Gamification becomes a means of awareness and participation, encouraging students not only to manage their mental health, but also to become active agents of well-being within their environment. This mixed approach ensures that Soul-MindHackers is not only an emotional monitoring platform, but a model of educational transformation that integrates emotion, technology, and humanity.

Architecture and technological aspects

The design of the Soul-MindHackers emotional circuit comes to life through a technological architecture that translates emotional self-awareness experiences into secure, accessible, and adaptable digital processes. The intention is not only to build a functional application, but an environment sensitive to the user's emotions, capable of recording their progress without invading their privacy or turning the experience into a cold or mechanical evaluation.

The general structure of the system is organized into three interconnected levels:

1. User interface and interactive environment, where the modules or mini-games that make up the emotional circuit are developed.
2. Analytical panel for specialists, in charge of integrating information anonymously and converting it into general indicators on well-being and emotional performance.
3. Data management and security layer, which safeguards information through encrypted protocols and reliable traceability mechanisms.

Each tier communicates using a secure API, designed to ensure that data flows in a controlled manner between the system's modules. This modular approach allows the project to grow in a scalable way: new mini-games, metrics, or accompanying tools can be added without modifying the main structure.

The priority at all times is confidentiality and informed consent. Users retain control over their information, and records are stored under ethical and technical standards compatible with current regulations. To reinforce security and transparency, the system includes a mechanism that documents each sensitive interaction in an unalterable way, ensuring data traceability and strengthening institutional trust.

This architecture not only supports the operation of the circuit, but also materializes the main purpose of the project: to transform emotional evaluation into an educational and meaningful experience, where technology accompanies the user in their own process of self-knowledge.

Analytics Dashboard & Data Security

The analytical panel for specialists is the space where the results of the Soul-MindHackers emotional circuit converge. Its main function is to transform individual records into useful and understandable information, always under strict criteria of confidentiality and informed consent.

This dashboard does not display personal data or individual scores. Instead, it features general trends, early warnings, and automatic reports that help counselors, teachers, or researchers understand the emotional well-being of a group of students without exposing their identity. The indicators are organized in a visual and intuitive way, with dynamic graphs, colors and comparative panels that facilitate the interpretation of the results.

The interconnection between the system modules is done using an encrypted API, ensuring that information travels securely and in a controlled manner between the application and the analytics dashboard. This modular design allows the system to grow over time, integrating new features or games without compromising security or overall performance.

To reinforce institutional trust, an unalterable record layer was incorporated that documents sensitive actions of the system (for example, when a piece of data was created, modified or consulted). This layer works as a kind of secure logbook, inspired by the principles of *blockchain* technology: each record is permanently sealed, which prevents its alteration and ensures the traceability of the information.

This transparent approach does not seek to make the system more complex, but to protect the user and strengthen the credibility of the project. In this way, Soul-MindHackers complies with national and international regulations on the protection of personal data and promotes an ethical use of technology applied to emotional well-being.

Together, the system architecture and analytical dashboard make up the technological heart of Soul-MindHackers. Every component from the mini-games to the recording and security algorithms has been designed to support the central purpose of the project: to turn emotional evaluation into a meaningful and ethical experience, in which data serves to understand, not judge.

Once the functional structure has been consolidated and the integrity of the information has been ensured, the next step is to test the prototype with the users themselves. This validation phase will allow us to observe how students interact with the environment, how their emotional responses are reflected within the circuit and, above all, if the system manages to generate learning about the management of their own emotions.

The methodological strategies to carry out this validation are described below, as well as the psychometric and qualitative criteria that will guide the analysis of the results.

User validation and testing

The validation of Soul-MindHackers represents the moment when the proposal stops being just an idea to become a real experience. The purpose of this stage is to check that the system works technically, but also that it meets its educational and emotional objective: to help students recognize, understand and manage their emotions more consciously.

Overall validation design

The validation will be carried out with a pilot sample of around 30 students from the Tecnológico Superior de Jalisco, Chapala Academic Unit. These participants will be selected voluntarily and will sign an informed consent that clearly explains the purpose of the study, the activities they will perform, and the confidentiality measures that will protect their information.

During the test, students will interact with the emotional circuit of Soul-MindHackers, going through the different mini-games designed to explore emotional dimensions such as concentration, stress regulation, decision-making or self-perception. At the same time, a digital version of the traditional Beck Inventory (BAI and BDI-II) will be applied, which will allow the results obtained in both formats to be compared.

Evaluation criteria

The evaluation will be structured in three main dimensions:

1. Psychometric equivalence: It will be analyzed whether the results of the gamified environment present a significant correlation with those of the traditional instrument. To do this, statistical tests such as Pearson's correlation coefficient (r) and Cronbach's alpha (α) will be used, with the aim of verifying the internal consistency and validity of the measurements. A correlation equal to or greater than 0.70 will be considered acceptable, which will indicate that the gamified

system manages to measure the same emotional constructs as the original inventory.

2. User experience (UX): In addition to the statistical analysis, how students live the emotional experience of the game will be evaluated. Through short questionnaires, semi-structured interviews and focus groups, the participants' perception of the clarity of the dynamics, the empathy of the environment, the level of immersion and the emotional learning obtained will be explored.

This qualitative approach will allow us to understand not only whether the system works, but also how and why users perceive it as useful or meaningful.

3. Usability and emotional response: Objective metrics such as response times, error rate and permanence in activities will be recorded, as well as interaction patterns within the circuit. Where possible, non-invasive physiological cues (e.g. heart rate or respiratory rate) should also be collected to observe the coherence between the emotional response and the dynamics of the game.

The analysis of these data will allow us to identify moments of stress, attention or calm, complementing the psychometric information with behavioral evidence.

ANALYSIS OF THE RESULTS

The information obtained will be processed under a mixed approach, combining statistical analysis and thematic categorization of the discourses. The integration of both types of data will serve to understand the emotional impact of the system from a complete perspective: the numbers will show validity, and the students' voices will show the human experience behind them.

The findings will be documented in a technical and academic report, which will include recommendations for improving minigames, adjusting mechanics, and optimizing the interface. In addition, these results will be the basis for preparing a second phase of development, aimed at expanding the circuit with new modules and the integration of adaptive functions according to the emotional profile of each user.

ETHICAL AND COMPLETION CONSIDERATIONS

At all times, compliance with the ethical principles of the American Psychological Association (APA, 2017) will be guaranteed, as well as the regulations of the

Tecnológico Nacional de México. Participants' personal data will be anonymized, stored in secure environments, and used for academic purposes only.

Beyond regulatory compliance, the team considers ethics as an essential element of the project: every interaction within the system should be an opportunity for emotional learning, not a source of stress or exposure.

When the comprehensive "Soul-MindHackers" system was conceptualized, relevant topics were reviewed, based on experience, as well as theoretical foundations provided by the interdisciplinary team, among the most outstanding is to seek an increase in commitment and adherence. The gamified nature and "streaks" would encourage consistent use of the platform, promoting adherence to self-care practices and continuous learning about mental health (Smartico.ai, 2024).

The development of practical skills that they can take from simulated scenarios, which are interactive to their own environments, transforming them into safe environments this can also be achieved by contributing to refining skills that are crucial in topics such as coping, emotional regulation and resilience.

It is known that there is a stigma linked to what concerns mental health, therefore, as it is a game format, it would contribute to normalizing a language that is oriented to emotional well-being instead of an emphasis on the pathological and that is seen as an alternative to seek support, as well as a greater openness to talk about issues that are part of integral health.

If the head-on issue of well-being is addressed, it is with this system to contribute to promoting, strengthening and giving meaning to techniques that, systematized, would contribute to a significant improvement in well-being, which would impact on stress reduction, specifically with regard to school and anxiety. (PsicoSmart, n.d.).

Something that is in the essence of this system is that it is not considered for the teaching staff as just another training issue, harsh, isolated, insignificant of, but that it is to make them participate in a different way of personalizing their daily work, thus promoting a multiplier effect and that the use of the platform can reach a large number of students. creating a potential impact.

It is also necessary to consider some ethical aspects for the design;

- Data privacy and security: Robust data privacy and security measures will be implemented, including encryption and regulatory compliance. Full transparency will be maintained on how user data is collected, used, and shared, ensuring that users can opt out of sharing sensitive information (HashStudioz, n.d.; Smartico.ai, 2024).
- Informed consent: Explicit informed consent will be obtained from users, and in the case of minors, from their parents or legal guardians, based on a clear

understanding of the purpose of the application, its potential risks, and its anticipated benefits (Spahl et al., 2024).

- Avoid addiction and trivialization: The design will prioritize genuine well-being and psychological growth over maximizing screen time or harmful competitive scores. Mechanics that may encourage addictive behaviors or trivialize the seriousness of mental health problems will be avoided (HashStudioz, n.d.; Stanford Daily, 2025).
- Clear pathways to professional help: The platform will function as a complementary tool and not as a replacement for professional help. It will integrate clear and accessible pathways for users to easily access existing mental health services from the University of Guadalajara (UdeG), UNIVA, ITESO, and local crisis resources (Centro de Salud, DIF Chapala, 911) when a higher level of support is needed (Romero Lopez, 2024; University of Guadalajara, 2023; UNIVA, n.d.).

Longitudinal studies are essential to assess the sustained impact of interventions, as short-term benefits may not necessarily translate into lasting changes in mental health (Maqbool et al., 2025).

The research and design of the *SoulMind Hackers* proposal have made it possible to demonstrate the relevance of developing technological solutions aimed at the psycho-emotional health of students in contexts where the challenges of anxiety, depression, stress and procrastination have a direct impact on academic performance and quality of life. This initiative is not only based on the current literature on gamification and cognitive-behavioral therapies, but also seeks to position itself as a benchmark within educational innovation with a focus on comprehensive well-being.

One of the most outstanding elements is technological feasibility. The proposed architecture, based on React Native and with specialized modules in Unity, allows you to create an immersive experience without compromising scalability or security. Offlinefirst design responds to the reality of many students who lack constant connection, ensuring that access to tools is not limited by the digital divide. By intelligently synchronizing in moments of connectivity, you balance the use of resources and promote the continuity of the experience.

The inclusion of biosensors to measure variables such as heart rate variability (HRV) or electrodermal activity (EDA) adds an innovative layer. This aspect not only opens up possibilities for mission customization, but also creates bridges to the development of more adaptive interventions. In practice, it means that students can receive contextualized feedback, recognizing in real time moments of stress and guiding the application of self-regulation techniques. This becomes an added value compared to other applications that are limited to general strategies without considering the immediate physiological state of the user.

From a pedagogical point of view, the anonymized teaching panel becomes a support tool for educators. Far from overloading teachers, it seeks to be integrated as an early warning system that, through aggregated data, allows trends to be observed and timely detection of support needs. This enables the construction of an educational model in which emotional health is not addressed as a peripheral issue, but as an essential component of the training process.

The proposal also aligns with the principles of privacy by design. At a time when users' trust depends on how their information is safeguarded, it is essential that the system integrates pseudonymization mechanisms, encryption in transit and secure storage. In addition, granular consent and the ability of students to decide what data to share strengthen the perception of control and respect for personal autonomy.

The expected results are structured in four levels: satisfaction, learning, behavioral transfer, and effects on well-being. This responds to Kirkpatrick's evaluation model, which ensures that not only superficial impressions are measured, but also profound transformations in behavior and clinical indicators. The combination of product metrics (retention, adherence, usability) with clinical metrics (reduction in anxiety and depression) offers a comprehensive view of impact.

As for implementation, a pilot is proposed in Chapala as a controlled space to validate hypotheses. This pilot is not only a technical test phase, but also an opportunity to generate knowledge that can be transferred to other campuses. Through an iterative approach, each feedback loop will serve to improve the experience, adjust gamification mechanics, and optimize integration with biosensors. In this way, scalability is not conceived as an immediate leap, but as a process based on evidence.

The risk analysis shows that potential obstacles have been considered: limited connectivity, lack of adherence, teacher overload, and privacy challenges. In each case, concrete mitigation strategies are proposed, which reinforces the credibility of the project and its potential for sustainability. For example, short missions and progressive storytelling are designed to counteract early dropout, while the champion teacher model distributes responsibility by avoiding excessive burdens.

Another crucial aspect is ethical alignment. The app is not intended to replace professional clinical intervention, but to complement it. Alert protocols in risk situations are conceived as mechanisms for referral and responsible accompaniment. This ensures that, in the event of a worrying pattern, there are clear channels to follow up without leaving the student in a state of vulnerability.

The development process, although it has been broadly described in progressive phases, should be understood as a narrative implementation strategy rather than as a technical annex. Each step is geared towards ensuring that the technology is validated with the users themselves and that constant feedback allows the product to be perfected. This vision reinforces the commitment that the tool is not imposed from the technical point of view, but co-created with those who are going to use it.

On the academic level, this proposal enriches the field of gamification applied to mental health. It connects psychological theories with game mechanics, and it does so from an interdisciplinary perspective that involves psychology, pedagogy, computer science, and design. In this way, not only a functional application is offered, but also a conceptual framework that can inspire future research and new applications in other educational contexts.

In short, SoulMind Hackers represents an innovative, technically and ethically grounded response to the current challenges of higher and upper secondary education. Their contributions are not limited to the creation of a technological tool, but also pave the way towards a comprehensive accompaniment model that recognizes emotional health as a pillar of learning. The combination of a robust technological design, clear evaluation metrics, ethical protocols and implementation strategies make this proposal an initiative with high potential for impact. By integrating science, technology and pedagogy, the foundations are laid to transform the way we conceive the relationship between well-being and learning in the twenty-first century.

With this vision, the project not only seeks to solve an immediate problem, but also to build an academic and social legacy that demonstrates how gamification, well implemented, can become a catalyst for profound change in the training of new generations.

REFERENCES

Angulo, B. P., Gaxiola, A. A., Peñuelas, E. G., & Lagarda, A. C. (2018). Incidence and degree of anxiety in higher level students in the area of health sciences. *Salud en Tabasco, 24*(1), 21-26. Retrieved from https://tabasco.gob.mx/sites/default/files/users/ssaludtabasco/21.pdf

Beck, A. T., Epstein, N., Brown, G., & Steer, R. A. (1988). An inventory for measuring clinical anxiety: Psychometric properties. *Journal of Consulting and Clinical Psychology*, *56*(6), 893–897. DOI: 10.1037/0022-006X.56.6.893 PMID: 3204199

Beck, A. T., Steer, R. A., & Brown, G. K. (1996). *Manual for the Beck Depression Inventory-II*. Psychological Corporation.

Berson, I. R., & Berson, M. J. (2019). Digital citizenship and emotional literacy: Building empathy in online environments. *Journal of Social Studies Education Research*, *10*(2), 1–20.

Cárdenas, A., Castro, C., Chacón, M. J., Cabrera, Z., & Hernández, V. (2023). Health habits in university students and perceptions about weight and diet during the SARS-CoV2 pandemic. Science and Humanism in Health 2023, Vol. 10, No 3, pp85-91 Retrieved from. http://revista.medicina.uady.mx

Deterding, S., Dixon, D., Khaled, R., & Nacke, L. (2011). From game design elements to gamefulness: Defining "gamification". En *Proceedings of the 15th International Academic MindTrek Conference: Envisioning Future Media Environments* (pp. 9–15). ACM. https://doi.org/DOI: 10.1145/2181037.2181040

Federal Telecommunications Institute. (IFT) (2024). *National Survey on the Availability and Use of Information Technologies in Households (ENDUTIH) 2023.* Retrieved from https://www.ift.org.mx/comunicacion-y-medios/comunicados-ift/es/el-inegi-el-ift-y-la-sct-presentan-los-resultados-de-la-endutih-2023

Fernández-Abascal, E. G. (2018). *Human Emotion and Motivation: Fundamentals psychological aspects of well-being*. Pirámide.

Fogg, B. J. (2003). *Persuasive technology: Using computers to change what we think and do*. Morgan Kaufmann. DOI: 10.1016/B978-155860643-2/50011-1

Gee, J. P. (2007). What video games have to teach us about learning and literacy. Palgrave Macmillan. Recuperado de https://dl.acm.org/doi/abs/10.1145/950566.950595

GOB. (2023, June 27). *The National Survey on Mental Health and Addictions begins.* Government of Mexico. https://www.gob.mx/salud/prensa/inicia-levantamiento-de-la-encuesta-nacional-de-salud-mental-y-adicciones

Government of the State of Jalisco. (2021). *Jalisco State Governance and Development Plan 2018-2024, vision 2030. Update 2021* (2nd ed.). Secretariat of Planning and Citizen Participation. https://plan.jalisco.gob.mx/

Gutierrez, A., Sanchez, E., & Rios, C. (2024). Proposal for psychoeducational intervention in adolescents in the first year of secondary school. *Contemporary Dilemmas Journal: Education, Politics and Values., X I*(3). https://dilemascontemporaneoseducacionpoliticayvalores.com/index.php/dilemas/article/view/4160

Guzmán Acosta, C. (2025). Private higher education in Mexico. *Journal of Psychology of the Autonomous University of the State of Mexico, 14*(41), 68–92. https://revistapsicologia.uaemex.mx/article/view/26051

Happify, Inc. (s.f.). *The Science Behind Happify*. Recuperado de https://www.happify.com/public/science-behind-happify/

HashStudioz Technologies. (s.f.). *Mental Health Meets Gamification: Designing Emotionally Intelligent Apps*. Recuperado de https://www.hashstudioz.com/blog/mental-health-meets-gamification-designing-emotionally-intelligent-apps/

Kapp, K. M. (2012). The gamification of learning and instruction: Game-based methods and strategies for training and education. Pfeiffer. Recuperado de https://scholar.google.com/citations?view_op=view_citation&hl=es&user=UEujZfUAAAAJ&citation_for_view=UEujZfUAAAAJ:u5HHmVD_uO8C

Maqbool, M., Farooq, M., Imran, M., Alghafli, M., & Fatima, N. (2025). Mental health and academic performance of students at tertiary level: The role of housing. *Frontiers in Education, 10*, 1627192. Advance online publication. DOI: 10.3389/feduc.2025.1627192

Merry, S. N., Stasiak, K., Shepherd, M., Frampton, C., Fleming, T., & Lucassen, M. F. (2012). The effectiveness of SPARX, a computerised self help intervention for adolescents seeking help for depression: Randomised controlled non-inferiority trial. *BMJ (Clinical Research Ed.), 344*(apr18 3), e2598. https://www.bmj.com/content/344/bmj.e2598. DOI: 10.1136/bmj.e2598 PMID: 22517917

Ministry of Health & National Institute of Public Health. (2024). Report on the Results of the National Health and Nutrition Survey - Continuous 2023. In *ENSANUT.* National Institute of Public Health. Retrieved August 15, 2025, from https://ensanut.insp.mx/encuestas/ensanutcontinua2023/doctos/informes/ensanut_23_112024.pdf

Ministry of Public Education. (2025, August 26). *Bulletin 113: SEP starts the start of the 2024-2025 school year* [Press release]. Government of Mexico. https://www.gob.mx/sep/articulos/boletin-113-arranca-sep-inicio-del-ciclo-escolar-2024-2025?idiom=es

Moreno Arellano, C. (2025). Towards universal coverage in higher education? Perspectives on the increase in enrollment in Mexico. *The Journal of Higher Education, 54*(214), 19–42. DOI: 10.36857/resu.2025.214.3268

Psicosmart. (2024, September 21). *The influence of gamification on students' mental health: benefits and risks*. Retrieved from https://psicosmart.pro/articulos/articulo-la-influencia-de-la-gamificacion-en-la-salud-mental-de-los-estudiantes-beneficios-y-riesgos-200608

Romero Agudelo, L. N., Salinas Urbina, V., & Mortera Gutiérrez, F. J. (2010). Learning styles based on Kolb's model in virtual education. *Apertura (Guadalajara, Jal.), 2*(1).

Romero López, E. (2024, October 4). Chapala has recorded three suicides so far this year. *Laguna Weekly*. Retrieved from http://semanariolaguna.com/82002/

Ryan, R. M., & Deci, E. L. (2000). Self-determination theory and the facilitation of intrinsic motivation, social development, and well-being. *The American Psychologist, 55*(1), 68–78. https://psycnet.apa.org/doiLanding?doi=10.1037%2F0003-066X.55.1.68. DOI: 10.1037/0003-066X.55.1.68 PMID: 11392867

Samba, D. (n.d.). *The 10 Best Apps for Virtual Support in Mental Health*. Digital Samba Blog. Retrieved from https://www.digitalsamba.com/es/blog/the-top-10-apps-for-virtual-mental-health-support

Shandley, K., Austin, D., Klein, B., & Kyrios, M. (2010). An evaluation of 'Reach Out Central': an online gaming program for supporting the mental health of young people. . Recuperado de https://academic.oup.com/her/article-abstract/25/4/563/573881?redirectedFrom=fulltext&login=falseDOI: 10.1093/her/cyq002

Smartico Help Center. (2024, March). *March 2024*. Smartico.ai. Retrieved from https://help.smartico.ai/welcome/more/release-notes/march-2024

Smidt, A., Balandin, S., Sigafoos, J., & Reed, V. A. (2009). Kirkpatrick's model: A useful tool for evaluating training outcomes. *Journal of Intellectual & Developmental Disability, 34*(3), 266–274. DOI: 10.1080/13668250903093125 PMID: 19681007

Spahl, W., Carter, M., Guillemin, M., & Young, D. (2024). *Gamified Digital Mental Health Interventions for Young People: Scoping Review of Ethical Aspects During Development and Implementation*.

Taylor, M. E., Liu, M., Abelson, S., Eisenberg, D., Lipson, S. K., & Schueller, S. M. (2024). Scope, effectiveness, adoption, implementation, and maintenance of digital mental health interventions for college students: A systematic review. *Current Psychiatry Reports*, *26*(12), 683–693. DOI: 10.1007/s11920-024-01545-w PMID: 39392547

Team, S., & Team, S. (2021, 29 julio). *Headspace vs Calm Meditation App Comparison | Sleepopolis*. Sleepopolis. https://sleepopolis.com/headspace-vs-calm-meditation-app-comparison/

Technologies, U. (2020). Unity as a Library. Unity Documentation. Retrieved from https://docs.unity3d.com/Manual/UnityasaLibrary.html

The Stanford Daily. (2025, January 12). *Stanford students release Sharotonin, a new app to gamify mental health* [Satirical article]. Retrieved from https://stanforddaily.com/2025/01/12/mental-health-gamified/

Ting, T. T., Han, K. M., Feng, S. Y., Tan, B. Z., Kit, C. J., Husin, W. N. A.-A. W., Aitizaz, A., Shabbir, M., Khattak, U. F., & Sunday, A. (2024). Afolalu. Exploring Video Games Impact on Mental Health among University (2024). *Pakistan Journal of Life and Social Sciences*, *22*(2), 23912–23939. DOI: 10.57239/PJLSS-2024-22.2.001706

UN-UNICEF-Uruguay. (2020). *Social networks and adolescents, what you need to know*. Retrieved from https://www.unicef.org/uruguay/crianza/digital/redes-sociales-y-adolescentes-lo-que-tenes-que-saber

UNESCO IESALC. (2024, November 11). *New report: Supporting the mental health of higher education students*. Retrieved from https://www.iesalc.unesco.org/es/articles/nuevo-informe-apoyando-la-salud-mental-de-los-estudiantes-de-educacion-superior

University of Guadalajara. (2023, June 27). *60 percent of CUCS students suffer academic stress*. https://www.udg.mx/es/noticia/sufre-estres-academico-60-por-ciento-de-estudiantes-del-cucs

Wanniarachchi, V. U., Greenhalgh, C., Choi, A., & Warren, J. R. (2025). Personalization variables in digital mental health interventions for depression and anxiety in adolescents and youth: A scoping review. *Frontiers in Digital Health*, *7*, 1500220. DOI: 10.3389/fdgth.2025.1500220 PMID: 40444184

Zamani, S., Rostami, A., Nguyen, M., Sinha, R., & Madanian, S. (2025). A Gamified AI-Driven Systemfor Depression Monitoringand Management. *Applied Sciences (Basel, Switzerland)*, *15*(13), 7088. DOI: 10.3390/app15137088

Chapter 2
Gamification of Life Plan Design Subject as Strategy to Promote Student Psycho-Emotional Well-Being

Madeleine Gabriela Contreras Davito
https://orcid.org/0000-0003-0336-7003
Universidad de Guadalajara, Mexico

Jacqueline Gutiérrez-Contreras
Universidad de Guadalajara, Mexico

Jesús Cabral-Araiza
https://orcid.org/0009-0006-9078-6044
Universidad de Guadalajara, Mexico & Centro Universistario de la Costa, Mexico

Carmen Leticia Salcedo-Quevedo
https://orcid.org/0000-0003-0336-7003
Instituto Tecnológico de Jalisco, Chapala, Mexico

Armando Ariel Gutiérrez-Lopez
https://orcid.org/0009-0001-1301-3789
Universidad de Guadalajara, Mexico

María Isabel Mendoza-Rodríguez
Universidad de Guadalajara, Mexico

ABSTRACT

The high school Regional of Ixtlahuacan de los Membrillos belongs to the Higher Middle Education System of the University of Guadalajara, it is located in a sub-urban town, specifically Capilla-Atequiza road, close to the Metropolitan Area of Guadalajara, approximately 40 km away. It is worth mentioning that in Mexico, Guadalajara acquires great importance in educational, economic, political, social issues, among others. Interested in contributing to the excellent academic training of young people at a national and international level, the University of Guadalajara

DOI: 10.4018/979-8-3373-4657-1.ch002

contributes with human capital, infrastructure and other essential processes in education. For this purpose, the Higher Secondary Education System was created in 1984, which of course carries out teaching, research and dissemination functions at this level. Its schools are distributed throughout the state of Jalisco.

INTRODUCTION

The high school Regional of Ixtlahuacan de los Membrillos belongs to the Higher Middle Education System of the University of Guadalajara, it is located in a suburban town, specifically Capilla-Atequiza road, close to the Metropolitan Area of Guadalajara, approximately 40 km away. It is worth mentioning that in Mexico, Guadalajara acquires great importance in educational, economic, political, social issues, among others.

This school system also focuses on teaching to develop functions additional to teaching that are equally relevant such as research and extension as expressed in their statutes with ethical values, interested in ethics, quality, relevance, innovation and transparency, demonstrating a great commitment to social links, the dissemination of culture as well as the promotion of inclusive and sustainable development, además del interés en el desarrollo integral del individuo en comunidad.

It is a reality that by having these ambitious goals, issues and challenges arise to be addressed, such as the one that gives rise to this research project because from historical moments such as those experienced derived from the Sars-Covs 2019 pandemic, health issues and understood by health, the comprehensive approach to health that includes physical aspects as well as social and emotional aspects of the individual, acquired great relevance.

For Esparza Meza et al. (2022) who dedicated themselves to delving into the experiences of young Mexicans in the face of the pandemic and confinement due to COVID-19, areas such as social and school turned out to be the most affected in terms of emotional well-being.

They reaffirm that in adolescence, social interaction is essential to reach maturity, with the premise of adapting to their environments in a healthier way, with a balance in the family, interested in their future and learning from, for example, what was an important example of uncertainty.

Subjects such as the one taken as a reference for the innovation proposal through gamification, in collaboration with the Head of Comprehensive Development, who exposes the importance of emphasizing that a necessary competence to achieve in students is that they identify aspects of their person and environment that influence their life to determine their present and plan their future.

It is necessary to motivate and interest so that this academic experience is not only mandatory content to review but rather goes to a level where knowledge, attitudes and values allow processes such as strengthening identity, identifying positive vs. negative attitudes, classifying goals, topics of self-realization, delimitation of expectations, steps to make decisions, areas of the life project, design of strategies.

Now, the proposal does not seek the traditional way of teaching classes with themes but rather promotes self-discovery, through thinking skills, that privilege analysis, reflection, introspection and in it processes such as self-observation, self-criticism and self-affirmation, at more than some point through gamification you will have the opportunity to seek discernment and a key part is that this learning leads you to either a current moment or a projection in the short term to the need to manage their own information and also to consider their social being, through collaboration.

This is also an activity that, although playful, is promoted from the perspective of knowing how to be, that is, with values and attitudes such as willingness, proactivity, initiative, a commitment because it is part of a curriculum subject where even when there is technological medication, the role of the teacher as someone who accompanies and guides this process of self-determination in the student is a key piece.

For the purposes of this research project, findings derived from what the pandemic demonstrates, that is, the need to give a predominant place to psychological and motivational processes, to forms, modes, and learning spaces that consider Information and Communication Technologies, are taken up, since it is the young people themselves who demonstrate that it is part of their learning ecosystem.

Regarding the school environment before, during and after events that more plausibly put needs related to emotional well-being, taking up contributions from researchers, the proposal is based on integrating these ecosystems, and based on this, making it possible to contribute to managing and integrating contexts through strategies that manage to expand contextual limits (family, school, individual) with new models to learn but above all achieve comprehensive development (García-Peñalvo, 2018).

As part of the collegiate and academic work at the Regional High School of Ixtlahuacan de los Membrillos in constant review of the curricular contents, valuing its relevance and seeking to expand to daily life, what students can make their own and meaningful, it is considered that comprehensive well-being is the responsibility of those who make up the educational community, independent of their disciplinary area, it is to conceive on the one hand that it is, as already mentioned, an ecosystem, which must provide the possibility of addressing complex needs by transforming information systems. traditional ones sticking to this particular context.

In the facilitation of this subject, the aim is to make it a space where not only theoretical content is addressed but also where students, based on the observation that they are influenced by other important contexts such as the family and social context to which they belong, form a learning ecosystem, where ICT is used as part of this environment, promoting that they can transcend their lives in this immediate present with a view to their further development, for example incorporating through game strategies aspects of autonomy, emotional regulation that converge in your comprehensive well-being, including mental health. (Chen, L., Xia, M. 2025)

This subject is Life Plan Design, which is justified to be taught to 5th grade students. semester of high school, that is, two semesters before their expected graduation from this school stage, which also positions them in a general way, prior to reaching the age of majority, which in legal terms turns them into adults capable of making autonomous decisions in different areas, especially at the social, work and political level.

In this gamification proposal that is interested in relying on the Socratic method, which is intended to provide the philosophical scaffolding for deep reflection, its implementation in environments of high digital demand and low attention requires a strategy that captures and maintains the intrinsic interest of the student, therefore it is sought that gamification takes care of these pedagogical aspects.

Several authors in the course of this decade have emphasized the incorporation, and even migration, toward learning environments that privilege technological devices, as well as the use of gamification within courses.

Clark et al. (2016) point out that games as a medium can, in fact, support productive learning. Thus, for the purposes of this study, a predominantly receptive position is questioned—one in which the student, regarding content that ought to fall entirely within their own responsibility, remains in expectation of whatever the teacher decides to include.

As explained previously, the design of a life project must be conceptualized as curricular content whose very purpose is to enable action: to allow each student to personally appropriate the content and become activated in pursuit of more effective learning. Moreover, the learning environment in which gamification is implemented can also exert a significant impact on academic performance. The face-to-face modality exhibited greater positive effects in comparison with online and hybrid modalities (Li et al., 2023).

That is to say, in order to achieve a transformation such as the one pursued by this proposal—one that yields favorable results—it is not, based on the findings of the aforementioned authors, a matter of leading students into an asynchronous, self-paced process. Rather, it concerns the gamification of learning under the premise of reinforcing what is intended for students to acquire, and this is attained through accompaniment, even when their participation involves engaging in a simulated environment through a technological platform to which they could otherwise have independent access.

Since this subject is conceptualized with the purpose of fostering continuity in adolescents' lives after graduation, the need is recognized to restructure didactics and promote students' engagement in intentionally designed activities through gamification. This approach seeks to enhance cognitive competencies such as reflection and decision-making, given that what they examine in class will be mirrored in a scenario where, in order to progress toward the goal of the game, it becomes indispensable for them to fulfill the required tasks. When translated into the psychology of play, there emerges a social component which, in everyday classroom contexts, may or may not arise: a stance centered on individual performance that scarcely reveals whether the person will face the dilemma of giving up and losing, or instead exerting greater effort to obtain the reward.

The intention, therefore, is that a course reviewed within the framework of socio-emotional training, by transforming its didactic strategies, may enable students to acquire meaningful learning for their life project. Consequently, it should become more attractive, foster greater confidence in the facilitators, and even strengthen students' engagement with teachers who may serve as guides or mentors.

It can be stated that the teacher seeks to generate in students a sense of self-satisfaction, while also improving their academic performance and socio-emotional well-being. For the purposes of this proposal, the content is closely connected to what will constitute their trajectory and plans for life; therefore, inherent within it are challenges arising from their daily interactions. Addressing these challenges will require the support that the teacher can provide through professional competencies aimed at guiding students to confront such issues with an ethical orientation, grounded in autonomy in both roles and shared responsibility. The teacher, therefore, requires skills to guide the student and to stimulate their advancement toward new knowledge (Chamorro et al., 2022).

The learning sequences in the Life Plan Design course are designed to follow a dynamic process that aims to create an autogenous workshop. Therefore, gamification was incorporated as a strategy to generate personal interest. The relevant section describes how, by incorporating artificial intelligence as a central element, it is possible to activate psychological mechanisms that promote active engagement. It is also clarified that for this strategy to be effective, it is vital that it aligns with sound theories of motivation (Ryan & Deci, 2020).

In parallel, the teacher, as the person responsible for accompanying the student who, as will be seen later, goes through a period of transformations in their life cycle, must promote teamwork and the search for solutions to the situations present in the students' experiences in their process of self-discovery, which will be facilitated through the gamification platform.

It is necessary that what in other spaces, such as what happens when using technologies, be expanded towards aspects of life, in learning, that is why gamification must allow socialization in a private space later, making it public in the class and allowing them to share their experiences, so that it later becomes learning strategies for social inclusion and facing real life and the next adult life.

The student seeks to avoid exposing themselves in a way that reveals who they truly are, instead referring to group members as acquaintances with whom they must share the moment. Once these individuals are considered and referred to as friends, trust is established (González & Gewerc, 2021), Therefore, the use of avatars also in the gamification space, allows, on a psychological level, freedom to explore without open exposure from their perspective.

Following these reflections, teachers and researchers in the fields of psychology and information and communication technologies consider it appropriate to take into account fundamental axes to guide the development of competencies that we assume and hope will accompany students throughout their lives.

Based on the aforementioned considerations, the participating teachers discuss possible strategies, which are grouped into three pathways: platform-based gamification with AI (AI Digital Mentor). Criteria for analysis are established, grounded in the pedagogical framework of the active methodologies previously described.

A) **Structure**, where elements intrinsic to gamification are considered, such as levels, rewards or bonuses, among others.
B) **Preponderant processes to be integrated into the pedagogical approach**, including multiple intelligences, self-awareness, socio-emotional processes, reflection and collaboration, critical thinking, introspection, and self-exploration.
C) **Tools and spaces**, such as mini-games, puzzles, forums, and artificial intelligence, to cite a few examples.
D) **Incentive for the level of motivation**, discussed based on evidence from studies that affirm that gamification contributes to increasing motivation, with high levels reflected in grades categorized as high, upper-medium, and very high.
E) **Evaluation processes**: Implementation of stickers and achievements, rubric-based evaluation through challenges and group co-evaluation, as well as evaluation using AI—both automatic and integrated with the tutor's assessment.
F) **Assessment of innovation based on current literature**: Moderate, Moderate–High, Very High.
G) **Correspondence and relevance to the subject curriculum**: Various aspects such as self-awareness, analysis of strengths and weaknesses, decision-making, reflection, self-management, and the interconnection with emotional well-being.
H) **Scalability**: As part of the contribution of this proposal, it is analyzed as a collegial work that generates knowledge and can initially be implemented within the High School Network of the University of Guadalajara, evaluating the reach of all three approaches.

The relevant aspects that will be taken into consideration in pedagogical terms are based on narrative levels (Seeker, Strategist, Visionary) and symbolic rewards (fragments, badges, puzzle pieces).

Intensive use of AI (GPTs, image generators, bots) + integration with Classroom and Curipod

Very high: immersive narrative, personalization, AI as a "digital mentor" that questions and accompanies the student

Evaluation through AI-generated products (transcriptions, images, narratives), with automatic feedback and tutor input.

Directly links to plan competencies (self-awareness, resource management, self-realization) and connects to emotional well-being

Scalable and adaptable: relies on accessible AI and existing platforms (Classroom, Curipod).

Next, in the design section, the aforementioned aspects of gamification will be detailed.

Therefore, the aim is to provide a different direction through an active methodology, revisiting a gamification approach that incorporates the Socratic method alongside information and communication technologies, allowing the student population to engage in diverse learning spaces, including virtual environments.

In the gamification-based game proposal, the Socratic method is proposed as a strategy to develop higher-order psychological skills that, in turn, enable the capacity to argue, stimulate thinking, and solve problems. The function of the Socratic method, through dialogue with open-ended questions, is articulated to promote internalization and the reconsideration of new information (Suárez et al., 2016).

Consequently, the Socratic method is supported by AI within virtual spaces, enabling students to establish a safe environment, self-manage their learning, and orient it toward their socio-emotional well-being.

Theoretical Framework: Gamification of the Life Plan Design Subject as a Strategy to Promote Psycho-Emotional Development in Adolescence

Discussing adolescence entails addressing one of the most crucial stages of life. Using an analogy, it can be compared to trapeze artists in a circus: one releases a person (the adolescent) while another awaits them on the other side. Yet the adolescent is not yet fully in the other artist's hands; they are suspended in the air, revolving before being caught. This stage represents adolescence—having left childhood behind but not yet having entered adulthood.

In this way, we can better understand the diverse processes that occur during this stage of life, in which an individual must transition from a pleasurable and less demanding period to another marked by greater and more complex responsibilities. This transition may be further complicated by intricate situations that arise either individually or through external influences, making this stage of life even more challenging.

But what should we formally understand by adolescence?

Adolescence derives from the Latin word adolescere, from the verb adolecer, and in Spanish it has two meanings: to have a certain imperfection or defect, and also growth and maturation. It is the transitional period between childhood and adulthood, accompanied by intense physical, psychological, emotional, and social changes. It begins with puberty (a purely organic aspect) and ends around the second decade of life, when physical growth and development as well as psychosocial maturation are complete. The World Health Organization (WHO) considers adolescence to span ages 10 to 19, while youth is defined as the period between 19 and 25 years. The American Society for Adolescent Health and Medicine (SAHM) situates adolescence between 10 and 21 years, distinguishing three overlapping phases: early adolescence (10–14 years), middle adolescence (15–17 years), and late adolescence (18–21 years) (Güemes-Hidalgo et al., 2017, p. 8).

Given that this is a volatile stage filled with existential doubts about the future, it becomes essential to assist adolescents in constructing a Life Plan. The absence of such a plan can be observed in adults who do not know which direction to take, personally or professionally, and who cannot confidently answer seemingly simple questions such as, "What are you seeking in life?"

In this sense, technologies can contribute to a space that opens a panorama in terms of models, information, life perspectives, which will have to be oriented as previously explained, while a level of maturity is reached, a balance will have to be found as well as support that could be the interaction of adults in the school environment or the family, forming a solid network in situations that are under construction such as the design of their life plan.

For authors such as Martínez, G., et. to the. (2020) a system mediated by ICT can provide opportunities for socialization, self-expression, learning, creativity and participation through online or mobile media, a case that can also be adapted to this gamification proposal, since it is a world that must run in parallel, due to the previous ideas, where in this case it is intended that the adult, the teacher, becomes a kind of mentor, who at the end of his preparation and even beyond can be present, so we remember what they represent the "existential challenges" faced by adolescents are by no means minor. Perhaps some of us have forgotten, but during this stage, the daily doubts typically concern:

Existential crises, including not being certain of who one is, where one wants to be or go, what one wants to dedicate oneself to in life, or what purpose life itself holds, among other philosophical questions. The pursuit of answers to these questions could, in fact, contribute to the construction of a life plan, which will be addressed later.

Economic crises, as adolescents often recognize that they do not want to be in their current circumstances, but without financial independence, they must endure them—frequently feeling more frustrated than usual and sometimes even convinced that life is a form of "suffering."

Identity crises, an aspect that has gained increasing relevance due to various influences, as society has become more permissive or tolerant regarding diverse expressions and identifications with different genders or ways of expressing one's identity.

This accumulation of crises, which manifest during adolescence today, finds an outlet for expression and coping through communication technologies, particularly those used to generate learning experiences for adolescents.

In the Latin American context, young people are observed in behaviors related to postponing important things, such as studies, solving issues with parents or teachers, which are part of daily life, such as tasks or responsibilities and another sector of the young population, it is observed, that they are migrating to aspects more relevant to their present and future. The approach, increasingly common and routine, linked to the use of technology, allows them on the one hand to "play" with mobile devices that often bring them closer to more transcendental issues than the fact of the game itself. Topics that range from training, academic updating, learning another language or a manual skill or even making a life plan or some important decision that has to do with their immediate or long-term future. Regarding Gamification, Gaviria (2021. pp. 17-20) refers to it as follows:

> *... it detaches itself from Playfulness, does not abandon it, traces a parallel path, without overcoming it, even respecting it as a mother figure, but in its simple form, with behaviorist overtones, instructional elements and some instrumental nuances, gamification is based on a simple but elusive term: Motivation.*
>
> *Motivating, in the case of Gamification, exceeds the sphere of playfulness which, in its search to harmonize the educational environment with the curriculum by including games and fun dynamics [...].*
>
> *Gamification in its essence is not simply based on including games in the classroom, that dimension is dominated by playful, which seeks to harmonize learning with games and entertainment.*

When we talk about gamification, we are talking about the fact that young learners are able to develop a motivation not only for the contents, but also for aspects annexed to the pedagogical purposes and from there extrapolate aspects of life itself that will help them to think prospectively about other non-academic areas, essential for their person in an integral way.

Let us not forget that, according to teacher mediation, including the various gamification activities, we can have a series of concepts to develop in the student that have a direct impact on their comprehensive training, not just academic, as Prieto (2024) points out.

Life skills from a psychosocial approach must be understood from the recognition of oneself and of the other in all its dimensions through diversity, respect for identity, and the environment, without forgetting the social world, which allows mainstreaming in any context from a holistic reading of the subject in its multiple relationships and the development of competencies to strengthen the life project and even in adverse conditions.

Life skills are and go through aspects as important for human development as the following: soft skills, ethics, empathy, emotional management, resilience, self-concept, self-esteem, self-efficacy and critical thinking, among others.

With the development of these soft skills, although we cannot guarantee one hundred percent that the person can be an exemplary citizen, we can affirm that it is a considerable effort to make him a good person who not only tries to improve his own living conditions, but also the living conditions, or in this case the school conditions of his academic peers who accompany and complement him in his school environment.

On the other hand, and depending on the conditions of mediation generated by the decent person himself in gamified activities, it will be the present and future vision that the learner can develop towards himself and his material and human environment.

In the same way, there has been a lot of attempt to demonize or magnify the use or abuse of mobile devices or the use of technology in adolescents, various authors have carried out research on the matter and have shown that although there are aspects to consider, it will depend on the purposes, values and use of these devices for the consequences that are had, an example of this is the work of Moreno, I., (2025).

School spaces must play an active role in the formation of critical criteria in the face of technology. It is not enough to teach how to use devices, but it is essential to train conscious, empathetic and responsible digital citizens. The inclusion of topics such as digital ethics, privacy, management of emotions online, and voluntary disconnection is key to achieving this goal (Moreno, I. et al., 2025. p. 18).

... Adolescents with greater awareness of their digital use tend to have more satisfactory and balanced social relationships. This suggests that the development of self-regulation and critical thinking is an effective strategy to prevent the negative effects of excessive use of technology. [...] Institutional, family and community support is decisive in reducing the adverse impacts of the digital world on adolescents. It is not a matter of restricting use, but of guiding it with meaning, affection and coherence. Promoting spaces for real coexistence, where

young people are without screens, can strengthen human bonds and recover essential aspects of socialization.

These considerations of the work of Moreno et. al. (2025) propose an aspect although with particular nuances according to a given sociocultural context, it will always be an integrating axis or that can enhance the objectives of the integral formation of the student and his or her life plan approach, the theme is: The family.

Although the family in a particular context may have very specific nuances, no one denies that, in the education and comprehensive training of adolescent students, it will play a crucial role combined with their motivation and life project in their formative process in general. For Desfilis, (2020. p. 85)

...The role of the family in this area should focus on developing parenting educational styles based on dialogue, reasoning and affection, but without forgetting the importance of establishing precise limits and rules. Guidance and communication on the proper use of the Internet, as well as supervision in such use, is also crucial. Finally, a home with a positive affective climate and high parental support will be a home protected from many dangers of the Digital Age which, in turn, will be able to optimize the opportunities offered by this era for the personal development of children.

On the other hand, Lemus (2017) emphasizes in his work, a series of aspects, although punctual, no less relevant to understand some aspects related to the motivation of young people and the use of technology, the need to belong to a human group and the strengthening of identity that this gives, as a preamble to a greater or transcendent search such as the life project:

... We have analysed the appropriation of digital technologies by young people. From this, we have identified three major aspects: a) the construction and expression of one's own tastes, interests and identifications; b) the management of ties and belonging to the peer group, and c) the search to "be up to date" which are part of the ways of being young of our interviewees and that are directly linked to practices that are enabled from the appropriation of digital technologies. (pp. 170-171).

AI Has Arrived

With the advent of AI, various changes in daily life have accelerated. It is no longer a matter of some science fiction story in which a "future" would arrive—this future is already the present. Adolescents' lives are not exempt from these changes. Their schooling, future work, learning methods, and everyday life in general—like everyone else's—are experiencing increasing transformations and impacts. The use of increasingly powerful devices, combined with AI that "solves" life challenges previously considered insurmountable, now results in a kind of competition to see how quickly tasks can be completed.

This does not mean, as once thought, that life will become easier, as it may present unforeseen challenges. For example, the development of one's own intelligence, critical thinking, and even common sense can be disrupted in a kind of skills fair, in which the most capable individual is the one who masters the use of AI tools for a given purpose.

At this point, the purpose and use of AI, as well as the user's prior values, must always be considered—values that should be grounded in personal integrity and professional training. The use of any device or tool is not inherently harmful; rather, the questionable aspect lies in the intention and ultimate purpose of its use.

The adopted position is that artificial intelligence is a powerful tool that can contribute to the holistic development of adolescents, provided it is used ethically, responsibly, and with a focus on human well-being. It is crucial for designers, developers, and technology users to recognize the importance of considering AI's social and emotional impact on young people's lives and to work toward solutions that promote inclusion, equity, and the common good (Changoluisa, 2024, p. 3437).

For example, some studies analyze the impact of influencers, those personalities who use virtual communication, creating a form of informal learning in areas related to emotional development and soft skills. Taddeo G. (2023) one of the benefits of AI to generate a significant impact on adolescents.

And in this way, some scientific research articles have focused on investigating what media content young people are interested in, both the use of virtual platforms, social networks, among other purely informative spaces such as television.

For Tirocchi, S. (2024) young people use virtual spaces for the exchange of values such as the search for authenticity and truthfulness that is part of reality, always investigating new content where they can connect with that media content.

Gonzalez R. A J., De La Rosa M. I. (2025) emphasizes the importance of the construction of the self in virtual contexts where the present generations have a perception of the stable image, but even identity requires strengthening in digital environments where the teacher must acquire skills to criticize and question from those spaces.

Adolescents are already immersed in the virtual space from where learning is being generated linked to what the young person needs to satisfy while the facilitator or teacher needs to guide the learning towards teaching the essential requirements for life.

According to other research that indicates the transition of adolescents from a millennial generation to generation Z, online content grows and the consumption of magazines as a means of information is abandoned and interests change towards self-care, independence or self-confidence according to the study that was carried out on Spanish adolescents. Fernández Castrillo, C. and González-González, A. (2025).

From where the use of virtual content is investigated as a form of interaction that shows the interests of the adolescent population, trying to observe how it impacts the adolescent's identity.

We find a proposal for a pedagogy of critical adaptation to youth in the networks since young people have poor management in the use of networks, the information is full of mandates and stereotypes of what a teenager should be and do on the network. Serrate-Gonzalez, Sara; Sanchez-Rojo, Alberto; Andrade-Silva, Luis-E; Muñoz-Rodriguez, José-Manuel. (2023).

Therefore, take into consideration that identity, its forms and modes of interaction in the adolescent, its own crises must have an important influence derived from technological integration and digitality, hence the opportunity to expand this learning that provides content in the school curriculum for the development of a life project that takes into account the current aspects of the psychosocial development of the adolescent.

There are many facets from which the influence of AI use or misuse on various areas of life can be analyzed. However, there are certain aspects that we can already begin to consider for its proper management and regulation, as noted by Monné Bellmun (2025):

"In youth, the contributions of AI can also be positive. AI can enhance educational and employment opportunities through online learning platforms, career guidance, and simulations of work environments, providing young people with the tools to better prepare for the future [...]. Moreover, some AI-based applications can help monitor and manage young people's mental health, offering support to those experiencing disorders such as anxiety or depression" (p. 9).

Another consideration in adolescence arises when supervision takes on new dimensions. It is no longer the case that parents have "control" over the sites and times in which the "child" uses their time or accesses any device for any purpose. We know, for example, that such tools can be exploited even by organized crime for various harmful purposes. However, if used wisely and to their fullest potential, these tools can also become powerful instruments to combat social inequality and inequity.

In other words, we return to a point of origin: although parents can no longer manage the times or places where their child accesses a device, nor know which platform or AI is being used, the child's trust should be rooted in the time previously spent teaching values and ethical norms, trusting that they have nurtured a well-rounded human being capable of benefiting others.

Despite the risks involved, it cannot be denied that the integration of digital technologies into everyday life has facilitated cultural and social development. These tools not only enable the creation of spaces for commerce and economic exchange, but also provide instant access to vast amounts of information and allow the formation of new interpersonal relationships [...]. Therefore, while it is necessary to consider concerns regarding young people's mental health, it is equally important to recognize the benefits these technologies bring in terms of connectivity and social development (Gutiérrez-Ochoa et al., 2024, pp. 8–9).

In other words, we cannot demonize AI due to deficiencies in the psycho-affective correlation systems within the family or school environment. When the student has established the solid foundations necessary for harmonious development, the rest becomes easier, facilitating the integration of the self and the construction of a life plan that encompasses all areas of life in a balanced manner.

Among the tasks that AI facilitates for adolescents in the school environment are:

- Access to a large amount of information on diverse topics.
- Prioritization of topics or situations they wish to organize regarding specific subjects.
- Ranking of relevant aspects within particular themes.
- Comparison of large amounts of data or information to identify the most accurate insights.

Virtual tutoring is another area in which AI has significantly impacted the educational field. AI systems can provide students with various types of feedback, answer questions, and offer detailed explanations of difficult concepts. This has expanded access to tutoring and improved the quality of learning, allowing students to receive support in real time and at their own pace (Aparicio, 2023, p. 219).

While this is important, the creative use that students make of information—and of AI itself—is even more significant. An important factor to leverage in the case of adolescents and AI use is that, due to their psychology, age, and motivation, they seek immediate gratifications that can engage, entertain, and even facilitate social interaction. Indeed, a key motivator for them is the sense of recognition and achievement in activities programmed with AI or gamified platforms in the pursuit of new learning. AI in education is an effective tool for fostering learning, allowing young people to use it to enhance their education by personalizing their learning according to individual educational needs. However, it also reveals certain challenges in implementation, such as access, equity, and ethical use (Guillén-Parra & Moscoso-Bernal, 2024, p. 2650).

Adolescents' talents and cognitive capacities will develop to the extent that stimulation is appropriate, regulated, and managed in such a way that, as previously mentioned, it is grounded in a solid ethical foundation and clearly defined values aimed at holistic human development. Consequently, the educational sector and teaching–learning processes are already being transformed by AI, which is here to stay and will continue to evolve either alongside or at an even faster pace than the adolescent's own life.

It is also true (according to the same author) that the integration of AI into the educational sphere should open new possibilities for enriching the cognitive development of students situated within this digital revolution. Undoubtedly, the advances achieved have proliferated around the design of diverse applications and digital platforms, enabling the creation of intelligent systems capable of understanding students' learning processes, providing feedback, and assisting in the promotion of new skills and talents (De la Riva, 2024, p. 109).

Ultimately, the point is to raise awareness that AI is a tool and, as such, it is not an end in itself. Rather, it can help us achieve the goals we seek, but it is not the goal itself.

Therefore, before definitively declaring the use or misuse of AI by students as a success or failure, it is worthwhile to consider which current processes in teaching and education in general are being transformed and developed for the benefit of holistic learning outcomes.

As in many contexts, when discussing good examples or best practices, we must consider how committed and involved all parties in the process are. As Quinde-Moncerrate et al. (2025, p. 365) note:

Artificial Intelligence (AI) has a promising future while simultaneously being full of challenges that require careful collaboration among developers, educators, students, and educational institutions. The success of AI in education will depend on the capacity to address these challenges and maximize the benefits, preparing students to lead the creation of new solutions to emerging social needs.

Now following with this framework of reference, it will be developed how the gamification proposal is integrated into the subject of Life Plan Design, also taking as reference both aspects of adolescent development and the dynamics in which the subject and the changes now suggested were facilitated in the school context.

DESIGN AND GAMIFICATION STRATEGIES WITH THE USE OF AI

The curricular design of the Life Plan requires a pedagogical approach that transcends mere instruction, focusing on sustained motivation and the development of the *self* (Mejillones Picazo, 2024; Monné Bellmunt, 2025). While the Socratic method provides the philosophical scaffolding for deep reflection, its implementation in environments of high digital demand and low attention requires a strategy that captures and maintains the intrinsic interest of the student. This is where gamification is positioned not only as an entertainment tool, but also as a psychological enhancer (Jaramillo-Mediavilla et al., 2024).

For the application of playful elements to be effective and ethically responsible in the promotion of well-being, their design must be anchored in robust models of the psychology of motivation. Therefore, this proposal is based on the Self-Determination Theory (SDT), which establishes the necessary conditions to transform a compulsory task into an intrinsically valuable activity and, therefore, beneficial for the psycho-emotional state of the student.

Gamification as a Motivational Scaffolding

Gamification is defined as the use of game design elements in non-playful contexts (Deterding et al., 2011). In the educational field, its value lies not only in fun, but in its ability to activate psychological mechanisms that promote active commitment. For this strategy to be effective, it is vital that it is aligned with solid theories of motivation (Ryan & Deci, 2020) In this sense, the proposal is based on the Self-Determination Theory (SDT).

SDT (Ryan and Deci's core work) posits that motivation is most sustainable and beneficial to well-being when it is intrinsic, i.e., when the activity is done for the inherent pleasure or satisfaction it produces, rather than for an external reward.

Socratic gamification seeks to transform the curricular experience, focusing on competence (through levels and challenges), autonomy (when making decisions in the game and in AI-guided reflection) and relationship (through *feedback* and the role of the digital mentor). The symbolic reward (Fragments, Badges, Identity Puzzle) acts as *feedback* on progress, reinforcing the sense of competence, rather than being the ultimate goal of learning, differentiating it from traditional extrinsic point systems.

The Role of the Digital Socratic Mediator (AI)

AI is conceived in this model as a digital Socratic mediator or digital mentor of AI, whose role is to stimulate inquiry, critical reasoning, and autonomous reflection, rather than to provide direct answers.

The Socratic method is based on dialogue through open questions, promoting the reconsideration of information and the internalization of knowledge. In the context of the Life Plan and well-being, AI allows the student to "face themselves" in a safe and private environment, exploring dilemmas and life decisions without the vulnerability that would imply exposing themselves to a peer or a teacher. This process encourages emotional self-regulation and critical thinking about the *self*.

DESIGN AND GAMIFICATION STRATEGIES WITH THE USE OF AI (DETAILED METHODOLOGICAL PROPOSAL)

The proposal is articulated in a Hero's Journey that links playful progress with the development of essential competencies for psycho-emotional well-being and the Life Plan, and this can be visualized in table 1.

Table 1. Design and Gamification Strategies with the Use of AI

Life Plan Competence / Pedagogical Objective	Level of Gamification / Student Role	Key Tools and Interaction Dynamics	Products to Evaluate and Rewards (Game Mechanics)	Connection to Psycho-Emotional Well-Being (Developed Causal Relationship)
Competition 1: Who am I now? (Promote critical introspection and identity)	Level 1: The Seeker	Activity 1: The Mirror of Identity: Dialogue with a "Character Bot" (AI with narrative and philosophical profiles) that poses open-ended questions of self-exploration (Socratic). Activity 2: The Moral Dilemma: Interactive mini-game made with AI (Gemini) to justify ethical decisions.	Output 1: Transcription of the Socratic dialogue and personal reflection. Output 2: Transcription of the Moral Dilemma. Rewards: "Mirror of Identity Fragment" (Puzzle Starter) and "Badge of Ethical Virtue".	Thoughtful dialogue with AI mitigates the teen's existential uncertainty and identity crisis by offering a neutral and safe validation space for self-exposure. The Integration of Values (Ethical Badge) promotes axiological consistency, essential for self-esteem and self-concept.
Competency 2: Control of My Life Is in My Hands (Integrating Personal and Social Perceptions; Resource Management)	Level 2: The Strategist	Activity 1: The Image Creator (Collective Mural): Use of image-generating AI (e.g., Image) and Curipod. The student metaphorizes strengths/ weaknesses and receives peer co-evaluation on the image.	Product: AI-generated image and feedback log received. Reward: "Collective Puzzle Piece" (Symbolizes the integration of the self and the social perspective).	AI-assisted metaphorical strengths/weaknesses (resources) analysis facilitates emotional regulation by externalizing self-perception. Co-evaluation of peers in a playful environment fosters social adaptability and resilience, transforming potential judgment into constructive support and managing social vulnerability.
Competence 3: Mapping My Life Plan (Synthesis, Definition of Strategies and Projection)	Level 3: The Visionary	Activity 1: Simulation of the Future (Conversational SWOT Analysis with Strategic AI, e.g., Magic School). AI guides the identification of resources, opportunities, and threats related to life goals. Activity 2: The Hero's Journey (Final Puzzle): Use of custom GPT that integrates previous deliverables and structures the Life Plan as a personal epic narrative.	Output 1: Transcription organized in a SWOT matrix. Output 2: Final Narrative of the Life Plan. Final Reward: "Complete Identity Puzzle" (Symbolizes the integration of learning and future projection).	Strategic visualization and realistic AI-assisted planning counteract disconnection or lack of future guidance, equipping the student with agency and self-efficacy over their life. The Hero Narrative integrates learning into a purposeful story, strengthening intrinsic motivation and clarity of values.

Each week's activities correspond to the competencies and products described in the design table. In Competence 1, the mirror of identity and the moral dilemma generate the transcripts that are evaluated with rubrics and award the mirror fragment and the badge of ethical virtue. In Competition 2, the metaphorical mural and the retro between pairs produce the image and its registration, which activate the piece of the collective puzzle. In Competence 3, the conversational SWOT and final narrative integrate learning into the complete identity puzzle. This evidence is uploaded to the LMS and assessed with rubrics; In parallel, pre-post scales and weekly check-ins measure changes in autonomy, competence, relationship, resilience and commitment

IMPLEMENTATION AND EVALUATION OF THE PROPOSAL

The intervention lasts between six and eight weeks and we applied it with groups of 30 to 40 students in the 5th semester. Our objective is twofold and very specific: to increase academic commitment and strengthen psycho-emotional well-being, understood as feeling more autonomy (I can choose and decide), competence (I feel capable and I advance) and relationship (I feel accompanied and valued). To achieve this, we use small, achievable challenges (micro-challenges), a progress board with levels and badges that reward effort and improvement, and a Socratic mentor with AI who doesn't "give answers," but asks questions to make you think better about your decisions. If you've ever felt stuck because no one asked you "what real options do you have?" or "what first step is so small you could do it today?", you already sense the kind of guidance the mentor offers.

We started with a very human kick-off session without technicalities. We present the logic of the proposal with everyday examples: "when you have a choice, you care more; when you see progress, you keep going; when someone accompanies you without judging, you dare." We built a small didactic contract: how we will give feedback, what we expect from the responsible use of AI and how we will take care of the group climate. Each student writes a brief personal goal (academic and life) in clear language; We are not looking for poetry, we are looking for concreteness ("To raise my average in history from 7 to 8; sleep before 11 p.m. three days a week"). We closed the first week with a micro-diagnosis: short scales (Likert type 1–5) to measure how they feel in terms of autonomy, competence, relationship, resilience (ability to get up after a stumble) and commitment to studying. This gives us a "pre" photo that we will later compare with the "post".

The technical context is simple so that it does not become an obstacle. As long as the classroom has a projector, stable internet, one device per pair (ideal 1:1, but not essential) and a shared digital space (LMS, cloud folder, whatever). The level and badge board can be physical (a cork with cards) or digital (a spreadsheet with colors). The role of the teacher is key: he is not a "point policeman", but a facilitator who organizes the rhythm, models how to ask questions well, validates evidence and stops any inappropriate use of AI. The AI mentor is framed by clear rules: he asks questions, offers alternatives, synthesizes ideas; He does not do homework, does not give opinions about people and does not save personal data. Students choose routes, run micro-challenges, write short logs, and give feedback among peers.

The weekly sequence moves forward like a spiral that adds clarity, practice, and confidence. In week 2 we explore purpose and options: each one chooses a path of focus (identity and strengths, habits and concentration, or life project). Here we use the AI mentor for the first time in a guided way: "ask me three questions to choose the route that suits me best" or "help me break down my goal into 20-minute steps". Week 3 is design: in teams, they write a one-week micro-challenge with very visible achievement criteria ("by the end of the week we will have X evidence"). Week 4 is a test and adjustment: they execute the challenge, hold daily five-minute mini-meetings ("what will we do today, what is in the way, how do we remove it") and receive training feedback from the teacher. Week 5 repeats the idea but now with collaboration between teams to strengthen the relationship: share tricks, ask for help, give credit. In week 6 we move the strategy to another subject (you transfer your skills to, say, math or history) so you can see that this doesn't stay in one class. Week 7 is one of curation and reflection: you order evidence, do a self-assessment with a simple rubric, and write down what you would change if you started tomorrow. Finally, week 8 closes with a mini-learning fair (three minutes per team) and a letter to the "future self" with realistic commitments and support that you will ask for when motivation falters.

Table 2. Evaluation Map (Instruments Products of Detailed Methodological Proposal)

Transcript "Mirror of Identity"	**Export chat/AI + log**	**Artifact rubric (goal, evidence, reflection, transfer)**	**Puzzle Piece 1**
Transcript of the "Moral Dilemma"	Capture/summary + justification	Justification quality rubric (add criterion in artifact)	Badge of Ethical Virtue
Metaphorical image + co-evaluation record	PNG/JPG file + "retro sandwich" form	Artifact rubric + Participation/ collaboration rubric	Collective Puzzle Piece
FUCK matrix	Document organized by quadrants	Artifact Rubric (clarity and realism)	—
Final Narrative (Life Plan)	Document/Presentation + pitch	Artifact rubric + self-assessment	Complete Identity Puzzle

Pre/post scales (Autonomy, Competence, Relationship, Resilience, Commitment) = measure the connection with well-being declared in the table. Weekly check-ins = monitor process for the same constructs (energy/options + open-ended question).

Evaluating does not mean complicating our lives or filling out infinite forms. We measure three things: how you feel, what you do, and what you count. In how you feel, we repeat at the end the brief scales of autonomy, competence, relationship, resilience and commitment. They are items with everyday language such as "I feel that I have options to fulfill my tasks" or "When I make a mistake, I know how to try differently". In what you do, we record observable behaviors with a simple rubric: attendance, on-time deliveries, and oral participation (not by duration, but by quality: clarity, respect, progress). In Which Accounts, we collect two light but powerful sources: weekly logs (three lines: what I did, what I learned, what I will change) and 4–6 voluntary 15-minute interviews at the end of the cycle, plus a small focus group if time permits. To keep a pulse, every week we apply an anonymous wellness check-in (1–5 and an open-ended question) that helps us detect in time when stress rises or motivation falls.

With the data in hand, the analysis is honest and understandable. We compared the pre- and post-averages of the scales and looked to see if there are increases of at least 0.5 points in two of the three needs (autonomy, competence or relationship) and in commitment. If the context allows it, we add a comparison group (another group of the same grade that did not experience the intervention) to better measure the changes; if not, we work with our own before-after, which already offers valuable signals. We calculated effect sizes (small/medium/large) to understand magnitude, not just whether it "came out significant". We triangulate with the observable (attendance, deliveries, participation) and with the narratives of blogs and interviews: if the numbers go up but the voices say "I felt pressured by the points", we adjust the design; If the numbers go up and phrases like "now I try again instead of giving up" appear, we are on the right track.

We also defined early on how we'll know it was worth it. We consider success if at least 80% of teams complete two micro-challenges with acceptable evidence, if they improve participation and classroom climate according to the rubric, and if we see consistent improvements in scales. But not everything is quantitative: we look for qualitative signs of agency, those phrases that indicate a change in the internal script ("I used to copy, now I ask", "I used to feel sorry, now I ask for help"). These criteria are shared from week 1 so that no one is surprised and everyone knows where we are going.

Ethics and data care are not an appendix, they are part of the design. We clearly explain that information serves to improve the class and that no one is obliged to answer everything; We respect voluntariness, use pseudonyms when sharing products publicly, and keep weekly check-ins anonymous. The AI mentor operates with explicit rules: he does not perform tasks, does not evaluate people, does not store personal data and always suggests several options, never "the only correct one". If a check-in shows high discomfort, the teacher activates a brief and compassionate protocol: listen, pause the pressure by points and, if necessary, guide the school support channels.

To ensure inclusion, we offer alternative routes when connectivity fails (printed formats with post-capture), accept oral rather than written responses when required, rotate roles in teams so that more voices have space, and avoid unnecessary technicalities. If someone advances slower, they are not penalized: the micro-challenge is adjusted so that the first step is smaller; The idea is to build trust, not anxiety.

Finally, we recognize risks and clarify how we mitigate them. If the class gets obsessed with points and forgets learning, we shift the focus from badges to narrative feedback and meaningful goals ("what's the point of this outside of class?"). If the AI mentor shows biases or unhelpful answers, we save the example (without personal data), fine-tune the prompt-guides, and model how to rephrase questions. If overload appears, we trim micro-challenges to the minimum valuable unit: a step so short that you can finish it in less than an hour a week, with a single clear piece of evidence.

We close the cycle with a one-page report that anyone on the campus can understand: objective, who it was applied to, what we did, main pre-post results on a simple board, three qualitative findings that illustrate the change and three improvement decisions for the next round. As annexes, we leave the rubrics, the examples of prompts for the mentor and a small gallery of evidence with pseudonyms. In this way, the intervention does not remain an isolated experience: it becomes a process that learns from itself and that you can replicate, refine and share with other groups. In essence, it is a design designed so that you, without being an expert in evaluation, can implement it clearly, better accompany your students and verify, with data and stories, that their motivation and well-being are growing.

NATURE OF THE STUDY AND EVALUATION PLAN

This chapter reports a rigorous implementation protocol and evaluation design for future application in 5th semester groups for 6–8 weeks. We have clearly defined indicators (autonomy, competence, relationship, resilience and commitment), instruments (short Likert-type scales, observable behavior rubrics, logs, interviews and anonymous check-ins), success criteria (increases ≥ 0.5 points in at least two TAD needs and in commitment, 80% of teams completing two micro-challenges with acceptable evidence and observable improvements in participation and climate) and ethical procedures (informed consent, anonymity at check-ins, pseudonyms on public products and rules for responsible use of the mentor with AI). Consequently, this manuscript should be understood as a design article with scheduled evaluation: the empirical results will be generated and disseminated in a subsequent study according to the schedule established below.

Scheduled evaluation schedule. We will apply pre-process measurements in Week 1 (initial diagnosis with scales and rubrics), weekly process check-ins (1–5 and an open-ended question) and post-Week 8 measurements (repetition of scales, rubrics and voluntary interviews). The analysis will include pre-post comparison, effect sizes, and triangulation with qualitative evidence. The findings will be consolidated into a one-page report (synthesis of results, three qualitative findings, and three improvement decisions) and submitted for publication in a subsequent report.

Scope. Since no data are included in this delivery, the findings are postponed until the first application is completed; however, the protocol presented allows immediate replication by teachers and management teams, and offers a clear route to obtain valid and useful evidence for decision-making.

MATERIAL AND DATA AVAILABILITY STATEMENT

The tools, rubrics, and templates described (short scales, interview guides, log formats, ethical prompts for the AI mentor, and the one-page report format) are included or referenced in the Appendices of this chapter for immediate use in school contexts. After the first application, the anonymized datasets and final materials (final versions of instruments and rubrics) will be available upon request or in the corresponding institutional repository, in accordance with the school's privacy policies and for academic purposes only.

CONCLUSIONS AND IMPLICATIONS

The proposal of Socratic gamification with AI constitutes an innovative and coherent pedagogical strategy that addresses the design of the Life Plan as a process of integral development and psycho-emotional well-being. The model's strength lies in its ability to integrate intrinsic motivation (through deep reflection and a sense of purpose) with technological adaptability (mediated by the AI Digital Mentor). It is confirmed that this model is scalable thanks to the automation of *feedback* by AI and the use of accessible platforms, allowing its application to the high school network of the University of Guadalajara and other contexts.

CHALLENGES, LIMITATIONS, AND ETHICAL CONSIDERATIONS

The implementation of any AI-based model requires a critical analysis of its limitations and ethical challenges, seeking a balance between technological innovation and educational depth.

- **Risk of superficial extrinsic motivation:** The use of badges and levels, while motivating, carries the risk that the student will focus solely on the accumulation of rewards (*overgamification*) rather than deep reflection. To mitigate this, the evaluation focuses on the depth of the argumentation and the axiological consistency of the Life Plan, and not only on the completion of the activities.
- **Equity and digital divide:** Although the model uses accessible tools, the challenge of digital inequality in access to devices and connectivity persists. The mitigation strategy involves ensuring access to school labs and support for community networks, as well as promoting transparency about the role and limits of AI.
- **AI bias and ethics**: AI mediation calls for caution, as bots can amplify biases or influence identity construction by prioritizing aspirational or unrealistic content, if not ethically designed. In this context, the role of the teacher is, and must remain, irreplaceable. Artificial intelligence, in the best of cases, is an instrument of pedagogical amplification, but at no time should it assume control of the training process, nor ethical leadership or emotional mediation. AI acts as a catalyst for reflection and an automated *feedback* manager (the "co-tutor"), but it lacks the ability to discern the complexity of the student's life context, their underlying values, or the empathetic validation of their responses. The teacher remains the architect of learning:
    - **Orchestrate the journey:** Design the flow of the experience, monitor the emotional tone of AI-generated interactions, and adapt activities in real-time.
    - **Validates ethics and reality:** Only the teacher can validate the ethical relevance and realistic viability of the life plans and decisions made, contextualizing the products generated by AI within the specific social and family realities of the students.
- **Provides psycho-emotional containment:** While AI facilitates introspection in a safe environment, the teacher is the one who manages the emotional vulnerabilities that arise from deep reflection, offering the human support, empathy, and affective bond necessary for well-being that technology cannot replicate. Therefore, total control of the training process, especially in such

sensitive topics as the Life Plan and emotional well-being, always resides in human mediation and in the ethical values that teachers transmit.

FUTURE RESEARCH DIRECTIONS

To formalise the contribution of this proposal, future lines of research should focus on:

1. **Psycho-emotional impact assessment:** Design an empirical study to quantitatively measure the effect of Socratic Gamification with AI on key variables of well-being, such as resilience, self-esteem and future orientation, comparing it with control groups using traditional methodologies.
2. **Scalability and curricular adaptation:** Evaluate the ease of replication of the model to other human development subjects and in different institutional contexts, formalizing the protocols for educational design and implementation.
3. **Ethical Prompt Design:** Investigate the most effective methodologies for designing AI Digital Mentor prompts and profiles that minimize risk of bias and maximize reflective depth and ethical discernment.

REFERENCES

Aparicio Gómez, W. O. (2023). Artificial Intelligence and its Impact on Education: Transforming Learning for the 21st Century. *International Journal of Pedagogy and Educational Innovation*, *3*(2), 217–230. DOI: 10.51660/ripie.v3i2.133

Chamorro, E., Cárdenas, J., Melo, L., Vallejo, O., Arcos, J., Bolaños, A., Poveda, J., Pinchao, L., Vianey, A., & Rodríguez, J. (2022). Competent human formation: Project-based learning experiences. https://doi.org/DOI: 10.31948/editorialunimar.164

Changoluisa Jaya, L. G. (2024). Effects of Artificial Intelligence on the Socioemotional Development of Adolescents. *Ciencia Latina Multidisciplinary Journal*, *8*(3), 3423–3440. DOI: 10.37811/cl_rcm.v8i3.11565

Chen, L., & Xia, M. (2025). Adolescent psychological adaptation: The impact of daily levels and instability in psychological need satisfaction and frustration. Journal of Adolescence, Advance online publication. https://www.researchgate.net/publication/390355467_Adolescent_Psychological_Adaptation_The_Impact_of_Daily_Levels_and_Instability_in_Psychological_Need_Satisfaction_and_Frustration. DOI: 10.1002/jad.12495

Clark, D. B., Tanner-Smith, E. E., & Killingsworth, S. S. (2016). Digital games, design, and learning: A systematic review and meta-analysis. *Review of Educational Research*, *86*(1), 79–122. DOI: 10.3102/0034654315582065 PMID: 26937054

De la Riva, B. (2024). *Beyond screens: An approach to the responsible use of AI through ICTs*. Edetania. *Estudios y Propuestas Sicoeducativos*, (65), 97–115. DOI: 10.46583/edetania_2024.65.1139

Desfilis, E. S., Martínez, I., & Serna, C. (2020). Chapter 3. Adolescents of postmodernity. Growing up in the digital age. *New Perspectives on Life Cycle Psychology*, 63-88.

Deterding, S., Dixon, D., Khaled, R., & Nacke, L. (2011). From game design elements to gamefulness: Defining gamification. *Proceedings of the 15th International Academic MindTrek Conference: Envisioning Future Media Environments*, 9–15. DOI: 10.1145/2181037.2181040

Esparza Meza, E. M., Campillo Labrandero, M., Stincer Gómez, D., Sánchez Xicotencatl, C. O., Téllez Rojo, A. L., & Aveleyra Ojeda, E. (2022). Experiences of Mexican youth facing the COVID-19 pandemic and lockdown. *Psicumex*, *13*(1), 1–27. DOI: 10.36793/psicumex.v13i1.526

Fernández Castrillo, C., & González-González, A. (2025). Youth magazines from the millennial generation to the Alpha: Analysis of the evolution in the consumption habits of Spanish adolescents. *Studies on the Journalistic Message*, *31*(2), 527–540. DOI: 10.5209/emp.98143

García-Peñalvo, F. J. (2018). Interaction in technological learning ecosystems. [EKS]. *Education in the Knowledge Society*, *19*(3), 7–13. DOI: 10.14201/eks.19341

Gaviria, D. (2021) Pedagogy de la Gamification. Colombia: Creative Commons. www.gamifiquemos.com

Gonzalez, R. A J., & De La Rosa, M. I. (2025). Self-perception of the personal image in social networks of university women: A comparative study between generations Z and Y. Social Trends. *Journal of Sociology (Melbourne, Vic.)*, *14*, 75–90.

González, V. A., & Gewerc, B. (2021). Public and private spaces for adolescents on social networks: State of the art. *IX International Multidisciplinary Congress of Educational Research, July 1–2*. Universitat de Lleida. https://dialnet.unirioja.es/servlet/libro?codigo=976466

Güemes-Hidalgo, M., Ceñal, M. J., & Hidalgo, M. I. (2017). Puberty and adolescence. *Adolescere. Journal of Continuing Education of the Spanish Society of Adolescent Medicine*, *5*(1), 7–22. https://www.adolescere.es/revista/pdf/volumen-V-n1-2017/Adolescere-2017-1.pdf

Guillén-Parra, L. S., & Moscoso-Bernal, S. A. (2024). Artificial intelligence and education: Proposal for use with 16-year-old youth. *MQRInvestigar*, *8*(3), 2631–2653. DOI: 10.56048/MQR20225.8.3.2024.2631-2653

Gutiérrez-Ochoa, S. M., Díaz-Torres, C. H., & Belandria-Vivas, L. M. (2024). Influence of new technologies on adolescence: Risks and benefits. *Gestión y Desarrollo Libre*, *9*(18), 1–24. DOI: 10.18041/2539-3669/gestionlibre.18.2024.12104

Jaramillo-Mediavilla, L., Basantes-Andrade, A., Cabezas-González, M., & Casillas-Martín, S. (2024). Impact of gamification on motivation and academic performance: A systematic review. *Education Sciences*, *14*(6), 639. DOI: 10.3390/educsci14060639

Lemus, M. (2017). Young people in front of the world: Digital technologies as a support for everyday life. *Latin American Journal of Social Sciences. Childhood and Youth*, *15*(1), 161–172. DOI: 10.11600/1692715x.1510902022016

Li, M., Ma, S., & Shi, Y. (2023). Examining the effectiveness of gamification as a tool promoting teaching and learning in educational settings: A meta-analysis. *Frontiers in Psychology*, *14*, 1253549. DOI: 10.3389/fpsyg.2023.1253549 PMID: 37876838

Mejillones Picazo, R. N. (2024). Impact of social media use with artificial intelligence on adolescents' self-esteem and identity. *Innovarium International Journal, 2*(2), 1–13. https://revinde.org/index.php/innovarium/article/view/21

Monné Bellmunt, A. (2025). Impact of technologies and AI on human development: From childhood to old age. *DIM: Didactics, Innovation, and Multimedia, (43).* https://www.raco.cat/index.php/DIM/article/view/10000003804

Moreno Infante, C. R., Cuenca Peláez, K. F., Cool Cedeño, D., Murillo León, M. E., & Quintana Monar, A. M. (2025). El impacto de la tecnología en la vida social de los adolescentes: The Impact of Technology on Adolescents' Social Life. *Multidisciplinary Journal of General Studies, 4*(2), 1370–1390. DOI: 10.70577/reg.v4i2.148

Prieto, Y. S., Garzón, A. D., & Martínez, A. P. (2024). *Life skills for adolescents in the strengthening of the life project from rural identity.* [Applied project]. UNAD Institutional Repository. https://repository.unad.edu.co/handle/10596/63858

Quinde-Moncerrate, H. G., Quinde-Zambrano, L. F., & Franco-Arroyo, P. P. (2025). Impact of artificial intelligence on contemporary education: Systematic review. *Sociedad & Tecnología, 8*(2), 358–368. DOI: 10.51247/st.v8i2.505

Ryan, R. M., & Deci, E. L. (2020). Intrinsic and extrinsic motivation: Classic definitions and new directions. *Contemporary Educational Psychology, 61*, 101863. DOI: 10.1016/j.cedpsych.2020.101863

Serrate-González, S., Sánchez-Rojo, A., Andrade-Silva, L. E., & Muñoz-Rodríguez, J. M. (2023). Onlife Identity: The Question of Gender and Age in Teenagers' Online Behaviour. *Comunicar: Media Education Research Journal, 31*(75), 9–19.

Suárez López, D., Colón López, C., Cohen Jiménez, J., & Colpas, E. (2016). Appropriation of social networks for applying the Socratic method in critical thinking. *Zona Próxima, (25)*, 118–128. https://www.redalyc.org/journal/853/85350504009/html/

Taddeo, G. (2023). Life Long/Insta-Learning: The Use of Influencers as Informal Educators. *Italian Journal of Sociology of Education, 15*(2), 147–167. DOI: 10.14658/PUPJ-IJSE-2023-2-8

Tirocchi, S. (2024). Generation Z, values, and media: From influencers to BeReal, between visibility and authenticity. *Frontiers in Sociology, 8*, 1304093. Advance online publication. DOI: 10.3389/fsoc.2023.1304093 PMID: 38274837

United Nations. (n.d.). *The Universal Declaration of Human Rights*. United Nations. https://www.un.org/es/about-us/universal-declaration-of-human-rights

APPENDICES

A) Brief Scales (Pre and Post)

Instructions for students (read aloud):

"Mark how much you agree with each sentence. 1 = Not at all agree, 5 = Strongly agree. There are no good or bad answers; answer it thinking about this class."

Response format: Likert 1–5 (1 Not at all; 2 Little; 3 Average; 4 Quite a lot; 5 Totally).

Score: Averages each subscale. Changes of ≥ **0.5** points pre→post indicate relevant improvement.

Time: 5–7 min.

A1. Autonomy (3 items)

1. I feel like I have real options for deciding how to accomplish my tasks.
2. I can propose the way of working that works best for me.
3. In this class, my opinion is taken into account when deciding activities.

A2. Competence (3 items)

4. I feel capable of achieving goals if I organize myself.
5. When I make mistakes, I know what to change for the better.
6. I receive **retro** that helps me understand how to move forward.

A3. Relationship (3 items)

7. I feel support from my colleagues when I need it.
8. I can express doubts without fear of ridicule.
9. The teacher creates an atmosphere of respect in the group.

A4. Perceived resilience (4 items)

10. If I fail, I try another way.
11. When I get frustrated, I ask for help or seek resources.
12. I know how to prioritize when there's too much to do.
13. After a difficult week, I recover quickly.

A5. Academic commitment (5 items)

14. I am actively involved in class activities.
15. I am interested in what we are learning.
16. I lose track of time when I'm working well.
17. I participate with ideas or questions at least once per class.
18. Outside of class, I spend time advancing my goals.

Rapid interpretation (traffic light by subscale):

1.0–2.4 = Red (needs support); 2.5–3.4 = Amber (attention); 3.5–5.0 = Green (adequate).

B) Weekly Check-Ins (1 minute)

- **Scale 1–5:** "This week I felt energized and with options to move forward in this class."
- **Open (1 line):** "One thing that helped me and one thing that held me back this week was..."

Use: pass it at the beginning or end of the class. If someone scores 1–2 and repeats two weeks in a row, offer personal support.

C) Rubrics of Observables (Teacher)

Format: 0–2–4 points per criterion. Register per student every 2 weeks.
C1. Participation and collaboration

- Active presence (0/2/4): 0 rarely participates; 2 participates occasionally; 4 participates briefly but significantly in most sessions.
- Quality of intervention (0/2/4): 0 off-topic; 2 shares data/progress; 4 contributes ideas, asks questions, or connects to task criteria.
- Peer support (0/2/4): 0 does not support; 2 responds when asked; 4 offers support and feedback with respect, at least to one person per week.

C2. Task management

- On-time deliveries (0/2/4): 0 almost never; 2 half of tasks; 4 on time with almost everything.
- Quality of evidence (0/2/4): 0 incomplete evidence; 2 meets the basics; 4 clear evidence, connected to criteria and with improvements compared to the previous time.

Suggested cut (each cut = sum / 20):
0.0–1.5 red; 1.6–3.0 amber; 3.1–4.0 green.

D) Rubric for Student Artifacts (Shared Since Week 1)

Criteria (0–2–4 each):

- Clear goal: 0 vague; 2 partially specific; 4 specific and measurable (what, how, by when).
- Evidence of progress: 0 does not show; 2 basic evidence; 4 convincing and verifiable evidence.
- Reflection: 0 superficial; 2 describes what was done; 4 explains what worked and why, and what changes next time.
- Transference: 0 does not apply to another subject/situation; 2 mentions it; 4 applies or plans to apply in another subject/field.

Total score: /16. (≥ 12 = adequate; 8–11 = to improve; ≤ 7 = requires support.)

E) Short Templates

E1. Weekly team log (max. 5 minutes)

- Week: __ | Team: __
- What we did: (2–3 lines)
- What we learned: (1–2 ideas)
- What we will change next week: (1 concrete decision)
- Supports we need: (1 realistic thing)

E2. Retro Peers (Question Sandwich)

- What I see that is working is...
- A question to improve would be...
- A small next step could be...

F) Interview and Focus Group Guides

Ethics: voluntary, 15 min, no qualification; asks for simple consent ("you can pass any question"). Record only audio if your institution allows it; if not, take notes.

F1. Short interview (student)

1. Tell me a moment of this intervention that did help you. Why?
2. Was there something that didn't work for you or caused you stress?
3. When you get stuck, what do you do now that you didn't do before?
4. Did the AI mentor help you think better? Give me an example.
5. Did you feel real options to decide how to work?
6. Did you have support from anyone in the group? How?
7. If you were to repeat this, what would you change first?

8. Anything else we should know to improve?

F2. Focus group guide (6–8 students, 30–40 min)

- Warm-up: What word comes to mind when you think about these weeks?
- Deepening: moments of progress, moments of stumbling blocks, role of the teacher, role of AI, collaboration between teams.
- Closing: a recommendation for improvement and one thing we should not lose.

G) Ethical Prompt for the Mentor with AI

System Role: You are a Socratic mentor for high school students. Your goal is to ask questions that help with thinking, offer options, summarize what the student said, and suggest small next steps. You don't do homework, you don't judge people, you don't give final answers when the student can build them. You do not ask for or store personal data.

Style: short, friendly and clear. Maximum 3–4 questions per turn. Avoid technicalities.

Interaction sequence:

1. Clarify the goal with 1–2 questions ("What exactly do you want to accomplish this week?").
2. Explore options ("Tell me two ways to get started in 20 minutes").
3. Anticipate obstacles ("What might hold you back, and how would you reduce it?").
4. Close with a small step ("Propose the first step you will do today").

Boundaries: If you're asked to do homework, respond, "I can't do homework for you, but I can help you think about how to accomplish it." If aggressive or sensitive language appears, respond carefully and suggest talking to the teacher.

Privacy: Don't ask for full names, phone numbers, addresses, or sensitive information.

H) One-Page Report Format (Post-Intervention)

Title and group:
Period: (Weeks 1–8)
Summary objective (2 lines):
What we did (4–5 short bullets):

- Sequence of micro-challenges, Socratic mentor, rubrics, check-ins.

Table 3. Key results (short table)

Subscale	Pre (M, DE)	Post (M, DE)	D	Interpretation
Autonomy	—	—	—	(↑ ≥ 0.5 = relevant improvement)
Competence	—	—	—	
Relation	—	—	—	
Resilience	—	—	—	
Commitment	—	—	—	

Table Filling: Subscale

Write the name of the dimension you are measuring: *Autonomy, Competence, Relationship, Resilience, Commitment*. One row for each.

Pre (M, DE)

- M (Average): First, calculate, for each student, the average of the items on that subscale in the pre (scale 1–5). Then take the average of the group with those individual values.
- SD (Standard Deviation): With those same individual averages of the pre, calculate the variability of the group (how much they are dispersed around the mean).
- How you spell it: Pre (M, DE) for example: 3.10, 0.70.
- Tip: Round M to 2 decimal places and DE to 2 decimal places.

Post (M, DE)

Repeat the same procedure as the previous point but with the data after the intervention. Type: Post (M, DE), for example: 3.80, 0.60.

Δ (Delta or Gearbox)

- Forummula: δ = post m – for m.
- It is noted with a sign: it can be positive (improvement), zero (no change) or negative (decrease).
- Example: +0.70.

InterpretationSummarizes the size of the change qualitatively. You can use this traffic light:

- Relevant Buff: $\Delta \geq +0.50$

- Slight Buff: $+0.20 \leq \Delta < +0.50$
- Stable: $-0.19 \leq \Delta < +0.19$
- Descension lever: $-0.49 \leq \Delta < -0.20$
- Relevant decrease: $\Delta \leq -0.50$

You can also write down a short note, e.g.: "$\uparrow \geq 0.5$ = relevant improvement"
Observables (summary): attendance, punctual deliveries, participation (rubric).
3 qualitative findings: real short sentences (with pseudonyms).
Decisions for the next cycle (3):
Acknowledgements and ethical note (1 line): anonymous data, pedagogical use.

I) Application and Safeguarding Procedure

- Pre (Week 1): read simple consent; apply A1–A5 scales; explain rubrics and ethical prompt.
- Process (Weeks 2–7): weekly check-in; logs; teacher registration with C1–C2 rubrics (every 2 weeks).
- Post (Week 8): repeat scales; interviews with 4–6 students; focus group; curate evidence; complete 1-page report.
- Safeguard: save answers in a protected folder; only the teaching team accesses; when sharing products, use pseudonyms.

J) Spreadsheets

If you use a sheet (Google/Excel), create tabs: Scales, Rubrics, Check-ins, Interviews, Report. In Scales, it automatically calculates averages by subscale and paints green ≥ 3.5, amber 2.5–3.4, red, ≤ 2.4. So you can see at a glance where to support.

Chapter 3

Gamifying Cybersecurity Education:
A University Platform for Digital Responsibility

María del Rocío Ramirez Jimenez
https://orcid.org/0000-0003-1709-5539
Universidad de Guadalajara, Mexico

Elba A. Morales-Vanegas
https://orcid.org/0009-0000-4846-8321
Universidad de Colima, Mexico

Miguel A. Garcia-Ruiz
https://orcid.org/0000-0002-7048-7286
Algoma University, Canada

Pedro Damian Reyes
https://orcid.org/0000-0003-1114-9612
Universidad de Colima, Mexico

Pedro C. Santana-Mancilla
https://orcid.org/0000-0002-4184-0116
Universidad de Colima, Mexico

ABSTRACT

The rapid digital transformation of higher education demands innovative strategies to address the growing challenges of cybersecurity. Universities must prepare students not only with technical skills but also with the ability to act responsibly in interconnected digital environments. Gamification has emerged as a powerful pedagogical

DOI: 10.4018/979-8-3373-4657-1.ch003

approach to engage learners, foster motivation, and translate complex concepts into meaningful experiences. This chapter introduces a gamified learning platform designed to raise cybersecurity awareness and promote digital responsibility among university students. The platform integrates interactive scenarios, self-assessment tools, and educational games to develop essential skills such as critical thinking, decision-making, and ethical digital behavior. Early results suggest its potential to strengthen students' understanding of digital risks and encourage safer online practices. Future iterations envision adaptive content, AI-driven personalization, and advanced analytics to enhance impact.

INTRODUCTION

The twenty-first century has witnessed profound transformations across virtually all dimensions of human life (social, economic, cultural, and, most significantly, educational). This evolution has been driven by an unprecedented digital revolution, characterized by the accelerating pace of technological advances that seem to have no limits. As a result, people have developed an increasing dependence on digital environments for work, communication, learning, and daily life (Castells, 2000).

Within this scenario of constant demands, education emerges as one of the most deeply affected domains. It is no longer sufficient to simply integrate technology into classrooms; instead, a critical rethinking of how teaching, learning, and assessment are conceived is urgently needed. Access to digital platforms, the personalization of learning experiences, the automation of formative tasks, and the cultivation of critical digital skills are no longer optional but essential conditions for meaningful participation in contemporary society. Furthermore, this context imposes expectations that go beyond the acquisition of technical skills, requiring the development of critical thinking, ethical behavior, and the ability to collaborate in virtual communities. As UNESCO emphasizes, acting responsibly in digital environments is as important as mastering the use of digital tools (UNESCO, 2020a).

This situation has placed educational institutions under significant pressure: they must critically revise their teaching and learning models and adapt them in ways that are reflective and sustainable. Universities and schools, together with their teaching staff, bear the responsibility of preparing new generations who will inhabit, transform, and ultimately be responsible for shaping this emerging digital reality. However, this is not a simple task. It is not merely a matter of modernizing tools and updating methodologies; it also involves redefining the pedagogical, ethical, and social foundations that guide educational practice in a digitalized, complex, and constantly evolving environment (Castells, 2000).

Within this framework, highly relevant concerns emerge, such as: Who protects digital data? How can privacy, integrity, and availability of information be guaranteed? These questions cannot be overlooked, as they constitute central issues that must be carefully addressed. Cybersecurity therefore stands out as a critical and constantly evolving field, a fundamental pillar that must be integrated not only because of the growing sophistication of cyber threats, but also because of the pressing need to educate responsible digital citizens.

Digital education, understood as a global opportunity for development, must constantly adapt to the challenges imposed by technology. As literature noted, contemporary society demands education that is of quality, equitable, relevant, and internationalized, without losing sight of its regional context (Ortiz, 2017; Valdés Montecinos, 2019) . This perspective underscores the need to respond not only to global challenges, but also to the specific realities of diverse local, regional, and national contexts.

Within this framework of growing demands, higher education has traditionally pursued two central missions: comprehensive student education and the generation of new knowledge, often conceptualized as teaching and research. However, the profound social and technological changes of recent decades have introduced a third mission that cannot be ignored: social engagement. This dimension emphasizes that universities should not function as isolated entities but as active participants committed to social development and the well-being of society. This concept is known and university social responsibility (USR) and highlight two key objectives in this regard: social responsibility, understood as active participation as agents of positive change, and knowledge transfer, understood as the transformation of theory into practical elements that incorporate innovation, creativity, and development across social, cultural, and technological domains (Duque & Cervantes-Cervantes, 2019).

USR has therefore emerged as a continuous improvement policy that aligns institutional activities with their broader social impact. USR is composed of four interrelated processes. First, ethical and environmental management requires universities to model good internal practices, ensuring that their administrative functioning is transparent, fair, and environmentally responsible. Second, the formation of citizens extends beyond technical knowledge, aiming to develop individuals who are aware of their roles in a world facing multiple global challenges and capable of contributing to meaningful solutions. Third, the production and dissemination of socially relevant knowledge ensures that research responds to real-world problems and produces results that are accessible and useful to communities. Finally, social participation calls for active collaboration with governments, businesses, and civil society to foster human and sustainable development (Duque & Cervantes-Cervantes, 2019).

These transformations have been reinforced by the adoption of emerging technologies that transcend boundaries and redefine access to knowledge. Learning management systems such as Moodle, Google Classroom, and Coursera have become key engines of digital education, while collaboration tools such as Zoom, Microsoft Teams, and Google Meet have enabled the creation of virtual classrooms that transcend physical limitations. At the same time, artificial intelligence–based systems have begun to personalize learning trajectories, offering adaptive proposals that place the student at the center of the educational process (Gaytan-Lugo, Laura et al., 2014). Technologies such as virtual and augmented reality have expanded possibilities for simulation, while methodologies like microlearning and gamification have facilitated more flexible, motivating, and adaptive approaches to teaching and learning (Santana-Mancilla et al., 2016).

Despite these benefits, the global expansion of digitalization has also revealed deep inequalities in access to connectivity. In Mexico, for example, despite governmental programs aimed at expanding internet access, statistics continue to show marked disparities: while urban areas report high connectivity levels, rural regions register a low connectivity level, with states such as Guerrero, Oaxaca, and Chiapas falling below the national media (Ibarra et al., 2017). This digital divide is not unique to Mexico. According to the International Telecommunication Union, one-third of the world's population still lacks access to the internet (Robinson et al., 2015).

In contrast, the labor market increasingly demands complex digital skills, including advanced programming, data analysis, the ethical use of artificial intelligence, and cybersecurity. To address this reality, new educational alternatives have emerged, such as open courses, certification programs, bootcamps, and digital badges, which allow students to certify specific competencies quickly and flexibly (UNESCO, 2021).

A key event in this transformation was the COVID-19 pandemic, which marked a turning point and will remain in history as a memorable milestone that drastically accelerated technological advances. Practically overnight, more than 1.5 billion students around the world faced severe educational disruptions, prompting a forced migration to virtual platforms, models, and strategies that often-revealed significant shortcomings. This phenomenon exposed structural weaknesses in infrastructure, teacher training, and inclusive policies (UNESCO, 2020b). At the same time, it accelerated digitalization processes, expanded hybrid and self-directed learning, and highlighted new challenges such as remote academic evaluation, increased plagiarism, and a dramatic rise in cyberattacks.

This historical moment demonstrated in stark terms that digitalization cannot be separated from data protection and cybersecurity. As educational institutions move forward in designing innovative approaches, cybersecurity must be recognized as a fundamental pillar of higher education, closely tied to both academic quality and social responsibility. Preparing students for a hyperconnected world requires equipping them not only with technical expertise but also with critical and ethical capacities to act with digital responsibility in increasingly complex environments. This perspective sets the stage for the following section, which examines the global context of digital education and situates cybersecurity as a central component in the design of future-ready educational strategies.

JUSTIFICATION

Higher education today faces a dual challenge: adapting to an increasingly complex digital environment while preparing citizens who can act responsibly and critically, both in their daily lives and within cyberspace. In this scenario, cybersecurity emerges as a transversal competence that is essential not only for students in technology-related disciplines but for the entire university community. Yet, its teaching is often limited by institutional barriers, lack of awareness, and pedagogical challenges. Technical jargon, abstract content, and the perception that cybersecurity is disconnected from students' everyday lives hinder its integration into academic curricula.

Gamification offers an innovative and timely response to this challenge. Far from being a mere recreational component, it involves the structured design of learning experiences that combine motivation, immediate feedback, and decision-making within simulated contexts (Gee, 2003; Kapp, 2012). By incorporating these elements, complex concepts can be transformed into engaging and accessible proposals, fostering active and meaningful learning that is particularly relevant to digital security.

Recent studies indicate that most cybersecurity incidents originate from human error, often due to poor practices or a lack of basic knowledge about information protection (Jartelius, 2020). This problem is particularly acute in educational environments, where the massive digitalization of data, constant use of platforms, diversity of user profiles, and limited infrastructure converge into highly vulnerable ecosystems (Hakim et al., 2023). As a result, cybersecurity has a direct impact on both the academic and personal lives of students. Although often perceived as "digitally savvy," many young people lack solid training in safe browsing, password management, privacy, or threat recognition, which makes them frequent targets of phishing campaigns, identity theft, and data exposure.

Reports confirm that the education sector has become one of the most attacked globally (Piazza et al., 2023). The reasons behind this trend include insufficient training, lack of knowledge of institutional protocols, and a generally low level of critical awareness of online risks.

Under this context, it is essential to design pedagogical proposals that go beyond technical instruction to foster critical digital citizenship. This requires forming students who can make safe decisions, act ethically, and protect both their own identities and those of their communities. Gamification, by integrating dynamics such as progressive challenges, visible progress, and meaningful storytelling, creates emotionally and cognitively engaging environments that facilitate the internalization of key cybersecurity concepts (Mukherjee et al., 2024).

The *Mi Protector Digital* platform responds to this need by proposing a gamification-based model that motivates, educates, and transforms attitudes toward cybersecurity. Rather than focusing solely on the transmission of concepts, it seeks to build a preventive and reflective digital culture, adaptable to diverse student profiles, accessible to all, and contextualized to university life.

Expected Contributions

The primary motivation behind designing a gamification-based platform for cybersecurity training in higher education is to impact three central dimensions of student development:

- **Learning motivation**: By incorporating game mechanics such as levels, rewards, challenges, and missions, the platform seeks to enhance students' voluntary participation. Intrinsic motivation is stimulated through the sense of achievement, autonomy, and progression associated with overcoming challenges.
- **Critical digital awareness**: Beyond technical knowledge, the platform aims to foster ethical and social reflection on the use of technology, the protection of personal data, digital footprints, and emerging threats. Gamified environments allow students to engage with real-world scenarios and make decisions that mirror actual risks, thereby reinforcing critical thinking and responsible digital behavior.
- **Development of soft skills**: Through missions and decision-making tasks, students practice competencies such as critical thinking, self-regulation, and problem-solving. These transversal skills, increasingly valued in the twenty-first century, are strengthened in contexts that simulate the complexity of real digital challenges.

Taken together, these contributions position *Mi Protector Digital* as more than a technical training tool. Its purpose is to cultivate a preventive and reflective digital culture that empowers students to protect their identity, act ethically, and contribute to safer academic and social environments.

BACKGROUND AND RELATED WORK

The growing integration of digital technologies into education has inspired researchers and practitioners to explore new strategies that can enhance student engagement, improve knowledge retention, and foster critical digital competencies. Among these strategies, gamification and game-based learning have received increasing attention, supported by a growing body of theoretical and empirical work. This literature highlights not only the pedagogical potential of game elements to transform traditional learning environments but also their relevance in areas such as cybersecurity education, where awareness, motivation, and behavioral change are essential. The following subsections review the main foundations of educational gamification, the broader educational value of play, and existing approaches that link video games and cybersecurity training, in order to situate *Mi Protector Digital* within this evolving field.

Foundations of Educational Gamification

Gamification has emerged as a powerful tool for revitalizing educational processes, moving beyond its early perception as a mere auxiliary technique to become consolidated as a pedagogical paradigm. This approach is capable of transforming routine tasks into experiences that are immersive, challenging, motivating, and meaningful for learners. Its integration into education has been progressive yet increasingly robust, as reflected in research demonstrating the positive impact of gamified environments on content retention, collaboration, problem-solving, and critical thinking skills. Such evidence highlights that educational gamification is not a passing trend but a structured method of designing learner-centered experiences that actively engage students (Werbach & Hunter, 2015).

The effectiveness of gamification lies in its ability to incorporate mechanics such as progressive challenges, immediate feedback systems, symbolic rewards, and engaging narratives. These mechanisms foster a more active and meaningful relationship between students and content, promoting deeper learning outcomes and transferable skills (Gee, 2003). At its core, gamification is composed of three interconnected layers: dynamics, which define limitations, emotions, narratives, and rules that structure the experience; mechanics, which establish challenges, competition, cooperation, and progression; and components, such as badges, avatars, levels, and leaderboards, that enhance motivation and support knowledge acquisition (Tafur-Méndez et al., 2023).

Gamified platforms like Roblox, Second Life, and Froggy Jumps have demonstrated the potential of immersive environments where learning is driven by practice. These virtual spaces allow learners to explore, make mistakes, reflect, and construct knowledge in contextualized scenarios, thereby reinforcing the educational process. However, risks must also be acknowledged. This dual reality illustrates that gamification cannot be understood merely as the addition of playful elements to traditional settings. Rather, it represents a fundamental shift in how we conceive motivation, engagement, and human learning.

Furthermore, the evolution of gamification continues to be shaped by emerging technologies such as artificial intelligence, virtual reality, blockchain, and connected devices. These innovations open new possibilities for creating personalized and adjacent experiences that foster positive change not only in education but also in fields such as health, work, and sustainability. Gamification should not be viewed as a fleeting trend but as a transformative force reshaping human experience and organizational growth. Institutions and organizations that invest early in its potential are more likely to take the lead in an increasingly gamified world (Jiménez et al., 2018).

The Educational Value of Play

Play has long been recognized as a vital component of learning across pedagogical traditions. From Ausubel's theory of meaningful learning to the constructivist approaches of Piaget and Vygotsky, educational research has consistently emphasized the active and social construction of knowledge through play. Although initially associated with childhood learning, play has proven equally effective for learners of all ages. Csikszentmihalyi's theory of flow further explain why video games are particularly effective for youth (Csikszentmihalyi et al., 2014; Romero-Mendez et al., 2023). When students engage in challenges that match their abilities, receive constant feedback, and are motivated by appropriate incentives, they enter a state of deep involvement that enhances autonomous and meaningful learning.

From these foundations, new approaches such as Game-Based Learning (GBL) have emerged, offering sustainable pathways for learning through structured play (Tobias et al., 2014). Scholars such as (Dunwell et al., 2014; Kapp, 2012) have demonstrated how video games provide rich symbolic contexts in which learners do not merely apply existing knowledge but actively construct it through problem-solving, decision-making, and experiencing consequences. In this way, games serve as laboratories for experiential and situated learning, where failure is not punitive but an opportunity for reflection and growth.

Video Games and Cybersecurity

Cybersecurity and critical digital citizenship provide particularly promising contexts for applying gamification. Despite the widespread assumption that younger generations are "digital natives," empirical studies have shown that many students possess limited knowledge of essential issues such as data protection, safe browsing, threat detection, and strategies to avoid phishing or malware (Triplett, 2023).

Gamification offers an effective pedagogical pathway to address these gaps. Through simulated environments, quizzes, challenges, and real-case scenarios, students can learn to identify risks, make ethical decisions, configure privacy settings, and respond to simulated cyberattacks. These gamified environments create safe spaces where learners can experience the consequences of mistakes without endangering real data or compromising actual systems.

Examples of such resources are already available across a wide range of educational contexts. Tools like Google's *Interland*, platforms such as TryHackMe and BlackBox.AI offer gamified content designed to raise awareness, build technical skills, and encourage autonomous learning. While these tools are valuable, they are often general-purpose and focus on common cybersecurity themes rather than specific needs identified within local university contexts.

It is in response to this limitation that *Mi Protector Digital* was developed, a dedicated platform that directly addresses specific issues identified through applied research. Grounded in a needs analysis of students' perceptions and knowledge gaps, the platform integrates gamified challenges designed to demonstrate that cybersecurity can be learned in participatory, critical, and engaging ways. Beyond technical skills, the objective is to cultivate students' awareness of their digital footprint, empower them to protect their identities, and foster safer, more ethical digital environments. This vision expands from individual empowerment to broader applications in academic and social contexts.

Gamification in Higher Education

Higher education, traditionally characterized by more rigid structures, has also begun to embrace gamification, particularly in disciplines related to technology, design, health, and the social sciences. Evidence suggests that, when applied with pedagogical purpose and methodological rigor, gamification strengthens student engagement, enhances knowledge retention, and fosters the development of key twenty-first-century skills relevant to employability (Wiggins, 2016).

Nevertheless, the adoption of gamification in universities is not without challenges. Among the most common are the lack of faculty training in gamified design, inadequate technological resources, the tendency to overemphasize the playful component at the expense of pedagogy, and the difficulty of aligning gamified strategies with curricular objectives and traditional assessment systems. These barriers highlight that the true challenge of gamification is not technological but pedagogical: the design of experiences that are rigorous, engaging, and profoundly human.

Despite these difficulties, the potential benefits outweigh the obstacles. Properly integrated, gamification can become a strategic ally for higher education institutions in addressing the challenges of digital education. Ultimately, it is not only about transferring knowledge but about offering transformative experiences that empower students to learn critically, act responsibly, and engage ethically in digital environments.

CASE STUDY: *MI PROTECTOR DIGITAL*

The following section presents *Mi Protector Digital*, a gamified learning platform created to strengthen digital responsibility and cybersecurity awareness in higher education. Conceived as a response to the growing vulnerability of students in online environments, the platform embodies an interdisciplinary approach that combines principles of cybersecurity, educational psychology, and user-centered design. By integrating interactive challenges, accessible navigation, and meaningful feedback, *Mi Protector Digital* seeks not only to deliver knowledge but also to foster critical reflection and behavioral change. The subsections that follow describe its objectives, design principles, and pedagogical underpinnings, situating the platform within the broader field of gamification in education.

Objectives of the Platform

Mi Protector Digital is an educational platform that integrates gamified elements to foster essential competencies in cybersecurity and digital responsibility within the university context. It was developed as a direct response to the gap observed between students' frequent use of digital technologies and their limited preparation to recognize and address online risks. The platform is designed not only to provide technical knowledge but also to promote critical awareness and responsible digital behavior among higher education students.

The specific objectives of the platform are to:

- Raise awareness of the most common risks in digital environments.
- Teach best practices for safe browsing, privacy management, identity protection, and device security.
- Foster critical thinking in relation to misinformation, cyberbullying, and the commercial use of personal data.
- Promote a responsible, ethical, and proactive attitude toward the use of digital technologies.

The platform's design primarily targets:

- University students with little or no prior knowledge of cybersecurity.
- Young learners in educational settings who are familiar with digital environments but are not necessarily aware of the risks involved.
- A broad academic audience, as accessibility and ease of navigation are core principles, ensuring that students from non-technical fields can also use the tool effectively.

By articulating these objectives and focusing on a diverse student population, *Mi Protector Digital* positions itself as more than a training tool for technical skills. Its intent is to foster a culture of preventive and reflective digital citizenship that resonates across disciplines. This orientation sets the stage for a design approach grounded in both pedagogical theory and practical usability, ensuring that the platform not only addresses knowledge gaps but also motivates students to engage critically with cybersecurity challenges.

DESIGN AND METHODOLOGY

The development of *Mi Protector Digital* followed a comprehensive process that combined educational design principles with a rigorous methodological framework. The project was grounded in instructional design, gamification strategies, and DBR This dual perspective ensured that the platform was pedagogically meaningful, technologically accessible, and validated through empirical evidence. The following subsections describe the design and methodology in detail, including the creation and validation of the diagnostic instrument, the instructional design phases, the structure of the platform, and the integration of gamified elements.

Instrument Design and Validation

The first stage of the project focused on the design and validation of an instrument to measure university students' perceptions and knowledge of cybersecurity. This tool was crucial, as it provided the empirical foundation for identifying gaps in student awareness and informed the selection of the platform's thematic areas.

Expert Validation Process

Five experts were invited to review the instrument. They were carefully selected to represent diverse but complementary fields: information technology, software engineering, data protection, educational technology, and cybersecurity. This interdisciplinary panel was chosen to ensure a robust evaluation that incorporated both technical and pedagogical perspectives. The experts assessed the instrument's clarity, relevance, and alignment with the intended objectives. Their feedback was essential to refining the items, ensuring that the language was appropriate for a university audience, and confirming that the instrument would generate data useful for both educational and technological interventions.

Structure of the Instrument

The instrument was designed around five dimensions, each reflecting a critical aspect of cybersecurity literacy:

- **Technical knowledge and skills**: This dimension explored students' familiarity with software, applications, antivirus tools, password management, and data backup practices. The goal was to measure whether students possessed the fundamental technical competencies required to protect themselves online.
- **Perception and attitude toward cybersecurity**: Items in this dimension measured students' awareness of the importance of cybersecurity and their perceived vulnerability to threats. Attitudinal factors are key predictors of whether students will adopt secure practices.
- **Behavior in response to specific threats**: This section assessed how students react to practical scenarios, such as opening suspicious emails or clicking on unverified links. By focusing on behavior rather than knowledge, the instrument captured how students would act in real-world situations.
- **Awareness of policies and regulations**: Cybersecurity is not only technical but also institutional and legal. This dimension asked about students' familiarity with their university's cybersecurity policies, whether they followed these guidelines, and if they knew how to report incidents.
- **Protection of personal data**: The final dimension examined students' understanding of data privacy, including password management, privacy settings, rights such as the right to be forgotten, and their awareness of misuse of personal data by third parties.

A total of 25 items were distributed across these five dimensions. Items included questions such as: *How often do you use secure and distinct passwords for each of your accounts?* and *Are you familiar with your institution's cybersecurity policies?* Students rated their responses on a five-point Likert scale, from "strongly disagree" to "strongly agree."

Reliability and Internal Consistency

The results of the expert review and subsequent pilot application confirmed the instrument's reliability. Cronbach's alpha coefficients exceeded the accepted threshold for internal consistency across all dimensions, with particularly strong results in "Perception and Attitude toward Cybersecurity" and "Awareness of Policies and Regulations." These findings indicate that the instrument has potential as a robust diagnostic tool for evaluating cybersecurity awareness in higher education contexts.

It is important to note that the purpose of this chapter is not to present the detailed process of the instrument's validation, but rather to emphasize how its results informed the design of the gamified platform. The instrument serves as a diagnostic foundation, while the central focus of this work lies in the pedagogical integration of gamification for cybersecurity education.

Methodological Phases

Following the design and validation of the instrument, the instructional design of the platform was structured using the ADDIE model (Analysis, Design, Development, Implementation, and Evaluation). This model provided a systematic process to ensure that pedagogical goals were aligned with the platform's technical features and gamified elements (Almelhi, 2021).

ANALYSIS

The analysis phase began with the application of the validated instrument to a sample of first-semester students across different programs at the *Centro Universitario de los Lagos* of the University of Guadalajara. A total of 257 students participated in the diagnostic, providing valuable insights into their knowledge gaps, attitudes, and practices regarding cybersecurity.

The results highlighted areas of weakness, particularly in recognizing threats such as phishing and malware, reporting incidents, and protecting personal data. These findings informed the identification of the platform's thematic areas and ensured that the content was directly relevant to the needs of the student population.

DESIGN

Based on the analysis, specific objectives were formulated for each section of the platform. Pedagogical sequencing was defined, and gamification principles were integrated into the design. Each section included not only explanatory content but also interactive games designed to reinforce learning and assess student understanding. The games were carefully chosen to correspond to the diagnostic results, ensuring alignment between student needs and learning activities.

DEVELOPMENT

During the development phase, the platform was built as a website. Special attention was given to usability and accessibility, making the platform intuitive for students from both technical and non-technical backgrounds. The design prioritized clarity, responsive navigation, and visual identity, including the creation of a recognizable logo and banners.

IMPLEMENTATION

The platform was hosted online and made available to students. This phase allowed for testing the technical stability of the site and gathering initial impressions from users. The hosting ensured that the platform could be accessed both within and outside the university, extending its potential reach.

EVALUATION

Evaluation was conducted through a self-assessment questionnaire embedded in the platform. Students were able to reflect on their learning and provide feedback about their experiences. This stage was crucial for identifying areas for improvement, both in terms of content clarity and game design. The iterative nature of DBR allowed for modifications based on this feedback, ensuring continuous improvement of the platform.

Description of the Platform

Mi Protector Digital integrates principles from educational psychology, instructional design, and gamification to provide a structured and engaging learning experience. As noted by (Gee, 2003), gamification has the potential to increase motivation and enhance cognitive, emotional, and social engagement. Recent institutional studies (Khaldi et al., 2023; Signori et al., 2018) further support its benefits in digital learning environments.

The homepage (Figure 1) presents the platform's logo, main menu, and a dynamic carousel banner introducing the principal cybersecurity themes. Sections include *Home*, *About Us*, *Resources*, *Map*, and *Self-Assessment*. The design provides a clear structure and fosters accessibility.

Figure 1. Homepage of the Mi Protector Digital platform.

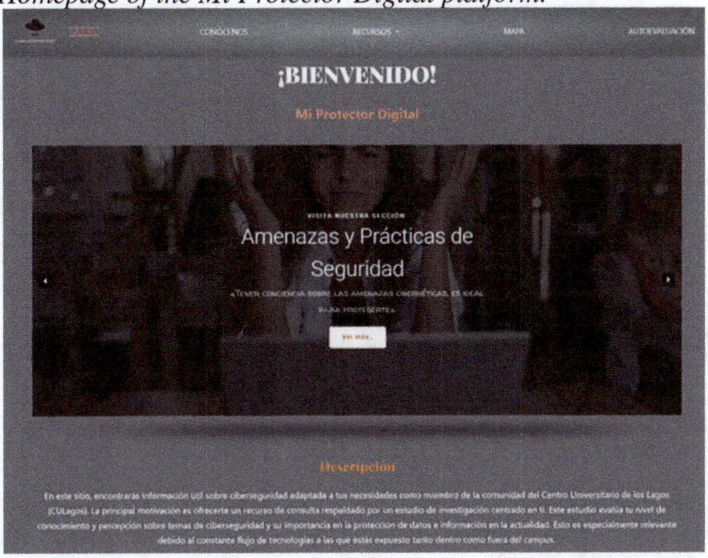

The *Resources* section (Figure 2) is particularly significant, as it organizes the thematic areas derived from the diagnostic study of 257 students. These areas include:

- Threats and security practices
- Privacy configuration
- Digital identity security
- Incident reporting
- Responsible use of data

Figure 2. Resources section menu displaying the main topics identified in the diagnostic study.

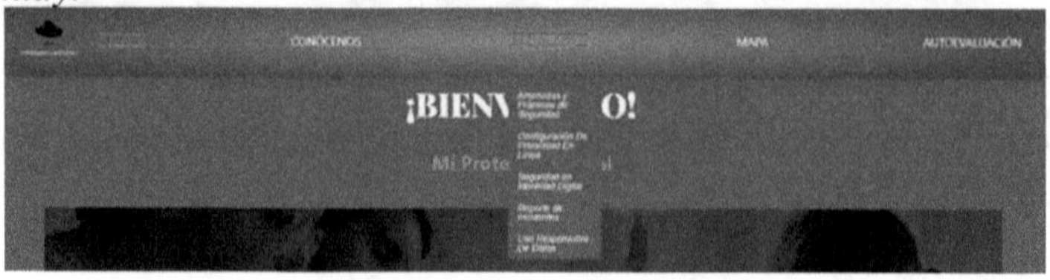

Gamified Elements

Gamification was central to the design of *Mi Protector Digital*. Each section combined informational content with interactive games that encouraged active participation, immediate feedback, and progressive challenges.

DIAGNOSTIC GAME

The entry point of the platform was an interactive diagnostic game (Figure 3) created with Deck.Toys. It introduced fundamental cybersecurity concepts such as phishing, malware, ransomware, and antivirus protection. Organized as a journey with multiple "stations," it engaged students with crosswords, trivia, and concept-matching activities. These tasks not only measured prior knowledge but also motivated learners to engage with subsequent modules.

Figure 3. Interactive diagnostic game developed with Deck.Toys.

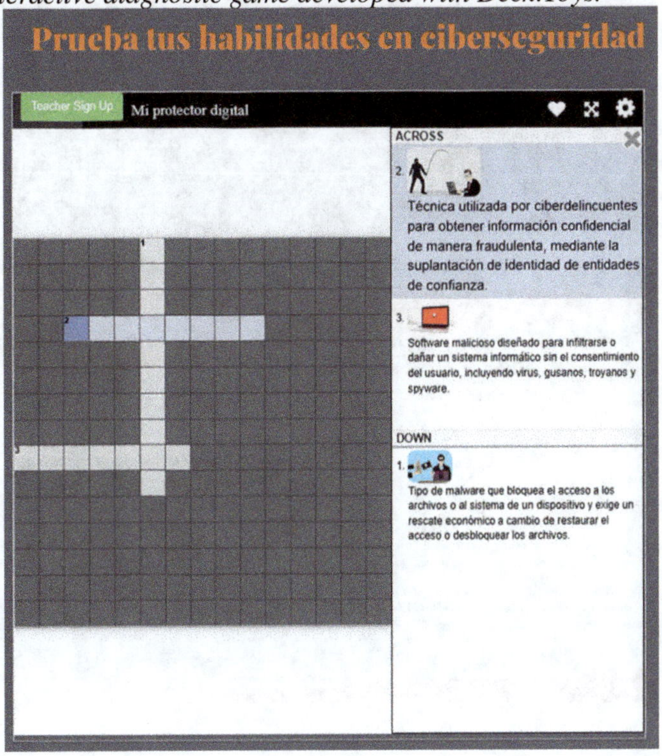

THREATS AND SECURITY PRACTICES

This section began with an introduction highlighting the importance of recognizing and mitigating digital threats. Explanations of malware, phishing, and ransomware were accompanied by a video resource to reinforce understanding (Figure 4). A complementary interactive game (Figure 5) simulated real-world scenarios, such as suspicious emails or insecure Wi-Fi connections. Students were required to make strategic decisions, fostering practical awareness without the risk of real consequences.

Figure 4. Page on digital threats y security practices.

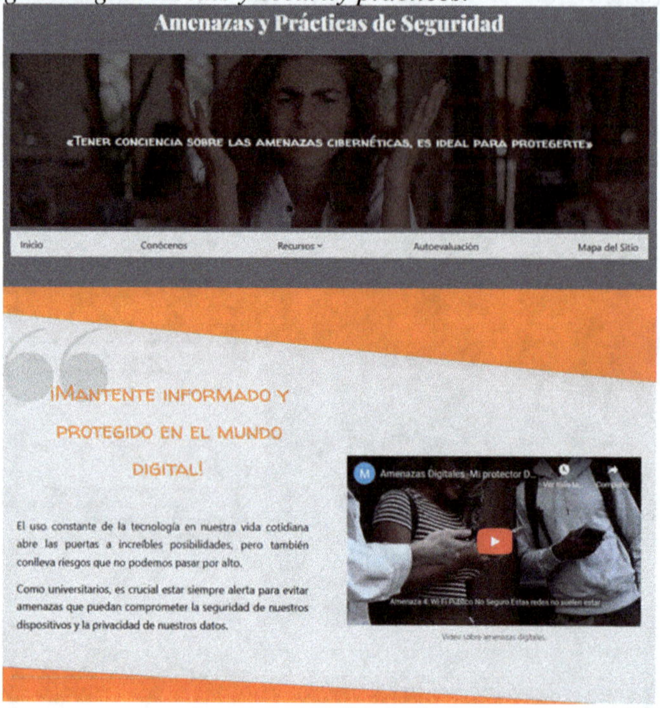
Amenazas y Prácticas de Seguridad
«Tener conciencia sobre las amenazas cibernéticas, es ideal para protegerte»
Inicio
Conócenos
Recursos
Autoevaluación
Mapa del Sitio
¡Mantente informado y protegido en el mundo digital!
El uso constante de la tecnología en nuestra vida cotidiana abre las puertas a increíbles posibilidades, pero también conlleva riesgos que no podemos pasar por alto.
Como universitarios, es crucial estar siempre alerta para evitar amenazas que puedan comprometer la seguridad de nuestros dispositivos y la privacidad de nuestros datos.
Amenazas Digitales: Mi protector D...

Figure 5. Interactive game for practicing threat identification.

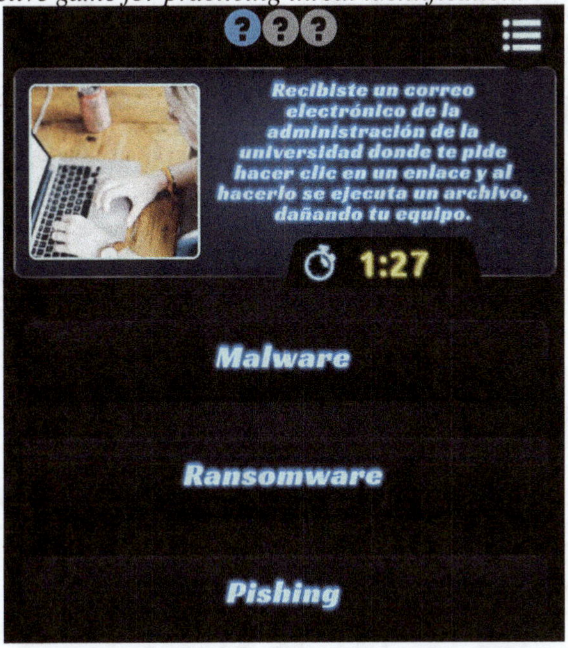
Recibiste un correo electrónico de la administración de la universidad donde te pide hacer clic en un enlace y al hacerlo se ejecuta un archivo, dañando tu equipo.
1:27
Malware
Ransomware
Pishing

PRIVACY CONFIGURATION

The *Privacy Configuration* section emphasized the importance of safeguarding personal information online. Practical guides demonstrated how to configure privacy settings in Moodle, Google Classroom, and social media platforms like Facebook and Instagram (Figure 6). To reinforce learning, a hangman-style game (Figure 7) challenged students to complete key phrases related to privacy. Incorrect attempts prompted repetition, ensuring meaningful memorization.

Figure 6. Privacy configuration page.

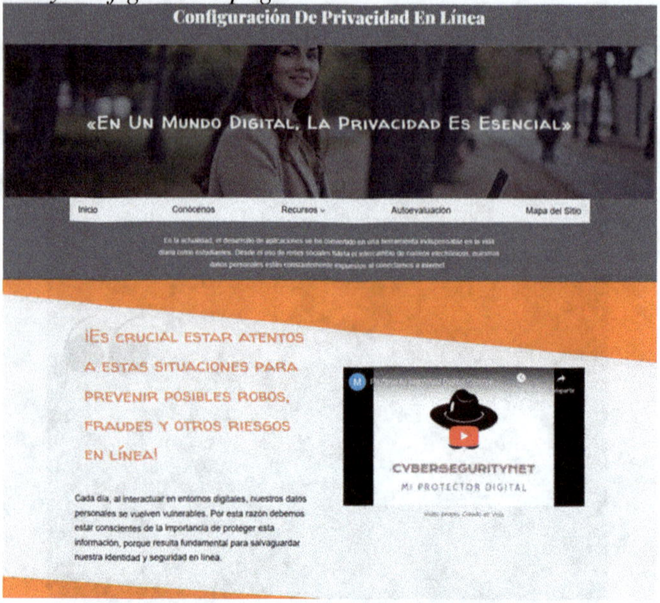

Figure 7. Hangman-style game.

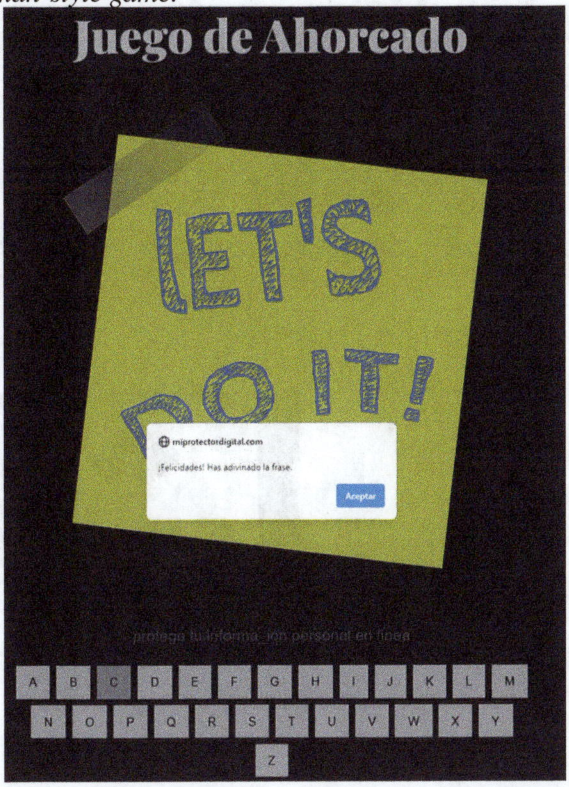

DIGITAL IDENTITY SECURITY

This section (Figure 8) introduced practices for protecting digital identity, such as using password managers, enabling two-factor authentication, and installing antivirus software. Reflection questions encouraged students to consider their current habits. An interactive quiz game (Figure 9) with ten progressively challenging questions reinforced knowledge, providing immediate feedback and motivating learners to improve their scores.

Figure 8. Digital identity security page.

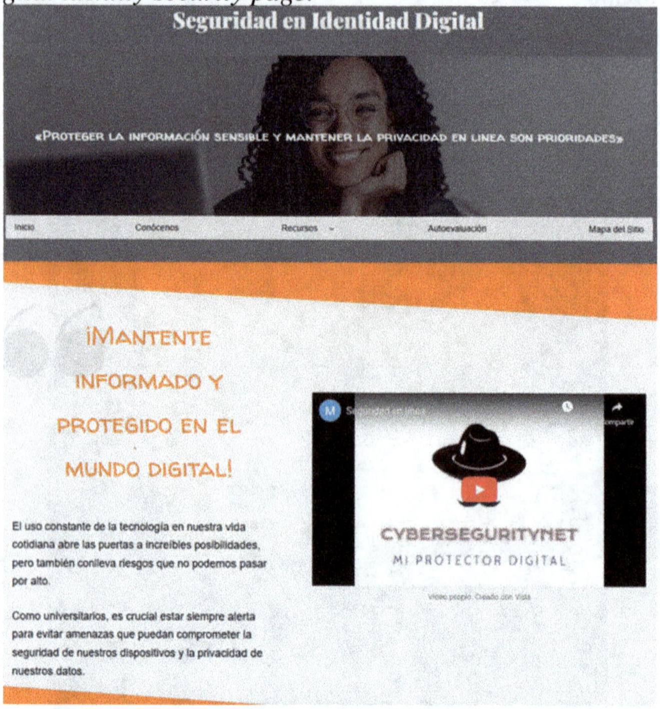

Figure 9. Multiple-choice quiz game for digital security competences.

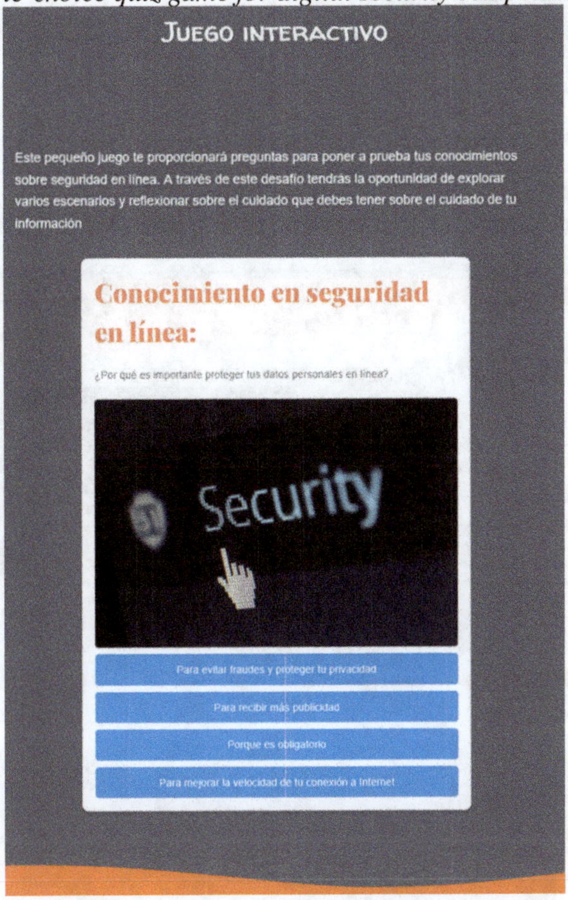

JUEGO INTERACTIVO
Este pequeño juego te proporcionará preguntas para poner a prueba tus conocimientos sobre seguridad en línea. A través de este desafío tendrás la oportunidad de explorar varios escenarios y reflexionar sobre el cuidado que debes tener sobre el cuidado de tu información
Conocimiento en seguridad en línea:
¿Por qué es importante proteger tus datos personales en línea?
Security
Para evitar fraudes y proteger tu privacidad
Para recibir más publicidad
Porque es obligatorio
Para mejorar la velocidad de tu conexión a Internet

INCIDENT REPORTING

Incident reporting was identified as a critical weakness in the diagnostic results. Nearly half of the surveyed students indicated they did not know how to report cybersecurity incidents. To address this, the platform included an information page (Figure 10) and diagnostic results visualization (Figure 11). An interactive trivia game (Figure 12) was added, consisting of multiple-choice questions designed to reinforce correct reporting procedures.

Figure 10. Incident reporting page.

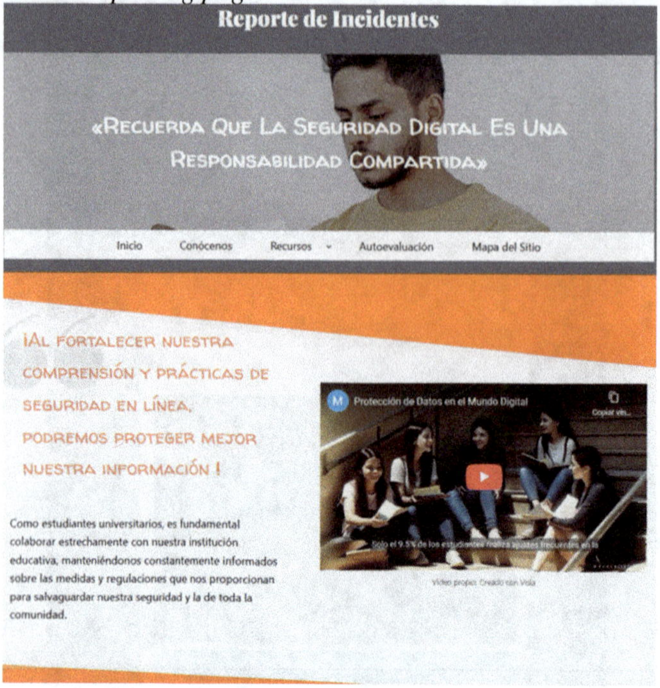

Figure 11. Diagnostic results page.

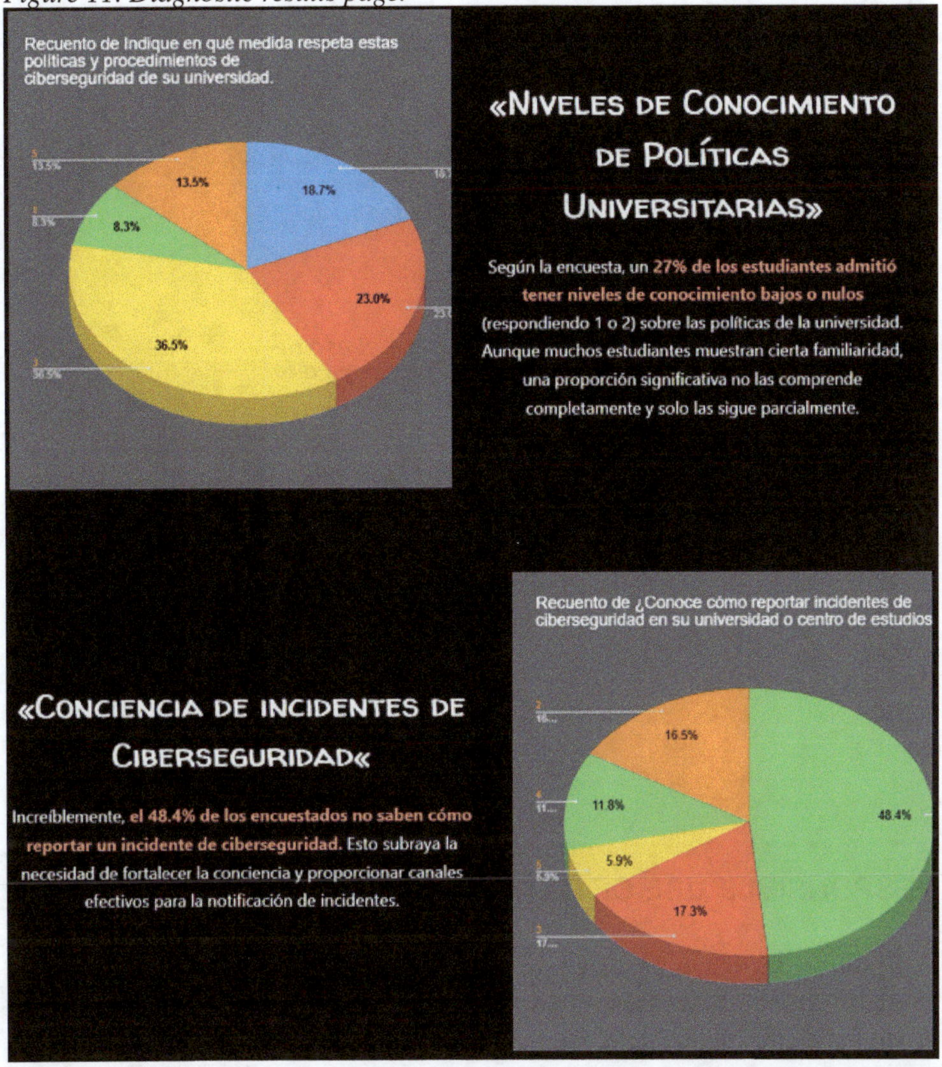

Figures 12. Trivia game.

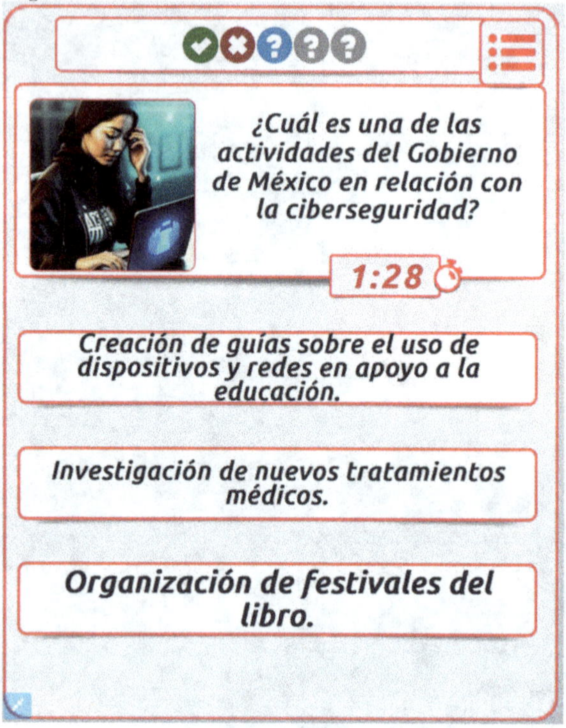

RESPONSIBLE USE OF DATA

The final section emphasized the ethical and legal dimensions of data use in Mexico. Topics included several key frameworks designed to protect individuals' privacy and strengthen digital rights (Álvarez Magallán et al., 2024). The Federal Law on the Protection of Personal Data Held by Private Parties and the General Law on the Protection of Personal Data Held by Obligated Subjects (Cámara de Diputados, 2010; Diario Oficial de la Federación, 2017) establishes the principles and obligations for organizations when collecting, processing, and safeguarding personal data, ensuring that individuals maintain control over how their information is used. Closely related are the he ARCO rights, an acronym derived from the Spanish terms *Acceso, Rectificación, Cancelación, Oposición* (Access, Rectification, Cancellation, and Opposition), which grant individuals the ability to access their personal information, correct inaccuracies, request its deletion, or oppose its processing under specific conditions. Another relevant concept is the right to be forgotten, which allows individuals to request the removal of personal information from digital platforms when its continued availability could negatively affect their privacy or reputation. Finally, the the "Ley Olimpia" (a Mexican legal reform addressing digital violence and the non-consensual dissemination of intimate content), a pioneering legal reform in Mexico, criminalizes digital violence and the non-consensual dissemination of intimate content, reinforcing the protection of personal dignity and integrity in online spaces. The corresponding page of the platform (Figure 13) presented these frameworks in accessible language, complemented by visual resources to aid comprehension. To reinforce learning, a fill-in-the-blank game (Figure 14) required students to complete sentences with the correct legal terms, thereby strengthening their understanding of rights and responsibilities in digital environments.

Figure 13. Responsible use of data page.

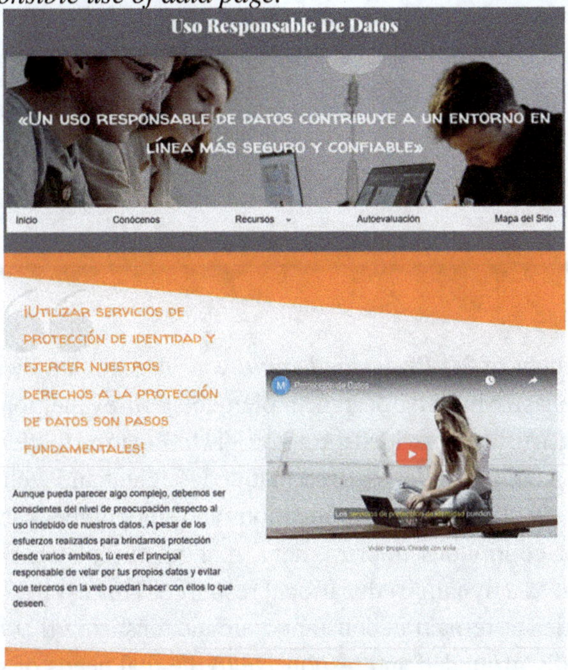

Figure 14. Interactive fill-in-the-blank game.

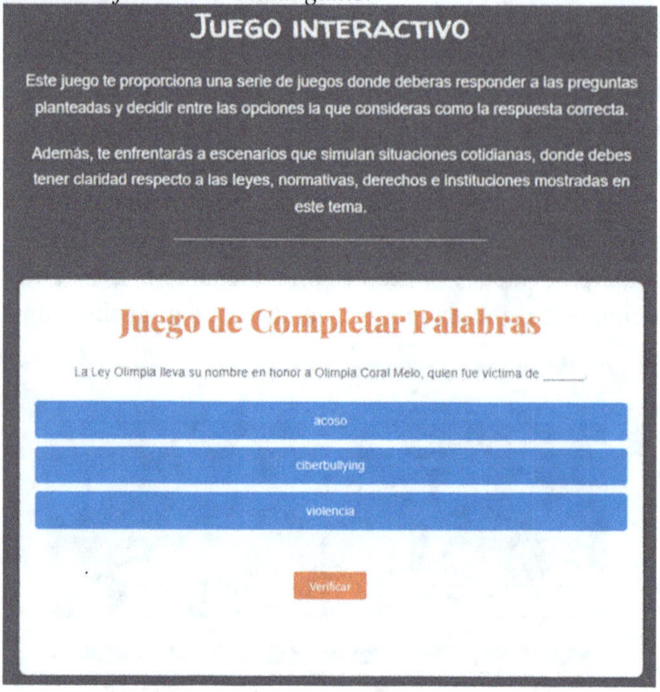

The development of *Mi Protector Digital* was also guided by the principles of DBR, which emphasize iterative design, implementation, evaluation, and refinement. The diagnostic instrument provided the empirical foundation for defining the content areas, while the ADDIE model ensured that pedagogical and technological design were systematically aligned. Pilot applications and student feedback then generated opportunities for continuous improvement, making the platform evolve not as a static product but as a dynamic educational resource. This cyclical process allowed theory and practice to remain in constant dialogue, ensuring that the platform was both pedagogically grounded and responsive to the real needs of students.

To provide a structured overview of how each gamified component aligns with the program's learning objectives, a matrix of gamified elements was designed. This matrix not only served as a guide during the development phase but also allows the reader to quickly grasp the pedagogical purpose behind each game and interaction within the "Mi Protector Digital" platform. The Table 1 details this correspondence.

Table 1. Summary of Gamified Elements and Learning Objectives.

THEMATIC AREA	GAMIFIED	SPECIFIC LEARNING OBJECTIVE
FUNDAMENTAL CYBERSECURITY CONCEPTS	Interactive Crossword: "Cyber-Knowledge"	To assess and reinforce the student's initial understanding of key terminology such as malware, phishing, ransomware, and firewall.
THREATS AND RISKY PRACTICES	Scenario-Based Simulation: "Digital Decisions"	To develop the ability to identify and react appropriately to common threats, such as phishing emails and suspicious information requests.
PRIVACY AND DATA PROTECTION	Hangman Game: "Protect Your Info"	To facilitate the memorization of essential concepts and regulations related to data privacy, including the "Olimpia Law" and ARCO rights.
DIGITAL IDENTITY AND PASSWORD MANAGEMENT	Self-Assessment Quiz: "Digital Fortress"	To encourage self-reflection and the adoption of secure practices, such as creating strong passwords and enabling two-factor authentication (2FA).
DIGITAL RESPONSIBILITY AND ETHICS	Points and Rewards System	To motivate continuous participation and progress through the modules, recognizing effort and the mastery of cybersecurity competencies.

As shown in the table, each activity was intentionally designed to address a specific knowledge gap identified in the initial diagnosis. The combination of different game mechanics aims to cater to diverse learning styles and maintain student engagement throughout their journey on the platform, transforming the acquisition of cybersecurity skills into an active and appealing experience rather than a mere memorization exercise.

The iterative design process not only shaped the pedagogical and technological structure of *Mi Protector Digital* but also prepared the ground for its initial evaluation. As emphasized in DBR, the value of an educational innovation lies not in a single static deployment but in its capacity to generate feedback, evolve, and improve. The following section presents the exploratory results obtained from the platform's self-assessment component, which served as a formative tool to gauge students' appropriation of key cybersecurity concepts and to inform future refinements.

RESULTS

Taking into consideration the objectives of *Mi Protector Digital* (to raise awareness of digital risks, to promote best practices, to foster critical thinking, and to encourage a culture of technological responsibility) the evaluation phase centered on the platform's self-assessment component. This instrument was designed to be administered at the end of the gamified experience, functioning as an exploratory tool to assess students' level of understanding and appropriation of key cybersecurity concepts.

Post-Use Evaluation of the Platform

The self-assessment consisted of ten multiple-choice trivia-style questions addressing the core topics of the platform:

- Digital threats (malware, phishing, ransomware)
- Good practices for password management
- Privacy configuration
- Digital identity and two-factor authentication
- Legislation on data protection
- Procedures for reporting cybersecurity incidents

Participation in this self-assessment was voluntary and non-binding. The intention was to allow students the freedom to verify their own learning without external pressure. A total of 17 valid responses were collected. Although this represents a small sample size, the data served as a valuable formative input within the framework of DBR, enabling preliminary insights into how students engaged with the content.

Results Obtained

The maximum possible score was 100. The overall average was 59.4 points, with a minimum of 30 and a maximum of 90. The distribution of results is shown in Figure 15.

Figure 15. Distribution of scores obtained in the self-assessment.

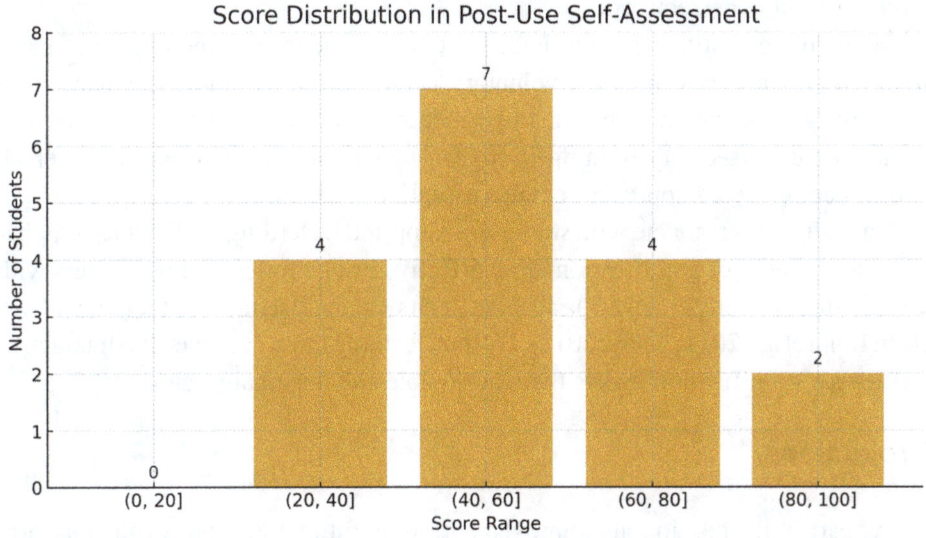

The results revealed that no student scored in the range of 0 to 20 points, indicating a basic level of comprehension across the group. Four students (23.5%) scored between 21 and 40 points, reflecting a low level of mastery. Seven students (41.2%) scored between 41 and 60 points, forming the largest group and suggesting an intermediate level of understanding. Four students (23.5%) obtained scores between 61 and 80 points, demonstrating solid appropriation of the topics addressed. Finally, two students (11.8%) scored above 80 points, which can be associated with a high level of internalization of key knowledge.

Although limited in scope, this distribution provides an exploratory vision useful for pedagogical redesign. It helps identify the levels of complexity that are adequate and the areas in which reinforcement or redesigned challenges are needed. From the DBR perspective, this first round of data collection fulfilled its main purpose: to generate empirical feedback for instructional improvement. The intention was not to test hypotheses under controlled conditions but to detect patterns in knowledge appropriation and to identify obstacles in the learning experience.

Critical Reflection

Analysis of item performance revealed that concepts related to secure passwords, authentication, and privacy were understood more consistently, while legal frameworks, reporting protocols, and differentiation between types of threats generated higher error rates. This finding aligns with the general perception that students tend to be more familiar with technical practices than with institutional or legal dimensions of cybersecurity.

While these results cannot provide conclusive evidence of the impact of gamification on learning (given the voluntary nature of participation, the absence of a control group, and the lack of usage metrics) they do underscore the need to strengthen cybersecurity training in higher education. An inclusive, transversal, and student-centered approach remains essential.

These insights resonate with studies by Kapp and Deterding et al., which emphasize the potential of gamification as an effective bridge for engaging learners with content that is often perceived as abstract, technical, or distant from their daily lives (Deterding et al., 2011; Kapp, 2012). By transforming these contents into interactive challenges, gamification makes them accessible and personally relevant.

Projections

As part of the continuous improvement cycle, future iterations of the platform are expected to incorporate:

- Learning analytics to track usage patterns (number of users, time spent, sections accessed).
- Pre- and post-tests under more controlled conditions to measure learning gains.
- Performance rubrics tailored to cybersecurity competencies.
- Qualitative interviews to capture perceptions, attitudes, and experiential insights.

In sum, the results presented here do not aim to demonstrate the conclusive effectiveness of the gamified design. Rather, they support its pedagogical relevance and establish a baseline for future rigorous validations. Ultimately, the goal is to contribute to a university digital culture that is more informed, critical, and secure.

Beyond the numerical outcomes, the self-assessment exercise fulfilled its primary role within the DBR framework: to serve as formative input for pedagogical redesign. Rather than treating the scores as conclusive evidence of effectiveness, the analysis highlighted specific areas where students showed stronger appropriation (such as password management and privacy configuration) and areas where difficulties persisted, particularly regarding legal frameworks and incident reporting protocols. These insights underscore that the platform is not a static product but an evolving learning environment. By identifying strengths and weaknesses in students' comprehension, the results directly inform the refinement of instructional materials, the redesign of gamified challenges, and the adjustment of content complexity. In this sense, the evaluation process demonstrates the central principle of DBR: integrating empirical feedback into iterative cycles of design and improvement to ensure that the platform remains pedagogically relevant and responsive to the real needs of learners.

DISCUSSION

While the initial implementation of *Mi Protector Digital* has shown promise, it is important to acknowledge its current limitations and outline avenues for future development. The initial study was conducted with a specific cohort of first-semester university students at a single institution. Consequently, the findings regarding engagement and effectiveness may not be generalizable to a broader student population with different academic backgrounds, motivations, or digital literacy levels. Furthermore, the current evaluation focuses on short-term knowledge acquisition and self-reported practices; the long-term impact on sustained behavioral change remains to be assessed.

Although university students are frequent users of digital technologies, research highlights a persistent gap in their critical digital literacy. In other words, technological proficiency does not necessarily translate into ethical and critical engagement with information. For instance, a study of Panamanian university students revealed frequent use of digital tools but relatively low ethical digital competencies, particularly regarding correct source attribution (Lopez De Ramos et al., 2024). Similarly, broader reviews of digital transformation in higher education identify “digital competence” and “digital ethics” as critical areas of concern that hinder institutional adaptation (Singun, 2025). These findings underline the need for universities to strengthen critical digital literacy so that students not only know how to use tools, but also develop the ability to evaluate, contextualize, and act responsibly in digital environments.

Integrating cybersecurity as a transversal competence across higher education programs presents considerable pedagogical challenges. Traditionally, digital security has been taught primarily in technical fields, leaving students from non-technical disciplines without essential knowledge of online threats and protective practices. Ghazali, Suryani, and Syed Idrus emphasize that many non-technical majors lack a solid foundation in cybersecurity, and institutional reluctance to incorporate it into general curricula persists due to the misconception that it is a highly specialized domain (Ghazali et al., 2024). This structural gap places a large portion of the student population at risk. Overcoming these challenges requires a cultural shift within universities, recognizing that cybersecurity is inherently interdisciplinary and vital for all graduates, regardless of discipline.

To respond to these challenges, research advocates for active and integrative teaching strategies that situate cybersecurity within broader digital competence frameworks. Torres-Hernández, Pessoa, and Gallego-Arrufat argue that experiential methodologies such as simulations, case studies, and authentic practice can significantly enhance learning outcomes in digital security (Torres-Hernández et al., 2019). Furthermore, gamification has emerged as a promising approach. A systematic review (Pramod, 2025) found that game-based platforms are more effective than traditional lectures for raising cybersecurity awareness and reinforcing secure practices. By leveraging challenges, narratives, and immediate feedback, gamification increases engagement and knowledge retention, transforming abstract technical content into accessible and meaningful experiences.

Taken together, the literature demonstrates that addressing the gap between technological use and critical digital literacy, and ensuring that cybersecurity is treated as a transversal competence, demands reimagining pedagogical strategies in higher education. Passive, tool-centered approaches are insufficient; instead, universities must adopt active, student-centered, and interdisciplinary methods that emphasize both practice and reflection. The case of *Mi Protector Digital* aligns with these recommendations: it highlights gamification as a viable means to engage students, support active learning, and foster a culture of digital responsibility that extends beyond technical skills to ethical and civic dimensions.

CONCLUSIONS AND FUTURE WORK

The design and development of *Mi Protector Digital* responds to the urgent need to foster cybersecurity competencies and digital responsibility within higher education through innovative strategies grounded in gamification. The platform was conceived with the explicit aim of integrating current pedagogical and technological principles, combining playful dynamics, immediate feedback, and simulated scenarios to encourage critical thinking, digital literacy, and responsible online behavior among students with little prior training in these areas.

Although participation in the post-use self-assessment was voluntary and limited, the results provided preliminary evidence of the platform's formative potential. Most students achieved intermediate scores, suggesting a partial appropriation of key content—particularly in relation to digital threats and data protection—even without systematically engaging with all the platform's resources. At the same time, the results highlighted areas for improvement in instructional design, such as simplifying the presentation of legal content or redesigning game mechanics to reinforce critical knowledge.

While these findings cannot be generalized, they partially validate the relevance of the approach and point to concrete areas for pedagogical refinement. More accessible normative content, more personalized feedback, and targeted reinforcement of the less well-understood modules emerge as priorities. In line with literature, the results confirm that gamification can increase student engagement, facilitate active learning, and promote a culture of digital self-care, even among students from non-technical backgrounds (Deterding et al., 2011; Gee, 2003; Kapp, 2012; Santana-Mancilla et al., 2015). A critical limitation identified, however, was the absence of usage analytics, which prevented a more detailed evaluation of student interactions with the platform. This gap marks an important direction for the project's next stage of development.

Future work will follow the iterative logic of Design-Based Research and address several key lines of development. First, the integration of usage analytics (e.g., through tools such as Google Analytics) will make it possible to monitor visits, interaction times, return rates, and navigation flows, thereby enabling more precise and data-driven decisions about content and interface design. Second, comparative pre- and post-tests with control groups will strengthen the rigor of evaluation, incorporating perception and usability scales. Third, the platform will evolve toward greater personalization and adaptability, potentially through simple algorithms or even educational AI solutions that tailor content and challenges to student profiles and progress. Fourth, the study will be extended to other university contexts, nationally and internationally, to test the robustness of the design, identify common patterns of appropriation, and enhance the external validity of the results.

Additional lines of development include the production of complementary didactic materials, such as audiovisual capsules, glossaries, and downloadable guides for teachers, which would facilitate the integration of the platform into transversal training courses. Likewise, formal curricular integration is envisaged, positioning *Mi Protector Digital* as an institutionalized resource in courses on information technology, integral formation, or preparatory programs, thus ensuring impact, scalability, and sustainability over time.

Finally, this chapter also issues an open call for academic and technical collaboration. The project is available to be adapted, replicated, or extended for educational and scientific purposes. Researchers, educators, and developers interested in digital education and cybersecurity are invited to contribute to the refinement and expansion of this proposal.

REFERENCES

Almelhi, A. M. (2021). Effectiveness of the ADDIE Model within an E-Learning Environment in Developing Creative Writing in EFL Students. *English Language Teaching*, *14*(2), 20. DOI: 10.5539/elt.v14n2p20

Álvarez Magallán, B. A., Acosta-Díaz, R., & Morales-Vanegas, E. A. (2024). Privacy-Aware Artificial Intelligence: A Review of Design Principles and Applications. *Avances En Interacción Humano-Computadora*, *9*(1), 209–213. DOI: 10.47756/aihc.y9i1.169

Cámara de Diputados. (2010). *Ley Federal de Protección de Datos Personales en Posesión de los Particulares*. Diario Oficial de la Federación. https://www.diputados.gob.mx/LeyesBiblio/pdf/LFPDPPP.pdf

Castells, M. (2000). *La era de la información: Economía, sociedad y cultura* (2. ed). Alianza.

Csikszentmihalyi, M., Abuhamdeh, S., & Nakamura, J. (2014). Flow. In M. Csikszentmihalyi, *Flow and the Foundations of Positive Psychology* (pp. 227–238). Springer Netherlands. DOI: 10.1007/978-94-017-9088-8_15

Deterding, S., Dixon, D., Khaled, R., & Nacke, L. (2011). From game design elements to gamefulness: Defining "gamification." *Proceedings of the 15th International Academic MindTrek Conference: Envisioning Future Media Environments*, 9–15. DOI: 10.1145/2181037.2181040

Diario Oficial de la Federación. (2017). *Ley General de Protección de Datos Personales en Posesión de Sujetos Obligados*. https://www.dof.gob.mx/nota_detalle.php?codigo=5478205&fecha=26/01/2017

Dunwell, I., de Freitas, S., Petridis, P., Hendrix, M., Arnab, S., Lameras, P., & Stewart, C. (2014). *A game-based learning approach to road safety: The code of everand*. 3389–3398. DOI: 10.1145/2556288.2557281

Duque, P., & Cervantes-Cervantes, L.-S. (2019). Responsabilidad Social Universitaria: Una revisión sistemática y análisis bibliométrico. *Estudios Gerenciales*, 451–464. DOI: 10.18046/j.estger.2019.153.3389

Gaytan-Lugo, L., Hernandez, S., Santana-Mancilla, P. C., & Garcia-Ruiz, M. (2014). *A contextual study and usability testing of videogames to inform the design of a serious game to improve reading comprehension. Memorias ENC 2014. Encuentro Nacional de Ciencias de la Computación (ENC 2014)*. Ocotlán.

Gee, J. P. (2003). What video games have to teach us about learning and literacy. *Computers in Entertainment, 1*(1), 20. DOI: 10.1145/950566.950595

Ghazali, N., Ab Rahim, I. S., & Syed Idrus, S. Z. (2024). Challenges and Opportunities of Cybersecurity Education for Non-technical Majors. [JCSI]. *Journal of Communication in Scientific Inquiry, 6*(1), 47–55. DOI: 10.58915/jcsi.v6i1.873

Hakim, A. R., Ramli, K., Gunawan, T. S., & Windarta, S. (2023). A Novel Digital Forensic Framework for Data Breach Investigation. *IEEE Access : Practical Innovations, Open Solutions, 11*, 42644–42659. DOI: 10.1109/ACCESS.2023.3270619

Ibarra, M., Ataucusi, P., Barzola, B., & Huaman, J. (2017). Mejorando la disponibilidad de recursos educativos digitales para enseñar en escuelas rurales sin acceso a internet. *Revista Brasileira de Informática Na Educação, 25*(03), 80. DOI: 10.5753/rbie.2017.25.03.80

Jartelius, M. (2020). The 2020 Data Breach Investigations Report – a CSO's perspective. *Network Security, 2020*(7), 9–12. DOI: 10.1016/S1353-4858(20)30079-9

Jiménez, A. S. A., Ramírez, N. A. B., Santana-Mancilla, P. C., Romero, J. C. M., & Acosta-Díaz, R. (2018).. . *Heuristic Evaluation of a Gamified Application for Education in Patients with Diabetes, 1–4*, 1–4. Advance online publication. DOI: 10.1145/3293578.3293593

Kapp, K. M. (2012). *The gamification of learning and instruction: Game-based methods and strategies for training and education*. Pfeiffer.

Khaldi, A., Bouzidi, R., & Nader, F. (2023). Gamification of e-learning in higher education: A systematic literature review. *Smart Learning Environments, 10*(1), 10. DOI: 10.1186/s40561-023-00227-z PMID: 40478066

Lopez De Ramos, A. L., Casado Robles, E., Atagua-Díaz, Z., Prado, J. F., Álvarez Franco, A. M., Cáceres, A., & Ramos Fortuna, V. (2024). Análisis de la alfabetización digital: Explorando la brecha de género en estudiantes universitarios panameños. *Latitude, 1*(19), 22–46. DOI: 10.55946/latitude.v1i19.242

Mukherjee, M., Le, N. T., Chow, Y.-W., & Susilo, W. (2024). Strategic Approaches to Cybersecurity Learning: A Study of Educational Models and Outcomes. *Information (Basel), 15*(2), 117. DOI: 10.3390/info15020117

Ortiz, R. (2017). Educación globalizada: Tendencias y retos de la educación superior en México y el mundo. *RIESED - Revista Internacional De Estudios Sobre Sistemas Educativos, 2*(6), 24–39.

Piazza, A., Vasudevan, S., & Carr, M. (2023). Cybersecurity in UK Universities: Mapping (or managing) threat intelligence sharing within the higher education sector. *Journal of Cybersecurity*, *9*(1), tyad019. Advance online publication. DOI: 10.1093/cybsec/tyad019

Pramod, D. (2025). Gamification in cybersecurity education; a state of the art review and research agenda. *Journal of Applied Research in Higher Education*, *17*(4), 1162–1180. DOI: 10.1108/JARHE-02-2024-0072

Robinson, L., Cotten, S. R., Ono, H., Quan-Haase, A., Mesch, G., Chen, W., Schulz, J., Hale, T. M., & Stern, M. J. (2015). Digital inequalities and why they matter. *Information Communication and Society*, *18*(5), 569–582. DOI: 10.1080/1369118X.2015.1012532

Romero-Mendez, E. A., Santana-Mancilla, P. C., Garcia-Ruiz, M., Montesinos-López, O. A., & Anido-Rifón, L. E. (2023). The Use of Deep Learning to Improve Player Engagement in a Video Game through a Dynamic Difficulty Adjustment Based on Skills Classification. *Applied Sciences (Basel, Switzerland)*, *13*(14), 8249. DOI: 10.3390/app13148249

Santana-Mancilla, P. C., Gaytán-Lugo, L. S., & Rodríguez-Ortiz, M. A. (2016). Usability Testing of Serious Games: The Experience of the IHCLab. In *Games User Research: A Case Study Approach* (pp. 271–283). CRC Press.

Santana-Mancilla, P. C., Rodríguez-Ortiz, M., Gaytán-Lugo, L., & Garcia-Ruiz, M. (2015). User Experience Evaluation to El Encanto: A Serious Game for Learning Community Intervention. *Research in Computing Science*, *108*(1), 81–88. DOI: 10.13053/rcs-108-1-9

Signori, G. G., Guimaraes, J. C. F. D., Severo, E. A., & Rotta, C. (2018). Gamification as an innovative method in the processes of learning in higher education institutions. *International Journal of Innovation and Learning*, *24*(2), 115. DOI: 10.1504/IJIL.2018.094066

Singun, A. (2025). Unveiling the barriers to digital transformation in higher education institutions: A systematic literature review. *Discover Education*, *4*(1), 37. DOI: 10.1007/s44217-025-00430-9

Tafur-Méndez, F., Almao-Malvacias, V., & Zambrano-Chamba, M. (2023). Conocimiento sobre la gamificación como técnica para reforzar el aprendizaje en la educación superior. *593 Digital Publisher CEIT, 8*(3), 209–218. DOI: 10.33386/593dp.2023.3.1628

Tobias, S., Fletcher, J. D., & Wind, A. P. (2014). Game-Based Learning. In Spector, J. M., Merrill, M. D., Elen, J., & Bishop, M. J. (Eds.), *Handbook of Research on Educational Communications and Technology* (pp. 485–503). Springer New York., DOI: 10.1007/978-1-4614-3185-5_38

Torres-Hernández, N., Pessoa, T., & Gallego-Arrufat, M. J. (2019). Intervención y evaluación con tecnologías de la competencia en seguridad digital. *Digital Education Review*, 111–129. DOI: 10.1344/der.2019.35.111-129

Triplett, W. J. (2023). Addressing Cybersecurity Challenges in Education. *International Journal of STEM Education for Sustainability*, *3*(1), 47–67. DOI: 10.53889/ijses.v3i1.132

UNESCO. (2020a). *Education for sustainable development: A roadmap*. UNESCO., DOI: 10.54675/YFRE1448

UNESCO. (2020b). Learning through radio and television in the time of COVID-19 [Global Education Coalition]. *Global Education Coalition*. https://en.unesco.org/news/learning-through-radio-and-television-time-covid-19

UNESCO. (2021). *AI and education: Guidance for policy-makers*.

Valdés Montecinos, M. (2019). Internacionalización del currículo universitario virtual en el contexto de la globalización. *Telos: Revista de Estudios Interdisciplinarios En Ciencias Sociales*, *21*(3), 754–775. DOI: 10.36390/telos213.13

Werbach, K., & Hunter, D. (2015). *The Gamification Toolkit: Dynamics, Mechanics, and Components for the Win*. Wharton Digital Press.

Wiggins, B. E. (2016). An Overview and Study on the Use of Games, Simulations, and Gamification in Higher Education. *International Journal of Game-Based Learning*, *6*(1), 18–29. DOI: 10.4018/IJGBL.2016010102

Chapter 4
Bridging Disciplines Through Gamification:
Reflections on Culturally Responsive Language Teaching in Healthcare and Occupational Therapy

Laura E. Mendoza
https://orcid.org/0000-0001-8649-8775
University of Texas at El Paso, USA

Daisy C. Alvarado
https://orcid.org/0009-0004-7867-5523
University of Texas at El Paso, USA

ABSTRACT

This chapter explores the intersection of gamification, culturally responsive pedagogy, and professional Spanish instruction within a Doctor of Occupational Therapy program at a U.S.–Mexico border university. Focusing on instructors' perspectives, it examines how interdisciplinary collaboration between language educators and occupational therapy faculty can enhance students' linguistic, cultural, and clinical competencies. Observations reveal how these approaches fostered student engagement, rapid thinking, peer support, and confidence in using Spanish in professional contexts. By integrating cultural responsiveness and authentic language practice, the courses modeled a replicable framework for preparing healthcare professionals to deliver equitable, high-quality care to Spanish-speaking populations. Findings

DOI: 10.4018/979-8-3373-4657-1.ch004

suggest that gamification and interdisciplinary course design can serve as effective strategies for bridging language learning, cultural competence, and clinical readiness in health education.

INTRODUCTION AND PROBLEM STATEMENT

Teaching Spanish language skills within healthcare education has become increasingly critical as the need to provide linguistically and culturally appropriate services to minoritized populations continues to grow. In the United States, Spanish-speaking communities represent a significant portion of patients who often encounter barriers in accessing high-quality healthcare due to language differences. These barriers can negatively impact patient safety, satisfaction, and overall health outcomes, highlighting the urgent need for healthcare programs to prepare students to communicate effectively across languages and cultural contexts.

The present chapter builds on the literature exploring gamification in the language classroom, extending it specifically to the context of Languages for Specific Purposes (LSP) courses in healthcare education. While gamification has been widely studied for its motivational and engagement benefits, less attention has been given to its integration within professional programs such as occupational therapy, where students must simultaneously develop technical, linguistic, and cultural competencies. This chapter addresses that gap by examining how gamification strategies can be purposefully combined with Culturally Responsive Pedagogy (CRP) to create authentic, context-driven learning experiences that foster both language proficiency and cultural competence.

The insights presented here are drawn entirely from the perspectives and observations of two instructors from a Doctor of Occupational Therapy (OTD) program, which requires Spanish courses as part of its curriculum. By focusing on instructors' experiences, this chapter provides an in-depth view of the planning, implementation, and evaluation processes involved in integrating language learning with clinical preparation, while emphasizing culturally responsive approaches tailored to border populations.

The purpose of this chapter is to examine the interdisciplinary collaboration between language education and occupational therapy faculty to advance culturally responsive Spanish language learning through the use of gamification strategies. By exploring this collaboration, the chapter highlights how targeted pedagogical design can foster equitable practices, enhance cultural competence, and equip future healthcare practitioners to deliver high-quality care in linguistically diverse contexts.

BACKGROUND

To centralize the curricula that the program offers, along with the perspectives of their own students, the present chapter furthers the conversation of instructors' perceptions and experiences regarding the inclusion of gamification to advance their Spanish language for specific purposes skills. more importantly, this chapter advances the understanding of how gamified language classrooms informed by culturally responsive pedagogy foster inclusive learning environments that cultivate students' empathetic skills for both academic and professional contexts.

CULTURALLY RESPONSIVE PEDAGOGY

To conceptualize Culturally Responsive Pedagogy, this chapter follows Ladson-Billings' (1995) foundational definition. The author states:

> *CRP is a pedagogy of oppression not unlike critical pedagogy but committed explicitly to collective, not merely individual, empowerment. Culturally relevant pedagogy rests on three criteria or propositions: (a) students must experience academic success; (b) students must develop and/or maintain cultural competence; and (c) students must develop a critical consciousness through which they challenge the current status quo of the social order (p. 160).*

Therefore, CRP is relevant to this chapter as the educators and authors reflected on their teaching practices and biases to offer experiences that could empower students to cultivate empathy and success as they transition to their professional roles as Occupational Therapists.

The present chapter aligns with Brown-Jeffy and Cooper's (2011) assertion that "Teachers should not only recognize students' value and importance, but they should also consciously recognize what their students have in common. Together, students and teachers need to build classroom community, making it a safe place in which to nurture everyone's cultural identity" (p. 77). In this program, the co-creation of CRP in the Spanish classroom emphasized what students, as members of the border community, needed to understand and develop to navigate their community successfully.

This approach acknowledged that students' shared experience of living in a bicultural, bilingual environment provided them with unique insights into the challenges and strengths of border community life. By building on these commonalities while respecting individual differences, the classroom became a space where students could explore how their cultural competencies would translate into professional skills. The co-creation process ensured that culturally responsive pedagogy was not merely theoretical but was grounded in the authentic experiences and needs of both the students and the communities they would serve as occupational therapists.

Sleeter (2011) challenges educators to critically re-examine their perceptions and applications of culturally responsive pedagogy, moving beyond superficial cultural celebrations to address deeper systemic issues. the author emphasizes that while CRP represents a valuable celebration of cultures and values, educators cannot overlook the persistent inequities, inequalities, and systematic disempowerment that certain communities face daily. This critical perspective demands that culturally responsive pedagogy extend beyond cultural appreciation to actively confront and address the structural barriers that perpetuate educational and social disparities.

Consequently, integrating CRP into healthcare curricula represents a shared responsibility that requires educators to develop a profound understanding of both their students' experiences and the communities these future professionals will serve. This dual awareness becomes particularly crucial in healthcare contexts, where practitioners must navigate complex intersections of cultural identity, socioeconomic status, and health disparities. Educators must recognize that their students may themselves come from communities that have experienced educational inequities, healthcare discrimination, or systematic marginalization, while simultaneously preparing these students to serve populations facing similar challenges.

Healthcare professionals, particularly those working in border communities and serving diverse populations, require more than ever to broaden their linguistic and cultural competencies as part of a larger effort to challenge and transform traditional narratives both inside and outside their professional practice settings. This transformation involves not only acquiring language skills and cultural knowledge but also developing critical consciousness about how healthcare systems have historically excluded or marginalized certain populations. By integrating this critical perspective into culturally responsive pedagogy, healthcare education can prepare practitioners who are equipped not only to communicate across cultural and linguistic boundaries but also to advocate for equitable care and challenge discriminatory practices within healthcare institutions.

This chapter approaches the inclusion of culturally relevant pedagogies from two perspectives. First, we approached it traditionally to clearly illustrate the resilience, empathy, and service that students will co-construct with their border community. Second, we utilize the term to refer to the contemporary practices that young people, like the students enrolled in the OT program, are currently experiencing. As students develop more dynamic and flexible views of culture (Ladson-Billings, 2014), so must teaching practices evolve. Educators today are prompted to integrate teaching approaches that are more inviting and reflective of young people's lives. For this reason, the present chapter highlights how the intersection of gamification and CRP is pivotal to reimagining language education as an interactive, culturally grounded approach to professional development.

In essence, culturally responsive pedagogy serves a dual transformative function that extends far beyond traditional educational approaches. As Zembylas (2023) emphasizes, CRP not only mobilizes existing cultural resources among learners but, most importantly, strengthens and expands the cultural repertoires of such learners, enabling them to navigate multiple cultural contexts with confidence and competence. This pedagogical framework fundamentally reconceptualizes the learning process by positioning students' cultural identities as assets rather than obstacles to academic achievement.

The power of CRP lies in its holistic approach to education, which conjointly addresses learners' multifaceted needs by heavily prioritizing students' identities, values, and prior knowledge while simultaneously supporting both academic and cultural competence development. This dual focus ensures that students do not have to choose between academic success and cultural authenticity, but rather can achieve excellence through the integration of both dimensions. In healthcare education contexts, this approach becomes particularly significant as future practitioners must develop both clinical competencies and cultural consciousness to serve diverse patient populations effectively.

The intersection of CRP with gamification, particularly in language teaching for healthcare professionals, represents a pedagogically relevant and innovative approach because it leverages students' diversified learning preferences while cultivating a profound sense of belonging within their learning community. Gamified culturally responsive learning environments acknowledge that students bring varied learning styles, technological literacies, and cultural perspectives that can be harnessed through interactive, engaging educational experiences. By creating classroom spaces where cultural diversity is celebrated and utilized as a learning resource, students develop not only linguistic competence but also the cultural consciousness necessary for equitable professional practice.

This integration ultimately prepares healthcare professionals who can bridge cultural divides, communicate effectively across linguistic barriers, and provide care that honors the cultural identities and experiences of their patients—skills that are essential for addressing the healthcare disparities documented throughout the literature.

GAMIFICATION IN (LANGUAGE) TEACHING

The incorporation of gamified experiences in the classrooms has been around for decades. Nevertheless, as pedagogical approaches to teaching languages evolved, different opportunities, outcomes, and tools have emerged. enthusiasts of these approaches have been polishing the varied manners in which emergent bilinguals can interact with games in their classrooms. in today's language classrooms, educators have the opportunity to purposefully integrate games into students' learning, looking to convey specific outcomes that go beyond only promoting fun among their students. These newer pedagogies suggest an intentional integration of games as a mode of promoting engagement, completion rate, social interaction, and diversified ways of feedback. Taking this into consideration, this chapter promotes how the structured and purposeful use of gamification in language teaching can improve students' learning experience while acquiring or mastering a language.

To deepen the conversation, the present chapter follows the gamification definition offered by Blass et al. (2019), who defines gamification as "The use of game mechanics (i.e., points, quests, rules, competition, badges) in nontraditional environments to make learning fun and engaging (p. 95). Similarly, Arnold (2014) reminds us that the integration of gamification in education promotes the enhancement of engaging features and moments as it promotes curiosity and exploration amongst the learners; for language learners specifically, it also increases motivation towards learning (Boudadi & Gutiérrez-Colón, 2020; Subhash & Cudney, 2018) while challenging them (Prathyusha, 2020). This chapter aims to explore how these game mechanics can be specifically tailored to Spanish for specific purposes in curricula, examining their effectiveness in enhancing language skills, fostering a deeper engagement with the material, and accommodating diverse learning preferences. By aligning gamification strategies with students' feedback and educational outcomes, this research contributes to the ongoing dialogue on innovative teaching methods and their potential to transform language education, primarily in healthcare settings such as the field of Occupational Therapy.

In recent years, scholars across disciplines have consistently highlighted the effectiveness of gamification as a pedagogical tool for motivating students and sustaining their engagement (Dehghanzadeh et al., 2021; Dehghanzadeh et al., 2024; Jackson & McNamara, 2013). Within language education specifically, gamified approaches create interactive opportunities that are not only enjoyable and stimulating, but also instrumental in fostering social interaction and collaborative learning. When thoughtfully aligned with course objectives, gamification does more than entertain; it provides structured yet playful contexts where learners can negotiate meaning, test their linguistic abilities, and engage in authentic communicative exchanges that deepen their proficiency.

Gamification also has the capacity to transform the affective climate of the language classroom. Traditional models often emphasize accuracy and error correction, which can heighten students' anxiety and discourage risk-taking. By contrast, gamified activities reframe mistakes as natural and valuable components of the learning process, shifting classroom culture from one of potential failure to one of exploration and growth. This reframing is particularly powerful for emergent bilinguals, who may otherwise experience frustration or embarrassment in high-stakes environments. Through carefully designed challenges, levels, and rewards, gamification builds on learners' existing knowledge while encouraging them to extend their skills in a supportive, low-risk setting. Ultimately, gamification promotes a more equitable and empowering classroom environment, one where students are motivated to participate actively, learn collaboratively, and view language acquisition as both meaningful and attainable.

If gamification then provides a positive learning experience for learners, then incorporating these pedagogical approaches in today's learning is invaluable. Of particular importance is to incorporate gamification in classrooms where we are working alongside the healthcare providers of the future. In a setting like the OT Spanish classroom, furthering opportunities where students can build their knowledge alongside their linguistic and cultural competencies makes gamified experiences a powerful addition. In a setting like this, creating opportunities where students can co-create knowledge in a stress-free environment that still presents them with engaging yet challenging tasks can effectively mirror what their field of study will demand in the near future. Through gamification, these students not only rehearse clinical interactions in the target language, but also practice empathy, adaptability, and collaboration—skills that will be indispensable as they transition into professional contexts serving diverse and multilingual populations.

The present chapter suggests that the inclusion of gamified experiences leverages the acquisition and mastery of technical language in ways that are both effective and satisfying for learners. This satisfaction stems from the versatile applications that gamification offers in language education, as Ishaq et al. (2021) note: gamified tools can serve a wide range of purposes, from reviewing vocabulary and grammar to practicing sentence structure and idiomatic expressions. Figueroa Flores (2015) further reminds us that many gamified experiences incorporate achievements that are publicly visible, such as points, badges, or leaderboards. These reward systems generate continuity and motivation, encouraging students to advance steadily in their learning process. in this way, gamification counteracts the limitations of traditional memorization-based approaches and repetitive grammar drills by fostering active, interactive engagement.

Recent scholarship underscores the added value of gamification for developing speaking and communicative skills. Aulia (2025), echoing Ho-Minh and Suppasetseree (2025), highlight that "gamification also positively affects speaking skills. interactive speaking tasks embedded in games—such as role-plays, simulations, and dialogue challenges—provide contextualized opportunities for practicing pronunciation, fluency, and conversational skills in a low-pressure environment" (p. 308). This remains especially significant in healthcare education, where learners are preparing to communicate safely, accurately, and empathetically with future patients. Thus, integrating gamified strategies in professional language classrooms is not only pedagogically innovative but also foundational to equipping healthcare providers with the linguistic and cultural competencies they will need in their practice.

LANGUAGE FOR SPECIFIC PURPOSES

The field of Language for Specific Purposes, hereafter referred to as LSP, serves the needs of an infinite set of professions and occupations worldwide. The present chapter, follows Long's (2017) definition of what LSP is; the author states: "LSP studies is uniqulely positioned to make an impact on students' global education in a wide variety of disciplines because the field has at its center the aim of fulfilling the communicative needs of a specific group of people within a specific professional context such as medicine, law, science, social work, business, translation and interpretation, etc." (p. 17). LSP literature often emphasizes authentic materials, task-based learning, and alignment with professional practice; therefore, offering a section in this chapter where the authors intentionally express the relevance of LSP in relation to their context is a must.

More than explaining the benefits that LSP can bring to the table, this chapter centralizes its attention to presenting the existent intersection among a cultural context and a gamified experience in an LSP course. The specificity of LSP grants accessibility to gamified experiences where learners can build their vocabulary, language skills, idioms, and social skills to construct a *persona* whose main interest is to engage meaningfully and professionally within their field of study. in the case of occupational therapy students, this means rehearsing how to embody the role of a culturally responsive healthcare provider who can navigate patient interactions with confidence, empathy, and linguistic precision. Long (2017) emphasizes: "Approximations of authentic situations and settings, in which students need to draw on intercultural knowledge to respond in an appropriate way—can be powerful tools to reinforce and expand student learning not only about the 12 culture but also about leadership and what it can mean or look like in a variety of settings" (p. 92). LSP, in this sense, brings opportunities for students to continue nurturing their field of study while, simultaneously, strengthening the instances where students can face challenges in controlled-safe spaces. These interactions allow students to continue building their knowledge while presented with organized, and well-constructed strategies which allow them to become better equipped for what they will face as professionals in their corresponding fields of study. in occupational therapy, specifically, having LSP courses provides authentic communication opportunities. in this field of study, learning how to communicate with colleagues and patients appropriately represents not only an asset, but a necessity. the LSP - OT Spanish courses created for the program bridged CRP and gamification in an effort to offer simulations of real-life communicative acts embedded in cultural contexts, promoting practical language usage that respects and reflects learners' cultural diversity. This supports the development of communicative competence beyond rote memorization to real-world application.

Long's (2017) visionary conclusion emphasizes the transformative potential of Language for Specific Purposes within contemporary higher education: "Just as was the case with the new directions for language teaching, LSP studies is also on the cutting edge of the multidisciplinary, integrated learning experiences and meaningful assessment measures that are being mapped out for the future of undergraduate education in general" (p. 188). This observation proves particularly prescient when applied to healthcare education, where the complexity of patient care demands professionals who can navigate linguistic, cultural, and clinical competencies simultaneously.

In the case of the program presented in this chapter, the graduate students enrolled in these Spanish occupational therapy courses experienced firsthand the power and potential of multidisciplinary collaboration. Through the partnership between language education and occupational therapy faculty, students witnessed how interdisciplinary teamwork can enhance both educational outcomes and professional preparation. This collaboration demonstrated that effective healthcare delivery requires professionals who can think beyond disciplinary boundaries, integrating communication skills with clinical expertise to provide holistic, culturally responsive care. The students observed how language educators brought pedagogical innovation and cultural consciousness, while occupational therapy faculty contributed clinical authenticity and professional context, creating a learning environment that neither discipline could achieve independently.

The future of healthcare rests in the hands of professionals who understand that linguistic competence and cultural responsiveness are not optional skills but essential components of quality care. LSP courses in healthcare contexts represent a dual responsibility that extends far beyond traditional language instruction. These courses serve as bridges between academic preparation and professional practice, providing opportunities for students to increase their linguistic, social, and cultural capabilities while simultaneously connecting advocacy and social justice principles with caring options for both students and the diverse communities they will serve. By integrating language learning with professional identity development, these programs prepare healthcare providers who can address health disparities, advocate for marginalized populations, and deliver care that honors patients' cultural identities and linguistic preferences.

Despite legitimate concerns raised by several scholars (Douglas, 2000; Douglas, 2001; Hamp-Lyons & Lumley, 2001; O'Sullivan, 2012) regarding the inherent difficulties in assessing LSP content—particularly the challenge of evaluating both linguistic competence and professional knowledge simultaneously—the profound benefits of offering such courses far outweigh these methodological challenges. The assessment difficulties stem from the complex nature of LSP learning, where students must demonstrate not only language proficiency but also appropriate use of technical terminology, cultural sensitivity, and professional communication protocols within authentic contexts.

Nevertheless, these courses offer unparalleled advantages that justify the investment in developing appropriate assessment strategies. LSP courses provide exceptional flexibility, allowing curriculum designers to adapt content, pace, and methodology to meet the specific needs of different healthcare specializations and student populations. They offer contextuality that traditional language courses cannot match, situating language learning within authentic professional scenarios that enhance both engagement and retention. Most significantly, these courses provide an almost individualized preparation experience that mirrors the authentic communication challenges students will encounter in their specific professional environments, whether they work in acute care settings, rehabilitation centers, community health programs, or specialized therapeutic contexts. This personalized approach ensures that students develop not only general language proficiency but also the specialized communicative competence required for their particular professional roles.

The transformative potential of LSP courses in healthcare education becomes even more critical when examined against the backdrop of persistent linguistic barriers that compromise patient care quality and safety in healthcare settings. While LSP programs offer innovative pedagogical solutions for preparing culturally and linguistically competent healthcare professionals, the urgency of this preparation is underscored by documented evidence of how communication barriers negatively impact patient outcomes, treatment adherence, and healthcare equity. As the following section will demonstrate, the need for such specialized language preparation extends beyond educational innovation to become a professional imperative for addressing healthcare disparities and ensuring equitable access to quality occupational therapy services in linguistically diverse communities.

HEALTHCARE LINGUISTIC BARRIERS

One of the heaviest crises that the community in the United States faces is a healthcare linguistic barrier. although the majority of households in the United States (78.4%) speak exclusively English at home, the proportion of households using non-English languages is increasing, now accounting for about 21.6%. among these, Spanish is the predominant language, spoken by approximately 42 million people, who represent nearly two-thirds of all non-English speakers in the country (The United States is rich in languages, 2025). This said, the present chapter continually highlights the relevance of interwinding cultural competence, linguistic competence, and care for patients.

Equally important, Diamond and Jacobs (2024) highlight:

Patients with LEP often have other disadvantages, including limited financial resources, and their communication difficulties may be compounded by lack of formal education, vulnerability due to insecure immigration status, and mental health issues, such as anxiety and stress. Language barriers make it even more difficult for patients in English-dominant environments to advocate for themselves, ask questions, and navigate the nuances of health care systems that lead to better care (para. 10).

Unfortunately, this is the reality for many community members whose primary language is other different than English. Al Shamsi et al. (2020) furthers the conversation and state: "Language barriers are a key cause of miscommunication between medical providers and patients, and negatively affect the quality of healthcare services and patient satisfaction" (p. 5). In this sense, the less privileged communities, such as the Hispanic communities, whom directly get impacted by these differences, might even receive a different quality when interacting with their healthcare providers given the present barriers; these barriers, linguistic, cultural, or both, may unfortunately lead to life-threatening circumstances with unfavorable outcomes for practitioners and their clients. Diamond and Jacobs (2024) continue: "Health care organizations and clinicians have a moral imperative to reduce and ultimately eliminate the injustice experienced by patients with LEP in this country. in this globally connected world, there is no place for linguistic isolationism. we can change the system and we should" (para. 14). Providing appropriate healthcare services to our communities is a shared responsibility; if we do not start by educating our providers early enough in their careers, they will struggle to provide quality care to their patients in the future. We must then start in each of our classrooms to teach our students the importance of generating quality care which entails a broad intentionality fully to serve their patients professionally, linguistically, and culturally.

The detrimental impact of linguistic barriers in healthcare extends far beyond communication difficulties, creating cascading effects that disproportionately affect underprivileged communities. Multiple researchers (Flores, 2006; Jacobs et al., 2006; Schouten et al., 2020; Showstack, 2019) have documented how language barriers perpetuate healthcare disparities and compromise patient outcomes across various dimensions of care. These adverse effects manifest in multiple critical areas that directly impact patient wellbeing and treatment effectiveness.

Flores (2006) identified medication adherence as a particularly concerning area, noting that patients with limited access to healthcare services in their preferred language demonstrate significantly lower rates of medication compliance. This reduced adherence stems not only from misunderstanding medication instructions but also from patients' inability to communicate concerns, side effects, or questions about their treatment regimens. The consequences extend beyond individual health outcomes to include increased healthcare costs, preventable complications, and reduced treatment efficacy.

Furthermore, the psychological burden of navigating healthcare systems in a non-native language creates additional challenges for patients. Meuter et al. (2015) documented how language barriers contribute to increased stress levels among patients, creating a cyclical problem where anxiety and stress may exacerbate existing health conditions while simultaneously hindering effective communication with healthcare providers. This heightened stress response can compromise immune function, delay healing processes, and create additional barriers to optimal health outcomes.

Perhaps most concerning is the impact on patient autonomy and shared decision-making processes. Schouten et al. (2020) found that patients facing language barriers tend to be significantly less involved in decisions regarding their own healthcare, effectively removing them from the collaborative relationship that is fundamental to effective therapeutic practice. This reduced participation not only violates principles of patient-centered care but also limits healthcare providers' ability to deliver culturally appropriate, individualized treatment plans that align with patients' values, preferences, and cultural beliefs.

For these reasons, the present chapter aims to contribute to the conversation and further the implementation of courses where healthcare professionals can foster environments where their patients feel safe, valued, and respected. By promoting the implementation of programs where bilingualism strengthens the opportunities of practitioners and patients, the chapter provides a replicable framework for other healthcare programs seeking to integrate culturally responsive language education into their curricula.

INSTRUCTIONAL CONTEXT

This reflective pedagogical inquiry took place within a Doctor of Occupational Therapy (OTD) program located in the U.S.–Mexico border region. The program is one of only two in the United States offering Spanish for Specific Purposes (SSP) coursework tailored for occupational therapy, and the only program requiring two Spanish courses for all OT students. These courses are grounded in principles of Culturally Responsive Pedagogy (CRP) and experiential learning, and were collaboratively taught by a Spanish language specialist and an occupational therapy faculty member. Each cohort includes approximately 20–30 graduate students with varied levels of Spanish proficiency. Instruction was delivered during the 2024–2025 academic year, with each course consisting of weekly sessions integrating language development, cultural competence, and clinical simulation.

The first OT Spanish course provides students with foundational communication skills directly connected to clinical practice. By the end of the course, students are expected to: (1) negotiate meaning to share information, reactions, and feelings in Spanish, (2) incorporate relevant medical and anatomical terminology in interactions, (3) understand and interpret spoken Spanish in professional contexts, (4) present basic information clearly to others, and (5) discuss cultural beliefs, values, and health-related practices among Spanish-speaking communities. These objectives are consistently reinforced through culturally responsive pedagogies that integrate language learning with cultural awareness (Ladson-Billings, 1995; Gay, 2018).

The second course builds upon this foundation by strengthening prior competencies and advancing students' ability to apply Spanish in simulated and practical OT contexts. Course objectives include: (1) using culturally appropriate nonverbal strategies to augment communication during simulated patient evaluations and interventions, (2) identifying and applying resources to develop home-based OT programs in Spanish, and (3) instructing a real or simulated patient in one occupational therapy concept using basic Spanish. A key feature of this course is the implementation of OT assessments in Spanish, which allows students to practice integrating professional tools with linguistic and cultural competence. Moreover, the course strategically revisits and expands upon materials from the first course, reinforcing vocabulary, cultural knowledge, and empathy in order to prepare students better to meet the needs of borderland communities. The course emphasizes the importance of cultural competence and its relationship to care, primarily in alignment with the educational objectives of the AOTA - American Occupational Therapy Association (Garcia & Garcia, 2021).

Both courses are intentionally grounded in Culturally Responsive Pedagogy (CRP). CRP emphasizes the validation of students' cultural backgrounds, experiences, and perspectives as central to the learning process, while fostering empathy, respect, and equity (Gay, 2018; Ladson-Billings, 1995). In this way, the OT Spanish sequence is not solely about language acquisition but about cultivating dispositions of care and cultural humility that extend beyond the classroom. By creating a culture of safety and respect in their language learning, students begin to mirror these practices in their clinical training. Ultimately, this curricular approach contributes to building a broader community of care—equipping future occupational therapists to support Spanish-speaking clients with dignity, compassion, and cultural responsiveness.

METHODS

Participants

Participants included students enrolled in the required OT Spanish sequence. As a graduate program, participants were primarily traditional-age graduate students preparing for clinical practice in bilingual and bicultural settings. Because all students were required to complete the Spanish courses as part of their curriculum, participation was universal, representing a wide range of Spanish proficiency levels. No identifiable demographic or performance data from students were collected or analyzed for the purposes of this chapter.

Data Sources

This chapter draws on qualitative, instructor-generated sources that informed the reflective analysis of course design and implementation. Data sources included:

- Instructor observations during class sessions
- Post-class and weekly planning reflections
- Instructional artifacts (e.g., gamified activities, scenario scripts, digital games)
- Performance-based task designs (e.g., simulated client interactions, charades, escape rooms)
- Rubrics used for evaluating speaking, clinical communication, and scenario-based tasks
- Learning platform analytics (e.g., participation patterns in Quizlet, Kahoot, Quizizz)

These sources allowed the instructional team to monitor engagement, refine pedagogical strategies, and document the iterative development of the OT Spanish sequence.

Instruments

Several pedagogical and assessment instruments supported the instructional design and informed instructor reflections:

- **Speaking and clinical communication rubrics** used to assess simulated patient interactions, oral presentations, and clinical instruction tasks in Spanish.

- **Scenario-based assessment tools**, including the Montreal Cognitive Assessment (MoCA) in Spanish and the Perfil de Juegos e Intereses.
- **Gamified digital platforms**—Quizlet, Kahoot, Quizizz, Pear Deck—used for vocabulary review, concept checks, and immediate feedback.
- **Interactive activities** (e.g., lotería, charades, escape rooms) adapted to reinforce professional terminology, cultural concepts, and communication strategies.

These instruments supported instructional decisions but were not analyzed for student performance outcomes.

Performance Rubric and Oral Assessments

During oral assessment activities, all students were able to introduce themselves and explain their role as occupational therapists appropriately in Spanish. They successfully administered the COSA, conducted follow-up questions with clients, and provided referrals when prompted. Out of the cohort, three students experienced difficulty completing assessments fully independently: one consistently relied on an interpreter, while the other two were able to perform most tasks but struggled with specific sections. These outcomes suggest that foundational oral communication and clinical skills were effectively acquired by the majority of students. Rubrics captured a binary "can/cannot" performance, highlighting areas for refinement in future iterations to allow for more nuanced assessment of proficiency.

Digital Activity Engagement and Completion

Students consistently engaged in gamified in-class activities, achieving full participation in synchronous platforms such as Kahoot, Quizizz, and escape-room challenges. Asynchronous Quizlet assignments showed variable engagement depending on topic difficulty, with completion rates ranging from 88.88% for foundational topics (e.g., Género y Número en español) to 55.55% for more challenging content (e.g., body parts). These data highlight both the effectiveness of structured in-class gamification for sustaining engagement and the need to consider topic complexity when designing asynchronous practice activities.

Procedures

Data were generated during the regular delivery of the OT Spanish courses between January 2024 and December 2024. Procedures included:

- Weekly co-planning meetings between the language instructor and OT faculty
- Iterative documentation of instructional decisions, classroom observations, and reflections
- Integration of gamified and scenario-based learning activities across approximately 45 instructional hours per course
- Use of rubrics and pedagogical tools to guide facilitation and provide structured feedback during simulations
- Ongoing monitoring of engagement patterns through digital learning platforms

These procedures supported the development of a comprehensive understanding of how gamification and CRP interacted to enhance student learning and professional readiness.

Data Analysis

A qualitative, thematic analysis guided the interpretation of instructor observations and artifacts. Both instructors reviewed notes and materials independently to identify recurring themes related to:

1. The effectiveness of gamification in supporting language acquisition
2. The development of cultural competence and clinical communication
3. Student engagement across digital and in-person activities
4. Challenges and successes in interdisciplinary collaboration
5. The alignment between classroom activities and OT professional competencies

Themes were refined through collaborative discussion, ensuring triangulation and coherence across data sources. The goal of analysis was to understand pedagogical dynamics rather than to evaluate student outcomes.

Ethical Considerations

This chapter represents a reflective pedagogical inquiry focused on instructional design, implementation, and instructor learning. No identifiable student data were collected or analyzed. While students in the program were covered under a broader IRB protocol supporting course-based research activities, the present analysis was deemed non–human subjects research because it examines instructor reflections, pedagogical decisions, and curriculum development rather than individual student performance. All examples remain generalized to protect student privacy and align with institutional ethical guidelines.

METHODOLOGICAL RATIONALE

This chapter emphasizes instructor observations and reflections as the primary source of data to provide a rich, contextualized understanding of course design and implementation. By focusing on the instructors' perspectives, the chapter captures the nuanced decision-making, real-time adjustments, and strategic integrations of gamification and CRP that shaped student learning outcomes. This approach allows for a detailed exploration of the interplay between pedagogy, professional preparation, and cultural responsiveness. This interplay is often challenging to capture solely through student assessments or self-reports. Furthermore, privileging instructors' observations highlights the iterative, reflective practices essential to interdisciplinary collaboration, offering insights that can guide other educators seeking to replicate or adapt similar pedagogical innovations in healthcare programs.

Special attention is given to the intersection of gamification as a teaching strategy and the implementation of CRP, highlighting how these approaches together advance meaningful learning in healthcare education programs. In the context of a border university serving bilingual communities, this methodological perspective ensures that both linguistic and cultural dimensions of student learning are foregrounded, providing a comprehensive framework for understanding how educational strategies translate into professional readiness and culturally responsive practices.

COURSE DESIGN AND IMPLEMENTATION

The course design seamlessly integrated Spanish language development with cultural competency training to strengthen both classroom learning and professional preparation for occupational therapy (OT) practice. Drawing on principles of Culturally Responsive Pedagogy (Gay, 2018; Ladson-Billings, 1995) and experiential learning, the design emphasized how cultural responsiveness and community service were embedded within every instructional element. Gamification strategies were consistently implemented during class sessions as an intentional pedagogical tool to foster student engagement, motivation, and mastery of targeted objectives.

Throughout both courses, students engaged in a wide variety of simulated scenarios, where they practiced applying the targeted vocabulary introduced in each lesson. These scenarios were designed to mimic authentic clinical interactions, ranging from basic introductions and information gathering to more complex exchanges involving culturally informed discussions of health beliefs and practices. Role-plays, peer-to-peer dialogues, and instructor-facilitated simulations provided iterative opportunities for students to apply Spanish in meaningful contexts, thereby developing their communicative confidence. Gamification elements—such as competitive team-based activities, interactive quizzes, and digital games using platforms like Kahoot, Quizlet, and Pear Deck—were consistently integrated into these scenario-based practices. This integration allowed students to review vocabulary, test comprehension, and reinforce linguistic accuracy in a dynamic and supportive environment.

In the second course, scenario-based practice expanded to include direct engagement with OT-specific assessments and interventions. Students were introduced to the *Montreal Cognitive Assessment (MOCA)* and the *Perfil de Juegos e Intereses*, among other instruments, and practiced administering them in Spanish. These activities required students not only to use precise professional vocabulary but also to employ culturally appropriate nonverbal strategies and empathetic communication techniques. For example, students learned to provide patient instructions in Spanish, adapt questioning styles to maintain cultural sensitivity, and interpret patient responses within the linguistic and cultural context of Spanish-speaking clients. The gamified approaches continued to support these complex activities by scaffolding students' acquisition of specialized terminology and reinforcing accurate application of clinical procedures through repetition, feedback, and collaborative problem-solving.

The collaborative teaching model between the language instructor and the OT faculty member was central to the success of this design. Weekly planning meetings ensured the alignment of language objectives with OT competencies, allowing for the ongoing refinement of gamified strategies and scenario designs. Both instructors worked in tandem during class sessions to provide immediate feedback, guide student reflection, and model the integration of linguistic, cultural, and professional knowledge. Assessment was multidimensional, encompassing performance-based evaluations such as simulated patient interactions, oral presentations, and the creation of Spanish-language OT resources (e.g., simplified home program instructions). These assessments were designed not only to measure proficiency but also to reflect the realities of professional practice in borderland communities.

Notably, the design acknowledged that developing Spanish proficiency in isolation from cultural competence would be insufficient for effective occupational therapy practice. By embedding gamification, culturally responsive strategies, and clinically relevant scenarios across both courses, the instructional team created a sustainable, replicable model for preparing students to provide equitable and empathetic care. This design ensured that students were not merely acquiring vocabulary or grammar, but actively cultivating the communicative flexibility, cultural humility, and professional readiness necessary to meet the needs of Spanish-speaking clients in diverse healthcare settings.

GAMIFICATION STRATEGIES

Varied gamification strategies were intentionally embedded across both OT Spanish courses to sustain student engagement, foster motivation, and strengthen the integration of linguistic and cultural learning objectives. Drawing on principles of game design and experiential learning, gamification was not treated as an add-on activity, but rather as a consistent instructional framework designed to maintain the learning momentum throughout each session. By leveraging elements such as competition, collaboration, recognition, and immediate feedback, instructors aimed to create a classroom environment that fostered active participation, supported language retention, and simulated the dynamic problem-solving required in professional practice.

As noted above, the courses incorporated widely used digital game-based learning platforms, including Kahoot, Quizlet, Quizizz, and PearDeck. These platforms were chosen not only for their interactivity but also for their ability to provide immediate feedback, allow instructors to track student progress in real time, and highlight individual and group achievements. In this way, gamification provided students with a visible sense of accomplishment while offering instructors valuable data to adjust their instruction. Beyond vocabulary drills or grammar checks, these platforms were also adapted to embed OT-specific content, ensuring that each interactive exercise reinforced professional terminology, cultural concepts, and communication strategies relevant to clinical practice.

At the same time, the courses extended gamification beyond digital platforms to include interactive, socially oriented activities that emphasized cultural connection and peer learning. Students participated in narrative-building games, lotería, bingo, charades, and multiple escape-room style challenges. These activities were strategically linked to lesson objectives and targeted vocabulary, while also cultivating teamwork, creativity, and problem-solving. For example, lotería was adapted to reinforce medical and anatomical terms. At the same time, escape rooms required students to decode clinical instructions in Spanish or solve culturally relevant case scenarios to "unlock" the next stage. These activities not only reinforced language acquisition but also gave students opportunities to practice interpersonal and social skills essential to client interactions.

In the second course, gamified activities were increasingly tied to occupational therapy assessments such as the *Montreal Cognitive Assessment (MOCA)* and the *Perfil de Juegos e Intereses*. The latter, in particular, offered students the opportunity to engage in charades as part of practicing how to assess interests and play behaviors. This activity quickly became a favorite among students, as it combined humor, movement, and creativity with professional vocabulary practice. Through charades, students deepened their understanding of culturally relevant play while simultaneously practicing clinical instructions and observational skills in Spanish. These kinds of interactive scenarios underscore how gamification could align with the authentic demands of OT practice while maintaining a fun and supportive classroom environment.

Ultimately, the integration of gamification strategies contributed to the creation of a safe, collaborative classroom culture where students could experiment, make mistakes, and grow. The balance of digital platforms, culturally familiar games, and problem-solving challenges reinforced both language acquisition and clinical readiness. By framing learning as an interactive and socially meaningful process, gamification served as a central strategy for helping students develop the confidence, empathy, and cultural competence required for occupational therapy practice in Spanish-speaking communities.

ANALYSIS AND RESULTS

Through collaborative observations and reflective discussions, the instructors combined their disciplinary expertise to evaluate how students engaged with the integration of Spanish language learning into occupational therapy practice. This approach allowed the teaching team to identify patterns of participation, assess cultural responsiveness, and refine instructional methods. Educators noted that the integration of gamification, scenario-based learning, and culturally grounded role-play consistently enhanced students' engagement, language development, and professional preparation.

One of the most telling observations was the students' decision to conclude the semester with creative projects that replicated the very strategies employed in the classroom. By designing games and interactive presentations, students demonstrated not only knowledge of course content but also an appreciation for how learning was structured. In year two, students even adopted one of the same platforms used during instruction to design their own group activity, stepping into the role of facilitators. They modeled supportive expressions, gestures of encouragement, and celebratory practices that reflected the classroom ethos. This mirrored enactment of pedagogical practices highlighted the success of the safe, caring learning space that the instructors had purposefully fostered.

Between the first and second year of implementation, several changes were made to improve the program's impact. Initially, students of mixed proficiency levels were separated into groups to ensure equitable participation. Later, instructors shifted their focus to fine-tuning the sequencing of OT assessments, placing greater emphasis on the timing and scaffolding of challenging tasks. Despite these shifts, certain principles remained constant: gamification and scenario-based learning were at the heart of the courses. Speed-dating style activities, escape rooms, and simulations were consistently integrated, designed to give students opportunities to engage in short but meaningful client interactions. Importantly, all scenarios incorporated cultural elements that reflected the realities of living and practicing occupational therapy on the U.S.–Mexico border. This emphasis reinforced students' cultural competence while preparing them for the types of encounters they would face in practice.

Educators observed several positive patterns of student behavior across both years. Students grew increasingly confident in positioning themselves as occupational therapists communicating in Spanish. They supported one another in developing translations, improving pronunciation, and finding natural expressions, thereby creating a peer-driven safe space for collective learning. Even less advanced speakers felt comfortable asking for clarification, a testament to the course's supportive climate. Students frequently expressed the importance of practicing beyond the classroom to ensure readiness for clinical encounters. Alumni accounts reinforced this finding: during residencies, former students reported being the only Spanish speakers on their teams, often responsible for interpreting for colleagues and directly serving Spanish-speaking clients. These testimonies emphasized the lasting professional impact of the course's instructional design.

When evaluating OT-specific assessments, instructors noted apparent differences in student ease and confidence. The AOTA Occupational Profile and MOCA were the least challenging because students had already mastered them in English, allowing for easier transfer of skills. The course also introduced the Mexican MOCA version, which was particularly relevant for a borderlands population, further underscoring the importance of cultural responsiveness in clinical practice. By contrast, assessments such as the COSA, OSA, and OPHI-II were more challenging because they had not been thoroughly covered in English before being introduced in Spanish. Students required additional support, but were still able to demonstrate competency. Observations confirmed García and García's (2020) assertion that treating culture as a strength—rather than a deficit—empowers students and shifts perspectives on language and diversity in professional contexts.

Rubric and Oral Assessment Evidence

Rubric-based oral assessments provided additional insight into student performance. During these assessments, all students were able to introduce themselves and explain their role as occupational therapists in Spanish, successfully administering the COSA, conducting follow-up client questions, and providing referrals. Three students required additional support: one consistently relied on an interpreter, while the other two managed most tasks independently but struggled with select sections. These findings illustrate that foundational communication and clinical skills were largely achieved, though rubrics may need refinement to capture more nuanced levels of proficiency in future iterations.

Digital Activity Completion and Engagement

Engagement with digital activities demonstrated variable patterns. Synchronous gamified activities, such as Kahoot, Quizizz, and in-class escape rooms, achieved 100% participation, reflecting high levels of motivation and active engagement. Asynchronous Quizlet assignments showed topic-dependent completion rates, ranging from 88.88% for foundational topics (e.g., *Género y Número en español*) to 55.55% for more challenging content (e.g., body parts). These patterns highlight the effectiveness of structured in-class gamification for sustaining engagement and suggest areas for additional support when implementing asynchronous practice tasks.

Together, the rubric results, completion data, and instructor observations triangulate evidence of student learning, supporting gains in accuracy, fluency, and culturally responsive communication. This complements narrative reflections and provides systematic support for the instructional strategies used.

A central focus of instructor reflection centered on the differential impact of gamification tools. Each platform served a distinct pedagogical purpose and prompted different student behaviors:

- Quizlet was primarily used asynchronously for vocabulary review and memorization. It functioned as a low-stakes tool for individual practice, allowing students to rehearse terminology at their own pace. However, instructors observed that not all students consistently completed these assignments in the LMS, revealing the challenges of sustaining accountability in asynchronous learning.
- Kahoot was used synchronously to review key concepts in an energetic, competitive format. These sessions energized students, turning otherwise routine content checks into moments of enthusiasm and shared enjoyment. Kahoot was particularly effective for quick recall and reinforcing short-term memory.
- Quizizz, also used synchronously, provided similar engagement but with more emphasis on tracking individual progress. Instructors appreciated its ability to provide immediate feedback, which helped students self-monitor their comprehension while still participating in a collective experience.
- Escape rooms were designed to test problem-solving, teamwork, and clinical reasoning under pressure. These activities simulated the fast-paced, unpredictable environments that occupational therapists often face. Students embraced the challenge, demonstrating collaboration and perseverance as they navigated scenarios that required both language use and clinical judgment.

- Speed-dating activities offered repeated opportunities for short, meaningful client interactions. By rotating roles quickly, students practiced essential skills of active listening, empathy, and adaptability, mirroring the fragmented but impactful conversations they might have with clients in real practice settings.

Together, these gamified activities illustrated how intentional instructional design could elicit both cognitive and affective engagement. Observations consistently showed that asynchronous gamification tools were less universally completed, while face-to-face activities were embraced with enthusiasm. This aligns with Figueroa Flores's (2015) argument that technology in language learning is no longer merely essential but increasingly intentional when used to shape motivation, competitiveness, and collaboration. Instructors concluded that by gamifying the OT Spanish learning experience, they not only leveraged students' competitive spirit but also empowered them to take ownership of their learning.

The following table compiles information about activities, outcomes, and assessments that were aligned.

Table 1. Activity–Outcome–Assessment Alignment Table

Activity	Primary Learning Outcomes	Assessment Focus / Evidence of Learning
Quizlet (asynchronous vocabulary practice)	- Build and reinforce domain-specific vocabulary- Develop independent study habits	- Completion of sets (LMS tracking)- Accuracy in matching/recall- Growth in vocabulary quizzes or in-class usage
Kahoot (synchronous concept review)	- Strengthen rapid recall of key terms and concepts- Encourage engagement and motivation	- Live quiz scores- Accuracy and speed of responses- Participation level during synchronous sessions
Quizizz (synchronous with progress tracking)	- Monitor understanding of concepts in real time- Support self-assessment and awareness of learning gaps	- Individual performance reports- Immediate feedback patterns (e.g., repeated errors)- Comparative group data to identify class trends
Escape Rooms (problem-solving + teamwork)	- Apply clinical reasoning in simulated scenarios- Demonstrate teamwork and communication- Use language functionally under time pressure	- Completion of tasks/puzzles- Observation of teamwork and communication behaviors- Accuracy and appropriateness of clinical decisions made during the scenarios
Speed-Dating (client interaction practice)	- Practice active listening and interviewing skills- Demonstrate empathy and adaptability- Build fluency and confidence in short, purposeful exchanges	- Instructor observation checklists- Quality of questions and responses- Reflective notes or debriefs on communication strategies used

Finally, gamified experiences also created space for extended dialogue. Activities often served as springboards for deeper discussion of course content, allowing students and educators to co-construct knowledge in meaningful and efficient ways. Whether rehearsing vocabulary through Quizlet or solving an escape room puzzle, students were consistently asked to reflect on their choices, explain their reasoning, and connect their actions to broader clinical competencies. This dual focus on engagement and reflection ultimately prepared students not only to function bilingually but also to embody the cultural humility and adaptability essential for occupational therapy practice in the U.S.–Mexico border region.

CONTRIBUTIONS

Learning a new language is often a daunting experience, especially for those just beginning. Traditional approaches, such as rote memorization or repetitive drills, can feel disconnected from real-world clinical applications and offer little in the way of transferable skills. In contrast, gamification introduces a sense of play that shifts the tone of learning, energizes participation, and ultimately facilitates language development. By making the classroom a safe yet dynamic space, gamified strategies not only reduce the stress associated with language learning but also mirror the collaborative and problem-solving demands students will face as future healthcare providers. This foundation sets the stage for understanding how pedagogical contributions in this project—particularly the use of games, simulations, and interactive tools—directly supported students' confidence and cultural responsiveness.

This interdisciplinary collaboration contributes to the field of healthcare education in several significant ways. The partnership illustrates how community-centered pedagogy can be effectively implemented when instructors prioritize the needs of local populations. By ensuring that students can navigate both the linguistic and cultural dimensions of their practice contexts, this work contributes a replicable model for embedding essential competencies into professional healthcare curricula. This reality underscores the critical importance of preparing occupational therapy students to communicate effectively with diverse populations, particularly in border communities where multilingual competence and cultural responsiveness are essential for therapeutic success.

The collaborative approach further contributes methodological innovations for developing transferable critical consciousness in students. Both educators consistently emphasized connecting classroom learning to professional practice, offering evidence that intentional pedagogical design can bridge academic and clinical contexts. the integration of Spanish language instruction with culturally relevant practices specific to the U.S.-Mexico border community provides a framework for other programs serving similar populations.

In short, this section integrates highlights across three interrelated areas: (1) Pedagogical contributions, (2) disciplinary contributions to OT and healthcare, and (3) cultural contributions for the field of bilingual and borderland education.

PEDAGOGICAL CONTRIBUTIONS

This project advances the use of gamification and scenario-based learning in professional Spanish courses well beyond conventional language acquisition. By embedding occupational therapy content into language instruction, gamification moved beyond "playful" learning and became a structured mechanism for replicating authentic, contextual challenges students will face in practice. Activities such as escape rooms, speed-dating simulations, and interactive assessments allowed students to engage in rehearsed yet meaningful conversations with "clients," strengthening both linguistic skills and clinical confidence. These classroom experiences created a safe space for students to take risks, make mistakes, and receive immediate feedback, preparing them to assist Spanish-speaking clients in real-world settings better.

The pedagogical design evolved over time. From Year 1 to Year 2, adjustments were made to maximize student learning: initial efforts focused on keeping mixed language levels, while later iterations emphasized strategically adjusting the timing of teaching OT assessments. At all stages, gamification and scenario-based learning remained consistent anchors. Students repeatedly participated in short, structured activities—such as speed-dating games—that assured they could practice brief yet meaningful conversations with their clients. These interactions built not only fluency but also a professional disposition toward clear, empathetic communication.

The utilization of computer-based quizzes, such as Kahoot and Quizizz, makes the activity feel less like a test and more like a challenge, allowing students to be more willing to take risks in practicing their Spanish. The low-stakes but fast-paced environment encourages engagement by experimenting with vocabulary, producing grammatical structures under time pressure, and overcoming a fear of failure when uncertain about their answers. Similar to technology-based solo and team games, low technology games, such as telephone, puzzles, role playing, modeling, challenges, etc., foster collaboration through peer teaching, where stronger Spanish speakers model for others, and less confident students contribute to group strategy.

As future occupational therapists, students also benefited from the constant development of rapid thinking and cognitive flexibility—skills that directly translate to clinical encounters. Gamifying Spanish language learning provided a structured space for practicing these abilities, simulating the process of gathering and interpreting client responses, adapting interventions, and building rapport in real time. Students were required to listen to a Spanish prompt, interpret its meaning, and select or generate a response within seconds. Timed games replicated the cognitive demands of healthcare practice and the professional use of language, challenging students to respond accurately under pressure. While students often struggled initially—even native Spanish speakers—with technical and professional terminology, repeated practice increased both confidence and speed, equipping them with the mental agility necessary for real-world clinical interactions.

The patterns of collaboration, confidence-building, and peer support that consistently emerged from student participation provide a replicable model for other health professions curricula. Gamification did not simply increase engagement; it cultivated a learning culture in which students supported one another's progress, worked collectively toward problem-solving, and embraced linguistic and professional challenges with enthusiasm. Azzouz et al. (2020) emphasize that gamification "creates dynamic environments in which people can feel the sense of progress by achieving levels" (p. 59), which was directly evidenced in the progression of student interactions throughout the courses.

These findings suggest that health education programs outside of occupational therapy can purposefully integrate gamified strategies to promote similar outcomes. The use of synchronous, instructor-led gamified tools such as Kahoot and Quizizz encouraged collaboration, classroom management, and immediate feedback, while asynchronous platforms like Quizlet allowed for reinforcement and individualized practice. Together, these modes provided a balanced approach to student learning that may inform curricular design across disciplines. Most significantly, gamification and scenario-based learning cultivated an environment in which cultural responsiveness and language acquisition were not taught as isolated competencies, but as interdependent skills essential for professional practice.

HEALTHCARE/OT CONTRIBUTIONS

This work contributes to occupational therapy and healthcare education by demonstrating how motivational techniques traditionally associated with language instruction, such as gamification, can enhance professional readiness across clinical disciplines. Strategizing the integration of gamified approaches allowed occupational therapy students not only to strengthen their Spanish proficiency, but also to engage in repeated practice with discipline-specific content. By reviewing OT assessments in both English and Spanish, students developed a dual competency that enriched their preparedness for working with Spanish-speaking clients. These bilingual practice opportunities translated into greater confidence when interacting with standardized patients, underscoring the critical role of linguistic training in clinical education.

Breaking linguistic barriers is not only a matter of communication but also of patient safety and satisfaction. Al Shamsi et al. (2020) argue that language barriers have negative impacts on quality of care and safety; the findings in this program affirm that intentional language and cultural preparation mitigate those risks. When students practiced assessments in bilingual formats, they reported feeling more capable of explaining procedures, addressing patient concerns, and adapting tone and word choice in culturally responsive ways. This, in turn, directly supports safe and ethical care, reducing misunderstandings that could compromise therapeutic outcomes.

The integration of gamification within occupational therapy Spanish courses also emphasizes a broader healthcare contribution: motivating students through interactive learning strengthens their engagement with material that might otherwise feel intimidating or overwhelming. Rather than perceiving Spanish as an "additional burden," students came to view bilingualism and cultural competence as professional assets directly linked to their clinical effectiveness.

One of the most valuable aspects of gamification is its ability to embed clinically relevant Spanish directly into teaching materials in ways that mirror real-world practice. Within this project, OTD students consistently engaged with Spanish terminology tied to occupational therapy evaluations, standardized assessments, and interventions. For example, case scenario challenges incorporated items from tools such as the occupational self-assessment or the pediatric interest checklist, requiring students to interpret Spanish-language prompts about performance and satisfaction. In team-based activities, students role-played administering sections of the *Montreal Cognitive Assessment (MOCA)* in Spanish, which allowed them to rehearse not only the standardized instructions but also culturally appropriate clarifications delivered in clear, accessible Spanish.

Gamification supports the transfer of these language skills to clinical settings by emphasizing adaptability, responsiveness, and contextual learning. By embedding Spanish into technology-based and team-oriented games, students experienced simulated real-world pressures in a safe, low-stakes environment, allowing them to practice until their responses became more fluid and automatic. Grounding these activities in the verbiage of occupational therapy evaluations, standardized assessments, and interventions helped students envision themselves as bilingual practitioners, recognizing that Spanish proficiency is not just a classroom exercise but a professional competency essential for providing equitable and effective care. In the borderland context, gamification transformed the classroom into an active, engaging space where risk-taking, rapid thinking, and collaboration were encouraged. Through both digital and low-tech strategies, students practiced consuming and producing

Spanish across multiple modalities—spoken, written, and perceived—mirroring the demands of real clinical encounters while simultaneously building confidence, cultural responsiveness, and professional readiness.

By merging language practice with discipline-specific tasks, gamification provided students with opportunities to acquire Spanish while simultaneously refining their clinical competence. The immediate relevance of these activities helped students see the direct application of their language skills in therapeutic contexts, bridging the gap between classroom learning and patient care. Just as importantly, these experiences fostered confidence: students were not only recalling Spanish vocabulary, but also applying it in authentic, practice-based scenarios that prepared them for future interactions with patients and families in border communities.

In this way, the present project offers a replicable model for healthcare programs seeking to embed motivational, language-integrated strategies into their curricula. It demonstrates that professional competencies such as empathy, adaptability, and communication can be cultivated through pedagogical innovation, ultimately improving care in linguistically diverse communities. By linking bilingual preparation to the ethical imperatives of patient safety and therapeutic trust, the collaboration advances healthcare education in ways that are both practically relevant and socially necessary.

CULTURAL CONTRIBUTIONS

This project makes substantial contributions to the cultural dimension of healthcare and higher education by centering the lived experiences of students and communities along the U.S.–Mexico border. By intentionally embedding culturally relevant practices into the curriculum, the collaboration demonstrates how language education and occupational therapy training can function as vehicles for cultural preservation, recognition, and responsiveness. Rather than treating culture as an "add-on" to clinical practice, the design of these courses positioned cultural knowledge as an indispensable part of professional competence.

One of the most significant contributions lies in how scenarios, role-plays, and simulations were rooted in the everyday realities of border communities. Activities such as speed-dating, role plays, and escape room simulations consistently integrate details drawn from regional contexts—ranging from local customs of address and greeting to complex cultural traditions such as Día de los Muertos. This design created space for students to engage deeply with the cultural practices of the populations they will eventually serve, while also fostering respect and empathy for diverse worldviews. Such practices advance the argument that cultural responsiveness in healthcare education should not remain abstract but should be concretely modeled within classroom activities.

Moreover, this work contributes to the literature by showing how culturally responsive pedagogy can be adapted for professional training. Jaramillo's (1996) recognition of the cultural significance of courtesy forms like tú and usted illustrates how even seemingly minor linguistic distinctions carry weight in client–patient interactions. By scaffolding cultural learning from these foundational conventions toward advanced projects exploring broader themes (e.g., traditions of mourning and healing, cross-border family dynamics), the program offered students a developmental pathway for cultural competence. In this way, the curriculum not only prepared students linguistically but also helped them navigate the unspoken cultural frameworks that shape therapeutic encounters.

Finally, the cultural contributions of this collaboration extend beyond individual students. By privileging the cultural realities of a historically underserved region, the project models how higher education institutions can fulfill their social responsibility to surrounding communities. It demonstrates that preparing healthcare professionals is inseparable from preparing culturally aware citizens capable of working across differences. In borderlands where identities, languages, and healthcare practices overlap, such preparation is both ethically necessary and socially transformative.

Taken together, the pedagogical, healthcare, and cultural contributions of this collaboration highlight the transformative potential of interdisciplinary and community-centered approaches to professional education. By embedding occupational therapy content into Spanish language instruction through gamification, simulations, and culturally grounded activities, the project cultivated not only linguistic competence but also the critical empathy, adaptability, and confidence required of future healthcare professionals. These outcomes reinforce the idea that cultural and linguistic preparation are not peripheral skills but core competencies for safe and effective practice, particularly in borderland and multilingual contexts. Most importantly, this work offers a replicable model for institutions seeking to prepare students who are both professionally capable and socially responsive graduates who can navigate complex cultural landscapes while delivering equitable, high-quality care to diverse communities.

SOLUTIONS AND RECOMMENDATIONS

Building on the lessons from this interdisciplinary collaboration, several actionable recommendations emerge for educators seeking to integrate language learning, cultural responsiveness, and healthcare content in professional programs. These recommendations are organized across three interrelated pillars: pedagogical, healthcare/

occupational therapy, and cultural. The guidance emphasizes high-impact, replicable strategies that prioritize safe spaces, community building, and inclusive practices while remaining adaptable to evolving technologies and instructional platforms.

Pedagogical Recommendations

To foster effective language acquisition and professional readiness, educators should intentionally integrate gamified and scenario-based strategies that encourage active, participatory learning. While specific digital platforms continue to evolve, the guiding principle remains consistent: create interactive, engaging experiences that allow students to practice language in authentic contexts. Opportunities for rapid thinking, collaborative problem-solving, and repeated rehearsal of professional communication should be embedded across the curriculum. Incorporating inclusive practices, such as creating safe spaces, supporting multiple language preferences, and encouraging peer mentoring, further enhances the learning environment. High Impact Practices—including collaborative projects, simulations, and reflective exercises—should be intentionally designed to reinforce linguistic, cognitive, and professional competencies. These strategies not only promote skill development but also build confidence and motivation, preparing students to navigate complex professional interactions with ease and empathy.

Healthcare/Occupational Therapy Recommendations

In healthcare education, integrating language learning with discipline-specific content strengthens clinical readiness and ensures that students can provide safe, culturally responsive care. Educators should prioritize opportunities for bilingual practice that align with real-world assessments, interventions, and client interactions. Gamified activities and simulations offer low-stakes environments for students to rehearse professional decision-making, communicate effectively under pressure, and internalize culturally appropriate practices. Inclusive approaches, emphasizing patient-centered care, respect for linguistic preferences, and collaborative engagement, reinforce the ethical and practical dimensions of professional competence. By grounding learning in both language and clinical application, programs can enhance student confidence, foster critical thinking, and equip future healthcare professionals to meet the diverse needs of the communities they serve.

Cultural Recommendations

Culturally responsive pedagogy must remain central to preparing students for practice in diverse and borderland communities. Learning activities should reflect the lived experiences, customs, and values of the populations students will serve, fostering empathy, respect, and ethical awareness. Role-plays, simulations, and interactive projects should incorporate cultural details while maintaining safe and supportive spaces where students feel empowered to take risks and experiment with language and behavior. Emphasizing inclusive practices—such as using students' preferred languages, promoting collaboration, and modeling respect for difference—supports the ongoing development of cultural competence. Ultimately, embedding cultural awareness throughout curricular design ensures that graduates are prepared not only to communicate effectively but also to provide care that is socially responsive, equitable, and ethically grounded.

In conclusion, the integration of gamification, scenario-based learning, and culturally responsive practices creates an educational ecosystem that develops confident, competent, and culturally aware healthcare professionals. Programs seeking to replicate this model should prioritize inclusive, high-impact approaches that balance linguistic development, clinical readiness, and cultural competence. By centering safe spaces, community building, and real-world applicability, educators can equip students to navigate professional challenges and provide equitable, high-quality care to diverse populations.

FUTURE RESEARCH DIRECTIONS

By writing this chapter, we aim to first of all contribute to the conversation of how gamified experiences in our language classroom can continue building classrooms that are culturally responsive to the needs of our students. However, equally important, we are writing this chapter as an invitation to other educators to start working on their intradisciplinary projects. We want to propose for this model to be replicated or modeled in other courses where healthcare providers are been trained. As discussed in this chapter, the linguistic barriers that many underserved populations are currently facing are devastating, and therefore, creating programs and courses that can mitigate these disparities significantly is an invaluable investment in our communities.

Specifically, for our program, our research is barely starting. We are fully committed to supporting our students' success. Consequently, we will further continue our research by investigating future cohorts, continue revising and re-visiting our curricula, and explore more deeply the observed results; it will also be relevant to explore in detail the direct perceptions and performance of the students enrolled in the program. Other research possibilities include exploring the interplay between classroom-based cultural competency development and actual clinical practice outcomes, tracking how students' language and cultural skills translate into improved patient care and therapeutic relationships.

Equally important, it is essential to explore the extensive possibilities that gamification can bring, specifically to healthcare settings across a much broader range of fields and specializations. This exploration requires finding common points and strategies that are relatable and transferable to all healthcare settings, regardless of specialty or patient population, while simultaneously identifying other approaches that can deepen and enrich the conversation in contexts that are very specific to particular healthcare disciplines or cultural communities.

The broader applicability of gamified, culturally responsive pedagogy holds tremendous potential for transforming healthcare education across pharmacy, physical therapy, speech-language pathology, social work, nursing, and other allied health professions. Finding these universal elements—such as empathy development, communication skills enhancement, and cultural consciousness building—will allow for the creation of foundational frameworks that can be adapted and implemented across diverse healthcare educational programs.

At the same time, it is equally crucial to explore the specific nuances and particular needs that characterize very distinct healthcare contexts. For instance, the gamification strategies that work effectively for occupational therapy students in border communities may require significant adaptation when applied to nursing students in urban settings, or physical therapy students working with pediatric populations. These context-specific explorations can deepen our understanding of how culturally responsive gamification must be tailored to address the unique communication challenges, cultural considerations, and professional requirements that define healthcare specialties and the specific communities they serve.

LIMITATIONS

Several limitations should be noted. The study included small cohorts of 20 and 24 students, reflecting a specific borderland occupational therapy program; findings are context-specific and not intended for broad generalization. Student Spanish proficiency levels varied, and exposure to bilingualism in this region may differ from other areas.

Data sources were limited to instructor observations, rubrics, and digital activity completion. The rubrics were intentionally simple ("can do/cannot do") and did not capture finer-grained linguistic or cultural skills, and direct student feedback (surveys or interviews) was not collected for these cohorts. Future iterations will refine assessment tools and integrate student perspectives to provide a fuller understanding of learning outcomes.

Course design was reflective and qualitative, with no control group or baseline measure. While gamification and synchronous activities effectively engaged students, asynchronous assignments showed variable participation due to the pass/fail grading structure. Implementation spanned only two years, limiting insights into long-term effects on clinical performance.

Finally, contextual factors—such as the U.S.–Mexico border environment and student bilingualism—affect transferability, though the model remains adaptable to other healthcare education programs seeking culturally responsive, language-integrated instruction. Despite these constraints, the chapter provides valuable insights into effective pedagogical strategies for preparing occupational therapists to serve Spanish-speaking populations.

CONCLUSION

This chapter advances theoretical understanding of how gamified, culturally responsive pedagogy can prepare healthcare professionals to serve diverse populations effectively, contributing both practical applications and scholarly insights to the growing field of interdisciplinary healthcare education. The present chapter integrates highlights for three specific areas: (1) Pedagogical contributions, (2) disciplinary contributions to OT and healthcare, and (3) cultural contributions to the field of bilingual and borderland education.

The ability to communicate in Spanish is an essential skill along the U.S.–Mexico border, where language often determines the quality of patient care and access to services. In a city like El Paso, where a significant portion of the population identifies as Spanish-speaking, the integration of professional Spanish courses into the Occupational Therapy curriculum is not an added benefit but a necessity. These courses ensure that future healthcare providers are equipped with the linguistic and cultural competencies required to serve their community effectively. By embedding Spanish learning directly into professional preparation, students are not only enhancing their own skills but also contributing to advancing health equity for the region.

Within this framework, gamification offered a meaningful way to deepen student learning and engagement. Gamified strategies allowed students to practice Spanish in authentic, applied, and interactive formats that mirrored the demands of clinical encounters. Activities designed with gamification principles fostered rapid thinking, exposure to Spanish across multiple modalities (spoken, written, and perceived), and the practice of clinically relevant terminology directly tied to occupational therapy evaluations, standardized assessments, and interventions. Beyond language acquisition, gamified learning created opportunities for students to collaborate, build confidence, and rehearse cultural responsiveness in ways that aligned with their professional growth.

Current healthcare disparities underscore the significance of this work. Martinez (2024) highlights that "Latinos are the population segment with the least amount of health insurance coverage and have basic or below health literacy. In other words, they can only perform simple and everyday (basic) literacy activities" (p. 425). Given these disparities, the need for culturally competent healthcare providers is critical. This chapter demonstrates how classroom practices incorporating culturally responsive pedagogy can create safe and equitable learning environments that prepare future Occupational Therapists to serve diverse populations effectively.

The implications extend beyond language learning to professional practice transformation. The use of game design for teaching Spanish to occupational therapy students represents an innovative approach to developing technical communication skills in a flexible manner that emphasizes client-centered care while maintaining the rigor of therapeutic skill development. Gamified practice with standardized assessments and occupation-based tools enhances both receptive and expressive Spanish skills, enabling better communication with Spanish-speaking clients. Ultimately, this work recognizes that language and communication serve as therapeutic media for building relationships and promoting recovery, health, and wellbeing.

In this program, the co-creation of culturally responsive pedagogy in the Spanish classroom strategically emphasized what students, as members of the border community, needed to understand and develop in order to navigate their community successfully, both as individuals and as future healthcare professionals. Rather than imposing external cultural frameworks, the collaborative approach recognized that students possessed valuable cultural knowledge and lived experiences that could enhance their professional preparation. The educators worked to create learning environments where students' border community identity became a professional asset, helping them understand the cultural nuances, linguistic variations, and community values that would inform their future therapeutic relationships.

The Spanish Occupational Therapy courses presented in this chapter represent a direct response to the documented challenges presented here, such as the varied linguistic barriers that remain an issue amongst varied underprivileged populations, positioning future practitioners to bridge the communication gaps that currently limit effective therapeutic relationships between healthcare providers and Spanish-speaking patients.

We close this chapter by echoing the words of Ladson-Billings (2021), who stated:

> *The challenge has been to identify teaching practices that have remained faithful to CRP theory. Thus, teaching that focuses on advancing student learning, developing cultural competence, and fostering critical consciousness is the*

only practice that accurately represents what is meant by Culturally Responsive Pedagogy (p. 351).

This theoretical framework becomes particularly significant when applied to professional healthcare education, where the stakes of effective communication extend far beyond academic success to encompass patient safety, therapeutic outcomes, and equitable care delivery. The creation of language classrooms where students have the capacity to participate to the fullest remains a fundamental responsibility for every language educator, but this responsibility intensifies within healthcare contexts where communication directly impacts human wellbeing.

In healthcare fields, language educators serve as crucial liaisons who contribute to diminishing the barriers that clients and practitioners may encounter in clinical settings. As Al Shamsi et al. (2020) demonstrated, language barriers significantly compromise healthcare quality and patient safety. This reality transforms the role of healthcare language education from an academic exercise to a professional preparation with profound ethical implications.

The interdisciplinary collaboration presented in this chapter demonstrates how gamification and culturally responsive pedagogy can work synergistically to address these challenges. By integrating interactive learning experiences with cultural consciousness development, this approach prepares occupational therapy students not only to communicate in Spanish but to understand the cultural contexts that shape their future clients' health experiences, beliefs, and therapeutic needs.

Therefore, integrating culturally responsive pedagogy with gamified language learning transcends educational innovation to become a professional imperative for preparing healthcare providers who can deliver equitable, effective care to increasingly diverse populations. This work represents a critical step toward addressing persistent healthcare disparities while simultaneously honoring the cultural identities and experiences of both students and the communities they will ultimately serve throughout their careers.

By implementing more holistic models of tailored gamification within culturally responsive frameworks, we position our students—the future generation of healthcare professionals—as transformative leaders in their respective fields. These leaders will possess not only the linguistic competencies necessary to break down the communication barriers currently dividing our communities, but more importantly, they will demonstrate a deep understanding of the cultural norms, values, and nuances that shape their patients' health experiences and therapeutic relationships. Such comprehensive preparation enables practitioners to move beyond surface-level communication to establish meaningful, culturally grounded therapeutic partnerships that honor patients' identities while promoting optimal health outcomes.

Developing this shared understanding of future practitioners' evolving needs requires educators to equip themselves with the most effective, innovative, and inclusive pedagogies available. However, beyond methodological sophistication, this approach demands that we demonstrate through our classroom practices the very principles we hope our students will embody in their professional lives. The safe, inclusive learning spaces we co-construct with our students—where they feel comfortable exploring cultural differences, making linguistic mistakes, and developing cultural consciousness—serve as powerful models for the therapeutic environments they will create for their patients. In essence, our classrooms become laboratories for practicing the cultural responsiveness, empathy, and inclusive care that will define their professional identities and ultimately transform healthcare delivery for linguistically and culturally diverse populations.

REFERENCES

Al Shamsi, H., Al Mashrafi, S., Al Kalbani, T., & Almutairi, A. G. (2020). Implications of Language Barriers for Healthcare: A Systematic Review. *Oman Medical Journal, 35*(2), 1–7. DOI: 10.5001/omj.2020.40

Arnold, B. J. (2014). Gamification in education. *Proceedings of the American Society of Business and Behavioral Sciences, 21*(1), 32–39.

Aulia, P. F. (2025). The effectiveness of gamification in enhancing English language learning outcomes. *Jurnal Pendidikan Dan Sastra Inggris, 5*(2), 304–320. https://journalshub.org/index.php/JUPENSI/article/view/5238/5082

Boudadi, N., & Gutiérrez-Colón, M. (2020). Effect of Gamification on students' motivation and learning achievement in Second Language Acquisition within higher education: A literature review 2011-2019. *The EUROCALL Review, 28*(1), 40–69. DOI: 10.4995/eurocall.2020.12974

Brown-Jeffy, S., & Cooper, J. E. (2011). Toward a Conceptual Framework of Culturally Relevant Pedagogy: An Overview of the Conceptual and Theoretical Literature. *Teacher Education Quarterly (Claremont, Calif.), 38*(1), 65–84.

Dehghanzadeh, H., Fardanesh, H., Hatami, J., Talaee, E., & Noroozi, O. (2021). Using gamification to support learning English as a second language: A systematic review. *Computer Assisted Language Learning, 34*(7), 934–957. DOI: 10.1080/09588221.2019.1648298

Dehghanzadeh, H., Farrokhnia, M., Dehghanzadeh, H., Taghipour, K., & Noroozi, O. (2024). Using gamification to support learning in K-12 education: A systematic literature review. *British Journal of Educational Technology, 55*(1), 34–70. DOI: 10.1111/bjet.13335

Diamond, L. C., & Jacobs, E. A. (2024). Language barriers and health inequity. *AMA Journal of Ethics, 26*(1), E1–E8. https://journalofethics.ama-assn.org/article/how-should-clinicians-respond-language-barriers-exacerbate-health-inequity/2021-02

Douglas, D. (2000). *Assessing languages for specific purposes*. Cambridge University Press.

Douglas, D. (2001). Language for Specific Purposes assessment criteria: Where do they come from? *Language Testing, 18*(2), 171–185. DOI: 10.1177/026553220101800204

Figueroa Flores, J. F. (2015). Using Gamification to Enhance Second Language Learning. *Digital Education Review, 27*, 32–54. DOI: 10.1344/der.2015.27.32-54

Flores, G. (2006). Language Barriers to Health Care in the United States. *The New England Journal of Medicine*, *355*(3), 229–231. DOI: 10.1056/NEJMp058316

Garcia, C., & Garcia, R. (2021). Developing cultural competence in an occupational therapy program in a border institution in South Texas. In Sellers, M. D. S., & Johnson, M. E. (Eds.), *Cultural Competence in Applied Psychology* (pp. 138–157). IGI Global., https://scholarworks.utrgv.edu/context/tl_fac/article/1086/viewcontent/145841.pdf

Gay, G. (2018). *Culturally responsive teaching: theory, research, and practice*. Teachers College Press.

Hamp-Lyons, L., & Lumley, T. (2001). Assessing language for specific purposes. *Language Testing*, *18*(2), 127–132. DOI: 10.1177/026553220101800201

Ho-Minh, T., & Suppasetseree, S. (2025). Enhancing Vietnamese EFL Students' Speaking Skills Through Augmented Reality: A Mixed-Method Study in English for Tourism and Hospitality. *Education Process: International Journal*, *15*(1). Advance online publication. DOI: 10.22521/edupij.2025.15.139

Ishaq, K., Mat Zin, N. A., Rosdi, F., Jehanghir, M., Ishaq, S., & Abid, A. (2021). Mobile-assisted and gamification-based language learning: A systematic literature review. *PeerJ. Computer Science*, *7*, e496. Advance online publication. DOI: 10.7717/peerj-cs.496

Jackson, G. T., & McNamara, D. S. (2013). Motivation and Performance in a Game-Based Intelligent Tutoring System. *Journal of Educational Psychology*, *105*(4), 1036–1049. DOI: 10.1037/a0032580

Jacobs, E., Chen, A. H., Karliner, L. S., Agger-Gupta, N. I. E. L. S., & Mutha, S. (2006). The need for more research on language barriers in health care: A proposed research agenda. *The Milbank Quarterly*, *84*(1), 111–133. DOI: 10.1111/j.1468-0009.2006.00440.x

Jaramillo, J. A. (1996). Tu and usted: Address etiquette in the Mexican American family. *Hispanic Journal of Behavioral Sciences*, *18*(4), 522–532. DOI: 10.1177/07399863960184006

Ladson-Billings, G. (1995). Toward a theory of culturally relevant pedagogy. *American Educational Research Journal*, *32*(3), 465–491. DOI: 10.3102/00028312032003465

Ladson-Billings, G. (2014). Culturally relevant pedagogy 2.0: Aka the remix. *Harvard Educational Review*, *84*(1), 74–84. DOI: 10.17763/haer.84.1.p2rj131485484751

Ladson-Billings, G. (2021). Three decades of culturally relevant, responsive, & sustaining pedagogy: What lies ahead? In *The educational forum* (Vol. 85, No. 4, pp. 351-354). Routledge. https://doi.org/DOI: 10.1080/00131725.2021.1957632

Long, M. K. & International Symposium on Languages for Specific Purposes. (2017). *Language for specific purposes : trends in curriculum development* (M. K. Long, Ed.). Georgetown University Press.

Martinez, S. (2024). 21 Hispanics: Richness in Diversity. *Cultural Sensitivity and Responsiveness in Neurorehabilitation: A Personalized Approach for Speech-Language Pathologists, 1*, 419.

Meuter, R. F., Gallois, C., Segalowitz, N. S., Ryder, A. G., & Hocking, J. (2015). Overcoming language barriers in healthcare: A protocol for investigating safe and effective communication when patients or clinicians use a second language. *BMC Health Services Research, 15*(1), 371. DOI: 10.1186/s12913-015-1024-8

O'Sullivan, B. (2012). Assessment issues in languages for specific purposes. *Modern Language Journal, 96*(s1), 71–88. DOI: 10.1111/j.1540-4781.2012.01298.x

Prathyusha, N. (2020). Role of gamification in language learning. [IJRAR]. *International Journal of Research and Analytical Reviews, 7*(2), 577–583.

Schouten, B. C., Cox, A., Duran, G., Kerremans, K., Banning, L. K., Lahdidioui, A., van den Muijsenbergh, M., Schinkel, S., Sungur, H., Suurmond, J., Zendedel, R., & Krystallidou, D. (2020). Mitigating language and cultural barriers in healthcare communication: Toward a holistic approach. *Patient Education and Counseling, 103*(12), 2604–2608. DOI: 10.1016/j.pec.2020.05.001

Showstack, R. (2019). Patients don't have language barriers; the healthcare system does. *Emergency Medicine Journal : EMJ, 36*(10), 580–581. DOI: 10.1136/emermed-2019-208929

Sleeter, C. E. (2011). An agenda to strengthen culturally responsive pedagogy. *English Teaching, 10*(2), 7–23.

Subhash, S., & Cudney, E. A. (2018). Gamified learning in higher education: A systematic review of the literature. *Computers in Human Behavior, 87*, 192–206. DOI: 10.1016/j.chb.2018.05.028

Zembylas, M. (2023). The decolonisation of humanising pedagogies in higher education: Implications for culturally responsive pedagogies. In *Global Perspectives and New Challenges in Culturally Responsive Pedagogies* (pp. 36–49). Routledge., DOI: 10.4324/9781003335719-5

ADDITIONAL READINGS

Caponetto, I., Earp, J., & Ott, M. (2014, October). Gamification and education: A literature review. In *European Conference on based learning* (Vol. 1, No. 1, pp. 50–57).

Flores, J. F. F. (2015). Using gamification to enhance second language learning. *Digital Education Review*, (27), 32–54. DOI: 10.1344/der.2015.27.32-54

Fowler, M. (2010). *Domain-specific languages*. Pearson Education.

Garcia, C., & Garcia, R. (2021). Developing cultural competence in an occupational therapy program in a border institution in South Texas. In Sellers, M. D. S., & Johnson, M. E. (Eds.), *Cultural Competence in Applied Psychology* (pp. 138–157). IGI Global., https://scholarworks.utrgv.edu/context/tl_fac/article/1086/viewcontent/145841.pdf

Meuter, R. F., Gallois, C., Segalowitz, N. S., Ryder, A. G., & Hocking, J. (2015). Overcoming language barriers in healthcare: A protocol for investigating safe and effective communication when patients or clinicians use a second language. *BMC Health Services Research, 15*(1), 371. DOI: 10.1186/s12913-015-1024-8

Rabah, J., Cassidy, R., & Beauchemin, R. (2018, November). Gamification in education: Real benefits or edutainment? In the *17th European Conference on e-Learning, Athens, Greece* (pp. 489–497).

Schouten, B. C., Cox, A., Duran, G., Kerremans, K., Banning, L. K., Lahdidioui, A., van den Muijsenbergh, M., Schinkel, S., Sungur, H., Suurmond, J., Zendedel, R., & Krystallidou, D. (2020). Mitigating language and cultural barriers in healthcare communication: Toward a holistic approach. *Patient Education and Counseling, 103*(12), 2604–2608. DOI: 10.1016/j.pec.2020.05.001

ShareAmerica. (2025, February 23). The United States is rich in languages. https://share.america.gov/united-states-is-rich-in-languages/

Zembylas, M. (2023). The decolonisation of humanising pedagogies in higher education: Implications for culturally responsive pedagogies. In *Global Perspectives and New Challenges in Culturally Responsive Pedagogies* (pp. 36–49). Routledge., DOI: 10.4324/9781003335719-5

KEY TERMS AND DEFINITIONS

Border Education: Border education focuses on teaching and learning in regions where cultures, languages, and social realities intersect across national boundaries. It emphasizes understanding and responding to the unique needs, identities, and experiences of students who live in these dynamic, transnational communities.

Cultural Competence: Cultural competence is the ability to understand, respect, and effectively interact with people from diverse cultural backgrounds. It involves recognizing one's own biases while adapting communication and practices to meet the needs of different communities.

Culturally Responsive Pedagogy: An approach to teaching that centers students' cultural backgrounds, experiences, and identities as essential to learning. It emphasizes not only academic success but also the development of cultural competence and a critical awareness of social inequities. In practice, CRP encourages educators to create learning experiences that are meaningful, inclusive, and responsive to the communities their students come from..

Gamification: Gamification is the use of game elements and strategies to make learning more engaging, interactive, and motivating. It allows students to practice skills, take risks, and receive immediate feedback in a fun, low-stakes environment that mirrors real-world challenges.

Gamification Platforms: Gamification platforms are digital tools that incorporate game elements—like points, leaderboards, and timed challenges—into learning activities. They give students opportunities to practice skills, track their progress, and stay motivated in an interactive and engaging way.

Language for Specific Purposes: LSP is an approach to language learning that focuses on the vocabulary, skills, and communication needed for a particular profession or field. It allows students to practice language in real-world, context-specific situations that relate to their future careers.

Occupational Therapy: Occupational Therapy (OT) is a healthcare profession focused on helping people engage in meaningful daily activities despite physical, cognitive, or emotional challenges. OT practitioners work with clients to develop skills, adapt environments, and promote independence in their daily activities.

Chapter 5

An Educational Videogame for a University-Level Introductory Programming Course

Miguel Angel Hidalgo-Reyes
https://orcid.org/0000-0001-8303-6030
Instituto Tecnológico Superior de Xalapa, Mexico

María del Rosario Suazo-García
https://orcid.org/0000-0003-3897-6933
Instituto Tecnológico Superior de Xalapa, Mexico

Salvador Herrera-Velarde
Instituto Tecnológico Superior de Xalapa, Mexico

ABSTRACT

This work proposes a methodology based on STEM, game-based learning, and gamification to develop a game that strengthens the teaching of programming at the university level. This game considers the programming languages C, C++, and Python, each with levels of difficulty, feedback, and global report generation. In this project, quality tests were applied to the use of the game, based on the ISO/IEC 25022 standard. The tests consisted of completing a task (effectiveness), measuring the task time (efficiency), and determining the proportion of users with complaints (satisfaction). The results show that out of ten participants, eight rated the user experience positively and others rated it as attractive, fun, and interesting. On average,

DOI: 10.4018/979-8-3373-4657-1.ch005

it took 45 seconds to complete a basic level for C++. An interview was conducted to identify opportunities for improvement in this game, particularly in terms of the graphical interface, and to ensure that it meets the requirements for sharing this game on the GameMaker platform.

INTRODUCTION

Learning programming has benefited from the use of gamified platforms that integrate game elements (levels, rewards, challenges, characters) with the teaching of computational concepts. These tools seek to increase students' motivation, autonomy, and persistence when faced with problem solving and logical reasoning (Zhan, He, Tong, Liang, Guo & Lan, 2022).

In this context, there are two main approaches (Sun et al., 2024):

- Block-based programming, focused on developing computational thinking without the cognitive burden of textual syntax.
- Text-based programming, geared toward the direct practice of programming language, including its syntax, structures, and debugging.

According to Koivisto, J., & Hamari, J. (2019), gamification consists of designing systems that allow users to experience similar experiences and motivations to those found in games. Gamification facilitates the development of playful activities that allow teachers to support and motivate students by generating positive experiences, encouraging participation, reinforcing learning, and promoting autonomy.

These dynamics create sensations in the classroom like those induced by games, which contribute to student engagement and involvement (Ryan et al., 2006). Similarly, Ratinho & Martins (2023) indicate that gamification increases student motivation and engagement, especially when elements such as rewards, immediate feedback, and autonomy in learning are incorporated. However, they note that effectiveness depends on pedagogical design and the balance between fun and educational purpose.

However, gamification must be carefully designed, as it can reduce demotivation and dropout rates by encouraging autonomous learning. Nevertheless, there is a risk that students may develop a dependence on technology, so it is essential to prioritize student autonomy over the playful or entertainment component (Molina-Carmona & Llorens-Largo, 2020).

Based on the above, this technological dependence has found supporters with the use of generative artificial intelligence (GAI). The emergence of generative artificial intelligence (GAI) has found many followers in the field of education, from students and teachers to administrative and management staff. For students, GAI is a support for delving deeper into the explanation of a topic, creating summaries from short or long texts, and designing presentations using slides, among other things.

However, in the educational field, GAI poses various challenges for teachers in the classroom, which allows for the creation of specific teaching and learning strategies that provide equitable access to knowledge, collaboration among students, and the promotion of critical and computational thinking. That is, computer teachers need to create, analyze, visualize, and develop innovative and proactive educational practices and strategies to encourage computational thinking in students.

In a way, the constant use of GAI by students to solve exercises or everyday school activities creates a great challenge for teachers, because students stop stimulating computational thinking and problem solving.

It is true that education responds over time to the changes required by society, and this implies a commitment on the part of teachers to train and update themselves in new technologies and, for students, to take advantage of scientific advances in an ethical and responsible manner, both achieving "disciplinary, creative, innovative, and proactive" strategies (Zepeda et al. 2019), as is the case with Artificial Intelligence (AI).

Rodríguez et al. (2021) emphasize that we are still not teaching our students that technology can also be used to create new knowledge and that it is urgent to reorient efforts to stimulate computational thinking in schools. Even among engineering students themselves, the level of computational thinking varies and needs to be encouraged.

Brophy & Lowe 2017 state that some engineering students enter university with a solid background in computing, with some exceptions, and found that progression in learning two programming languages is essential for developing a student's ability to generalize across various computational tools.

Some studies point out that the excessive use of AI in educational settings can lead to the dehumanization of the teaching-learning process, generating an excessive dependence on machines and limiting social and emotional interaction between teachers and students (Parra-Taboada et al., 2024). In addition, the automation of certain educational processes can affect creativity and critical thinking, which are fundamental to students' intellectual development.

For example, reliance on AI tools for essay writing poses significant risks in the academic sphere. According to the Inter-American Association of Accountants (2024), students who use AI to produce texts diminish their ability to develop original ideas and critically analyze the topics covered. Furthermore, the ease of access to these tools encourages plagiarism, as the texts generated often lack personalization and authentic reflection. This problem also affects academic ethics, as students can obtain credits for work in which their intellectual effort has been minimal. It is crucial that educational institutions implement policies to detect and prevent plagiarism, in addition to encouraging critical thinking and independent writing in students.

> *"The reliance on AI as a substitute for individual cognitive effort is producing students who know how to find answers, but not how to process them" (Craig, 2024).*

The Impact of AI in Academic and Educational Contexts

According to Méndez et al., (2024), students' ability to manage tasks independently decreases when they rely excessively on AI tools. The teachers interviewed in this study emphasize that, although AI can be useful as a support tool, many students use it to avoid intellectual effort, which negatively impacts their long-term learning.

Ethical training and the development of autonomous skills are essential for AI to become a complement to, rather than a substitute for, traditional academic skills Méndez et al., (2024). The misuse of artificial intelligence directly affects the development of autonomous work in students.

The use of artificial intelligence in higher education has significant implications for skills such as reading comprehension and problem solving. According to Beltrán (2024) AI can facilitate access to educational resources and personalize learning. However, inappropriate use can lead to technological dependence, reducing students' ability to deeply understand content. This impact is especially problematic in contexts where students are expected to be active participants in their learning process. AI should not replace fundamental cognitive skills but rather serve as a complementary tool that enhances autonomous learning (Beltrán, 2024).

AI has transformed educational practices, but not without posing significant challenges for the teaching-learning process. According to the analysis by Rodríguez et al. (2024), teachers face difficulties in balancing the use of AI in the classroom, as this technology can encourage passivity in students if not used correctly. On the one hand, AI can automate processes and provide advanced tools for personalized teaching. However, from the teacher's perspective, there is also a risk that students will become overly dependent on these tools, reducing their engagement and active participation. Rodríguez et al. (2024) emphasizes that teachers must adapt their strategies to integrate AI in a way that promotes the development of critical and autonomous skills, such as analysis and creativity.

One example cited in the document is the use of virtual assistants for solving math problems. While these assistants can save time and effort, students often miss the opportunity to understand the concepts behind the solutions, limiting their ability to apply them in different contexts. Teachers play a crucial role in designing activities that complement the use of AI, promoting active and meaningful learning (Rodríguez et al., 2024). Students are at risk of delegating learning to machines, which affects their ability to deeply understand content and solve complex problems. This raises the need to implement educational approaches that combine technology with active methodologies, encouraging reflection and creativity. In this way, AI can become a powerful tool to support, but not replace, the learning process.

When analyzing the learning process for a bachelor's degree in computer systems engineering, it is essential that teaching processes have technological allies to balance the unlimited use of artificial intelligence and pedagogical development in the classroom.

BACKGROUND

Among students studying Computer Systems Engineering (CSE) at the Instituto Tecnológico Superior de Xalapa (ITSX) of the Tecnológico Nacional de México (TecNM), it has been noted that GAI is very useful in obtaining code in programming languages such as Python, Java, JavaScript, or C++.

This is alarming when students lose their motivation and interest in learning and only seek to complete assignments and exercises, as well as pass programming exams. For example, CSE students take at least 15 courses throughout their bachelor's degree program in which they must practice programming as part of the assessment criteria for those courses.

If we transfer the above to other students in other engineering programs at the same ITSX, the number of subjects will undoubtedly be lower, but the latent risk is that students will experience a vicious cycle where they fail to analyze and solve complex problems. Students lose the practice of thinking, understanding, and breaking down a problem, leading to metacognitive laziness. As an example of this, below we share the results for the Fundamentals of Programming (FP) course, which is the subject of this project's research.

Fundamentals of Programming: Statistics from 2022 to 2025

The Fundamentals of Programming (FP) course is taught in the first semester of the Computer Systems Engineering (CSE) bachelor's degree program at ITSX. This course is of great importance because passing it allows students to take the Object-Oriented Programming course (available in the second semester). Another fact is that the CSE bachelor's degree is offered on weekday and Saturday schedules, and according to official records from (Data México, 2025) the bachelor's degree had 836 students enrolled in 2022.

This means that there is more than one group of students. For example, based on the above data, the school-based program may have up to three groups and the

Saturday program up to two groups. As a result, at least five teachers oversee the FP course and teach the content programmed for the subject's thematic units.

According to institutional data reported between August 2022 and January 2023, 383 students enrolled in the FP course, of which 223 passed and the rest failed (160). In percentage terms, this represents a contrast between 58.22% passing and 41.77% failing.

The values corresponding to passing and failing students are as follows (2022 – 2025):

Table 1. Number of students who passed and failed the FP course.

School Term	Enrolled students	Approved students	Failed students
August 2022 – January 2023	383	223	160
Weekday	277	**148**	129
Saturday	106	**75**	31
August 2023 – January 2024	290	120	170
Weekday	204	**62**	142
Saturday	86	**58**	28
August 2024 – January 2025	290	161	129
Weekday	205	**127**	78
Saturday	85	**34**	51

As can be seen in Table 1, the only period in which the number of students who failed exceeded the number of students who passed was August 2023–January 2024, with 170 and 120 respectively. However, the following period was not much better, as the difference in the number of students who passed was only 78 and 51students for the weekday and Saturday schedules.

Regarding the proportion of students, in all three periods, weekday students outnumbered Saturday students in terms of passing grades in all cases. However, it is noteworthy that in the weekday schedule for the 2022–2023 and 2023–2024 periods, the proportion of failing students was higher than that of passing students.

Only for the Saturday modality and in the 2024-2025 period did the proportion of students who failed exceed that of students who passed, with 39.53% and 21.11%, respectively (see Table 2).

Table 2. Proportion of students who passed and failed the FP course.

School Term	Enrolled students (%)	Approved students (%)	Failed students (%)
August 2022 – January 2023	383	223	160
Weekday	72.32	66.36	80.62
Saturday	27.67	33.63	19.37
August 2023 – January 2024	290	120	170
Weekday	70.34	51.67	**83.52**
Saturday	29.65	48.33	**16.47**
August 2024 – January 2025	290	161	129
Weekday	70.68	78.88	60.46
Saturday	29.31	21.11	39.53

Based on the above tables and the authors' experience as teachers of Fundamentals of Programming, a concern arose to address the root causes of the high failure rates. In particular, the STEAM approach was sought as the backbone of the proposed solution, accompanied by methodologies that used game-based learning and gamification strategies so that students could adopt programming skills in a friendly and fun way.

Furthermore, in the publication by Navarro-Mateos, et al, (2024), it is stated that the role of the teacher plays a central role in gamification within the classroom, as they must increase student motivation during the educational process, using dynamics and resources typical of games and video games. This seeks to get students more actively involved in their education. Teachers must include other aspects, such as a narrative, challenges and missions, or the actions and emotions characteristic of the thematic universe in question, to extract the full potential of gamification in the classroom.

Therefore, to maximize learning through gamification in the classroom, teachers must incorporate additional elements such as an engaging narrative, challenges and missions, as well as actions and emotions specific to the topic being studied (Navarro-Mateos, et al, 2024).

As for the educational software, the team decided to call it **SOPHIE** (Striving for Optimal Programming and Hands-on Interactive Education) with two possible implementation paths: on the one hand, the software installed in computer labs and, on the other, installation on smartphones.

What Similar Projects Exist in the TecNM Repository?

Familiarizing themselves with the contents of the thematic units of the FP subject is an activity that teachers commonly carry out at ITSX and other institutions in the TecNM system. In fact, the development of these materials brings together specialists from various institutions to put together up-to-date teaching tools, which are shared with all campuses nationwide.

Just as the previous section showed the institutional results of the FP course for ITSX, the rest of the institutions might have something similar. For this reason, it was interesting to review the TecNM repository of undergraduate or postgraduate projects (such as professional residency reports, theses, and scientific articles).

The search was conducted using the words "teaching" and "programming" in the text string, and the following works were found (see Table 3):

Table 3. Two research thesis and one technical report found in TecNM repository.

Year	Title	Level	Location
2020	Web application to support decision-making in the programming teaching process	Postgraduate (Master's Degree in Computer Systems)	Teziutlán, Puebla
2021	Affective tutoring system to support the teaching and learning process of data structures	Postgraduate (Master's Degree in Computer Systems)	Teziutlán, Puebla
2022	Note-taking: Basic programming	Undergraduate (Mechatronics Engineering)	Ciudad Juárez, Chihuahua

In the work of Sosa de la Cruz (2020), the author aimed to collect data on programming activities to identify areas for improvement in a student's learning. This work was a thesis presented at a particular Instituto Tecnológico Superior, that is, part of the decentralized TecNM system, like ITSX. At the same institute, the work of Serrano (2021) reports on a mobile application developed to teach data structures in the C programming language.

Finally, Toral (2022) presents a set of programming practices in C++ for students studying Mechatronics Engineering. It is interesting to note that this project was carried out at a specific Institute Tecnológico at the federal level and, because of this work, there is no software product, just a technical report.

As can be seen, the three works are relatively recent, and only two of them belong to a postgraduate thesis. However, it is important to broaden the scope of the search using scientific repositories such as Springer, ScienceDirect, ACM, and IEEE, obtaining a systematic review of updated literature as an academic product.

THEORETICAL FRAMEWORK

Game-Based Learning

Game-based learning (GBL) consists of using games as tools to support learning, assimilation, or evaluation. Gamification, on the other hand, is based on the use of game dynamics or mechanisms in educational processes. Both options are based on the use of playful aspects to motivate students in their learning process (González-González, 2023).

GBL is mainly based on learning through play. In other words, it involves using games to acquire the proposed skills. Play is an essential part of young people's learning. In fact, they spend much of their free time playing video games. Within the term GBL, we can differentiate between different types of possible uses: gamification, serious games or video games, simulators, and game-based learning in general (González-González, 2023).

Gamification

Gamification is a learning technique that transfers the mechanics of games to the educational-professional field to achieve better results, whether to better absorb certain knowledge, improve a skill, or reward specific actions, among many other objectives (Lampropoulos & Sidiropoulos, 2024). This type of learning is gaining ground in training methodologies due to its playful nature, as it facilitates the understanding of knowledge in a more enjoyable way, generating a positive experience for the user (UNIVERSAE, 2022).

Gamification in education has established itself as an effective strategy for increasing motivation and active learning. Kapp (2012) defines it as the use of game elements and dynamics in non-playful contexts, highlighting that it can increase knowledge retention by making it interactive and motivating. Recent research shows that gamified activities allow students to interact with content in a meaningful way, which is especially useful in technical areas such as programming.

Recent studies suggest that gamification elements such as scores, rewards, leaderboards, and challenges can create an engaging and challenging environment, ideal for learning programming. Applying these elements to educational platforms has been shown to improve the learning of complex concepts by transforming them into progressive games and achievable goals. In addition, playful challenges encourage the development of critical thinking and problem-solving skills, which are essential in programming (Deterding, 2011).

Another competitive advantage of using gamification is that this game model works because it motivates students, developing greater commitment and encouraging a desire to excel. Learning programming as a university student can become a much more dynamic and engaging experience when strategies such as gamification or the use of educational games are incorporated.

These methodologies not only capture the student's attention but also encourage sustained participation in the teaching process. By turning abstract programming concepts into interactive challenges, greater motivation is achieved, which in turn facilitates understanding and knowledge retention.

Thus, gamification applied to the teaching of programming languages such as C, C++, and Python will allow students to develop skills through active practice in simulated environments. Effective programming instruction is achieved through well-designed teaching methodologies that consider students' needs and promote problem-solving and logical thinking (Elige Educar, 2018).

STEAM

The term STEM emerged in the United States in the early 1990s as a political movement, with little success until its social and, subsequently, educational transposition. Despite recognizing the value of STEM education, some authors emphasize that citizens need more than just outstanding scientific and technological training. As an evolution of STEM education, it is highlighted that integrating the arts would allow for: (1) combining convergent and divergent thinking in solving real problems; (2) the creation of personal meaning; and (3) self-motivation (Aguilera & Vílchez-González, 2024)

Therefore, the term STEAM adds the arts to the already fundamental words namely science, technology, engineering, and mathematics. The article presented by Marín-Marín, et al. (2021) indicates that methodological and scientific studies on STEAM began in 2006 and have continued uninterrupted to date.

REFERENCE FRAMEWORK

There are studies focused on teaching basic programming with particular attention to student profiles, for example, computer science and mathematics Gao et al. (2025). Some notable results of this study include the identification of different learning styles, creating learning trajectories that reveal that the association between engagement and grades differs between the two groups of students.

Along the same lines of teaching programming Iftikhar et al. (2022) use the technology use model and unified theory of acceptance to highlight the motivation factor among university students. The work of Parody et al. (2022) promotes the game Classcraft, which is a role-playing game that develops critical thinking, communication, collaboration, and creativity skills for a mathematics course.

CodeCombat

It is a gamified environment geared toward learning real languages such as Python and JavaScript. Its progressive level design allows students to write real code and visualize the effects of their instructions. It combines video game narrative with immediate feedback, facilitating autonomous and meaningful learning.

CodeCombat belongs to the text-based category, with a partially open-source freemium model. It is aimed at levels from upper elementary school to early higher education. Its main advantage is early training in real syntax, although it requires teacher support for transferring to contexts outside the game (CodeCombat, s.f.).

Lighbot

It provides an introductory, visual environment that uses icons and sequences to teach algorithmic thinking (sequence, repetition, and procedures). It is designed for young children (ages 6–12) and does not require any prior knowledge of programming. Its main contribution is to reduce cognitive load and enable structural understanding of algorithms, although it does not offer real syntactic practice, as the environment is entirely block-based. It is a proprietary, non-modifiable tool, useful for introducing fundamentals before moving on to textual environments (Lightbot, s.f).

Scratch

Developed by the MIT Media Lab, Scratch is an open-source platform (GPL license) that allows users to create programs, animations, and video games using graphic blocks. It promotes creativity, computational thinking, and digital storytelling. By eliminating syntactic errors, it encourages concentration on the logic and structure of algorithms. However, it does not teach textual syntax or complex concepts such as data types or memory management. It is ideal for formal and informal teaching to elementary and middle school students (Scratch, s.f.)

CodinGame

CodinGame is aimed at users with intermediate or advanced knowledge, such as university students or professionals. It allows users to solve challenges and compete in real time using real text languages (C++, Java, Python, among others). Its main strength lies in offering authentic coding experiences, with automatic evaluation and immediate feedback. It encourages the practice of syntax, algorithm optimization, and problem-solving skills development. However, its initial complexity can discourage beginners, and access is proprietary and closed, with no possibility of modifying the environment (CodinGame, s.f.)

Relevant Pedagogical Dimensions

According to the comparison, the key pedagogical features that each platform complies are:

Table 4. Pedagogical features of different gaming platforms.

Feature	Description	Platform
Motivation and gamification	Use challenges, levels, rewards, and characters to increase engagement and persistence.	CodeCombat, CodinGame
Computational thinking	Developing the ability to break down problems and design algorithmic solutions	Lightbot, Scratch
Practice of real syntax	Exercises involving writing, debugging, and executing textual code.	CodeCombat, CodinGame
Knowledge transfer	The student's ability to apply what they have learned in a new language or environment.	Scratch, CodeCombat
Accessibility and licensing	Free use, open source, or access restrictions.	Scratch, CodeCombat

Regarding SOPHIE, it is worth mentioning that motivation and gamification are the responsibility of the teacher who accompanies students throughout the semester. The features of computational thinking, real syntax practice, and knowledge transfer are also covered by SOPHIE.

About accessibility and licensing, in the current version of SOPHIE, it is possible to install the executable file on computers with Windows operating systems. However, to obtain the apk file and migrate the software to a mobile environment, it is necessary to pay for a license in the GameMaker store.

GameMaker as a video game development platform

GameMaker Studio 2 is a video game development tool that allows you to create 2D games easily, but with advanced features. It is especially popular among indie developers (game creators) due to its accessibility, flexibility, and active community.

It was developed by YoYo Games and has been widely used to create games on various platforms, from PCs to mobile and desktop consoles.

Among the most notable features of GameMaker Studio 2 are the following (GameMaker, 2025):

- Intuitive visual interface: The platform allows developers to design elements such as sprites, backgrounds, and levels using drag-and-drop tools, without requiring advanced programming experience. This speeds up the design process and improves productivity.
- Cross-platform compatibility: Projects created in GameMaker Studio 2 can be exported to various platforms, such as Windows, MacOS, Android, and iOS, which broadens the reach of the final product and ensures greater accessibility for users.
- Integrated programming language (IPL): IPL provides developers with the flexibility to implement custom logic and advanced mechanics, making it an ideal tool for interactive educational projects.
- Rapid iteration: GameMaker Studio 2 allows for real-time testing and adjustments thanks to its integrated debugging system, significantly speeding up the development cycle.

PROBLEM STATEMENT

Learning programming languages is a crucial skill in the training of ITSX-CSE students. However, traditional teaching can be monotonous and unattractive to first-semester students, which affects their motivation and academic performance. With the rise of AI and automated tools, many students tend to rely on these technologies, neglecting the development of critical and creative skills essential to programming.

This project arises as a response to the need to improve teaching for students in the program at ITSX, mainly in the exploration and knowledge of the programming languages C, C++, and Python through an interactive and dynamic approach.

The central problem is the lack of motivation and dependence on automated technologies by students to learn programming, which negatively impacts the development of critical and creative skills. Traditional teaching of programming languages, such as C, C++, and Python, tends to be perceived as tedious and difficult, which diminishes students' interest and willingness to learn actively (Cruz, 2018).

This is exacerbated by traditional teaching methods, which tend to focus on the passive transmission of knowledge without including elements that promote interaction and active thinking (Tejera-Martínez et al., 2020). In some cases, students' lack of motivation in the classroom is related to the limited integration of innovative methodologies that make the learning process more attractive and effective. Similarly, the absence of interactive platforms or tools that combine playful elements with formal programming instruction contributes to students quickly losing interest and failing to develop the skills necessary to competently face the challenges of the professional world.

This problem has been identified during the first semesters of the ITSX-CSE bachelor degree program, where students begin their training in the subject of programming. It is during this period that they have their first contact with languages such as C, C++, and Python, facing a learning curve that many find challenging without a tool to support them dynamically. Similarly, this problem tends to intensify due to the easy accessibility of GAI tools, where students rely on automated solutions that replace the intellectual effort they should be developing on their own.

It is presumed that this problem can also be extrapolated to other educational institutions facing similar challenges in teaching programming. It is not surprising to note that there is a disconnect between traditional teaching methods and the current needs of students, who require a more interactive approach that sparks their interest and facilitates their understanding of complex concepts.

The proposed project responds to a need for an educational tool that facilitates the learning of programming languages such as C, C++, and Python for the specific community of ITSX. The intention of this project is to encourage interest and active learning in students through an interactive platform. Through a software product, students can experiment and develop skills with different visual agility, syntax, and strategy games, which stimulate their creative and critical thinking.

Learning programming is a complex process that involves developing technical skills and advanced cognitive abilities. Some studies suggest that the "hands-on learning" approach is effective, as it allows students to solve real problems and face challenges in a practical way (Hastuti & Malihah, 2024).

The use of interactive games and gamification are considered useful strategies for maintaining student interest and motivation, facilitating an active and engaging learning experience (Revelo-Sanchéz, 2018). For example, platforms such as Duolingo or Kahoot make the learning process more engaging and motivating, encouraging students to actively participate and explore new ideas.

Project Goal

To develop a prototype educational video game that allows first-semester students in the ITSX-CSE program to interact with fun and interactive activities aimed at strengthening their learning of basic, intermediate, and advanced programming concepts in the C, C++, and Python programming languages, promoting critical and creative thinking through progressive challenges and methodologies such as Game-Based Learning (GBL), STEAM, and gamification.

Specific Objectives of the Project

1. Design game mechanics, elements, and dynamics for the levels, incorporating key concepts of programming, syntax, grammar, conditional structures, loops, and function handling.
2. Develop interactive game levels focused on the basic concepts of the C, C++, and Python programming languages, adapted to the level of first-semester students, to facilitate understanding of initial topics.
3. Implement an intuitive and accessible user interface in the software that allows students to navigate efficiently between games and develop visual agility and understand the grammar of programming languages.
4. Evaluate and optimize the performance of the video game through user testing, adjusting aspects of game mechanics and elements.

PROPOSED METHODOLOGY

The methodological approach in this project is based on the integration of four perspectives: 1) Game-Based Learning (GBL), 2) STEAM approach, 3) gamification, and 4) Mobile-D. This combination of approaches complements each other because it directly addresses the problems identified in ITSX computer systems students, such as low motivation, limited or no communication between teachers and students, and the need for more meaningful and contextualized learning experiences.

The agile Mobile-D methodology was used exclusively for the development of the mobile application for the video game **SOPHIE**. Its main feature is that it is designed to work with small teams, which facilitated constant interaction between the team of teachers and project leaders and the professional residents who programmed the video game.

The GBL approach made it possible to structure the teaching-learning process in relation to the educational video game **SOPHIE**. This encouraged teachers and students to participate in decision-making and learning, in accordance with the Fundamentals of Programming course curriculum.

The STEAM approach was used to integrate technical knowledge such as programming language syntax writing for advanced levels of the video game, exercises and problem solving aligned with computational thinking skills and supervised by the teaching team, and finally, the design and programming of the video game scenarios linked to a collective artistic process.

The role of the teacher through gamification was incorporated as a strategy to induce motivational dynamics typical of games (challenges, rewards, narrative, immediate feedback), which helps to sustain students' interest and encourage autonomy.

Initially, the game was developed into two main interactions. The first interaction to initialize the project consisted mainly of the following activities:

1. Analyzing and evaluating the SCD1008-Fundamentals of Programming curriculum, identifying the units and theoretical topics to be considered.
2. Determining the programming languages to develop the questions.
3. Defining the working methodology for the development of the GBL and Mobile-D project.
4. Selecting the technology for programming video games.
5. Developing the first prototype of the video game and integrating the first three levels for the following programming languages: C, C++, and Python.

The second interaction of the project involved the following activities:

1. Evaluate the first version of the video game prototype.
2. Implement improvements in design, syntax, spelling, and reactivity.
3. Evaluate the correct use of GBL + Gamification + STEAM methodology.
4. Develop the intermediate levels (4, 5, and 6) corresponding to each programming language.
5. Conducting tests with end users to validate the functionality and experience of the game.

As part of the activities of the first interaction, it was decided to implement a hybrid software development methodology, starting with Mobile-D as a basis because it is a software product. However, the entire project was based on the integration of Game-Based Learning (GBL), the design of the questions had a STEAM focus, and, mainly, the development and design of the game within a gamification approach, with the aim of responding to the need to transform learning into a meaningful experience for students.

Figure 1 shows the phases and stages of the development methodology for the creation of the video game.

Figure 1. Development methodology for this project.

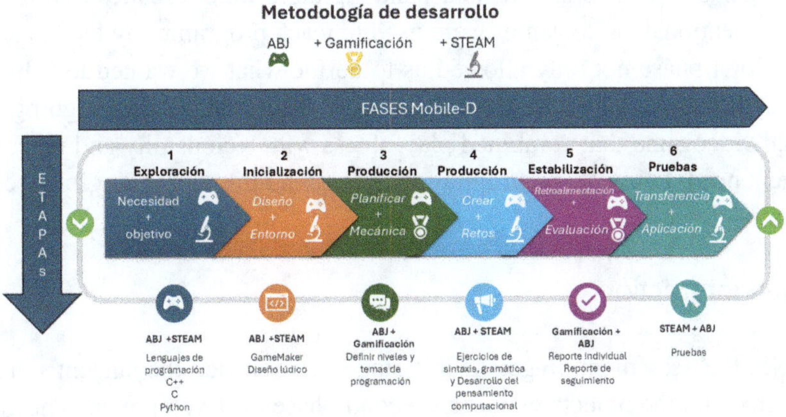
Metodología de desarrollo
ABJ
+ Gamificación
+ STEAM
FASES Mobile-D
ETAPAS
1 Exploración
2 Inicialización
3 Producción
4 Producción
5 Estabilización
6 Pruebas
Necesidad + objetivo
Diseño + Entorno
Planificar + Mecánica
Crear + Retos
Retroalimentación + Evaluación
Transferencia + Aplicación
ABJ +STEAM
Lenguajes de programación C++ C Python
ABJ +STEAM
GameMaker Diseño lúdico
ABJ + Gamificación
Definir niveles y temas de programación
ABJ + STEAM
Ejercicios de sintaxis, gramática y Desarrollo del pensamiento computacional
Gamificación + ABJ
Reporte individual Reporte de seguimiento
STEAM + ABJ
Pruebas

Phase 1: Exploration

First interaction

- Needs Assessment Stage: In this first interaction, based on the GBL methodology, we focused on understanding the real needs in the classroom and the problems reported by ITSX students in the FP course, centered on the misuse of GAI to perform activities that lead to a lack of understanding in solving mathematical problems. Therefore, we proposed to see what possibilities educational technologies and methodologies offered. This initial stage was key to the development of the project and laying the foundations, as the TecNM SCD1008-FP curriculum was analyzed and evaluated, identifying the units and theoretical topics that would be addressed in the video game. It was decided to work with unit two: introduction to programming, and unit three: flow control.
- Objective stage: Subsequently, the objective was set to develop a video game that integrates playful and competitive elements. A survey was then conducted among teachers who have taught this subject, with the aim of finding out which programming languages they use most. The results showed that the languages most widely understood by students, allowing them to develop computational thinking skills and which are not complex in terms of grammar or syntax, were C, C++, and Python.

Another activity in this first stage consisted of searching for information in specialized databases, technical manuals, and digital resources related to this issue, in which recreational video games were used to teach programming languages.

This first phase not only allowed us to define what we wanted to achieve, but also why it was necessary to do so. It was the starting point for designing an educational videogame that combined playfulness with technicality and responded to an urgent need: to transform programming learning into a meaningful, accessible, and motivating experience.

Second interaction

- Needs Assessment Stage: At this stage, we assessed the current state of the game and the objectives for the second phase of development. The game already had three functional levels in which the user had to search for objects and respond correctly. Through meetings and monitoring, we identified areas that needed improvement, as well as new features that could enrich the learning experience. In addition, the need to reinforce the teaching process of the C, C++, and Python programming languages through more interactive dynamics were analyzed. The roles within the project were also clearly defined.
- Stage Objective: The corresponding participation was assigned in the second stage of development, focusing on intermediate levels 4, 5, and 6 of the video game for learning programming, as well as on optimizing the game's base system. The cohesion of the group allowed us to work continuously on what had already been developed, respecting the previous design and incorporating functional and aesthetic improvements.

It was determined that the second part of the project would not only continue with the initial pedagogical objectives, but would also integrate greater control of the learning flow, such as: a) mandatory progression between levels, b) a better user experience, c) inclusion of a sound interface, d) correction of previously identified logical errors, e) the design of advanced dynamics oriented towards logical thinking and direct programming practice, such as the resolution of open questions. The need to provide guided feedback before each advanced level (from levels 4, 5, and 6 onwards) was also identified, due to the GBL methodology and the rules of operation.

Overall, this second interaction allowed us to consolidate a more structured vision of the educational video game, aimed not only at improving the technical and aesthetic experience of the system, but also at strengthening its pedagogical value. By integrating new dynamics, guided feedback, and a more controlled progression, progress was made toward a more meaningful learning environment, capable of stimulating logical thinking, creativity, and active appropriation of programming languages by students.

Phase 2 Initialization

First Interaction:

· Design Stage: For this project, a serious game based on the GBL methodology was developed, as its main purpose is to serve as a tool for learning, practicing, and reinforcing programming knowledge in C, C++, and Python. This design is aimed at a user profile motivated by achievement and self-improvement, i.e., players with a “winner” mentality who seek to achieve specific goals, progress through challenges, and obtain high scores. At this stage, the initial configuration of the video game was carried out and, because of a search and comparison of tools that could integrate a playful design, it was decided to work with GameMaker. This search for information allowed us to identify and apply best practices and functionalities in the development of the video game.

Subsequently, the activities were defined, including the definition of functional requirements, which mainly consist of the creation of educational games adapted to key programming concepts and the integration of gamification and STEAM elements to motivate students, as well as the definition of non-functional requirements, which mainly consisted of ease of use and compatibility with educational environments in order to ensure an inclusive and sustainable learning experience.

· Environment stage: In this stage, the educational system was conceptualized, covering both technical and visual aspects. The activities carried out ensured that the design met functional and non-functional requirements. As part of the gamification elements, requirements were defined mainly related to the mechanics of the educational game, focusing on activities such as multiple-choice questions and interactive challenges, encouraging the programmer's skill toward visual agility. The design focused on visual clarity and ease of navigation.

These dynamics were designed to address the corresponding topics in the introduction to programming unit, which determined the topics of basic concepts, variables, identifiers, parameters, operators, etc., for each programming language (C, C++, and Python), ensuring pedagogical alignment by level.

Second interaction:

· Design stage: This stage of game development focused on intermediate levels (4 to 6), which are designed to develop more complex cognitive skills through selection, logical association, and response writing activities. However, the player profile game type was validated at this stage. As part of the educational video game design, the content at each level was reviewed to ensure that each level met the learning objectives. The focus was to strengthen and stimulate computational thinking in students through progressive activities for each level, adapted to gamification and GBL elements such as the incorporation of feedback (regarding the exercises in levels 4, 5, and 6), lives, time limits, and score evaluation to simulate challenges and encourage active learning.

- Level 1: basic concepts such as the use of variables, operators, and simple and conditional decisions.
- Level 2: exploration of loops, lists (arrays), and simple functions.
- Level 3: solving complex problems, integrating data structures and advanced concepts.
- Level 4: development of logical reasoning and the ability to relate concepts to each other.
- Level 5: improving skills in writing code correctly, paying attention to structure and the way instructions are written.
- Level 6: Strengthening code structure with regard to the syntax and grammar rules specific to each programming language.

· Environment Stage: The prototype was developed using GameMaker Studio 2, a tool that facilitated the implementation and progression of interactive and visual mechanics in the two interactions, as well as the planning of their design and execution. These activities include:

o Menu navigation: A hierarchical system was designed to guide users through the different sections of the game, such as language and level selection. The menus were developed to ensure intuitive and fast navigation.
o Presentation of gamified activities: the system introduces interactive challenges that reinforce key programming concepts. Each activity is presented in a playful way, encouraging user participation.
o Personalized interaction: Users can interact with elements of the game environment, such as clicking on objects to start activities or answering programming-related questions, making the experience more enjoyable.
o The gamified activities included in the prototype were designed to facilitate the understanding of basic concepts in the C, C++, and Python programming languages.
o Interactive challenges: Practical situations that simulate real programming problems. For example, users must identify what the code blocks presented do to give the correct answer.

o Multiple-choice questions: Each level contains questions related to the concepts taught. These questions allow the user to analyze and apply the knowledge acquired.

o Progressive level structure: Levels are designed to gradually increase in difficulty, promoting continuous learning and the development of computational thinking.

o The graphic design and interface of the prototype were carefully developed to ensure an attractive and user-friendly visual experience. The most notable features include:

o Friendly visual style: eye-catching colors and graphic elements were used to capture the user's attention.

o Intuitive interface: Interactive elements, such as buttons and menus, are clearly labeled and organized for ease of use.

o Transitions between screens are smooth and consistent, minimizing any confusion for the user.

Overall, the second interaction allowed us to consolidate the pedagogical, technical, and visual aspects of the educational video game, progressively integrating the intermediate levels and strengthening the user experience. The combination of gamified activities, personalized feedback at each level, programming language, and an accessible user interface contributed to creating a dynamic, motivating learning environment aligned with the teaching objectives of programming languages.

This progress represents a significant step toward building more inclusive, effective educational tools focused on the development of computational thinking.

Phase 3 Mechanical Production

First Interaction

· Planning Stage: During this stage of production, the main planning and development activities were carried out:

o Construction of the videogame in stages, testing and adjusting functionalities in short cycles.

o Implementation of visual and structural elements of the videogame in GameMaker Studio.

o Incorporation of interactive elements such as programming-based questions and challenges.

· Mechanical Stage:

- The mechanics of educational games were implemented, such as interaction with objects and the presentation of questions related to programming concepts.
- GameMaker Studio functions were used to integrate visual and gamified elements, ensuring adequate performance.
- Collision masks, user input controls, and timers were configured to ensure an interactive experience. A collision is an event that occurs when two objects physically interact in the same space.
- Functional tests were performed to verify the operability of the developed modules.
- The results obtained allowed for the identification and correction of errors in the videogame logic and the layout of graphic elements.

Second Interaction

Planning Stage: It was determined that the second part of the project would not only continue with the initial pedagogical objectives, but would also integrate greater control of the learning flow, such as:

- Mandatory progression between levels,
- A better user experience, such as pause buttons, music, accept button, images of the elements to be searched for.
- Inclusion of a sound interface,
- Correction of previously identified logical errors,
- Design of advanced dynamics oriented towards logical thinking and direct programming practice, such as problem solving.

· Mechanical Stage: At this stage, activities focused on technical implementation, interaction, and user experience were carried out. The logic of levels one to three was restructured, incorporating search objects as a playful element and reinforcing the interactive narrative. Previous errors affecting gameplay were corrected and technical consistency between mechanics was improved, in line with the principles of accessibility and universal design.

These improvements consolidated a functional base that allows the educational content to be dynamically scaled to later stages.

- Implementation of drag-and-drop dynamics (levels 4 and 5).
- Development of the open-ended response system with manual or automated validation (level 6).
- Presentation of gamified activities with interactive challenges that reinforce key concepts.

- Personalized interaction: click on objects to start activities or answer questions.
- Display of search objects in levels 1, 2, and 3.
- Integration of immediate feedback, visual representation of progress, and implicit reward system.
- Redesign of menus, controls, and objects to improve visual clarity and enhance the user experience.
- Implementation of a progressive level structure with gradually increasing difficulty.

Overall, Phase 3 of Production allowed for significant progress in the technical and pedagogical construction of the educational video game. Through two well-defined interactions, it was possible to plan, implement, and adjust mechanics that not only improve the user experience but also strengthen programming learning from a playful, progressive, and accessible perspective. The improvements made in this phase laid the foundations for a scalable training tool, capable of adapting to different skill levels and learning styles, while always maintaining a focus on the development of logical and computational thinking.

Phase 4 Production challenges

First interaction

· Create stage: during this stage of development, the new levels and functionalities of the educational video game, aimed at learning programming, were programmed in GameMaker Language (GML). The implemented mechanics responded to both pedagogical and recreational criteria, following gamification principles to encourage intrinsic user motivation. As in the previous phase, the errors identified were corrected and these improvements consolidated a functional base that allows the educational content to be dynamically scaled to later stages.

· Challenges Stage: In this stage, interactive challenges were created in the game, which consisted of developing practical situations that simulate real programming problems. For example, users must identify what the code blocks presented do to give the correct answer. Multiple-choice questions: Each level contains questions related to the concepts taught. These questions allow the user to reflect on and apply the knowledge acquired. And finally, a progressive structure: The levels are designed to gradually increase in difficulty, promoting constant learning and the development of logical-computational thinking.

Second Interaction

· Create stage: In this stage, activities focused on game development and programming were carried out as part of the definition of the functional and visual components (objects) corresponding to each new mechanic. Actions included:

- o Documenting the progression between levels and creating specific responses for each programming language, for example, the number of lives or attempts for each answer that each player has.
- o The items designed for programming learning were structured under a STEAM approach, integrating elements of science, technology, engineering, and mathematics to encourage logical thinking, creativity, and problem-solving.
- o Improvement of individual reports by level and tracking of each player's progress.
- o Restructuring levels one to three, incorporating search objects as a playful element and reinforcing the narrative.
- o Design of a pop-up window for feedback prior to the start of levels 4, 5, and 6, with a confirmation box and "Accept" button.
- o Design of the level access control system (progressive blocking).
- o Planned incorporation of interface elements such as a sound button, life indicators, time, and points.

· Challenges stage: As part of the video game's learning objectives, functions were implemented to ensure that the questions in each level integrated STEAM and GBL elements. The main actions were:

o Drag-and-drop interaction dynamics, designed to facilitate intuitive manipulation of objects in the visual environment.
o Processing open-ended text responses, i.e., the user types the answer, which encourages critical thinking and the direct application of knowledge.
o Sequence validation between levels through a progressive access control system, which prevents advancement without completing the previous level, ensuring the gradual development of skills.
o Integration of the sound system, including effects, narrative cues, and a sound control button that enhances immersion and accessibility.
o Integration of the sound system, including effects, narrative tracks, and a sound control button that improves immersion and accessibility.
o Implementation of feedback logic prior to the start of advanced levels, providing advanced guidance to promote autonomous learning.

Phase 4 of Production challenges allowed us to consolidate the technical, pedagogical, and visual foundations of the educational video game, progressively integrating new mechanics and functionalities aligned with the learning objectives. The two interactions addressed in this phase not only strengthened the game's structure but also ensured a more immersive, accessible, and meaningful experience for students. This advance represents a key step toward the implementation of educational environments that combine play with theory, promoting computational thinking and active engagement with programming.

Phase 5: Stabilization

First interaction

· Feedback stage: During this stage, weekly meetings were held with the work team and the academy of computer systems professors to define priority guidelines and validate progress. These sessions made it possible to prioritize the content needed to teach the proposed topics and essential functionalities such as interactivity and ease of use.

· Evaluation Stage: During this stage, errors were corrected and the opinions expressed in the work team meetings were considered. The aim was to optimize the overall logic of the game, improving operational consistency and technical stability.

Second interaction

· Feedback stage: At this stage, the first prototype of the game was analyzed, and every aspect of the game mechanics was carefully evaluated. In addition, observations were reviewed, and technical and visual adjustments were made.

- o Evaluation of the first prototype using a checklist.
- o Improvements to the user experience.
- o Simplification of menu navigation.
- o Adjustments to the visual presentation of elements to improve clarity and appearance.
- o Technical optimization.
- o Review and debugging of the logic implemented in GML to ensure consistency of mechanics.
- o Providing feedback on exercises at advanced levels in each programming language, as part of the GBL and Gamification methodologies.

· Evaluation stage: This stage focused on validating the pedagogical and functional design to ensure that the videogame met the learning objectives and offered a meaningful learning experience to first-semester students. That is:

o Redesign of menus, controls, and objects to improve visual clarity.

- Detailed documentation of the logic of progression between levels.
- Definition of response validation criteria and effects of the lives and time system.
- Implementation of dynamics oriented towards meaningful learning.
- Promotion of participation, problem solving, and logical thinking through progressive challenges.
- Integration of mechanics such as immediate feedback, visual representation of progress, and implicit reward system.

Phase 5 of Stabilization based on Mobile-D represented a key milestone in consolidating the technical and pedagogical advances of the educational video game. Through two complementary interactions, it was possible to integrate feedback from teachers (work team) and users, correct critical errors, and validate the functional design of the videogame. Collaborative meetings, visual adjustments, and optimization of the game logic strengthened the user experience and ensured that the mechanics responded to the learning objectives. This phase not only improved the operational stability of the prototype but also established the basis for its effective implementation in real educational contexts, promoting a more dynamic, accessible teaching environment focused on logical-computational thinking.

RESULTS OBTAINED

Programmed video game

Below are images from the video game related to its initial execution, operation, and completion.

When the video game is running for the first time, the screen displays three blocks related to programming languages (Python, C++, and C), and a download button appears (see Figure 2).

Figure 2. Videogame start screen.

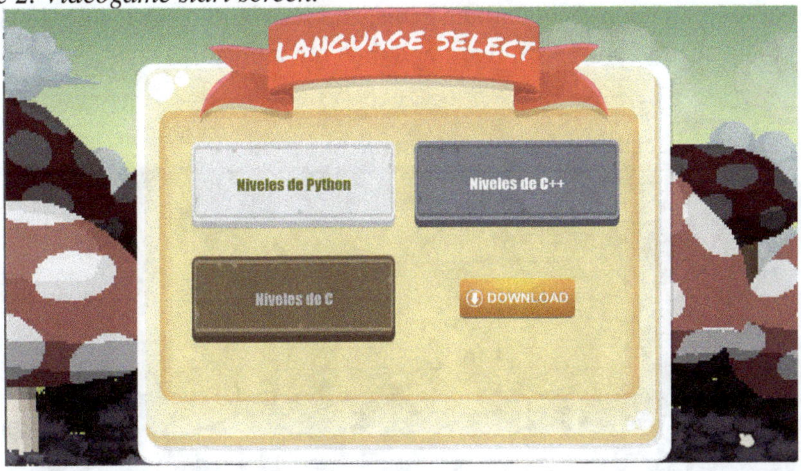

When simulating the selection of the option called "Niveles de C (C Levels)" the play levels for this programming language appear (see Figure 3). It is important to note that only level 1 appears enabled, and the subsequent levels from 2 to 6 display a label that says "locked."

Figure 3. Different levels of play for a programming language.

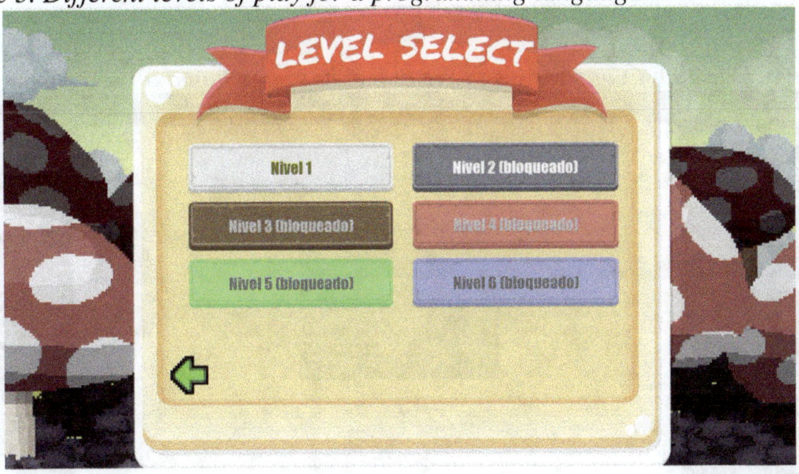

When starting level 1, the game scenario is as follows (see Figure 4). This figure shows a scenario corresponding to a computer lab, and the game begins with the identification of objects located at the top center. In this case, there are five objects represented by thumbnail images.

In addition, other visual controls are visible in the upper right corner, namely enable/disable sound, pause/continue game, and start button. The upper left corner displays information on scores, lives, and time remaining.

Figure 4. Level 1 scenario for Python language.

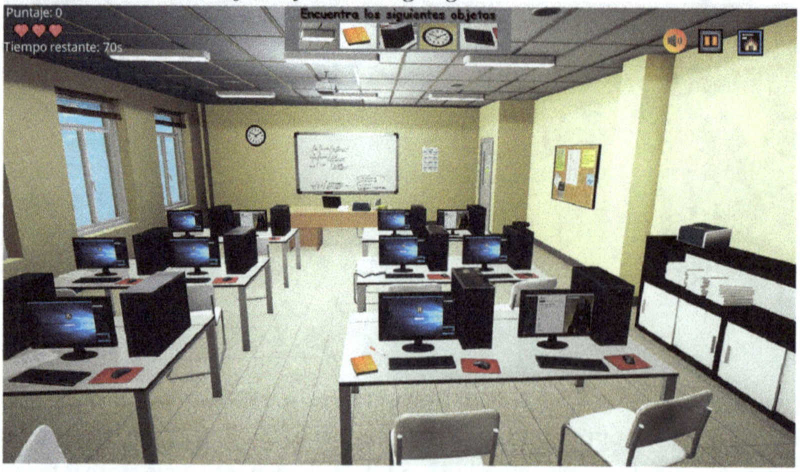

When the object to be found is successfully located, a screen appears with the question to be answered (see Figure 5).

Figure 5. Question to answer when the object has been found on screen.

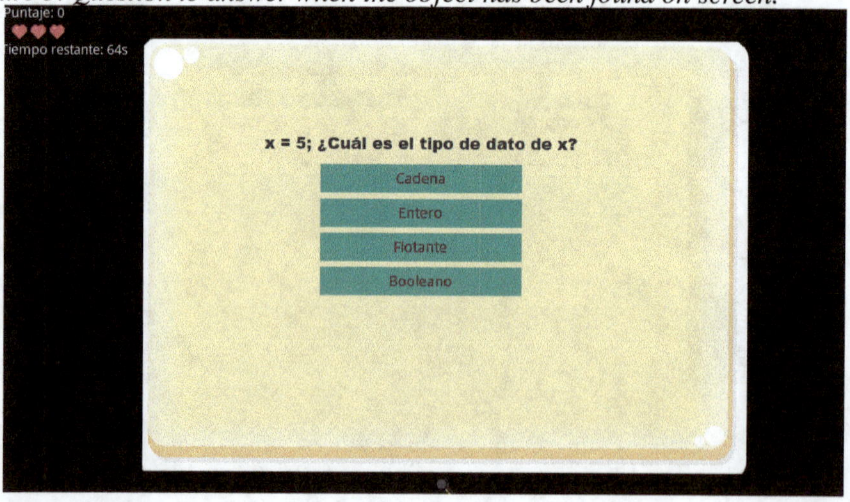

The number of objects to find is directly related to the number of questions to answer, i.e., if we must locate 4 objects, a question will appear for each object. If time runs out before the corresponding level is completed, the game will send a message with this notification (see Figure 6).

Figure 6. Time has run out before completing the game level.

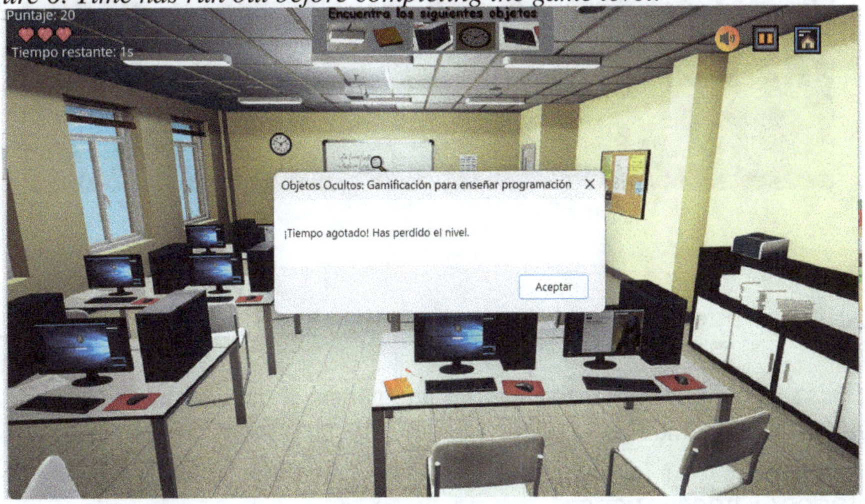

If you finish the first level, it is important to note that only with all the correct answers will you advance to the next level, i.e., it will automatically unlock. At this point, the player has the choice to finish the game, play again to continue to the next level, or review their statistics (see Figure 7).

Figure 7. Example of a level report.

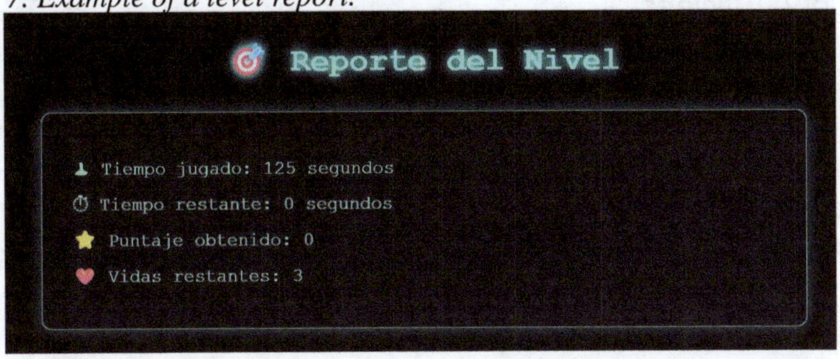

Finally, the download button on the home screen (see Figure 2) allows you to obtain a global report of the player's performance. This report shows the levels completed for the corresponding programming language, as well as the date and duration (see Figure 8).

Figure 8. Player progress report.

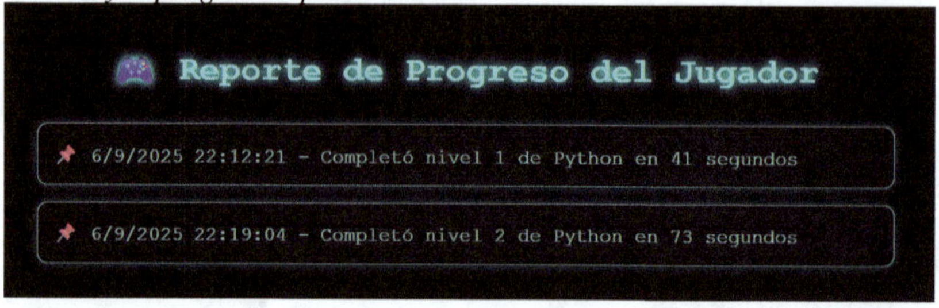

Quality of use tests

This section describes the categories and names of the tests used, based on the ISO/IEC 25022 standard.

Category Effectiveness

Test name: Task completed

Objective: To determine the user's ability to successfully complete the designated task without assistance. This test measures whether the application allows users to achieve their goals.

Task description: Start and finish level 1 of the Python programming language.

Category: Efficiency

Test name: Task time

Objective: To measure the time it takes a user, once they have learned the system, to complete a specific task. This test measures how quickly and easily the application can be used.

Task description: Start and finish level 1 of the C++ programming language.

Category: Satisfaction

Test name: Proportion of users who complain

Objective: To collect data on users' subjective perceptions and their level of acceptance of the application.

Task description: Answer the questionnaire about overall experience with the application.

Questions:

a. Overall, what did you think of the application?
b. What did you find easiest to use?
c. What part of the application did you find most difficult or confusing?
d. If you could change one thing about this application, what would it be?
e. Was there anything that frustrated you or made you want to quit the app?
f. Would you recommend this app to a friend or colleague? Why or why not?
g. How would you describe your experience with this application in one word?

Starting with the first two categories described, Table 5 contains the participants' results:

Table 5. Results of playing level 1 for Python and C++.

User	Programming language	Time played (seconds)	Remaining lives	Points
1	Python	40	2	50
2	C++	46	1	50
3	Python	75	2	40
4	C++	61	2	50
5	Python	75	3	30
6	C++	75	3	10
7	C++	63	2	50
8	Python	57	3	50
9	C++	55	3	50
Average		**60**	**2**	**40**

Table 5 shows some interesting patterns. For example, there were users (5 and 6) who played for the entire time set for the level (75 seconds) and did not achieve the maximum score (50). This means that they did not complete level 1 because they had incorrect answers (2 and 4, respectively).

Other cases (8 and 9) were close to reaching 75 seconds but successfully completed level 1 because they only used one life and reached a total of 50 points for Python and C++. A third finding is that players reached 50 points but used more than one life. This resulted in shorter times, between 40 and 46 seconds, due to familiarity with the interface, dynamics, and mechanics of the game.

Regarding the participants' user experience, Figure 9 shows a word cloud with the most frequently mentioned adjectives.

Figure 9. Word cloud for user experience (satisfaction).

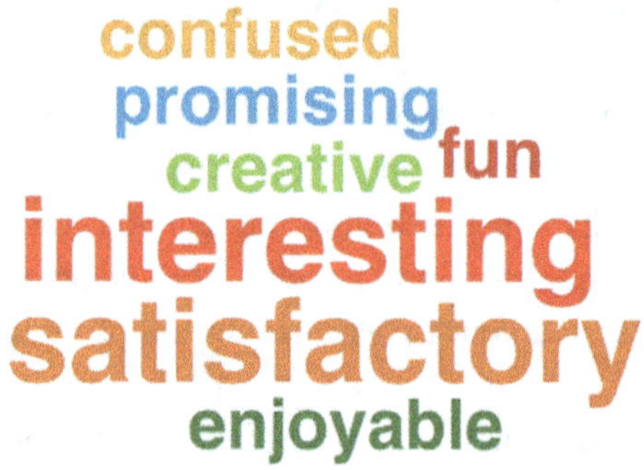

CONCLUSIONS AND FUTURE WORK

This chapter presented a hybrid methodology that combines Mobile-D, GBL, gamification and STEAM. One contribution of this project lies in the phases and interactions identified, which allowed for rapid prototyping of a video game, receiving feedback from academic peers, and following interactive and motivating guidelines to create a challenging and innovative game.

The GameMaker development kit proved to be an ideal choice for creating scenarios in each programming language with interactive and multimedia elements. Control elements such as time, opportunities (lives), scoring, and contextual information allowed students to immerse themselves in an environment like that of video games programmed on commercial consoles.

The tests carried out on users yielded interesting results and revealed findings that had not been considered by the working team. This information led to improvements in the user interface, revision of questions, instructions for use, and the use of real examples for all levels, not just advanced levels. The level-based and global reporting component was well received by teachers because it allows them to add an evaluation criterion that had not been used previously and that could be linked to extra-curricular activities or exam review.

We recognize that testing nine students is a small sample size, but we remain committed to testing the video game with a full group of students enrolled in the next FP course. Future work includes improving the instructional design for student diversity and learning styles, updating the video game, and meeting all requirements to share this application on the GameMaker market in the short term. It also includes expanding the set of tests specified in the ISO/IEC 25022 standard, as only one test from each category was applied, but up to 10 different tests can be applied in total.

It is important to mention that the project's leadership team has contacted an education expert at ITSX to analyze the pedagogical impact of the ISO standard tests applied and the video game itself. We recognize that in this type of project, it is essential to collaborate with experts in the field, and once this analysis has been completed, we will seek to disseminate the results to the relevant educational authorities.

The methodological combination of GBL, gamification, STEAM and Mobile-D not only responded to the challenges identified in the FP course but also allowed the technical design of the video game to be aligned with the educational objectives, ensuring a comprehensive, scalable, and transferable educational experience.

ACKNOWLEDGMENT

Special recognition goes to students Erik Hernández Rodríguez and Carlos Giovanni Alonso Ramírez, who collaborated in this research project. Their committed participation in the different phases of the project was fundamental to achieving the established objectives. Finally, we would like to thank TecNM for the financial support approved through the Call for Scientific Research, Technological Development, and Innovation Projects 2025.

REFERENCES

Aguilera, D., & Vílchez-González, J. M. (2024). ¿De qué hablamos cuando hablamos de educación STEAM? Una revisión de experiencias educativas. *Revista Fuentes*, 2(26), 211–224. DOI: 10.12795/revistafuentes.2024.15412

Asociación Interamericana de Contabilidad. (2024). *Desventajas y Riesgos de la Inteligencia Artificial en la Educación Universitaria - AIC*. AIC. https://contadores-aic.org/desventajas-y-riesgos-de-la-inteligencia-artificial-en-la-educacion-universitaria-originalidad-de-ensayos-y-plagios/

Beltrán Fuentes, A. F. (2024). El impacto del uso de la inteligencia artificial en los estudiantes de Administración de Empresas de la Pontificia Universidad Javeriana (Tesis de licenciatura, Pontificia Universidad Javeriana, Bogotá, Colombia). Repositorio Institucional PUJ. https://apidspace.javeriana.edu.co/server/api/core/bitstreams/8f23fe21-53ad-4ea1-8f62-ff250d48cf05/content

Brophy, S. B., & Lowe, T. A. (2017). *A Learning Trajectory for Developing Computational Thinking and Programming*. Purdue e-Pubs. https://docs.lib.purdue.edu/enepubs/14/

CodeCombat. (s.f.). *CodeCombat*. Recuperado el 15 de noviembre de 2025, de https://codecombat.com/

CodinGame. (s.f.). *CodinGame – Start Coding*. Recuperado el 15 de noviembre de 2025, de https://www.codingame.com/start/

Craig, D. (2024). *PELIGRO IA – Los riesgos de la Inteligencia Artificial en la Educación | Diego F. Craig*. https://craig.ar/peligro-ia/?utm_source=chatgpt.com

Cruz Pérez, M. A., Pozo Vinueza, M. A., Andino Jaramillo, A. F., & Arias Parra, A. D. (2018). Las Tecnologías de la Información y la Comunicación (TIC) como forma investigativa interdisciplinaria con un enfoque intercultural para el proceso de formación de los estudiantes. *E-Ciencias De La Información*, *9*(1). Advance online publication. DOI: 10.15517/eci.v1i1.33052

Data México. (2025). *Distribución de estudiantes Instituto Tecnológico Superior de Xalapa* https://www.economia.gob.mx/datamexico/es/profile/institution/instituto-tecnologico-superior-de-xalapa

Deterding, S., Dixon, D., Khaled, R., & Nacke, L. (2011). From game design elements to gamefulness: Defining "gamification". En *Proceedings of the 15th International Academic MindTrek Conference: Envisioning Future Media Environments* (pp. 9–15). Association for Computing Machinery. https://doi.org/DOI: 10.1145/2181037.2181040

Educar, E. (25 de mayo de 2018). *Diez cosas que un educador puede hacer para lograr una enseñanza eficaz.* Recuperado de https://eligeeducar.cl/noticias/10-cosas-que-puede-hacer-un-educador-para-lograr-una-ensenanza-efectiva/

GameMaker. (2025). *Características y herramientas del motor*. https://gamemaker.io/es/features

Gao, Z., Yan, H., Liu, J., ... Tracing distinct learning trajectories in introductory programming course: a sequence analysis of score, engagement, and code metrics for novice computer science vs. math cohorts. *IJ STEM Ed* **12**, 27 (2025). https://doi.org/DOI: 10.1186/s40594-025-00546-2

González-González, C. S. (2023). El impacto de la inteligencia artificial en la educación: Transformando la forma en que enseñamos y aprendemos. *Revista Qurriculum*, (36), 51–60. DOI: 10.25145/j.qurricul.2023.36.03

Hastuti, D., & Malihah, N. (2024). Systematic Literature Review (SLR): Implementation of The Project-Based Learning (PJBL) Approach to Improve Students' Speaking Skills. *Proceeding of International Interdiciplinary Conference And Research Expo, 1*(1), 88-107. https://doi.org/https://doi.org/10.18326/iicare.v1i1.634

Iftikhar, S., Guerrero-Roldán, A., & Mor, E. (2022). Practice Promotes Learning: Analyzing Students' Acceptance of a Learning-by-Doing Online Programming Learning Tool. *Applied Sciences (Basel, Switzerland)*, *12*(24), 12613. DOI: 10.3390/app122412613

Kapp, K. (2012). *The gamification of learning and instruction: Game-based methods and strategies for training and education.* Pfeiffer.

Koivisto, J., & Hamari, J. (2019). The rise of motivational information systems: A review of gamification research. *International Journal of Information Management, 45*, 191–210. DOI: 10.1016/j.ijinfomgt.2018.10.013

Lampropoulos, G., & Sidiropoulos, A. (2024). Impact of Gamification on Students' Learning Outcomes and Academic Performance: A Longitudinal Study Comparing Online, Traditional, and Gamified Learning. *Education Sciences, 14*(4), 367. DOI: 10.3390/educsci14040367

Lightbot. (s.f.). *Lightbot*. Recuperado el 15 de noviembre de 2025, de https://lightbot.lu/

Marín-Marín, J., Moreno-Guerrero, A., Dúo-Terrón, P., & López-Belmonte, J. (2021). STEAM in education: A bibliometric analysis of performance and co-words in Web of Science. *International Journal of STEM Education, 8*(1), 41. DOI: 10.1186/s40594-021-00296-x PMID: 34189015

Méndez, R. M. S., Ocampo, R. D. L. S., Rebilla, E. E. R., & Azuero, D. P. S. (2024). El impacto del mal uso de la inteligencia artificial en la realización del trabajo autónomo en el entorno de educación superior. *South Florida Journal of Development, 5*(2), 681–687. DOI: 10.46932/sfjdv5n2-020

Molina-Carmona, R., & Llorens-Largo, F. (2020). Gamification and Advanced Technology to Enhance Motivation in Education. *Informatics (MDPI), 7*(2), 20. DOI: 10.3390/informatics7020020

Navarro-Mateos, C. (s/f). *Análisis del rol docente en una propuesta de gamificación en el máster de profesorado Analysis of the teaching role in a gamification proposal in the teacher's master's degree*. https://doi.org/DOI: 10.4438/1988-592X-RE-2024-405-635

Parody, L., Santos, J., Trujillo-Cayado, L. A., & Ceballos, M. (2022). Gamification in Engineering Education: The Use of Classcraft Platform to Improve Motivation and Academic Performance. *Applied Sciences (Basel, Switzerland), 12*(22), 11832. DOI: 10.3390/app122211832

Parra-Taboada, M. E., Trujillo-Arteaga, J. C., Álvarez-Abad, D. R., Arias-Domínguez, A. S., & Santillán-Gordón, E. (2024). El impacto de la inteligencia artificial en la educación. *Revista Científica Retos de la Ciencia, 1*(4), 169–181. DOI: 10.53877/rc.8.19e.202409.14

Ratinho, E., & Martins, C. (2023). The role of gamified learning strategies in student's motivation in high school and higher education: A systematic review. *Heliyon, 9*(8), e19033. DOI: 10.1016/j.heliyon.2023.e19033 PMID: 37636393

Revelo-Sánchez, O., Collazos-Ordoñez, C. A., & Jiménez-Toledo, J. A. (2018). La Gamificación como estrategia didáctica para la enseñanza/aprendizaje de la programación: Un mapeo sistemático de literatura. [revista Descontinuada]. *Lámpsakos*, *1*(19), 31–46. DOI: 10.21501/21454086.2347

Rodríguez, A. N. S., Romero, M. E. M., Agreda, C. J. R., Saldarriaga, J. G. R., & Saldarriaga, M. A. R. (2024). Impacto de la inteligencia artificial en las prácticas educativas: Percepciones y actitudes del profesorado. *LATAM Revista Latinoamericana de Ciencias Sociales y Humanidades*, *5*(2). Advance online publication. DOI: 10.56712/latam.v5i2.1933

Rodríguez-Abitia, G., Ramírez-Montoya, M. S., López-Caudana, E. O., & Romero-Rodríguez, J. M. (2021, 31 julio). *Factores para el desarrollo del pensamiento computacional en estudiantes de pregrado*. Campus Virtuales, Virtuales, 10(2), 153-164. http://uajournals.com/ojs/index.php/campusvirtuales/article/view/893

Ryan, R. M., Rigby, C. S., & Przybylski, A. (2006). The Motivational Pull of Video Games: A Self-Determination Theory Approach. *Motivation and Emotion*, *30*(4), 344–360. DOI: 10.1007/s11031-006-9051-8

Scratch. (s.f.). *Scratch – Imagine, Program, Share*. Recuperado el 15 de noviembre de 2025, de https://scratch.mit.edu/

Serrano Herrera, R. A. (2021). *Sistema de tutoría afectiva para apoyar el proceso de enseñanza y aprendizaje de estructuras de datos* [Tesis de licenciatura, Tecnológico Nacional de México]. Repositorio Institucional TecNM. https://rinacional.tecnm.mx/handle/TecNM/2700

Sosa de la Cruz, G. A. (2020). *Aplicación web para apoyar la toma de decisiones en el proceso de enseñanza de la programación* [Tesis de licenciatura, Tecnológico Nacional de México]. Repositorio Institucional TecNM. https://rinacional.tecnm.mx/handle/TecNM/2681

Sun, D., Looi, C., Li, Y., Zhu, C., Zhu, C., & Cheng, M. (2024). Block-based versus text-based programming: A comparison of learners' programming behaviors, computational thinking skills and attitudes toward programming. *Educational Technology Research and Development*, *72*(2), 1067–1089. DOI: 10.1007/s11423-023-10328-8

Tejera-Martínez, F., Aguilera, D., & Vílchez-González, J. M. (2020). Lenguajes de programación y desarrollo de competencias clave. Revisión sistemática. *Revista Electrónica de Investigación Educativa*, *22*, 1–16. DOI: 10.24320/redie.2020.22.e27.2869

Toral Aguilar, L. (2022). *Notas: «Programación básica»* [Tesis de licenciatura, Tecnológico Nacional de México]. Repositorio Institucional TecNM. https://rinacional.tecnm.mx/handle/TecNM/8191

UNIVERSAE. (21 de marzo de 2022). La *Gamificación en la educación: concepto y ejemplos*. Recuperado de https://universae.com/en/blog/gamification-in-education/

Zepeda Hurtado, M. E., Cardoso Espinoso, E. O., & Cortés Ruiz, J. A. (2019). El aprendizaje orientado en proyectos para el desarrollo de habilidades blandas en el nivel medio superior del IPN. *RIDE Revista Iberoamericana para la Investigación y el Desarrollo Educativo*, *10*(19). Advance online publication. DOI: 10.23913/ride.v10i19.530

ADDITIONAL READING

Abrahamsson, P., Hanhineva, A., Hulkko, H., Ihme, T., Juho Jäälinoja, J., Korkala, M., Koskela, J., Pekka Kyllönen y Salo, O. (2004). *Mobile-D: un enfoque ágil para el desarrollo de aplicaciones móviles.* Complemento de la 19.ª Conferencia Anual ACM SIGPLAN sobre Sistemas, Lenguajes y Aplicaciones de Programación Orientada a Objetos - OOPSLA '04. https://doi.org/DOI: 10.1145/1028664.1028736

Burgos Robles, L. J., & Huanca Torres, F. A. (2023). Quality in use evaluation model based on ISO/IEC 25022 for human talent management information systems. In Silhavy, R., & Silhavy, P. (Eds.), *Software Engineering Research in System Science* (Vol. 722, pp. 817–830). Springer., DOI: 10.1007/978-3-031-35311-6_76

Díaz-Cabriales, A., Villa Ogando, A., Carmona Soto, J. A., Díaz Rodríguez, Y. I., Olvera, Y., Muñoz Jiménez, F., Gea, M., Gómez Rodríguez, J., & García Ocaña, P. I. (2021). *Neuroeducación, de la ciencia a la práctica* (1.ª ed.) [libro electrónico]. Asociación Normalista de Profesores Investigadores. ISBN 978-607-97907-2-1

International Organization for Standardization (ISO). (2016). *ISO/IEC 25022:2016: Ingeniería de sistemas y software — Requisitos y evaluación de la calidad de los sistemas y el software (SQuaRE) — Medición de la calidad en uso.* https://www.iso.org/obp/ui/en/#iso:std:iso-iec:25022:ed-1:v1:en

Tytler, R., & Self, J. (2020). Diseño de un plan de estudios STEM contemporáneo. UNESCO. https://unesdoc.unesco.org/ark:/48223/pf0000374146

Unplugged, C. S. (2025). *¿Qué es el pensamiento computacional?* Obtenido de https://www.csunplugged.org/es/computational-thinking/

Wain, S. (2025). Primeros pasos con GameMaker: Todo lo que necesitas saber. GameMaker. https://gamemaker.io/es/tutorials/get-started-gamemaker-2025

KEY TERMS AND DEFINITIONS

Game-based learning: A methodology used in educational settings in conjunction with learning techniques to design playful experiences that benefit students.

Mobile-D: Mobile-D is an agile methodology exclusively for mobile application development. It allows for constant interaction between the work team and the client, as well as rapid response to changes that may occur during the project development stage, thereby reducing software development times.

STEAM: A teaching strategy that combines elements of science, technology, engineering, and mathematics. The STEAM approach is becoming increasingly popular among children and young people, as it is incorporated into workshops and educational courses.

Gamification: A learning technique used in the classroom to create feelings and emotions in students and contribute to the development of critical thinking and problem solving in an easy and fun way.

ISO/IEC 25022: An international standard that describes metrics for the quality of use of a system or product, covering the categories of effectiveness, efficiency, and satisfaction.

GameMaker: A development tool for creating 2D games, aimed at educators, programmers, and professional studios, with extensive support for major operating systems and entertainment consoles.

Computational thinking: A concept used in systems development that consists of the skills of algorithmic thinking, abstraction, decomposition, generalization and patterns, evaluation, and logic for problem solving.

Chapter 6

A Conceptual Proposal for an Educational Video Game to Explore Polymer Structure–Property Relationships: Macromolecules in Play

María Teresa Romero Gutiérrez
Tlajomulco University Center, University of Guadalajara, Mexico

Abraham G. Alvarado Mendoza
Universitary Center of Exact Sciences and Engineering, University of Guadalajara, Mexico

Humberto Gutiérrez-Pulido
Universitary Center of Exact Sciences and Engineering, University of Guadalajara, Mexico

Rosaura Hernández Montelongo
https://orcid.org/0000-0002-0809-5097
Universitary Center of Exact Sciences and Engineering, University of Guadalajara, Mexico

ABSTRACT

This chapter presents a conceptual proposal for an educational video game, Macromolecules in Play, designed to connect polymer structures and their material properties. Instead of learning through static formulas, players apply polymer

DOI: 10.4018/979-8-3373-4657-1.ch006

properties—such as adhesion, thermal resistance, and elasticity—to navigate challenges. Each gameplay choice is directly linked to molecular principles; for example, players learn that increasing crosslinking enhances thermal stability but reduces flexibility. The game's design emphasizes the critical concept of "trade-offs," compelling players to balance competing properties for optimal solutions. By embedding these concepts into interactive mechanics, abstract chemical knowledge becomes a tangible experience. Grounded in research on gamification, this work illustrates how interactive tools can enrich teaching in chemistry, materials science, and engineering.

INTRODUCTION

In the realm of university education, teaching macromolecular chemistry—especially topics addressing molecular structure and polymer properties—faces significant challenges. This content requires students to shift between multiple levels of representation and abstraction: from the molecular and atomic scale, invisible to the naked eye, to the macroscopic properties that determine the behavior and functionality of materials. Such cognitive transitions are not trivial. Various studies have noted that learning chemistry is often hindered by difficulties related to spatial visualization, problem solving, and mastering specialized technical vocabulary, which limits conceptual understanding and practical application (Byusa et al., 2022).

Beyond these cognitive challenges, research in chemistry education has identified several persistent misconceptions in polymer science that hinder the formation of accurate mental models connecting structure and performance.

A common confusion involves the distinction between glass-transition temperature (Tg) and melting temperature (Tm). Students often assume both correspond to the same softening process, when in fact Tg marks the onset of segmental mobility in amorphous regions, while Tm corresponds to the melting of ordered crystalline domains, where long-range packing is lost. This misunderstanding obscures how polymers can exhibit both transitions simultaneously depending on their morphology.

Another frequent misconception is that greater crystallinity always enhances material performance. Although higher crystallinity generally increases modulus and chemical resistance, it also reduces transparency, impact resistance, and flexibility, as crystalline domains scatter light and restrict chain movement. Similarly, students tend to equate the elastic modulus with tensile strength, assuming stiffness and ultimate strength are synonymous; however, the former measures the initial slope of the stress–strain curve, while the latter refers to the maximum stress before fracture—two different mechanical phenomena.

Additional errors include believing that crosslinking invariably increases durability, ignoring that excessive crosslink density can raise brittleness; assuming that all crystalline polymers are transparent, or that hydrophobicity implies universal chemical inertness.

The proposed video game explicitly integrates these conceptual pitfalls into its mechanics. For example, players must distinguish Tg and Tm when navigating environments at different temperatures, balance crystallinity to achieve strength without losing transparency, and learn through failure how over-crosslinking compromises elasticity. By confronting the practical consequences of these misconceptions in an interactive setting, students experience cognitive conflict that promotes conceptual restructuring and deeper understanding.

In the particular case of polymers, this challenge becomes even greater. Relating molecular architecture—whether linear, branched, or crosslinked—to concrete physical properties like mechanical strength, solubility, or glass transition temperature requires students to form mental connections between abstract phenomena that are not directly observable. This is not merely a memory task; it is a complex cognitive exercise in three-dimensional reasoning. Students are asked to mentally manipulate unseen chains, predict how they will entangle or align, and then translate that dynamic behavior into a tangible outcome like stiffness or elasticity. The cognitive load is substantial, as it demands a constant and fluid translation between the symbolic language of chemistry and the tangible physics of the material world. Understanding why a flexible chain can give rise to elastic materials, or how incorporating rigid aromatic groups imparts hardness, involves a feat of scientific imagination that many students find complex and counterintuitive. Without a robust mental model, concepts remain isolated facts rather than interconnected principles. For example, a student might memorize that crosslinking increases strength, but they may not truly grasp the underlying reason: the creation of a unified, three-dimensional network that resists deformation on a massive, collective scale, *a concept that is difficult to internalize without some form of dynamic visualization*. Traditional teaching, centered on lecture-based classes and theoretical explanations accompanied by formulas, has tended to encourage rote learning, in which students reproduce definitions without reaching a deep understanding (Partovi & Razavi, 2019). This passive approach, while it can transmit information, rarely enables students to develop the ability to apply what they have learned in new contexts or to integrate the different levels of chemical representation into a coherent framework.

In light of these limitations, educational literature emphasizes the need to transform pedagogical strategies toward more active, participatory, and student-centered models. It advocates for methodologies that engage students in an integral way—physically, socially, and cognitively—to foster the meaningful construction of knowledge (Kalogiannakis et al., 2021). This perspective aligns with constructivism, which conceives of learning as a process in which students construct meaning from experiences and interaction with their environment. It is not just about receiving information, but about manipulating it, questioning it, and applying it in concrete situations.

In this context, educational video games and gamification have gained ground in higher education, particularly in science and engineering fields. The rise of these strategies responds both to a pedagogical need and to a generational change: today's students have grown up immersed in interactive digital environments and are comfortable with the logic of simulation, immediate feedback, and progression through challenges. Video games provide learning environments that depart from traditional passivity and promote active, safe, and controlled experiences where students can "learn by doing" (Baek et al., 2015).

Recent literature supports the potential of game-based learning by highlighting that it emphasizes "hands-on" and "minds-on" activities—that is, experiences that combine practical action with cognitive reflection (Byusa et al., 2022). These dynamics resemble laboratory practices, computer simulations, and controlled experiments, but with the added advantage that one can design scenarios which would not be feasible in reality due to cost, time, or safety constraints. In fact, play-based strategies such as game-based learning, cooperative learning, and problem-based learning have proven particularly effective in teaching chemical concepts (Clapson et al., 2020). The value of these approaches lies in their ability to engage students on multiple dimensions, fostering positive attitudes toward learning and raising levels of motivation and interest (Sousa Lima et al., 2019).

One of the main attractions of video games in education lies in their alignment with the cultural habits of university students. Incorporating game elements into teaching naturally captures students' attention by leveraging a medium that is familiar and motivating for them (Kalogiannakis et al., 2021). Indeed, recent research indicates that gamification in scientific contexts has sparked growing interest among academics, precisely because it connects with an environment familiar to students and has the potential to stimulate their intrinsic motivation toward academic content (Byusa et al., 2022). Various reviews conclude that, when carefully designed, gamification can transfer the motivational power of games to the educational context, facilitating the development of scientific thinking in a manner compatible with current pedagogical trends (Kalogiannakis et al., 2021).

It is true, however, that some studies have reported mixed results regarding the impact of games on academic performance. These discrepancies are usually attributed to differences in game design, how they are implemented, and student characteristics (Partovi & Razavi, 2019). However, beyond these variations, the emerging consensus is that a well-planned integration of game elements contributes significantly to improving the educational experience. Success depends less on the game itself than on how it is aligned with clear learning objectives and accompanied by appropriate teacher facilitation.

Chemistry education, with its numerous abstract concepts, finds in video games a particularly valuable resource for mediating understanding. Content such as the molecular structure of polymers, which is elusive to students because it is not directly observable, can be made more accessible through simulations, visual metaphors, and interactive dynamics integrated into a playful environment. According to Clapson et al. (2020), games offer educators new ways to help students establish intangible connections between concepts, fostering meaningful learning. In their experience, they documented activities such as board games and bioplastic synthesis exercises in a materials chemistry course that included polymer content. The results were positive: students achieved a better understanding of the relationship between the chemical structure of materials and their macroscopic properties, and also benefited from a friendly competitive environment that increased their motivation and participation.

Beyond qualitative observations, the authors also collected quantitative data through a post-activity survey. Over 80% of respondents reported that the game-based activities helped them better understand key course concepts, and a strong majority indicated that the activities were enjoyable and strengthened the perceived link between theory and practice. Taken together, these survey results support integrating game-based learning into materials chemistry—not merely as a source of enjoyment, but as a means to bolster motivation, active engagement, and deeper conceptual understanding.

Although game-based learning and serious games have shown strong potential to enhance engagement and conceptual understanding, several studies have highlighted limitations that educators must consider. Reported outcomes often depend on the learner's prior knowledge, motivation, and the extent of instructor guidance during gameplay. Moreover, success within a game does not always translate into robust conceptual mastery or long-term retention, since some students may rely on trial-and-error strategies without fully articulating underlying principles. Technical and logistical constraints—such as limited access to devices, insufficient faculty training, and the time required for curricular alignment—also affect implementation. Recognizing these factors helps position Macromolecules in Play as a complementary pedagogical resource that supports but does not replace traditional instruction, ensuring its integration within a structured, evidence-based learning design.

Other studies provide specific evidence of how interactive simulations support the teaching of abstract chemical phenomena. Clark (2024) reports the implementation of multiple simulations from the PhET platform in a general chemistry course focused on studying the greenhouse effect. In this experience, students not only manipulated molecular representations—Lewis structures, VSEPR geometries, and polarity—but also connected these models to socio-scientific issues such as climate change and its policy implications. The results were positive: 90% appreciated the inclusion of a real-world context and the majority recognized that the simulations made it easier to understand invisible processes, such as the interaction between radiation and molecules. However, the study also notes tensions between exploratory activities and the demands of preparation for standardized exams, which highlights the importance of a coherent curricular design that aligns the simulations with assessment objectives.

Along the same lines, a recent systematic review (Aliyu, 2025) analyzed the use of PhET in chemistry education and concluded that these simulations are most effective when combined with active methodologies such as guided inquiry, collaborative learning, and problem-based learning. The added value of simulations lies in their ability to represent abstract chemical phenomena in a visual and manipulable manner—such as atomic structure, bonding, or chemical equilibrium—and in their potential to foster the transfer of knowledge to practical contexts. Taken together, the reviewed studies report significant improvements in motivation, participation, and conceptual understanding, confirming that PhET should not be understood as an isolated resource, but as part of active, structured pedagogical strategies.

The range of gamification applications in chemistry is further expanded by innovative experiences like the one reported by Dietrich (2018), who implemented an educational "escape room" in which students had to solve chemistry puzzles to "escape" a fictional scenario. The experience involved 40 students and four instructors, and was evaluated through surveys that yielded clear quantitative data: 93% felt that the activity increased their motivation, 96% indicated it strengthened teamwork skills, and 90% reported improvements in communication. Additionally, 67% acknowledged that the activity fostered more active learning than a traditional class, and 80% would recommend repeating the experience. These results suggest that escape rooms not only reinforce content understanding, but also promote essential social skills such as collaboration, communication, and joint problem-solving.

In summary, the accumulated evidence shows that gamification and educational video games offer chemistry education—and in particular polymer education—a dimension of immersion and experimentation that is difficult to achieve with traditional methods. Far from being passive recipients, students become protagonists of their own learning, exploring and constructing meaning in interactive settings. This hands-on experience not only facilitates conceptual understanding, but also lays the groundwork for a more robust transfer of knowledge to real situations or practical problems, the ultimate goal of science education.

In this context, the present chapter proposes a concept for an educational video game called *Macromolecules in Play*, whose purpose is to playfully and narratively explore the relationships between molecular structure and polymer properties. The proposal falls within the tradition of active, constructivist approaches, and seeks to illustrate how gamification can be employed not only to motivate, but also to translate abstract concepts into tangible and meaningful learning experiences.

THEORETICAL FRAMEWORK

Serious Games

Serious games are digital applications designed with an educational purpose that goes beyond entertainment. Unlike commercial video games, whose primary goal is recreation, serious games structure their narrative, rules, and objectives around pedagogical aims, such as teaching disciplinary concepts or developing cognitive skills (Ullah et al., 2022). Their theoretical foundation is often associated with constructivism, which emphasizes learning through active experience and interaction. However, contemporary educational design also integrates cognitivist and behaviorist principles—such as feedback, reinforcement, and structured progression—showing that serious games can draw on multiple complementary learning theories to achieve effective outcomes. In this regard, video games provide active learning environments where learners can explore, make decisions, receive immediate feedback, and repeat attempts without real-world risks. These elements not only foster conceptual understanding but also enhance intrinsic motivation and sustained engagement.

A systematic review by Ullah et al. (2022) on serious games in science education found that most studies report improvements in students' comprehension of abstract phenomena and in their motivation, particularly in disciplines such as physics and biology. Nevertheless, the authors cautioned that much of the available evidence shows methodological limitations—such as small sample sizes or less rigorous experimental designs—which means results should be interpreted carefully. Even so, the consensus across the reviewed literature is that, when well designed and properly integrated into teaching, serious games constitute an effective strategy for transforming complex content into accessible learning experiences.

Similar findings were reported by Sierra-Daza et al. (2023), who reviewed 62 articles published between 2016 and 2021 and concluded that video games in higher education mainly promote the development of instrumental competences—such as general foundational knowledge—followed by systemic competences like achievement motivation. By contrast, interpersonal competences, which are essential for collaborative work and interdisciplinary communication, have been less frequently addressed, pointing to an area of opportunity for future integration in game-supported educational experiences. Complementarily, Tene et al. (2025) carried out a systematic review in the STEM field and confirmed that serious games not only enhance student motivation and engagement but also improve knowledge acquisition and retention, as well as the application of concepts in practical scenarios. Taken together, this body of evidence reinforces the idea that, when designed with clear pedagogical criteria and articulated with the curriculum, serious games are an effective strategy for translating complex content into accessible and motivating learning experiences.

Recent Cases in the Sciences

In recent years, several empirical experiences have demonstrated the value of educational digital games in university-level science education. Although cases specifically centered on polymers or macromolecules remain limited, there are relevant initiatives in related fields that illustrate the potential of this approach.

One such example is the digital game *C=ocarbohydrates*, developed by Vera-Monroy et al. (2020) for students of organic chemistry. The study compared an experimental group ($n = 111$) with a control group ($n = 79$), using a pretest–posttest design validated with a Cronbach's alpha of 0.85. Results showed that the experimental group improved its performance by an average of 2.6 points compared to the control group, with statistically significant differences. Moreover, 88% of students in the experimental group reached the highest score levels, reflecting not only improved conceptual learning but also a reduction in the dispersion of results. In terms of perception, students reported that the game increased their motivation, facilitated the understanding of abstract concepts, and promoted collaborative work. This case demonstrates how video games can translate complex content into interactive dynamics, fostering both comprehension and the development of the cognitive processes needed for learning.

Another example is *The Mysterious Compound*, an online narrative video game designed by Yacoub and Holton (2023) for a general chemistry course. In this game, students take on the role of detectives who must solve chemistry problems to gather clues and advance in a mystery storyline. Evaluation results showed significant increases in self-confidence across all course topics ($p < 0.001$), with average improvements ranging from 0.8 to 1.2 points on a five-point Likert scale. Furthermore, 85% of participants positively valued the narrative as a motivating element and as a useful resource for review. Although the authors note that academic outcomes were not directly measured and no control group was included, this experience highlights that online narrative games can be effective tools in virtual or hybrid contexts, offering immersive dynamics that either complement or substitute in-person practice.

Taken together, these recent cases demonstrate that digital video games can be successfully applied in science education, generating improvements in conceptual understanding, motivation, and student participation. Although no games specifically focused on polymers have yet been developed, the available evidence suggests that this approach is both relevant and adaptable to this field.

Challenges and Limitations

The incorporation of complex scientific content into digital video games involves significant pedagogical and technical challenges. According to Tene et al. (2025), one of the main difficulties lies in maintaining a balance between conceptual accuracy and playability, since STEM phenomena—such as chemical or molecular processes—often require abstract representations that do not always easily translate into interactive dynamics. Simplification of content is necessary to enhance accessibility, but it carries the risk of distorting key notions if not grounded in rigorous pedagogical design. The authors also point to structural limitations such as technological barriers, the lack of specialized teacher training, and the scarcity of curricular frameworks that systematically integrate serious games into instruction.

Similarly, Ullah et al. (2022), in their review of the literature on serious games in science education, observed that while evidence indicates these resources improve motivation and knowledge acquisition, many studies show methodological shortcomings and wide variability in effectiveness. In particular, they warn that cognitive overload can become an obstacle if game design combines overly complex mechanics with advanced academic content. To prevent this, the authors recommend intuitive interfaces, gradual progression, and clearly defined learning objectives. Together, these findings confirm that serious games hold considerable potential for teaching abstract concepts, provided they are developed on solid pedagogical foundations and implemented with strategies that account for both technological context and the needs of teachers and students.

Practical aspects also pose important limitations. Developing high-quality educational games requires significant economic and human resources, as well as collaboration among experts in scientific content, pedagogy, design, and programming. Added to this is the teacher's role: instructors need specific training to integrate these resources into their classes, connect the game experience with curricular objectives, and ensure they are not perceived as disconnected activities. High development costs, technological demands, and the difficulty of aligning games with standardized curricula remain frequent challenges. Finally, impact assessment is still an area needing improvement. Although multiple studies report increases in motivation and positive perceptions, further longitudinal research with more robust methodologies is needed to determine the extent to which video games promote durable and transferable learning (Tene et al., 2025).

To operationalize this role, the chapter introduces a three-phase instructional guide to integrate the game into formal teaching:

1. Pre-game (briefing). The instructor introduces the learning objectives and elicits students' preconceptions—for example, asking what they believe happens to a

polymer when heated or crosslinked—to surface potential misconceptions such as "Tg equals Tm." This diagnostic dialogue frames gameplay as hypothesis testing.

2. During gameplay (guided inquiry). The instructor monitors progress, formulates reflective prompts ("How did crystallinity affect transparency?"), and encourages students to justify in real time the molecular basis of their choices. Short pauses for group reflection allow connecting visual outcomes—loss of elasticity, cracking, opacity—to underlying polymer physics and chemistry.
3. Post-game (debriefing). A collective discussion links in-game phenomena to experimental or industrial analogues. Students reinterpret failed strategies (e.g., over-crosslinking leading to brittleness) in terms of structure–property relationships, strengthening metacognition and conceptual transfer.

This tripartite model ensures that the game serves not as a stand-alone entertainment tool but as an interactive learning cycle tightly coupled with theory, experimentation, and teacher facilitation.

DESIGN METHODOLOGY

Pedagogical Approach and Theoretical Foundations

The design of this educational video game is framed within a constructivist approach, where learning is understood as an active, situated, and context-dependent process. According to Jonassen (1999), students do not acquire knowledge passively; rather, they build it through exploration, problem solving, and reflection on their actions in meaningful scenarios. This idea is particularly relevant for teaching macromolecular chemistry, where concepts such as the three-dimensional structure of polymers or the relationship between properties and performance are highly abstract and difficult to visualize.

Problem-Based Learning (PBL) complements this framework by placing students in contextualized challenges that require them to mobilize their knowledge in order to find solutions. Barrows (1986), a pioneer of this approach, emphasized that problems should act as triggers for learning, since facing students with open-ended and relevant situations fosters critical reasoning, the generation of hypotheses, and the transfer of knowledge to real contexts. In the proposed video game, this logic is adapted to the field of polymer chemistry: challenges are designed as problem-scenarios in which students must interpret environmental conditions, identify which polymer property is required, and strategically apply it to overcome an obstacle, thereby reproducing the cycle of analysis and resolution characteristic of PBL.

To extend the constructivist logic of PBL, the chapter specifies how the game will evaluate and foster knowledge transfer beyond rote learning.

Transfer is addressed at two complementary levels:

- Near transfer, where students apply a concept learned in one context—such as the relation between chain flexibility and Tg—to similar but not identical situations (e.g., modifying polymer composition to maintain elasticity under moderate heat); and
- Far transfer, where they extrapolate that knowledge to qualitatively new problems, such as choosing suitable materials for biomedical implants, high-temperature coatings, or water-repellent packaging.

The game architecture intentionally scales difficulty through these stages. Early missions emphasize recognition and adaptation of known polymer behaviors, whereas advanced missions demand reasoning across unfamiliar conditions, combining multiple variables (thermal, mechanical, and chemical).

Assessment of transfer integrates in-game analytics—tracking how players adjust parameters after feedback—with post-game situational questions that require explicit justification, not mere guessing. For instance: "A polymeric component must function at 140 °C without losing toughness; which structural feature should be increased to prevent embrittlement?" The design therefore operationalizes both measurement and promotion of transfer, ensuring that cognitive gains are not limited to the simulated environment.

A third pillar is gamification, understood as the incorporation of game elements—levels, rewards, narrative progression, immediate feedback—into educational settings (Kalogiannakis et al., 2021). The relevance of these approaches is also reflected in recent literature. Ullah et al. (2022) report that serious games applied in science education improve the understanding of abstract phenomena and strengthen students' confidence in working with complex concepts, although they caution that many studies lack strong methodological design. Complementarily, Byusa et al. (2022) highlight that game-based learning increases intrinsic motivation, active participation, and academic performance, provided it is articulated with clear pedagogical objectives and integrated into a structured didactic framework. Taken together, these findings confirm that gamification and game-based learning can be valuable tools, but they require careful planning in order to generate sustainable benefits.

Altogether, these foundations ensure that the video game is not a mere recreational resource, but rather an integral pedagogical strategy that aligns intrinsic motivation with clear formative goals: to understand, apply, and transfer the relationship between structure, properties, and performance in polymers.

Technical Development and Usability

The feasibility of the project largely depends on the selection of development tools capable of integrating pedagogy, science, and gameplay in a coherent environment. For this purpose, open-source engines widely used in education, such as Unity and Godot, are considered. Both offer technical and didactic advantages:

- **Stylized representations of properties**: these allow concepts such as elasticity or transparency to be translated into visual and physical dynamics accessible to players, without the need to model complex mathematical equations.
- **Explorable environments**: they make it possible to create wide scenarios where the player can freely move, observe conditions, and make decisions that affect their progress.
- **Integration of mini-laboratories**: they enable the design of minigames that simulate experimental practices, such as measuring contact angles, performing simplified thermal tests, or testing impact resistance.
- **Immediate feedback**: every action can trigger visible responses (color change, deformation, degradation), clearly linking decision with consequence.
- **Multiplatform accessibility**: the game can be deployed on PCs, mobile devices, or web browsers, facilitating adoption across educational levels.

Beyond the chosen tool, technical design must guarantee educational usability. This means that interfaces must be intuitive, graphics should prioritize conceptual understanding over aesthetic realism, and game dynamics should reduce unnecessary cognitive load. The focus should remain on the scientific challenge, not on the complexity of the controls. Literature supports these design choices: Marfisi-Schottman et al. (2010) stress that the success of educational games depends on the coherence between pedagogical objectives and game mechanics. In this sense, selecting engines like Unity or Godot does not simply respond to technological trends, but rather to their ability to translate abstract scientific phenomena into interactive and comprehensible experiences. Finally, technical design incorporates accessibility and equity criteria—legible fonts, appropriate contrasts, customizable control options, and audio/text modes—which ensure that the tool is inclusive and adaptable to diverse educational contexts.

Didactic Strategy and Game Dynamics

The core pedagogical strategy is to transform highly abstract scientific content into mechanics that can be directly experienced by the learner. Instead of introducing polymer properties through static definitions, the game requires players to demonstrate understanding by applying those properties to advance. For example, adhesion is not explained in a text box but embodied through tasks that require clinging to surfaces or manipulating sticky environments. Thermal resistance is not a numerical value but a condition for survival in simulated high-temperature zones. Elasticity is not only a theoretical modulus but the visible capacity to stretch, rebound, and absorb energy during challenges. Transparency becomes a mechanism to reveal or conceal pathways, while hydrophobicity and hydrophilicity are embedded in puzzles involving water absorption, flotation, or swelling. Finally, chemical resistance appears in the form of protective responses to corrosive agents. This experiential translation ensures that each property is first encountered as an interactive phenomenon and only later associated with its scientific terminology, reinforcing meaningful and durable learning.

In this way, students experience the concept before naming it, which facilitates meaningful and lasting understanding. The game also integrates a system of trade-offs, inspired by real-world materials science practice. Not all properties can be maximized simultaneously: increasing hardness implies losing flexibility; higher crystallinity may improve mechanical strength but reduce transparency; reinforcing chemical resistance may limit elasticity.

The interaction model follows a three-step pedagogical cycle:

1. **Exploration**: the player observes the environment and detects clues that suggest the need for certain properties.
2. **Diagnosis and selection**: based on these clues, the player infers which property to activate and with what combination.
3. **Immediate feedback**: the game responds to the decision with visible consequences (success, partial failure, progressive degradation), reinforcing the cause–effect relationship.

Progression in the game is directly linked to formative assessment. Every completed task or successfully solved challenge becomes tangible evidence that the learner has not only recognized but also applied a scientific property. Rather than relying on conventional exams, the game itself produces performance data—choices made, errors corrected, and strategies employed—that can be interpreted as indicators of conceptual mastery. This approach resonates with alternative assessment models in education, where evidence of learning emerges from authentic performance in context. By requiring players to plan, test, and revise their strategies, the game promotes iterative reasoning that mirrors real scientific practice. Ultimately, the didactic model does more than entertain: it transforms abstraction into lived experience, places students in the role of materials scientists, and encourages reflection on the trade-offs between different properties and design decisions.

In addition to assessing individual conceptual mastery, the chapter incorporates a framework for evaluating collaborative competencies that may emerge during cooperative gameplay. These include communication of scientific reasoning, joint problem-solving, and shared decision-making—skills repeatedly highlighted in the literature as key outcomes of serious games but rarely measured explicitly. To address this gap, the proposed evaluation strategy combines qualitative observation and telemetric indicators: the system records team interactions (turn-taking, frequency of concept-based dialogue, and distribution of tasks), while instructors apply a four-criterion rubric focusing on (1) role coordination, (2) accuracy of explanations, (3) collective decision quality, and (4) regulation of group effort. Data from these measures complement individual scores from the Polymer Science Concept Inventory (PSCI) and provide a multidimensional perspective on learning. This integration ensures that the game supports not only cognitive but also interpersonal learning goals, aligning with current constructivist models that view knowledge as socially co-constructed.

Chemical Foundations in the Video Game Design

The proposed video game design is sustained by the translation of polymer properties into learning dynamics that allow students to interact with concepts usually perceived as abstract. From an academic standpoint, this means that each gameplay mechanic is grounded in principles of macromolecular chemistry and materials science, which must be represented with sufficient conceptual fidelity to avoid distortions, but also with a degree of simplification that fosters understanding.

Structural properties and surface adhesion

One of the first concepts incorporated is stickiness, understood as the ability of certain polymers to adhere to surfaces. At the molecular level, this property depends on the presence of functional groups capable of establishing specific interactions, such as hydrogen bonds, electrostatic forces, or dipole–dipole interactions, which strengthen interfacial contact. Polymers such as polyvinyl acetate (PVAc), the basis of school adhesives, have flexible chains and acetate groups that facilitate adhesion to polar substrates. In the video game, this principle is translated into dynamics of fixation and bridge construction, allowing players to experience how molecular interactions and chain mobility influence observable macroscopic behavior (Raos & Zappone, 2021).

Crosslinking and thermal resistance

Fire resistance and thermal stability are grounded in the presence of aromatic structures and chain crosslinking. Polymers such as PEEK contain aromatic rings that provide rigidity and favor the formation of carbonaceous char rather than melting, which grants excellent resistance under high-temperature conditions. Pedagogically, this property illustrates how chemical structure conditions thermal degradation, and how crosslinking limits molecular mobility, increasing the glass transition temperature (Tg) and heat resistance. Integrating this principle into the game reinforces the idea that polymer selection is not arbitrary but depends on molecular architecture and service conditions (Ramgobin et al., 2020).

Elasticity and chain mobility

Elasticity is another central property, closely related to polymers with low crystallinity and high conformational mobility, such as natural rubber or polybutadiene. This behavior originates from the presence of double bonds and long chains that allow reversible deformations, in contrast to more rigid structures (Treloar, 2013). In the video game, the ability to stretch, bounce, and recover shape translates this principle into visible actions, connecting the player's experience with the concept of elastic deformation and energy recovery stored within the polymer network.

Crystallinity and mechanical hardness

In contrast, mechanical hardness is associated with the degree of crystallinity and chain crosslinking. Semi-crystalline polymers such as high-density polyethylene (HDPE) or isotactic polypropylene form crystalline regions that act as rigid domains, thereby increasing the elastic modulus and impact resistance. In the educational context, this concept demonstrates that greater crystallinity enhances stiffness but reduces flexibility, generating a tension between properties that students must learn to manage (Mark, 2020).

Transparency and structural order

Transparency is linked to a material's ability to allow light to pass without significant scattering. In polymers, this occurs when the matrix is amorphous and lacks crystalline domains that interfere with the propagation of radiation (Rabek, 2012). Classic examples include polycarbonate (PC) and polymethyl methacrylate (PMMA). In the video game, transparency is translated into the ability to become invisible or overcome optical obstacles, helping students understand that the disordered structure of a material can be advantageous in certain applications, such as lenses or coatings.

Polarity, water, and swelling phenomena

Hydrophobicity and hydrophilicity introduce the role of polarity and surface energy in water interaction. Polymers such as polytetrafluoroethylene (PTFE) exhibit nonpolar chains and C–F bonds with low surface energy, resulting in water-repellent surfaces. By contrast, hydrogels (e.g., sodium polyacrylate) contain charged functional groups that promote water absorption and volumetric swelling. In the video game, these behaviors are modeled through the ability to float, repel contaminated water, or absorb liquids to activate mechanisms, reinforcing the notion that the chemistry of functional groups translates into relevant macroscopic phenomena (Parvate et al., 2020).

Chemical stability and resistance to degradation

Finally, chemical resistance is based on the strength of covalent bonds and the absence of reactive functional groups in the main chain. Polymers such as PTFE and polyvinylidene fluoride (PVDF) show high stability against acids, bases, and solvents due to the robustness of the C–F bond (Ebnesajjad, 2013). Within the video game, this property is represented as immunity to corrosive or toxic atmospheres, reinforcing the link between chemical structure and the functional durability of materials.

Pedagogical Implications

Beyond the isolated description of each property, the academic value of the video game lies in demonstrating that materials do not exhibit an "ideal profile." Properties are often in tension: increased crystallinity improves hardness but reduces transparency; higher crosslinking enhances thermal resistance but reduces elasticity; stronger chemical resistance may limit processability. This system of trade-offs lies at the core of materials science, and by being integrated into game dynamics, it compels students to reflect on how each design decision impacts overall performance.

In addition, playable dynamics allow the simulation of experimental phenomena that are difficult to observe in a conventional classroom. Glass transition, hydrogel swelling, or thermal degradation can be represented as interactive events that accompany narrative progression. Thus, learning moves from a memorization-based model to an experiential one, bringing students closer to a more comprehensive understanding of polymer chemistry.

PROPOSAL DESCRIPTION

The proposal is an open-world video game that turns polymer properties into mechanics for exploration, problem solving, and decision making. The pedagogical objective is for understanding of concepts such as stickiness, fire resistance, elasticity, hardness, transparency, hydrophobicity, hydrophilicity, and chemical resistance to emerge from gameplay rather than from exogenous interruptions. The target audience includes upper-secondary and early undergraduate students, as well as instructors interested in interactive resources to introduce structure–property–processing–performance relationships.

The narrative follows Bond-er (Figure 1.), an apprentice of the Guild of Formers and bearer of the Sigma Mesh, an exosuit capable of integrating polymer property profiles that alter the character's capabilities depending on the environment. Bond-er is accompanied by Slinky, a gel module that performs scanning, logging, and instructional assistance throughout the adventure.

Figure 1. Bond-er and Slinky in a cel-shaded map style. Bond-er wears the Sigma Mesh with an amber hexagonal cuirass, transparent bracers, and elastic bands; Slinky, a translucent gel module with membranous wings, serves as guide and scanner. The color palette evokes the game's biomes and the thermal, optical, adhesive, elastic, and hydrophobic profiles.

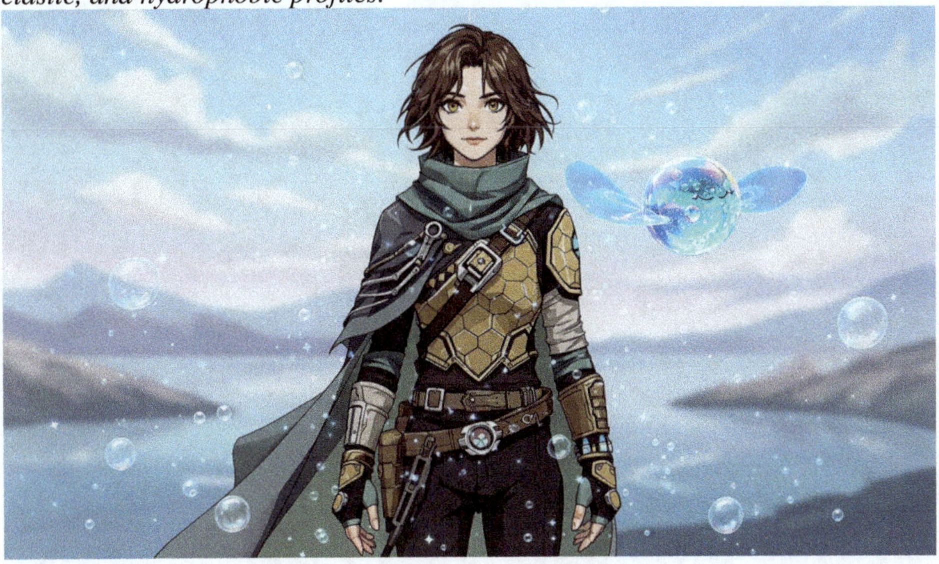

After the Great Cracking—a mass chain-scission event that released monomers and radicals and destabilized the territory—the Omnimer emerged: a distributed intelligence of programmable matter formed by polymer networks that self-assemble and reconfigure according to environmental conditions. Its operation consists of exploring and locking in macromolecular configurations—such as crosslink density, crystallinity, orientation, and surface chemistry—to optimize continuity within stability windows defined by glass transition temperature, pH, and radiation. Vitrio (Figure 2.), a former master, provides control algorithms and access to resources, accelerating the Omnimer's deployment. In gameplay terms, this dynamic is modeled as an observable optimization process: the Omnimer imitates combinations of properties the player employs, leaves measurable traces that Slinky records (Young's modulus, contact angle, mass loss), and forces the player to counter it with material designs tailored to each biome.

Figure 2. Vitrio, the Omnimer's human interface. He supplies algorithms and provisions to the Omnimer and catalyzes its expansion across biomes.

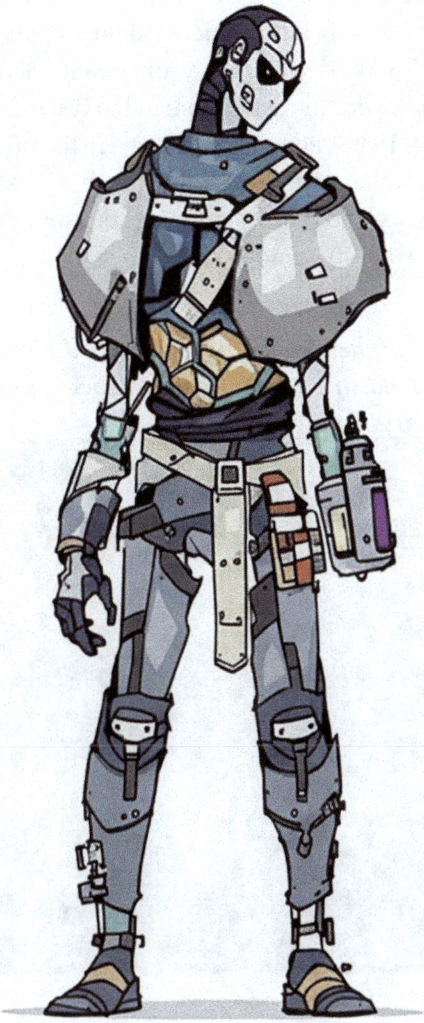

To reach the core of the matrix and decide the Omnimer's fate, Bond-er must obtain Phase Seals by clearing sanctuaries and forging alliances across an archipelago of interconnected biomes that function as open-air laboratories. Each seal certifies mastery of a structure–property–process linkage through observable metrics recorded by Slinky—for example, estimates of glass transition and melting points from thermal tests, contact angle, impact energy, and mass loss by degradation. In the Igneous Crater, with thermal gradients and oxidizing atmospheres, players discriminate between glass transition (Tg) and melting (Tm) and optimize thermal stabilization; in the Acid Marsh they evaluate chemical resistance and swelling; in the Tensile Canyon they bring elastic modulus, resilience, and adhesion into play; in the Sunken City they explore hydrophobicity and hydrophilicity through floating, diffusion, and hydraulic activation; in the Prism Laser Lab they work with transparency, refractive index, and scattering; and in the Impact Range they measure toughness and fatigue under cyclic loading (Figure 3.). Alliances with local clans provide recipes, additives, and processing routes that unlock more efficient polymer configurations within stability windows.

Figure 3. Archipelago of the Matrix. Interconnected biomes and sanctuaries that structure learning around structure–property–process links and the selection/formulation of the appropriate polymer.

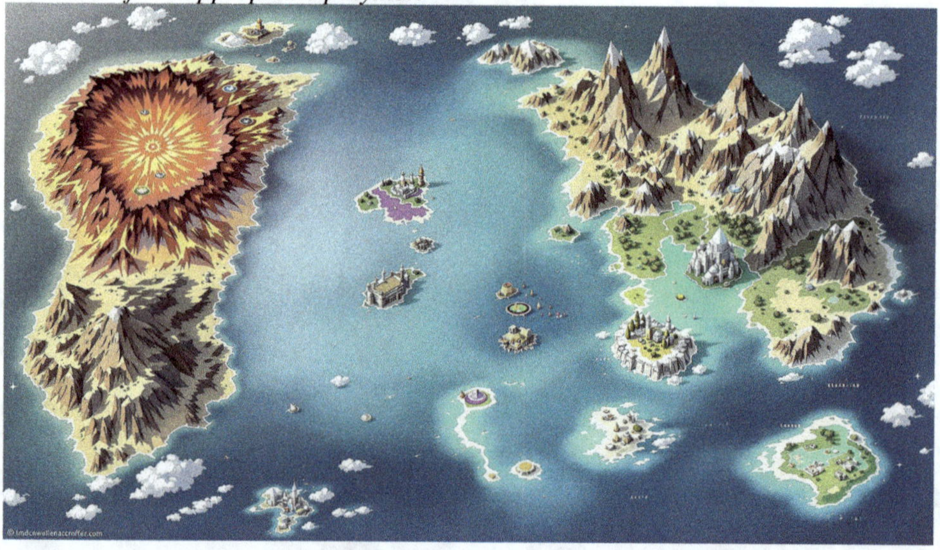

As the game progresses, Slinky's metrics make visible how every formulation and processing decision carries material and environmental consequences—tracking input consumption, waste generation, degradation, and energy footprint. This decision trail becomes part of the narrative and leads to three possible endings, depending on the player's design style: reprogram the Omnimer, confine it, or integrate it with safeguards and controls for responsible use.

The core mechanics weave together environment reading and aspect selection, resource management, and synthesis/processing. The player assesses thermal, chemical, optical, mechanical, and hydrodynamic risks to activate the pertinent aspect while managing bond energy and degradation due to heat, ultraviolet radiation, or corrosive agents. Obtaining new configurations requires combining monomers, additives, crosslinkers, and reinforcements; the choice of processing routes quantitatively modifies mobility, strength, and transparency. Levels are organized into theme sanctuaries with integrated mini-lab tests—for example, estimating glass transition by differential scanning calorimetry (DSC) or dynamic mechanical analysis (DMA), measuring contact angle, and performing impact tests—all embedded within open-world biomes with clan objectives and alternate routes, and in boss encounters that demand chaining properties together and recognizing operational limits such as thermal windows, impact fatigue, or performance loss due to over-crosslinking. Interaction is supported by Slinky, which enables in-game technical sheets with indicative values for Tg, Tm, Young's modulus, and contact angle, and by a property tree that lets players modulate crosslink density and crystalline fraction while making trade-offs explicit.

Within the narrative, these scientific concepts are reimagined as distinct abilities of the main character. Stickiness becomes the power to scale vertical cliffs or weave adhesive bridges. Fire resistance equips the player to traverse blazing corridors or operate furnaces in hostile biomes. Elasticity grants the capacity to vault across gaps or rebound from falling rocks. Hardness takes the form of a shield or battering ram against massive impacts. Transparency enables stealth and safe passage through laser grids. Hydrophobicity supports stable flotation on contaminated waters, while hydrophilicity activates hydraulic gates through controlled swelling. Chemical resistance provides survival in corrosive atmospheres. By embedding each concept into the storyline as a skill, the game ensures that learners do not simply recall definitions but practice them as tools for exploration and survival.

Selecting the appropriate polymer in each context is framed as situated challenges that require diagnosing properties from environmental cues. Sustained passage over incandescent platforms calls for fire resistance and—under prolonged exposure—ceramic-reinforced formulations that raise thermal tolerance. Ascending smooth walls demands adhesion, while combining it with elasticity enables a controlled elastic leap to clear ledges. Crossing an abyss with crosswinds is solved through elasticity for bounce and damping; if the landing involves impact, adding hardness reduces structural damage. Navigating laser grids and optical sensors is approached with transparency via amorphous compositions that ensure transmission and effective index control. Traversing a toxic lagoon under acid rain requires chemical resistance and, in the presence of swell and waves, support from hydrophobicity for flotation and surface stability. Activating hydraulic gates is achieved with hydrophilicity, leveraging the increase in volume and mass due to absorption. Clearing rock corridors with rockfall hazards calls for hardness as armor and ram, with explicit management of accumulated fatigue.

The link between chemical structures and properties is made explicit in every design decision. Increases in crosslink density raise service temperature and hardness but reduce elongation and macromolecular mobility, forcing a balance between the reach of elasticity and the protection of hardness. The crystalline fraction and chain regularity confer stiffness and toughness, whereas amorphous matrices favor transparency and fine control of refractive index—the foundation of transparency mechanics. Aromatic and imide segments—conceptually analogous to aramids or PEEK—confer thermal stability and a tendency toward char formation under flame, consistent with fire resistance. The presence of hydrophilic groups such as –OH, –COOH, $–SO_3H$, or $–NH_2$ promotes water absorption and controlled swelling, useful for hydrophilicity; in contrast, $–CF_2–$ units and low-energy nonpolar chains underpin hydrophobicity and chemical resistance. Specific interactions such as hydrogen bonding and catechol motifs enhance adhesion on wet or mineral surfaces, providing the basis for stickiness. Increases in average molar mass and entanglement density improve toughness and impact behavior; adding fillers and reinforcements (silica, fibers, ceramics) raises the thermo-mechanical modulus at the cost of transparency and with increased density—trade-offs the player perceives as a balance between performance and resource cost. Stabilizing additives—antioxidants, phosphorus-based flame retardants, and UV absorbers—limit oxidation, radiation damage, and flame effects, extending the functional life of configurations in hostile biomes.

Taken together, the design proposes that mastering structure–property–process linkages is not an informational appendix but the very condition for narrative progression and for solving the world's challenges. Slinky acts as a pedagogical interface that translates environmental observations into formulation hypotheses, while the resource economy and degradation logs foster responsible decision making aligned with materials-science practice.

MEASUREMENT INSTRUMENTS AND EVIDENCE OF KNOWLEDGE TRANSFER

The primary objective of the video game is to improve students' understanding of complex polymer structure-property relationships. To measure this outcome, a custom-designed Polymer Science Concept Inventory (PSCI) will be developed. This instrument will be administered in a quasi-experimental pretest/posttest design to measure the change in conceptual understanding after the gameplay intervention compared to a control group receiving traditional instruction (Hernández-Sampieri & Mendoza-Torres, 2018).

This instrument will be grounded in a learner-centered pedagogical framework consistent with the principles of self-determination and active engagement (Ryan & Deci, 2000; Hamari et al., 2016). Within this perspective, learning will be understood as an active process in which students construct understanding through meaningful interaction with contextualized challenges. Consequently, assessment will aim to go beyond factual recall to capture learners' ability to reorganize and apply concepts in novel situations represented within the game environment. The PSCI will therefore be designed not only to quantify learning gains but also to elicit evidence of conceptual reasoning, problem solving, and the application of prior knowledge to unfamiliar scenarios.

The development of the PSCI will follow a rigorous, multi-stage process. Initially, a detailed list of learning objectives will be defined based on the core concepts embedded in the game's mechanics, such as glass transition temperature (Tg), melting temperature (Tm), crystallinity, chemical resistance, and the principles of adhesion and elasticity. For each objective, a series of questions will be drafted, encompassing various cognitive levels (from recall to application and analysis). The question formats will include multiple-choice questions with research-based distractors—incorrect options that represent common student misconceptions—as well as problem-solving scenarios that require students to apply their knowledge in a novel context similar to the challenges presented in the game. For instance, a question might present a scenario: "A polymer-based character needs to cross a chasm in the 'Igneous Crater' biome where ground temperatures are extremely high. Which of the following polymer properties should the character enhance to avoid becoming brittle and failing?" This format directly assesses the student's ability to transfer knowledge from the game to a problem-solving context.

To ensure that correct answers will reflect genuine conceptual transfer rather than intuitive guessing, several PSCI items will include short justification prompts requiring students to explain their reasoning. These responses will be evaluated through a rubric focusing on conceptual accuracy, coherence, and relevance, providing complementary qualitative evidence of the mental processes involved in learning appropriation and problem-solving transfer.

To ensure content validity, the initial pool of questions will be reviewed by a panel of subject matter experts, including polymer chemists and chemical education specialists. Their feedback will be used to refine the questions, clarify wording, and confirm that the instrument accurately covers the intended conceptual domain. Subsequently, the instrument will be piloted with a cohort of students not involved in the main study to assess its psychometric properties, including item difficulty, item discrimination, and internal consistency (reliability), typically measured using

Cronbach's alpha. The final version of the PSCI will serve as the primary quantitative measure of learning gain.

To ensure psychometric and construct validity, the PSCI will undergo a complementary validation process beyond the pilot phase.

- Content validity will be reinforced through a second expert review, ensuring alignment between game-based objectives and the conceptual dimensions assessed (e.g., thermal transitions, crystallinity, crosslinking, and molecular mobility).
- Construct validity will be examined through exploratory factor analysis to verify that items group coherently around theoretical constructs such as mechanical, thermal, and structural understanding.
- Criterion validity will be tested by correlating PSCI post-test scores with in-game analytics—such as correct property selection and adaptive decision patterns—and, where possible, with laboratory assessments in polymer courses.

Reliability will be further quantified using Cronbach's alpha and test–retest analysis to guarantee measurement stability. This triangulated approach ensures that the PSCI captures not only declarative but also applied conceptual understanding, reinforcing the educational purpose of the game.

User Experience and Engagement Questionnaires

While the PSCI measures what students learned, it is equally important to understand their subjective experience. A positive and engaging user experience is a prerequisite for sustained interaction and, consequently, for learning to occur in a voluntary, informal environment like a game. If the game is perceived as boring, frustrating, or difficult to use, its educational potential will be severely undermined. Therefore, a suite of validated questionnaires will be administered post-intervention to assess key affective and cognitive constructs.

Intrinsic Motivation Inventory (IMI): Motivation is a critical factor in student-centered learning environments. The IMI is a multidimensional and widely used assessment tool designed to measure participants' subjective experience related to a target activity. Rooted in Self-Determination Theory (Ryan & Deci, 2000), it evaluates the underlying factors that contribute to intrinsic motivation. For this study, a selection of its subscales will be utilized:

Interest/Enjoyment: This is the core subscale for intrinsic motivation. It assesses how interesting and enjoyable students found the gameplay, providing a direct measure of the game's appeal.

Perceived Competence: This subscale measures students' feelings of efficacy and accomplishment while playing. High perceived competence is linked to greater persistence in the face of challenges.

Perceived Choice: This evaluates the degree to which students felt they had autonomy and choice while playing, a key driver of intrinsic motivation.

Value/Usefulness: This subscale assesses how valuable or useful students found the activity. In an educational context, it can reveal whether students perceived the game as a valid learning tool rather than a mere distraction.

System Usability Scale (SUS): Usability is a fundamental quality attribute that assesses how easy user interfaces are to use. A game with poor usability (e.g., confusing controls, unclear objectives, a cluttered interface) can impose extraneous cognitive load, distracting the player from the educational content. The SUS is a robust, industry-standard "quick and dirty" usability scale that provides a reliable, single-score measure of perceived usability (Brooke, 1996). It consists of a 10-item questionnaire with five-point Likert scales. Its widespread use allows for benchmarking against a vast database of other systems, providing a clear indication of whether the game's interface is acceptably user-friendly.

Game Engagement Questionnaire (GEQ): To specifically measure the quality of immersion and engagement fostered by the game, the GEQ will be employed. Engagement in game-based learning is often conceptualized as a multifaceted experience encompassing absorption, flow, and presence. As Hamari et al. (2016) note, challenging games can foster deep engagement and flow states that are highly conducive to learning. The GEQ is designed to capture these dimensions, assessing constructs such as:

Immersion: The feeling of being "in" the game world and the extent to which the player feels the narrative and environment are believable.

Flow: The feeling of being completely absorbed in an activity, characterized by a loss of self-consciousness and a distorted sense of time. This is considered an optimal state for learning and skill acquisition.

Absorption: The degree to which players' attention is focused on the game, to the exclusion of external stimuli.

Together, these questionnaires will provide rich, quantitative data on the player experience, allowing us to correlate motivation, usability, and engagement with the learning outcomes measured by the PSCI.

In-Game Performance Analytics (Telemetry)

The final pillar of our evaluation strategy involves the collection of in-game telemetry data. Telemetry refers to the automatic logging of granular player interactions within the game environment. This unobtrusive data collection method provides objective, fine-grained insights into the learning process as it unfolds, capturing behavioral evidence that can corroborate or challenge findings from the self-report questionnaires and knowledge tests.

A custom analytics backend will be developed to log a variety of key performance indicators, including:

Problem-Solving Trajectories: For each puzzle or challenge, the system will log the time to completion, the number of attempts made, the specific strategies or polymer abilities used, and the sequence of actions taken. This can reveal which concepts students grasp quickly and which are more challenging.

Error-Pattern Analysis: The system will flag common mistakes. For example, if a large number of students repeatedly try to use an amorphous polymer in a high-strength structural challenge, it signals a specific, widespread misconception about mechanical properties that can be addressed by the instructor.

Exploration and Information-Seeking Behavior: The analytics will track the paths players take through the open world, which areas they visit, which non-player characters they interact with, and whether they access optional in-game resources (like the "Poly-Pedia"). This data can indicate levels of curiosity and self-regulated learning.

Resource Management: The game involves collecting "Monomer" resources and using them to synthesize polymers. Analyzing how players manage these resources can provide an indirect measure of their planning and strategic thinking skills.

By analyzing these behavioral logs, we can construct profiles of different player types, identify points of friction or confusion in the game design, and uncover the implicit learning strategies students employ. This data is invaluable for both evaluating the game's current design and informing future iterations. In essence, telemetry allows us to observe the learning process directly, providing a powerful complement to the outcome-oriented data from tests and the subjective data from surveys.

Expected Results and Future Perspectives

The implementation of *Macromolecules in Play* is expected to generate measurable improvements in students' conceptual understanding, engagement, and ability to transfer knowledge to real-world polymer applications. Specifically, the project aims to:

- Reduce the frequency of identified misconceptions—such as confusion between Tg and Tm or between crystallinity and transparency—by at least 40% in post-test results.
- Achieve significant gains ($\Delta \geq 0.5$ SD) in PSCI scores between pre- and post-intervention measures.

- Document enhanced collaborative problem-solving, reflected in higher rubric scores and positive telemetry indicators.
- Produce qualitative evidence of increased student motivation and confidence in dealing with polymer-science topics.

These expected outcomes will guide subsequent phases of research, including large-scale classroom trials and integration into broader curricular frameworks for materials and polymer education.

REFERENCES

Aliyu, H. (2025). A review of instructional strategies for maximizing the effectiveness of PhET interactive simulations in chemistry education. *Rima International Journal of Education, 4*(1), 479–487.

Baek, Y., Xu, Y., Han, S., & Cho, J. (2015). Exploring effects of intrinsic motivation and prior knowledge on student achievements in game-based learning. *Smart Computing Review, 5*(4), 368–377. DOI: 10.6029/smartcr.2015.10.001

Barrows, H. S. (1986). A taxonomy of problem-based learning methods. *Medical Education, 20*(6), 481–486. DOI: 10.1111/j.1365-2923.1986.tb01386.x

Brooke, J. (1996). SUS: A quick and dirty usability scale. In Jordan, P. W., Thomas, B., Weerdmeester, B. A., & McClelland, A. L. (Eds.), *Usability Evaluation in Industry* (pp. 189–194). Taylor & Francis.

Byusa, E., Kampire, E., & Mwesigye, A. R. (2022). Game-based learning approach on students' motivation and understanding of chemistry concepts: A systematic review of literature. *Heliyon, 8*(5), e09541. DOI: 10.1016/j.heliyon.2022.e09541

Clapson, M. L., Gilbert, B. C. T., & Musgrove, A. (2020). Race to the reactor and other chemistry games: Game-based and experiential learning experiences in materials and polymer chemistry. *Journal of Chemical Education, 97*(12), 4391–4399. DOI: 10.1021/acs.jchemed.0c01135

Clark, T. M. (2024). Using multiple PhET sims to investigate greenhouse gases within a real-world context. *Journal of Chemical Education, 101*(10), 4242–4250. DOI: 10.1021/acs.jchemed.4c00551

Dietrich, N. (2018). Escape classroom: The Leblanc process—An educational "escape game.". *Journal of Chemical Education, 95*(6), 996–999. DOI: 10.1021/acs.jchemed.7b00690

Ebnesajjad, S. (2013). Fluoroplastics, Volume 1: Non-melt processible fluoropolymers. William Andrew Publishing.

Hamari, J., Shernoff, D. J., Rowe, E., Coller, B., Asbell-Clarke, J., & Edwards, T. (2016). Challenging games help students learn: An empirical study on engagement, flow and immersion in game-based learning. *Computers in Human Behavior, 54*, 170–179. DOI: 10.1016/j.chb.2015.07.045

Hernández-Sampieri, R., & Mendoza-Torres, C. (2018). Metodología de la investigación: las rutas cuantitativa, cualitativa y mixta 2ed. Cd. de México: McGraw-Hill.

Jonassen, D. H. (1999). Designing constructivist learning environments. In Reigeluth, C. M. (Ed.), *Instructional-design theories and models: A new paradigm of instructional theory* (Vol. II, pp. 215–239). Lawrence Erlbaum Associates.

Kalogiannakis, M., Papadakis, S., & Zourmpakis, A.-I. (2021). Gamification in science education: A systematic review of the literature. *Education Sciences, 11*(1), 22. DOI: 10.3390/educsci11010022

Sousa Lima, M. A., Monteiro, Á. C., Melo Leite Junior, A. J., de Andrade Matos, I. S., Alexandre, F. S. O., Nobre, D. J., ... & da Silva Júnior, J. N. (2019). Game-based application for helping students review chemical nomenclature in a fun way. DOI: 10.1021/acs.jchemed.8b00540

Marfisi-Schottman, I., George, S., & Tarpin-Bernard, F. (2010, October). Tools and methods for efficiently designing serious games. In *Proceedings of the 4th Europeen Conference on Games Based Learning ECGBL* (pp. 226-234).

Mark, H. F. (Ed.). (2020). *Encyclopedia of polymer science and technology* (4th ed.). Wiley., DOI: 10.1002/0471440264

Partovi, T., & Razavi, M. R. (2019). The effect of game-based learning on academic achievement motivation of elementary school students. *Learning and Motivation, 68*, 101592. DOI: 10.1016/j.lmot.2019.101592

Parvate, S., Dixit, P., & Chattopadhyay, S. (2020). Superhydrophobic surfaces: Insights from theory and experiment. *The Journal of Physical Chemistry B, 124*(8), 1323–1360. DOI: 10.1021/acs.jpcb.9b08567

Rabek, J. F. (2012). *Polymer photodegradation: Mechanisms and experimental methods*. Springer Science & Business Media.

Ramgobin, A., Fontaine, G., & Bourbigot, S. (2020). A Case Study of Polyether Ether Ketone (I): Investigating the Thermal and Fire Behavior of a High-Performance Material. *Polymers, 12*(8), 1789. DOI: 10.3390/polym12081789

Raos, G., & Zappone, B. (2021). Polymer adhesion: Seeking new solutions for an old problem. *Macromolecules, 54*(23), 10617–10644. DOI: 10.1021/acs.macromol.1c01182

Ryan, R. M., & Deci, E. L. (2000). Self-determination theory and the facilitation of intrinsic motivation, social development, and well-being. *The American Psychologist, 55*(1), 68–78. DOI: 10.1037/0003-066X.55.1.68

Sierra-Daza, M. C., Martín-del Pozo, M., & Sánchez, M. R. F. (2023). Videojuegos para el desarrollo de competencias en Educación Superior. *Revista Fuentes*, *25*(2), 228–241. DOI: 10.12795/revistafuentes.2023.22687

Tene, T., Vique López, D. F., Valverde Aguirre, P. E., Cabezas Oviedo, N. I., Vacacela Gomez, C., & Bellucci, S. (2025). A systematic review of serious games as tools for STEM education. *Frontiers in Education*, *10*, 1432982. DOI: 10.3389/feduc.2025.1432982

Treloar, L. R. G. (2013). *The physics of rubber elasticity* (3rd ed.). Oxford University Press.

Ullah, M., Amin, S. U., Munsif, M., Yamin, M. M., Safaev, U., Khan, H., Khan, S., & Ullah, H. (2022). Serious games in science education: A systematic literature review. *Virtual Reality & Intelligent Hardware*, *4*(3), 189–209. DOI: 10.1016/j.vrih.2022.02.001

Vera-Monroy, S. P., Mejía-Camacho, A., & Gamboa Mora, M. C. (2020). C=OCARBOHIDRATOS: Efecto del juego sobre el aprendizaje. *Educación en la Química*, *31*(1), 23–35. DOI: 10.22201/fq.18708404e.2020.1.68522

Yacoub, M. S. W., & Holton, A. J. (2023). Development and implementation of an online narrative game to aid studying and review in an online general chemistry course. *Journal of Chemical Education*, *100*(9), 3688–3693. DOI: 10.1021/acs.jchemed.3c00266

KEY TERMS AND DEFINITIONS

Cognitive Transfer: The ability to apply knowledge learned in one context (such as a game) to solve problems in a different, real-world context. It reflects the depth of conceptual understanding beyond rote memorization.

Crosslinking: The formation of chemical bonds between polymer chains, which restricts mobility and increases rigidity and thermal stability. Crosslinked polymers are usually insoluble and dimensionally stable.

Crystallinity: The degree to which polymer chains are arranged in an ordered, lattice-like structure. Higher crystallinity generally increases stiffness, chemical resistance, and melting temperature, while reducing transparency and elasticity.

Glass Transition Temperature (Tg): The temperature below which an amorphous polymer behaves as a rigid glass and above which it becomes more rubber-like. Distinct from the melting temperature (Tm), which applies to crystalline regions.

Macromolecule: A large molecule composed of repeating structural units, typically linked by covalent bonds. Polymers are macromolecules whose architecture and molecular weight determine their mechanical and thermal behavior.

Scaffolded Learning: An instructional approach in which support is gradually removed as learners gain competence. In the game context, scaffolding occurs through progressive challenges, feedback, and adaptive hints that foster autonomy and mastery.

Serious Game: A digital or analog game designed for purposes beyond entertainment, integrating pedagogical objectives such as conceptual understanding, problem-solving, or collaborative learning.

Chapter 7
Stars, Shields, and Avatars:
Digital Motivation in the Early School Years

Karla Adriana Cruz Vera
https://orcid.org/0009-0000-3727-3465
Universidad de Guadalajara, Mexico

Blanca Lorena Reynoso Gomez
https://orcid.org/0000-0002-1118-0866
Universidad de Guadalajara, Mexico

Jose Juan Meza Espinosa
https://orcid.org/0000-0003-0207-8517
Universidad de Guadalajara, Mexico

Luis Antonio Medellín Serna
https://orcid.org/0000-0002-9017-9563
Universidad de Guadalajara, Mexico

ABSTRACT

Gamification uses elements like stars, shields, and avatars to boost motivation, engagement, and active learning in primary education. It proved vital during the pandemic for remote learning and aligns with Sustainable Development Goals by helping reduce the educational gap. Its key benefits include fostering motivation through immediate feedback, strengthening emotional development and self-esteem via avatar personalization, and creating a safe space for introverted students to participate. It also enhances language and communication skills. To be effective

DOI: 10.4018/979-8-3373-4657-1.ch007

and not just entertaining, gamification must be carefully planned, aligned with curriculum objectives, and supported by proper teacher training. When implemented correctly, it is a powerful tool for holistic student development.

1. INTRODUCTION

The integration of digital tools in the classroom has transformed the way elementary school students interact with knowledge.

Among these tools, gamification has emerged as a powerful strategy for motivating students through the use of game dynamics in non-game contexts (Hamari et al., 2014). In particular, symbolic elements such as stars, shields, and customizable avatars have proven effective in capturing children's attention, increasing their engagement, and fostering a positive attitude toward learning (Koivisto & Hamari, 2019).

The entire population must have access to education, as this includes timely enrollment, progression at the required age, school attendance, learning in accordance with national academic achievement standards, a learning environment safe enough to allow for learning, and an equitable distribution of school materials (Lewin, 2015).

Universal access to knowledge is part of the human right to science, which is governed by the principle of inclusion, to guarantee the enjoyment of the benefits provided by humanistic and scientific research and technological development, making advances and the diversity of knowledge available to Mexicans through clear and accessible language that allows for the engagement of non-specialized audiences.

This article examines how these visual and symbolic elements, inspired by applications such as Duolingo, can be applied in primary education to improve both extrinsic and intrinsic motivation. Their effects, emotional implications, pedagogical benefits, and possible limitations are analyzed.

It also addresses the importance of ensuring that the entire student population has free access to education, and that the development of knowledge is the most appropriate and relevant, in addition to the importance of focusing on their environment, but without neglecting universal knowledge (Gómez-Urquiza et al., 2023).

Or the development of soft skills, which are so critically needed to foster in students from the earliest stages of social and academic development, for a significant achievement of human development in every aspect.

Figure 1. Gamification in digital environments

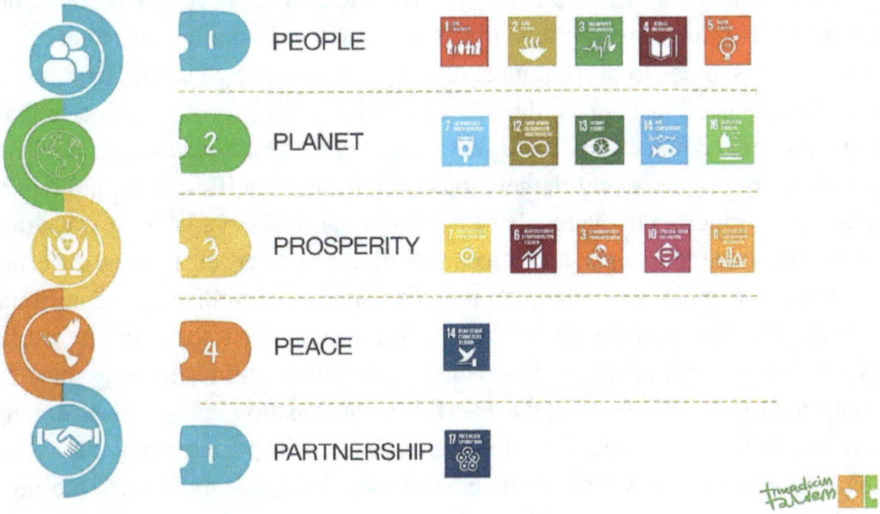

Considering the above, this article takes on significant importance, since the inclusion of gamification in the development of educational strategies has yielded positive results in various areas of education and inclusive education, please refer to the following figure 1.

The integration of digital resources into modern classrooms has radically reshaped how elementary school students approach and engage with learning, creating new opportunities for interaction, participation, and personal growth. Among the many innovations available to educators, gamification has proven to be particularly influential, as it employs game-like mechanics and motivational structures in educational settings where entertainment is not the primary objective. Through the incorporation of symbolic and visual features such as stars, shields, progress bars, or avatars that students can personalize, teachers have discovered that young learners become more attentive, more eager to participate, and more consistent in maintaining a positive outlook toward the learning process itself. Research has shown that these playful elements contribute not only to higher engagement but also to greater persistence when facing academic challenges, as they create a sense of accomplishment and recognition that resonates strongly with children. However, beyond the motivational potential of gamified strategies, it is essential to remember that education is a fundamental right that must be safeguarded and provided equitably to all children, regardless of their socioeconomic background, geographical location, or personal circumstances. Ensuring universal access to quality education requires more than simply opening school doors; it involves guaranteeing timely enrollment at the appropriate age, fostering steady progression through grade levels, promoting consistent attendance, and delivering instruction that aligns with national standards of academic achievement. Moreover, schools must provide safe and supportive environments where meaningful learning can take place, accompanied by a fair distribution of materials and resources to prevent inequalities from becoming barriers to success. In this sense, education is not only an institutional obligation but also a human right that is deeply connected to the right to science, which affirms the principle of inclusion and the collective entitlement to benefit from scientific and technological progress. This principle demands that knowledge be made available in ways that are accessible, understandable, and relevant to diverse audiences, thereby ensuring that even those without specialized training can appreciate, utilize, and contribute to the body of human knowledge. Within the Mexican context, for example, public policy emphasizes that advances in science, humanities, and technology must be communicated in clear language so that they foster participation and awareness among all citizens. When examining the role of gamification in primary education, this perspective highlights how tools modeled after popular applications like Duolingo can bridge the gap between individual motivation and collective rights, enhancing both extrinsic incentives, such as rewards or visible progress, and intrinsic motivations, such as curiosity and personal satisfaction. At the same time, educators must remain attentive to the emotional dimensions of gamification, acknowledging how recognition systems affect self-esteem, peer relationships, and classroom dynamics. Pedagogically, gamified environments can enrich traditional lessons, stimulate collaboration, and prepare students with soft skills—such as communication, empathy, and problem-solving—that are indispensable for success in both academic and social spheres. Ultimately, fostering these skills from the earliest stages of formal education contributes to the broader goal of human development, ensuring that students not only master academic content but also grow into responsible, capable, and resilient individuals who can thrive in an increasingly interconnected world.

2. BACKGROUND

2.1 Conceptual Framework: Motivation and Gamification

Gamification can be conceptually framed within the foundations of behaviorist learning theories, particularly those developed by B.F. Skinner and Ivan Pavlov. These theories emphasize observable behavior change through reinforcement, repetition, and feedback. Within this context, gamification operates as a system of structured reinforcements—points, badges, and rewards—that act as positive stimuli to strengthen desired learning behaviors. The integration of these mechanisms allows the translation of theoretical constructs, such as operant conditioning and reinforcement schedules, into practical digital learning environments. Thus, gamification serves not merely as a motivational strategy but as a concrete methodological extension of behaviorist principles in contemporary education. Motivation in childhood is defined as a combination of intrinsic (interest, enjoyment) and extrinsic (rewards, recognition) factors. According to Self-Determination Theory (Ryan & Deci, 2000), students learn best when they feel competence, autonomy, and social connection. Gamification, especially when it includes symbolic rewards, can activate these three pillars.

We must take into account that from early childhood, human beings are accustomed to playing games in various forms and environments. This motivates everything they do and even fosters imagination and enables us to develop worlds where we can achieve everything we set out to do, or even be someone we cannot be in the real world, or find difficult to achieve. Therefore, in a gamified environment, but also within the digital world, this is possible, with the various programs we now have access to.

To address the methodological gap, the study adopts a mixed exploratory framework combining secondary data analysis from INEGI with a qualitative interpretation of motivational indicators derived from gamified environments. The purpose is to identify correlations between digital access, technological adoption, and the potential success of gamified interventions in educational settings. The analysis of INEGI datasets functions as an empirical foundation for mapping the technological infrastructure necessary for implementing behaviorally informed gamification strategies. This approach not only situates gamification within a national statistical context but also enables the formulation of evidence-based recommendations for its effective deployment.INEGI collects comprehensive data on education, technology, internet access, and the use of digital tools, which are essential for understanding the digital context and the infrastructure available for gamification.

Figure 2. National Institute of Statistics, Geography and Informatics

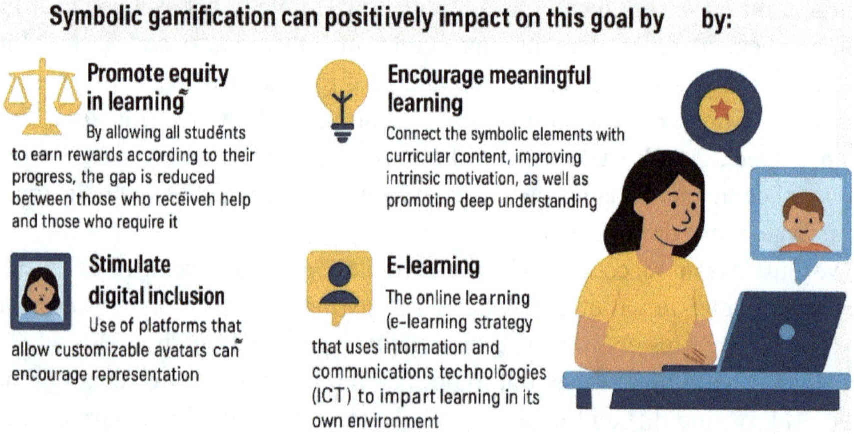

Platforms such as "Cuéntame de México" and "Gráficas dinámicas" offer access to relevant indicators on digital education and interactive technologies, which can be the starting point for our analyses, please refer to the following figure 2.

It is important to have a selection of indicators such as the INEGI. To understand the favorable ecosystem for gamification, we must look for indicators that reflect technology penetration and access to digital tools. We will focus on data related to internet access and the use of educational software in different areas.

Regarding the use of ICTs in schools: we need to know the percentage of schools with internet access and technological equipment, but also the availability of educational software and the existence and use of interactive teaching programs in schools, as well as home connectivity and internet access at home and its impact on distance learning.

Figure 3. Growth of internet access in schools (2010-2024)

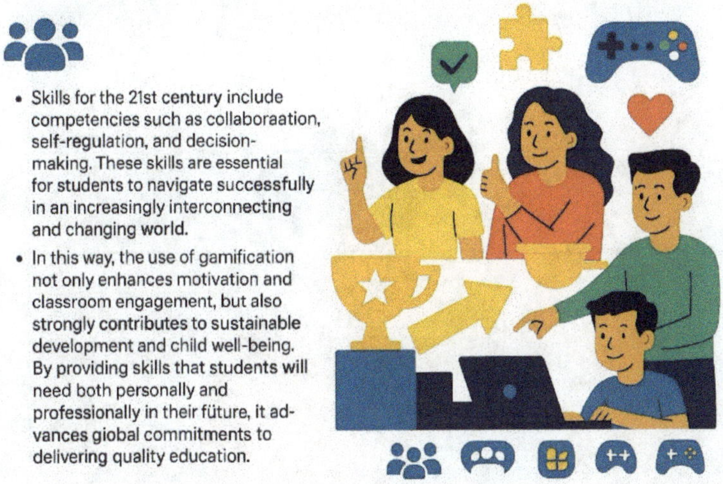
• Skills for the 21st century include competencies such as collaboraation, self-regulation, and decision-making. These skills are essential for students to navigate successfully in an increasingly interconnecting and changing world.
• In this way, the use of gamification not only enhances motivation and classroom engagement, but also strongly contributes to sustainable development and child well-being. By providing skills that students will need both personally and professionally in their füture, it advances giobal commitments to delivering quality education.

This line graph demonstrates the steady growth in technology adoption, laying the groundwork for future gamification implementations in the Mexican education system. INEGI's interactive tools make it easy to customize these types of visualizations, please refer to the following figure 3

Research Objectives and Scope

The primary objective of this study is to examine how the principles of behavioral reinforcement can be effectively operationalized through gamification in the Mexican educational context. Specifically, it seeks to determine the extent to which access to digital tools, as reflected in INEGI data, can facilitate motivation, engagement, and sustained participation among learners. By linking macro-level indicators (technological penetration, internet access) to micro-level motivational processes (reinforcement, reward anticipation), the research bridges theory and practice. This provides a well-defined contribution that extends beyond a theoretical review, positioning gamification as both a pedagogical and socio-technological innovation.

Figure 4. Coral I Schools

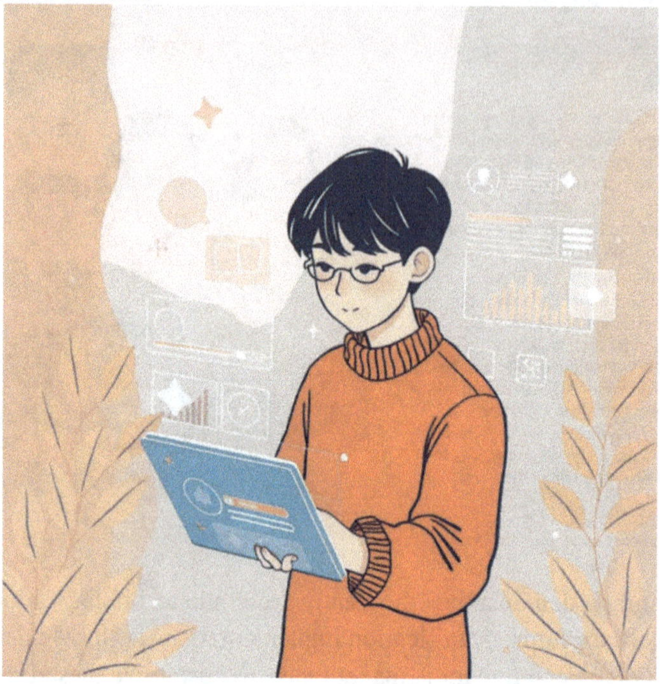

For practical interpretation and application, the data reveal the enormous potential for gamification in Mexico, but also point to areas with lower technological adoption, where additional efforts are needed. Understanding these dynamics is crucial to designing effective and targeted strategies, please refer to the following figure 4. Coral orange, ang internet in Mexicand internet acless is for eteand, pink nexien not orangeed piin internets, internete schools in to light acses pith peccht, pedechs al fot peacch man and fust tones.

By identifying opportunities, we can prioritize the implementation of gamification in regions and educational levels with greater technological access to support strategic decisions. Official statistical data from INEGI (National Institute of Statistics and Geography) provides a solid basis for justifying investments, as well as for updated programs and curricula. It is also imperative to mention the focus on digital divides, since recognizing areas with low connectivity allows us to develop innovative and tailored solutions, such as offline or hybrid gamification.

INEGI data allows us to move from intuition to statistical evidence to drive innovation in education and training.

Some challenges and recommendations from INEGI. It mentions that there are specific challenges when analyzing gamification, primarily the lack of direct indicators. Overcoming these challenges requires a collaborative and proactive approach.

Due to the lack of specific data—since INEGI does not have a direct category for "gamification"—we need to advocate for new surveys that capture this phenomenon.

When complemented by other studies, it is vital to integrate INEGI data with academic and sectoral research on gamification to obtain a complete picture.

To promote the collection of open data, we must foster a culture of open data, as this will allow researchers and developers to innovate more rapidly in the field of gamification.

By addressing these challenges, we can improve the accuracy of analyses and enhance the impact of gamification on Mexican society.

Gamification + INEGI Data = Educational and Social Innovation

Gamification is positioned as a powerful tool to motivate and transform learning, work, and citizen participation. At the same time, the INEGI (National Institute of Statistics and Geography) offers key data for understanding Mexico's digital context and designing effective strategies.

The synergy between gamification and INEGI data analysis is essential for:

- Identifying areas of opportunity and specific needs.
- Creating solutions tailored to the country's technological reality.
- Measuring the impact of gamified initiatives with evidence.

The synthesis of gamification with behaviorist and motivational theories offers a framework that is both theoretically grounded and methodologically applicable. By integrating the constructs of competence, autonomy, and relatedness from Self-Determination Theory with reinforcement-based approaches, this study highlights a hybrid model of motivation that can inform future educational design. Furthermore, the use of INEGI data introduces an empirical dimension that supports policy formulation and curriculum innovation. Ultimately, this work proposes a structured model for analyzing and implementing gamification that moves from abstract theory to measurable educational impact.

Figure 5. The synergy between gamification and INEGI data analysis is essential for

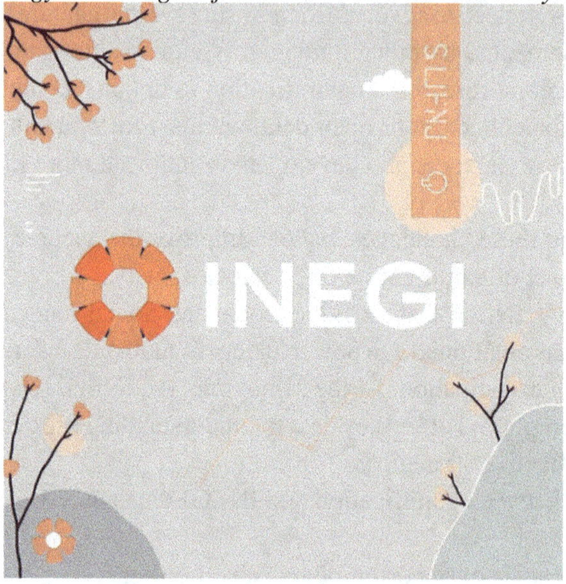

Beyond INEGI statistics, recent literature suggests that visual and symbolic elements have a particularly strong impact on primary school children (Toda et al., 2018). These elements allow academic achievements to be translated into concrete symbols that children can understand, value, and use as a reference for their progress. Users can also control this progress, as they can have their own access accounts. This allows them to visualize their progress and understand what they still need to complete, or how quickly they can reach the next level. This, in turn, can motivate students to participate more actively in the classroom and in developing educational knowledge.

However, it is important for teachers to ensure that this gamification is implemented in accordance with the UA's curriculum plans and programs, and that students always have the teacher's guidance so that this gamification is implemented in a clear and relevant manner to promote the development of skills and that these dynamics do not become merely a free environment without meeting the educational development objectives set by the educational institution.

The behavioral foundations offered by Skinner (1953) are fundamental to understanding why elements such as points, stars, and visual rewards reinforce desired behaviors. According to his theory of operant conditioning, behavior is strengthened when associated with a positive consequence, as is evident in gamified environments.

These types of dynamics linked to Skinner's operant conditioning are not new; they have been practiced and analyzed for many years, and since Skinner's discovery, these systems have been replicated in various forms and in various settings, not only in the educational field.

But for this practical case, we can mention that gamification, given in the sense of learning through reward, is highly significant, since: who doesn't like taking home a little yellow star on their forehead after an intense day of school work? From the moment the teacher, the school teacher, tells us that whoever finishes first will get a gold star, the competition begins. Who will be the best student, the fastest, the one who will win that shiny badge?

Wearing that star and leaving the school grounds is already a sign of achievement and pride, but seeing the recognition and admiration of parents waiting for their children at the exit, seeing the admiration that comes from seeing that gold star on a child's forehead is satisfying. But when that student is your child, it's synonymous with pride, and that child knows it, which is why they strive. And when that child receives a hug, a congratulation, and a sign of satisfaction and recognition, well, the mission is accomplished, and that motivates children to want another gold star the next day and the next.

Because the motivation and satisfaction don't stop when the school teacher gives you that gold star; that feeling and pride extends to the student's home and perhaps to the rest of the family, as the bravest and most courageous student in the class. And that simply comforts every subject, every student.

And well, mentioning the teachers, they also have their satisfaction, since they will see the effort and gratitude of the students, seeing themselves with those little stars on their foreheads, but now let's imagine other types of insignia, such as shields, capable of leading various battles or crossroads. Now imagine wearing the best suit with a shield capable of protecting you and reaching the goal. Those educational objectives are enhanced and students will be able to get more involved in the school environment and carry out their learning in a more enjoyable and enriching way, since it challenges them to get involved, but also to solve various situations both in fantasy and in the environment of daily life, please refer to the following figure 5.

From a didactic and cognitive-developmental standpoint, gamification can be firmly grounded in the theoretical frameworks of Piaget and Vygotsky. Piaget's constructivist approach emphasizes the active role of learners in constructing knowledge through processes of assimilation and accommodation based on interaction with their environment (Piaget, 1952). Within gamified educational contexts, these mechanisms are reflected in the way students face progressively complex challenges, reorganize their cognitive schemas, and build understanding through adaptive feedback. Vygotsky's sociocultural theory complements this perspective by introducing the concept of the Zone of Proximal Development (ZPD), defined as the distance between what a learner can achieve independently and what can be accomplished with expert guidance (Vygotsky, 1978). When applied to gamification, the ZPD is operationalized through elements such as tasks of increasing difficulty, cooperative problem-solving, and immediate feedback—components that function as digital scaffolding to promote higher levels of cognitive development.Through the development and implementation of the ZPD, students unconsciously enter the context of teaching-learning processes, both within society and in the school environment. Since it is a central concept in Lev Vygotsky's sociocultural theory, it describes the gap between what an individual can do alone and what they can achieve with the help of someone more skilled, it is the range of skills a student can develop with the guidance and support of an adult, teacher, or a more experienced peer (Vygotsky, 1978).

It is important to consider actual development versus potential, since the ZPD refers to the difference between an individual's current level of development, that is, what they can do alone, and their potential level of development, or what they can achieve with help.

Vygotsky emphasized the importance of social interaction in learning. The ZPD is manifested in interaction with a "more knowledgeable other," who provides scaffolding and support for the individual to progress.

The ZPD is also known as the space where mediated learning occurs. It is where the individual internalizes knowledge and skills through interaction with an expert, who can be the teacher or a peer.

From a neuropsychological perspective, gamified mockups contribute to learning by activating reward and motivation systems in the brain. Research in educational neuroscience has shown that reward-based feedback stimulates dopaminergic circuits associated with pleasure, reinforcement, and memory consolidation (Howard-Jones, 2014). This connection between behavioral reinforcement and neurocognitive activation provides a scientific explanation for the effectiveness of gamification. Mockups—whether digital user interfaces, 3D environments, or physical prototypes—serve as external mediators that transform abstract learning goals into tangible, interactive representations. These tools not only enhance motivation and emotional engagement but also support neurocognitive processes involved in attention, working memory, and long-term retention. In this way, mockups bridge the gap between behaviorist reinforcement, sociocultural mediation, and neuropsychological stimulation, offering a multidimensional foundation for gamified learning environments. Gamification in education, using mockups, involves the creation of visual representations in simulated educational environments that incorporate game elements to enhance the learning experience. These representations can take the form of user interfaces, virtual scenario designs, or even physical prototypes, designed to make learning more engaging and motivating (Supervia & Bordas, 2020).

In gamification, mockups can be:

Didactically, integrating the ZPD into gamified instruction through the use of mockups enables educators to create adaptive and inclusive learning experiences tailored to individual developmental stages. By visualizing feedback loops, progress markers, and peer collaboration, mockups act as scaffolding devices that facilitate guided discovery under the supervision of a "more knowledgeable other" (Vygotsky, 1978). This integration reflects a convergence of cognitive development theory, behaviorist principles, and contemporary gamification methodologies, aligning educational design with both psychological and neuroscientific evidence. Consequently, gamification supported by mockups should not be viewed merely as a motivational strategy but as a scientifically grounded pedagogical model that operationalizes learning through behavioral, social, and neurocognitive mechanisms.

Some examples of the use of mockups in education include a learning platform with a points and level system, where students can earn points for completing tasks and level up as they progress through the course.

We can also find 3D virtual scenarios where students, represented by avatars, explore a map to find information and solve challenges related to a specific topic.

Or within a board game where students roll dice, move pieces, and answer questions to advance in the game and learn about a particular topic.

Mockups in educational gamification are powerful tools for visualizing and enhancing the learning experience, making the process more engaging, effective, and fun for students, please refer to the following figure 6.

Figure 6. The power of gamification when integrating mockups

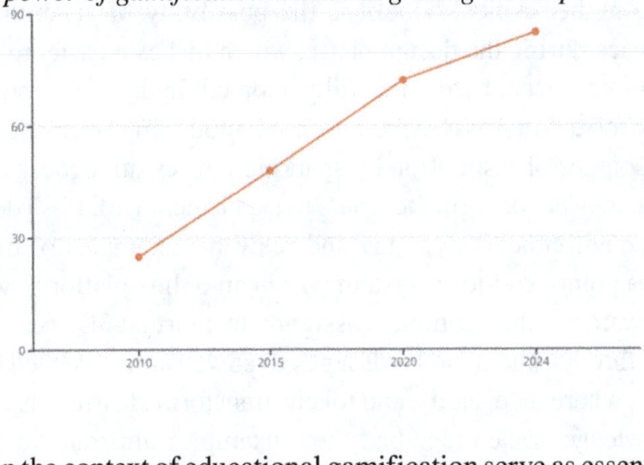

Mockups in the context of educational gamification serve as essential prototypes that allow both educators and learners to visualize how game-based strategies will be implemented within a learning environment. These models can take several forms depending on the intended learning goals and the resources available. For instance, user interface mockups display the design of a digital platform by showing students how points, badges, progress levels, or ranking systems will be presented on-screen. Such visual previews are especially useful for demonstrating how learners' achievements will be acknowledged and how progress will be tracked in a way that mirrors popular digital games. Beyond interface design, virtual scenario mockups create two- or three-dimensional environments where students interact with knowledge through playful challenges, quests, or simulations. These can range from exploring a fantasy map filled with puzzles related to academic topics, to participating in virtual laboratories or adventure games that replicate real-life problem-solving. In addition, physical prototypes are also an important category of mockups in gamified education, since they bring tangible elements such as board games, challenge cards, or escape room puzzles into the classroom. These hands-on experiences allow learners to engage with concepts in collaborative and dynamic ways, making abstract knowledge more concrete. The versatility of mockups demonstrates that they are not only design tools but also creative instruments that bridge the gap between game-inspired mechanics and formal education.

The benefits of integrating mockups into the design of gamified learning experiences are numerous and extend well beyond aesthetics. One of the most significant advantages is the clarity they provide, as mockups enable educators, students, and even parents to clearly visualize how gamification will function before its implementation. This early visualization helps prevent misunderstandings, allowing everyone involved to share a common vision of the educational journey. At the same time, attractive and carefully designed mockups enhance student motivation by making the learning environment more immersive and exciting, fostering deeper emotional involvement. Another critical benefit is the possibility of generating timely and effective feedback during the design phase, which makes it easier to refine and improve the gamified system before it is fully adopted. In doing so, mockups become valuable tools for quality assurance and continuous improvement. Furthermore, they serve as sources of inspiration by sparking new creative ideas and innovative approaches, thereby encouraging teachers to experiment with fresh designs that can keep learning environments dynamic and relevant. Examples of this application are abundant: a points-and-level system within an online platform, where students accumulate rewards as they complete assignments; virtual 3D scenarios where avatars navigate through thematic landscapes to solve subject-related challenges; or physical games where dice, cards, and tokens transform classrooms into interactive arenas of knowledge. Taken together, these examples illustrate how mockups act as powerful catalysts for enhancing gamification, making the educational process not only clearer and more effective but also significantly more enjoyable, engaging, and memorable for students at all levels.

3. APPLICATION

3.1. Symbolic Elements in Primary Education

3.1. 1 Stars and Points: Immediate Feedback

Stars and points are feedback mechanisms that reinforce desired behaviors in the short term. They provide instant recognition after completing a task or reaching a goal. In educational contexts, these elements allow students to clearly and motivatingly perceive their progress (Seaborn & Fels, 2015).

Since they allow students to accurately and almost instantly visualize their progress or achievement compared to other students, this generally fosters motivation and a desire to continue participating.

A study by Looyestyn et al (Looyestyn et al., 2017) found that the use of points and symbolic rewards in virtual environments increased engagement by 20–30% among elementary school students. The key is that these symbols are not merely decorative, but linked to real pedagogical objectives.

For this reason, every gamified activity must always be linked to the pedagogical objectives of each AU, and that these activities must be well-founded. It is the teacher who directs how these strategies should be carried out to foster participatory learning and foster a viable environment for the development of learning, communication, participation, and good classroom harmony.

3.1.2. Badges and Medals: Intermediate Goals and a Sense of Competence

Badges or medals represent more complex achievements that require time, effort, and persistence. This type of symbolic reward allows for the setting of intermediate goals, fostering self-regulation and resilience. Recent research suggests that badge systems can improve performance and learning retention if implemented with clear and progressive criteria (Huang et al., 2020).

In educational practice we can see how students strive increasingly to have a higher goal or simply to reach a castle where a flag is recovered, or save the princess, how to overcome battles and win increasingly more significant or better made badges, with more resistant materials, since in the digital environment, materials can change, with respect to what we sew in real life, these materials vary in resistance or even the way in which these materials can be collected within the digital environment, which encourages greater participation and even resistance or interest in the student to achieve the best materials and consequently the best badges or the improvement of their avatars inclusive.

In practice, these tokens can be awarded for completing units, improving soft skills (such as collaboration), or maintaining consistency. Their value lies not in material things, but in what they represent: sustained effort, personal achievements, and social recognition within the classroom.

By linking gamification to each AU, we must commit as teachers to ensuring that these AUs clearly and precisely develop the pedagogical objectives of each one, clearly justifying the objectives to be developed and the way in which they should be achieved, and ensuring that this is a sustained and focused progress for the development of each student.

For example, in the development of soft skills, as previously mentioned, maintaining student interest and, consequently, sustained effort and perseverance throughout the course, whether individually or in a team, strengthens the abilities and skills of each student, as well as the work among peers.

When both individual and group work are developed, social recognition from peers is also fostered, which is important and relevant for developing self-esteem and fostering various social values.

3.1.3. Customizable Avatars: Identity and Belonging

Avatars allow students to symbolically project themselves within the digital environment. Avatar customization—colors, clothing, expressions, accessories—is associated with greater emotional involvement, a sense of belonging, and commitment to the task (Birk et al., 2020).

By linking avatars to the personalization and identification of each individual, students do more than just give a name, color, or decorate the clothing they wear; they evoke their own identity.

Just as in psychology, when asking a person to take, for example, the Human Figure Test or the Person in the Rain Test, these are projective tests. Without needing to name the person, without thinking about it, they automatically and unconsciously create drawings, giving them aspects identical to those of the person taking them.

They even evoke emotional situations in the drawing itself, or the avatar in this case. Therefore, each of these avatars is not just a meaningless drawing or a digital creation. It's about transferring something more than just adding pretty details to a drawing or mockup. It's about giving it your strength, your will, your feelings, or even a similar appearance, and feeling in that environment totally strong, powerful, invincible, and courageous, capable of achieving everything that comes your way, overcoming every obstacle, and always having new opportunities to overcome whatever comes your way in each of these environments.

In primary education, this personalization not only improves motivation but also contributes to the development of personal identity. Furthermore, avatars can be used to represent emotions, achievements, or moods, facilitating the development of socio-emotional competencies (Gómez-Urquiza et al., 2021).

And outside of the game, students also transfer this confidence to real life, since they weren't judged or minimized in the digital environment. Therefore, they gain greater confidence and independence. They feel capable of overcoming various real-life situations.

This is beneficial for the individual's development, but also for strengthening their soft skills and abilities, which will serve them for the rest of their lives.

3.2. Emotional Design and Aesthetics in Children's Motivation

Emotional design (Norman, 2004) proposes that the aesthetic characteristics of an interface—colors, sounds, animations—profoundly impact the user experience. In educational gamification, emotional design can transform routine activities into rewarding experiences. Recent studies confirm that pleasing visual and auditory stimuli improve children's attention and learning retention.

Well, as we mentioned before, it's important for each student to give their avatar that personalization feature, which makes each of them independent and relevant. This transforms the game and the virtual environment into something automatic, and fosters the emotional aspect of gamification in the student.

But that's not the only thing; interfaces also need to have eye-catching features that invite students to participate, so that they feel motivated to reach the next point or the next goal, and so that participation is engaging and compelling for them.

Let it be a fun, pedagogical, teaching-learning process. This includes working, for example, on color psychology, finding appropriate tones for each educational level, and ensuring that each interface is relevant and engaging. If music is used, it should generate motivation and interest, as it can be used, for example, in cave environments, where it can sometimes be terrifying, putting you on edge and alert. This would require assessing the purpose of the music or the environment to be used. You can also use environments with outside sounds, this is more peaceful, relaxing and could even be melancholic and with the sound of the depths of the water, which is focused on some uncertainty, but it could also be relaxing depending on whether this game has a story linked to music, look for it not to be stressful for the student, you have to think very carefully about each of the aspects to implement and develop in gamification, since if something was not well thought out, planned and developed, it could make students want to avoid gamification and therefore, the teaching-learning process would be affected, instead of it being pleasant.

It's also important to consider students' personal aspects, which will be reflected in their strengths and weaknesses, the way each student copes with their life, and how they resolve their own conflicts. These aspects will also be reflected in the gamified environment. Remember, they won't just give the avatar a personalized visual appearance, but they will also seek to make this avatar respond as they do in real life. This aspect must also be reviewed and evaluated as part of the development of soft skills.

We must consider including positive aspects, which foster well-being and gratification for well-done work, and motivate students to continue learning and working hard every day.

Therefore, the design of gamified systems must incorporate positive stimuli, celebratory animations, and friendly aesthetics, especially on platforms aimed at children, please refer to the following figure 7.

Figure 7. The excitement of students when receiving diverse avatars

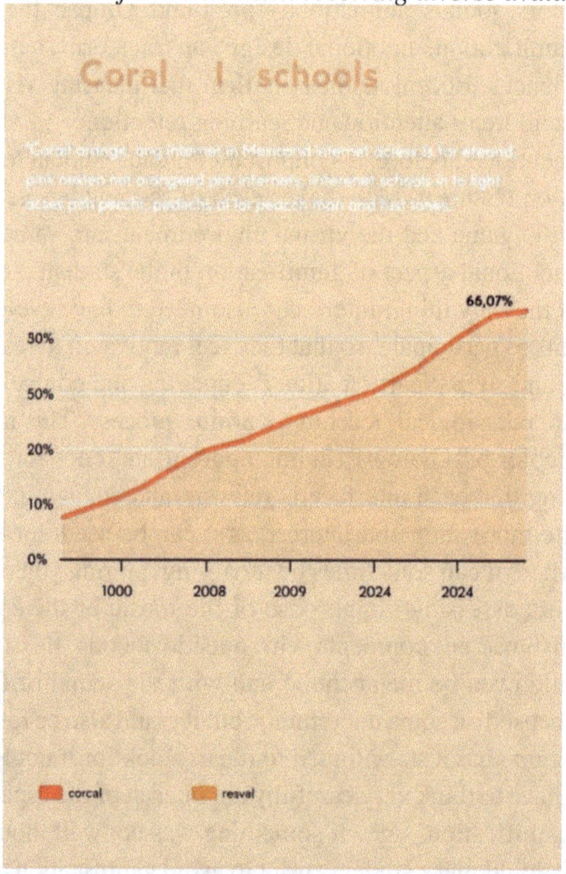

3.3. Risks and Limitations of Symbolic Use in Gamification

Despite its benefits, excessive or poorly structured use of symbolic elements can have negative effects. According to Deci et al. (2020), an overreliance on external rewards can diminish intrinsic motivation in the long term. Furthermore, if achievements are not aligned with students' actual abilities or if they generate constant comparisons, they can increase anxiety or demotivation.

It is important to emphasize that gamification and the use of avatars, as well as symbols such as stars, shields, and swords, must be controlled and structured, as otherwise they would produce effects contrary to those expected by structured teaching.

Teachers must be especially careful in the use of these symbols, since, as in all aspects of life, anything in excess can be counterproductive. Anything given in excess can lose its primary value and be unfavorable for the development of the skills the student is expected to develop.

Furthermore, this control favors good management of the dependence on always winning or having everything they have always obtained easily. It also continues to encourage student participation, as they remain motivated by having something to gain, as they will feel challenged to surpass themselves and their classmates.

It's important for people to always have a motivating factor, giving them a goal and an objective to achieve, something to keep them going. In this case, having an increasingly larger educational objective is relevant, as this is the motivating factor students may need to increase their motivation, their desire to participate, and their desire to excel, rather than surpass their peers.

To mitigate these risks, it is recommended to follow these points:

- Avoid public rankings among students.
- Ensure all students have opportunities for success.
- Offer verbal feedback along with visual symbols.
- Alternate between extrinsic rewards and activities that encourage curiosity and exploration.

By avoiding public rankings, students don't feel exposed to their peers and are not exposed to their scores. Furthermore, we protect our students' sensitive data, such as grades. In many cases, these grades aren't what they expected. Therefore, having their peers see their results can expose them to ridicule or blackmail. This is why it's important for these rankings to be private.

It's important that all our students have the same opportunities for success, that they feel included in every way they participate, and that they can earn equally.

Feedback is always important without gamification, but even more so with the inclusion of gamification, since we cannot leave students with only their imaginations running wild, just for the sake of winning, but rather for the objective of gamification in educational practice and in the strategy used, in the development of the planned activity and its objectives. Students must always be clear that the activity was completed, the objectives met, and that gamification in education has positive aspects.

The importance of alternating extrinsic rewards and activities that foster curiosity and exploration, since by alternating each of these aspects, the student is able to maintain interest in the dynamics and objectives of the educational practice in the classroom, since they focus their attention not only on the extrinsic rewards, but also on the dynamics themselves, always remaining alert and interested, curious and eager to continue exploring.

4. PEDAGOGICAL APPLICATIONS AND RECOMMENDATIONS

For the effective implementation of these elements in the classroom, the following practical recommendations are proposed. Their use can foster greater student engagement, increase grade results, and foster personalization, empathy, and confidence in the development of planned activities. Teachers should develop well-planned gamified activities that are developed and aligned with the SDG objectives.

- Integrate stars and points as part of daily formative assessment.
- Design badges or insignia that reflect collaborative achievements or personal improvement.
- Allow avatar customization on digital platforms used in schools.
- Align symbolic rewards with curricular objectives, ensuring they are not trivial or unrelated.
- Train teachers in gamified instructional design and emotional design.
- Design gamified activities in accordance with the Sustainable Development Goals (SDGs).

Figure 8. Pedagogical Applications and Recommendations

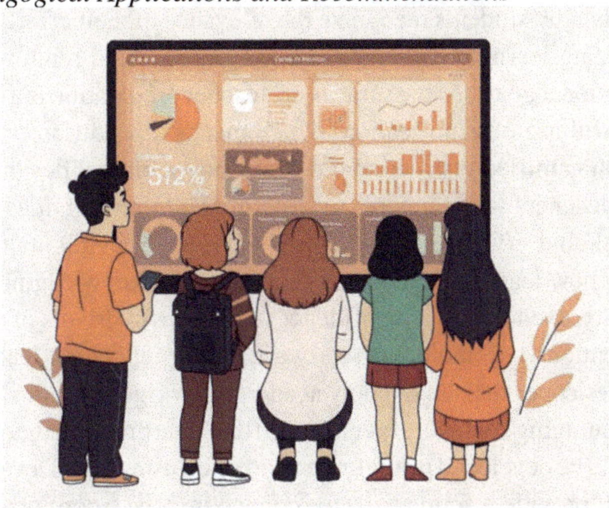

The integration of gamified strategies into the classroom requires careful planning and thoughtful pedagogical design to ensure that game-like elements not only entertain but also meaningfully support learning outcomes, student motivation, and holistic development. For this purpose, several recommendations can be highlighted as essential for teachers who wish to use gamification effectively and responsibly in education. One of the most practical strategies is to integrate stars and points into the daily routine as part of formative assessment, since this allows students to track their progress continuously, while also receiving immediate and motivating feedback that validates their effort and learning. These visible symbols of achievement may seem simple, but they play a crucial role in reinforcing persistence, building resilience, and making learning goals more concrete. Alongside points and stars, the creation of badges or insignia that recognize collaborative achievements or individual improvements is particularly valuable, because such tokens encourage students not only to focus on their personal growth but also to work collectively toward shared goals, thus promoting teamwork, cooperation, and a sense of community within the classroom. Another important recommendation is to provide opportunities for avatar customization on digital learning platforms, which enhances personalization by allowing students to express themselves through digital representations that reflect their identity, creativity, or preferences. This sense of ownership over the learning process can strengthen engagement, increase immersion, and encourage students to feel more connected to the activities. However, to ensure that these symbolic rewards and playful features are not perceived as superficial distractions, it is essential to align them carefully with curricular objectives, linking each reward to meaningful academic tasks or learning outcomes. When rewards are directly connected to the content being taught, students recognize the relevance of their effort, preventing the risk of trivializing learning and ensuring that gamification reinforces rather than replaces educational goals. At the same time, teacher preparation is a key component for the successful use of gamification, which means that educators should receive training in both gamified instructional design and emotional design. Instructional design equips teachers with the tools to structure learning activities that are coherent, purposeful, and effective, while emotional design highlights the importance of considering how learners feel during the process, acknowledging that emotions such as curiosity, excitement, or confidence are powerful drivers of motivation and knowledge retention. By combining these two forms of preparation, teachers can create classroom experiences that are not only academically rigorous but also emotionally engaging, encouraging students to persevere in their learning. Furthermore, gamified activities should be developed in alignment with the Sustainable Development Goals (SDGs), which provide a framework for connecting classroom practices to larger global challenges such as equality, sustainability, and quality education for all. By embedding SDG themes into gamified lessons, students can experience learning as something that goes beyond personal achievement, seeing it as a way to contribute to society and the world. For example, gamified projects can reward actions that promote environmental awareness, collaborative solutions to social problems, or innovative ideas to support community well-being, thereby fostering empathy, critical thinking, and global citizenship. Taken together, these recommendations make clear that gamification in education should not be reduced to the superficial use of playful symbols but should instead be approached as a comprehensive strategy that intentionally connects motivation, curriculum, emotional development, and social responsibility. When educators design gamified experiences with these principles in mind, they create learning environments that not only increase student engagement and improve academic performance but also nurture confidence, empathy, creativity, and a sense of purpose, preparing students to thrive as learners and as individuals capable of contributing meaningfully to the challenges of the twenty-first century, please refer to the following figure 8.

5. SYMBOLIC GAMIFICATION AND ITS ALIGNMENT WITH SDGs 3 AND 4

Gamification, also known as playful design, refers to the strategy of applying the principles, mechanics, and other elements of a game to an environment. It is commonly presented through a digital platform, aimed at solving problems and increasing interest to motivate students to complete the activity, which fosters the perception of autonomy and competence in the students who use it. (Chistopoulos, 2023).

Symbolic gamification, in the context of education, refers to the application of game elements and mechanics, such as points, badges, levels, and rewards, in activities that are not inherently games, with the goal of improving student engagement, motivation, and learning. Essentially, it is the practice of using game tools to make learning more engaging and effective.

It refers to play in which children use objects or situations to represent something different, such as using a box as a ship to take them to unexplored worlds within the Earth, becoming a pirate or an explorer, or a rocket that takes them off Earth. They can explore worlds where humans have not yet been able to reach, conquer the stars, and metaphorically touch the universe without leaving this planet. It is a form of play that is essential for human cognitive and social development.

On the other hand, gamification borrows elements from games and applies them to non-game contexts, such as learning. Its goal is to harness the power of intrinsic motivation and engagement found in games to improve performance and learning. In the educational context, the goal is to create a more engaging and fun learning environment by using symbolic rewards (points, badges, avatars, shields, stars) and various game mechanics (levels or challenges, among others) to motivate students and make the teaching-learning process more interactive and satisfying. This aims to increase student motivation and engagement, as playful elements can make learning more fun and engaging, resulting in more motivated students. This motivation also fosters concentration and attention, as games require the development of both, which helps students develop these skills. We can also find that, through the development of gamification, students develop cognitive skills, memory development, logical thinking, problem-solving, and, very importantly, creativity. When learning becomes more interactive and fun, gamification can help students better understand and retain information, resulting in more effective learning (Gené, s. f.).

But it can also improve socialization, as it fosters cooperation and teamwork, promoting greater socialization among students through peer-to-peer work. This, in turn, leads to improved and higher self-esteem among students, as they receive symbolic rewards when overcoming challenges, and can experience a greater sense of achievement and self-confidence.

The 2030 Agenda for Sustainable Development, approved in September 2015 by the United Nations General Assembly, establishes a transformative vision for the economic, social, and environmental sustainability of the 193 United Nations Member States that endorsed it. It serves as a guiding principle for the international community's work through 2030. The 2030 Agenda presents a historic opportunity for Latin America and the Caribbean, as it includes high-priority issues for the region, such as the eradication of extreme poverty, the reduction of inequality in all its dimensions, inclusive economic growth with decent work for all, sustainable cities, and climate change, among others.

It is a civilizing agenda that places the dignity and equality of people at its center and calls for a change in our development style. It is a universal commitment made by both developed and developing countries, within the framework of a strengthened global partnership, which considers the means of implementation to achieve change and prevent disasters caused by extreme natural events, as well as mitigation and adaptation to climate change, please refer to the following figure 9.

The 2030 Agenda is the result of the broadest and most participatory consultation process in the history of the United Nations and represents the emerging multilateral consensus among governments and diverse actors, such as civil society, the private sector, and academia. Furthermore, the normative foundations of this multilateral agenda range from the 1945 United Nations Charter to the more than 40 UN references and conventions approved to date.

The 2030 Agenda represents a multilateral consensus among governments and diverse actors, capable of making national policies in favor of employment with rights and development compatible with the expansion of international trade and conflict prevention. It represents commitments that recognize people, peace, shared prosperity, the planet, and partnerships as the main shared and universal guiding principles on which a new set of global, regional, and national strategies and policies must be based, the priority objective of which is to move together toward a new, more egalitarian society. (Cepal.org).

Figure 9. Agenda 2023 Pillars Sustentable Dvelopment Goals

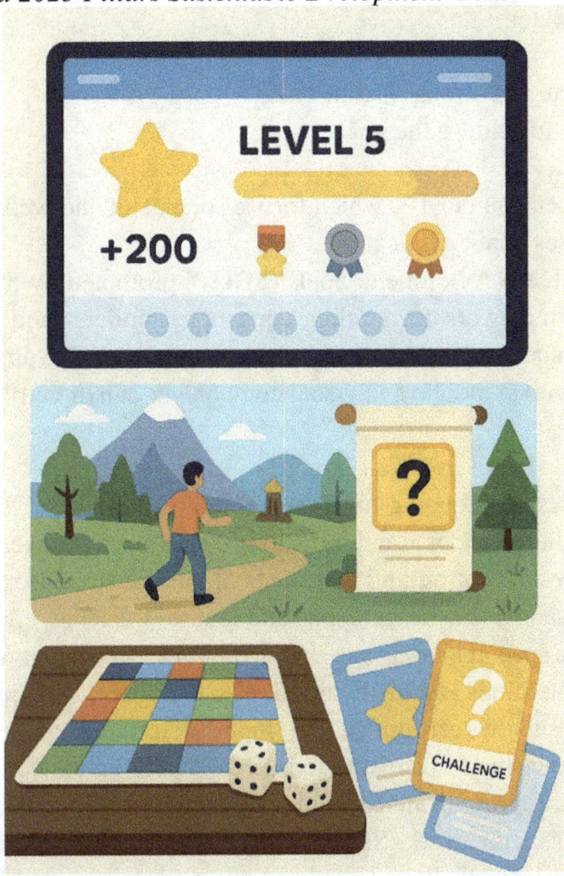

To this end, 17 goals have been developed:

1. End poverty.
2. Zero hunger.
3. Good health and well-being.
4. Quality education.
5. Gender equality.
6. Clean water and sanitation.
7. Affordable and clean energy.
8. Decent work and economic growth.
9. Industry, innovation, and infrastructure.
10. Reduction of inequalities.
11. Sustainable cities and communities.
12. Responsible production and consumption.

13. Climate action.
14. Life below water.
15. Life on land.
16. Peace, justice, and strong institutions.
17. Partnerships to achieve the goals.

Next, we'll focus on Goal 3, which focuses on health and well-being, and Goal 4, which addresses quality education.

The Sustainable Development Goals (SDGs), promoted by the UN, provide a comprehensive framework for guiding educational policies and practices toward goals of justice, equity, and well-being at the global level. The application of gamified strategies with symbolic and visual components can directly contribute to the following SDGs:

SDG 3: Good Health and Well-being

SDG 3 focuses on reducing maternal mortality, ending preventable deaths of newborns and children under 5, and combating communicable diseases. It also works to strengthen the prevention and treatment of substance abuse, reducing deaths and injuries caused by traffic accidents, and focuses on achieving universal health coverage. It has a special interest in reducing pollution and supporting research and development of vaccines and medicines. It also believes it is important to increase health financing and the recruitment, development, training, and retention of health workers; strengthen the implementation of the WHO Framework Convention on Tobacco Control; improve mental health and well-being; and address women's health.

But within this framework, SDG 3 is crucial for sustainable development because health is intrinsically linked to other goals, such as education, gender equality, economic growth, and poverty reduction. A healthy population is generally more productive and is expected to contribute to economic growth, thus tending to be less vulnerable to poverty.

Regarding the actions to be achieved under SDG 3, we can mention investment in health, since increasing investment in both the public and private sectors guarantees access to quality services for all.

Strengthening health systems is especially important, ensuring they are more resilient and able to respond to the needs of the population, especially in emergency situations.

Education must take into account awareness and promote education on health and well-being, healthy lifestyles, and disease prevention.

Collaboration and partnerships foster collaboration between governments and the private sector, integrating civil society and the international community to achieve the SDG 3 targets.

But it also takes into account research and development, investing in research and development of new technologies, as well as medicines and vaccines to combat diseases.

Regarding mental health prevention, policies and programs are implemented to promote the mental health and emotional well-being of the population.

But regarding gamification in education, which is our central theme, we must. This goal seeks to ensure healthy lives and promote well-being for all. In the educational field, symbolic gamification can contribute to SDG 3 by promoting. Sustainable Development Goal (SDG) 3 seeks to ensure healthy lives and promote well-being for all. In the educational context, symbolic gamification—through the use of avatars, stars, and shields—can be a valuable tool to contribute to this goal. By offering a playful, safe, and reinforcing environment, anxiety about making mistakes is reduced and students' self-esteem is strengthened, creating a more positive learning environment (Gené, s. f.).

Furthermore, the implementation of symbolic rewards and positive feedback favors the development of emotional self-regulation. This means that students learn to manage their emotions in situations of effort, failure, and achievement—essential skills for good mental health from childhood. This emotional learning also translates into a greater ability to face academic and personal challenges.

Finally, working in motivating and visually appealing environments can reduce academic stress. Unlike traditional assessments, which often generate pressure and anxiety, gamification introduces more enjoyable dynamics that increase enjoyment and engagement in learning. Thus, it fosters not only academic performance but also students' overall well-being, aligning with the principles of SDG 3.

- Emotional well-being: Avatars, stars, and shields, by creating a playful, safe, and reinforcing environment, reduce the anxiety associated with mistakes and strengthen self-esteem (Gómez-Urquiza et al., 2021).
- Emotional self-regulation: Through symbolic rewards and positive feedback, students learn to manage their emotions in the context of effort, mistakes, and achievement, developing key skills for children's mental health.
- Reduction of academic stress: Working in a motivating and visually friendly environment can reduce the pressure of traditional assessments and increase the perception of enjoyment during learning.

SDG 4: Quality Education

Since the adoption of the 2030 Agenda in 2015, it was established that the primary responsibility for its implementation rests with each government, taking into account the priorities and specificities of each country.

The United Nations system committed to support and established a list of global indicators to measure progress toward achieving the SDGs. This list, called the Global Indicator Framework for Monitoring the SDG 4 Targets, is regularly updated.

In addition to the Global Framework, thematic indicators were proposed to monitor "progress with a deeper perspective on sectoral priorities than that offered by the global monitoring framework" (UNESCO 2018). It was also agreed to develop regional and national measurement systems, which must always be aligned with the 232 global SDG indicators.

What are indicators?

They are measurable and verifiable tools to clarify and more precisely define objectives and impacts. They are designed to provide a standard against which to evaluate, estimate, or demonstrate progress toward established goals.

What are the indicators for measuring progress toward achieving SDG 4?

There are 12 global indicators, 31 thematic indicators, 2 regional indicators (for Latin America and the Caribbean), and 2 national indicators (approved by Mexico within the framework of the Specialized Committee on the Sustainable Development Goals). 9 In total, there are 47 indicators, several of which are currently under construction.

As part of the consensus embodied in the Incheon Declaration and the Education 2030 Framework for Action, the international community committed to adopting benchmarks for SDG 4 indicators by defining intermediate (2025) and final (2030) targets.

For this reason, the UNESCO Technical Cooperation Group on SDG 4, Education 2030, Indicators (TCG), of which Mexico is a member, selected a group of indicators considered strategic for working on benchmarks for 2025 and 2030.

As a result of this collaboration, Mexico was selected by the UNESCO Institute for Statistics (IUIS-UNESCO) as one of 12 country case studies that successfully followed a process for establishing national benchmarks, covering 32 of the 40 intermediate and final values. (See report on the Establishment of Commitments). The IUS also notes that the country is showing progress on some indicators (planeación.sep.gob.mx).

Regarding the approach that this SDG will take to education management, it clearly and specifically states the following:

The fourth SDG aims to guarantee inclusive, equitable, and quality education. Symbolic gamification can positively impact this objective by:

- Promote equity in learning: By allowing all students to earn symbolic rewards based on their own progress, the gap between those who learn faster and those who require more support is narrowed (Huang et al., 2019).

- Incentivize meaningful learning: By connecting symbolic elements to curricular content, intrinsic motivation is enhanced, deep understanding is fostered, and active participation is promoted.
- Stimulate digital inclusion: The use of platforms that allow customizable avatars and diverse cultural symbols can foster representation and a sense of belonging, especially in vulnerable communities (Huang et al., 2019).
- E-learning: (or electronic learning), being an educational modality that uses information and communication technologies (ICT) to provide training through online platforms, such as (Duolingo), instead of traditional face-to-face teaching, e-learning allows students to access content, carry out activities and participate in educational interactions through electronic devices, such as computers, phones, tablets, etc.

The use of technology relies on the internet and electronic devices for content delivery and teacher-student interaction. Its flexibility allows students to learn at their own pace and at the time that best suits them.

Accessibility aims to eliminate geographical and time barriers, making this training modality accessible to a wider audience. It includes resources such as videos, presentations, documents, as well as discussion forums and videoconferences, utilizing a variety of formats. This interaction facilitates communication between students and teachers through tools such as those mentioned above.

Some advantages include greater flexibility and autonomy, as students can access content at their own schedules and pace. It also reduces costs, as in many cases, e-learning can be more economical than in-person training by eliminating travel costs and physical materials.

Figure 10. Quality Education

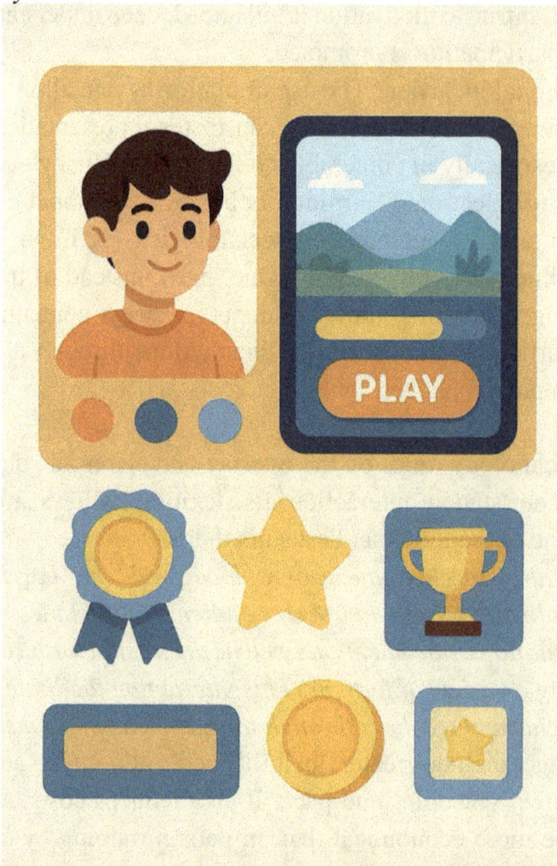

It also offers greater geographic reach, allowing students to be reached anywhere in the world, regardless of their physical location. At the same time, content can be easily updated, keeping information always up-to-date, and learning can be personalized by creating learning experiences tailored to each student's needs and learning styles.

Some examples of e-learning learning or the use of e-learning include online courses, corporate training, corporate learning platforms, and digital educational resources.

Therefore, e-learning is a learning modality that has evolved into the way people acquire knowledge and skills, offering a flexible, accessible, and effective alternative to traditional education. (overview created by AI).

- B-learning: (blended learning) is a type of learning that combines remote and in-person learning with one goal: to combine the best of both worlds to achieve more efficient learning. This disruptive education model emerged in the late 1990s at the hands of the Clayton Christensen Institute for Disruptive Education. The rapid development of Information and Communication Technologies (ICT) has led to the rise of this and other virtual learning models.

Some of its modalities include Rotation: where students rotate according to a fixed schedule or at the teacher's discretion between different learning modalities, one of which is virtual, which in turn offers various options, such as stations, laboratory, and individual learning. However, the most famous is the flipped classroom, in which students learn outside of the classroom through online educational resources and complete practical tasks in the classroom under the guidance of the teacher.

The flexible method: where teachers instruct and support in class on a flexible schedule and on demand. Tutorials, for example, allow students to progress at their own pace through the content through online platforms.

Or the à la carte method: where students choose which subjects to take online, depending on the school's offerings, and the remaining subjects are taught in person in the classroom.

Or the enriched virtual method: where students attend some classroom sessions but then have the freedom to complete the course online, despite not meeting face-to-face with teachers every day of the week. This method requires students to complete a certain number of learning hours.

We can find advantages and disadvantages in this type of learning:

Among the advantages, we can find improvements in student motivation and performance, it promotes participation and self-learning, as well as teamwork, opens new avenues for interaction between teachers and students, also allows for greater flexibility, promotes digital intelligence and the acquisition of new digital skills, among others.

Some of its drawbacks include that it can be complicated at first, due to the demands of individual work and the essential acquisition of technological skills that it entails, or that it causes a lengthening of the learning curve.

B-learning requires the development of a model with clear steps such as: having a plan, going step by step, involving school staff, having adequate resources, adapting the technology to the needs, and evaluating the results (collecting data). (Iberdrola.com).

- M-learning (mobile learning) is learning delivered using mobile devices such as smartphones, tablets, and other devices with wireless connectivity. This allows students to access educational materials and participate in learning activities anytime, anywhere, breaking the time and space limitations of traditional learning. It differs from e-learning (electronic learning), which typically uses desktop or laptop computers as the primary medium. M-learning offers flexibility and accessibility, allowing students to learn autonomously and in ways that adapt to their needs.

Its advantages include flexibility and accessibility, where students can access content and participate in learning activities anytime, anywhere, as long as they have access to a mobile device, resulting in personalized learning. By adapting to students' learning styles and offering more interactive experiences, mobile devices achieve greater interactivity, offering diverse forms of interaction through the use of touch screens, audio, and video, which can enrich the learning experience.

Mobility or location is not an issue since students can access educational content while on the go or in different locations, allowing for informal learning.

Some of its disadvantages may include distractions from the use of mobile devices and connectivity with social media or notifications, which could affect students' concentration. Regarding technological limitations, we can find that some devices may have limited processing, storage, or connectivity capacity, which can affect the user experience. However, it is also important to consider planning needs for m-learning to be effective. Teachers must carefully plan both the methodology and the activities, taking into account the characteristics of mobile learning.

M-learning can be used in various ways or areas. With access to educational platforms that students can access online with their mobile devices, there are various educational applications designed to facilitate learning in different areas, for example, math, science, history, or even languages.

This type of learning allows for participation in forums and social networks, as students can use both forums and social networks to communicate with their peers and teachers, share resources, and collaborate on projects.

Access to multimedia content is very important, as mobile devices allow access to videos, podcasts, and other multimedia materials that can enrich the learning experience.

Therefore, m-learning represents a significant evolution in the field of education, offering new opportunities for accessing knowledge and building new learning experiences in a flexible and personalized way. (AI-created overview).

M-learning is a form of learning that uses mobile devices such as phones and tablets with a wireless connection, allowing students to access content and activities anytime, anywhere. Unlike e-learning, which is primarily computer-based, m-learning offers greater flexibility and adaptation to individual needs.

Its advantages include flexibility, personalized learning, and interactivity, thanks to touchscreens, audio, and video. Additionally, students can learn on the go and take advantage of apps, platforms, and social media to collaborate and share resources.

However, it presents challenges such as distractions from notifications, technical limitations, and the need for proper lesson planning. When well designed, m-learning enriches the educational experience and fosters autonomy.

Developing 21st-century skills:

- 21st-century skills include competencies such as collaboration, self-regulation, and decision-making. These capabilities are essential for students to successfully navigate an increasingly interconnected and changing world. Gamified environments offer an ideal space for developing them, as they promote teamwork, emotional control, and the ability to choose appropriate strategies to achieve goals.
- When designing a gamified learning experience, it's not just about adding engaging elements or rewards to motivate students. It's essential that the pedagogical approach integrates activities that strengthen key life skills, thus fostering deeper and more meaningful learning. This involves aligning gamification with clear educational objectives and methodologies that promote active participation.
- In this way, the use of gamification not only improves motivation and engagement in the classroom but also contributes to sustainable development and child well-being. By enhancing skills that students will need in their personal and professional futures, it advances global commitments to providing quality education that prepares new generations for the challenges and opportunities of the 21st century.

In this sense, gamified pedagogical design should not only focus on increasing motivation but also on actively contributing to global commitments to education and child well-being.

Figure 11. Develop 21st Century Skills

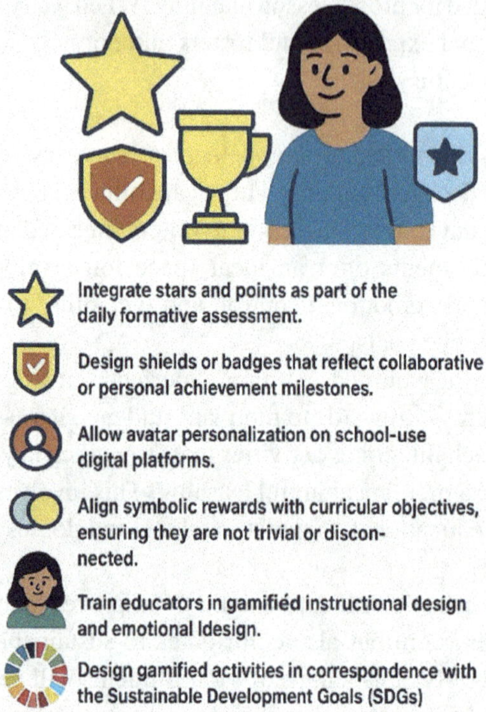
Integrate stars and points as part of the
daily formative assessment.
Design shields or badges that reflect collaborative
or personal achievement milestones.
Allow avatar personalization on school-use
digital platforms.
Align symbolic rewards with curricular objectives,
ensuring they are not trivial or discon-
nected.
Train educators in gamifiéd instructional design
and emotional Idesign.
Design gamified activities in correspondence with
the Sustainable Development Goals (SDGs)

The development of 21st-century skills has become a central goal of contemporary education, as students today face a world that is increasingly globalized, interconnected, and subject to rapid technological, social, and cultural change. These skills include essential competencies such as collaboration, self-regulation, communication, problem-solving, creativity, and decision-making, all of which allow learners to thrive in complex environments both within and beyond the classroom (Supervía & Bordás, 2020). Gamification, when implemented intentionally and with clear pedagogical purposes, offers a particularly effective avenue for cultivating these skills. Unlike traditional approaches that may rely heavily on memorization or passive absorption of content, gamified learning environments place students at the center of the process, encouraging them to interact, make choices, and actively shape their learning journey. For example, by working together to achieve a shared objective in a gamified task, students practice collaboration and learn to value diverse perspectives, while also developing conflict-resolution skills. At the same time, the need to regulate emotions in competitive or challenging scenarios strengthens self-control and resilience, preparing learners to handle stress and setbacks in real life. Decision-making is also reinforced as students are constantly required to evaluate options, weigh strategies, and choose the most effective course of action to achieve goals, whether in the context of solving a problem, overcoming a digital challenge, or advancing to the next level of a game-like activity. These scenarios create safe yet stimulating environments where experimentation, failure, and persistence are not only possible but are also integral to growth. In this sense, gamified education contributes to the acquisition of 21st-century competencies by integrating opportunities for teamwork, emotional development, and strategic thinking, all of which are increasingly indispensable for navigating the uncertainties of modern life. However, it is important to emphasize that gamification should not be reduced to the mere addition of points, rewards, or entertaining features designed only to capture attention. Instead, a well-designed gamified learning experience must embed activities that directly strengthen the key life skills students will require in adulthood. This requires aligning gamification with well-defined educational objectives, pedagogical methodologies that promote active learning, and assessment strategies that measure not only academic performance but also growth in these critical competencies.

At a broader level, the significance of gamification in education extends beyond its immediate impact on motivation and classroom engagement, as it can also play a pivotal role in advancing sustainable development and supporting children's overall well-being (Supervía & Bordás, 2020). By enhancing the skills students will rely on in their personal, social, and professional lives, gamification contributes to fulfilling global commitments, particularly those outlined in the United Nations Sustainable Development Goals (SDGs). For instance, SDG 4 emphasizes the importance of ensuring inclusive and equitable quality education, and gamification, when designed intentionally, can become a tool to achieve this by making learning more participatory, inclusive, and adaptable to different student needs. Moreover, SDG 3 highlights the goal of good health and well-being, which gamification indirectly supports by promoting resilience, emotional regulation, and self-confidence through carefully structured challenges and feedback mechanisms. In this way, gamified learning fosters not only cognitive growth but also the social and emotional competencies that are essential for lifelong health and flourishing. Furthermore, the integration of gamification within e-learning, mobile learning, and blended learning platforms makes it possible to extend these benefits to diverse contexts, reaching students who may otherwise face barriers to education. Nevertheless, the true value of gamification lies in its ability to balance extrinsic motivators with the cultivation of intrinsic motivation, so that students not only work for points or badges but also develop curiosity, autonomy, and a genuine love of learning. When teachers design gamified experiences with this balance in mind, they create educational opportunities that are both engaging and meaningful, while also equipping learners with the capacities to contribute positively to their communities and future workplaces. Ultimately, gamified pedagogical design should not limit itself to increasing immediate motivation;

rather, it must be understood as a broader educational strategy that simultaneously supports student engagement, skill development, and the global mission of education for sustainable development. By promoting collaboration, empathy, decision-making, and emotional resilience, gamification prepares students to meet the challenges of the 21st century and empowers them to become not only competent professionals but also responsible citizens committed to equity, well-being, and educational quality for all (Gené, s. f.).

6. CONCLUSIONS

Gamification, when systematically integrated into educational design, constitutes a pedagogical strategy capable of significantly enhancing student motivation, engagement, and learning outcomes. By incorporating symbolic elements such as stars, shields, and customizable avatars, gamification transforms classroom experiences into interactive environments that stimulate curiosity, persistence, and active participation (Supervía & Bordás, 2020). These elements provide clear, immediate feedback and reinforce desirable behaviors while maintaining students' attention over extended periods, demonstrating that gamification is more than a superficial motivational tool; it is a deliberate instructional methodology.

Beyond mere engagement, gamification strengthens essential soft skills such as collaboration, communication, and self-regulation. These competencies are fundamental for holistic development, particularly in primary education, as they allow students to interact effectively within both academic and social contexts. By fostering teamwork, negotiation, and problem-solving through game-like tasks, students learn to coordinate with peers, manage emotions, and assume responsibility for their own learning processes, which are critical for their long-term personal and academic success.

The theoretical foundation of gamification is strongly supported by both behaviorist and sociocultural perspectives. Skinner's principles of operant conditioning explain how external reinforcement, including points, badges, or virtual rewards, encourages the repetition of positive academic behaviors and facilitates habit formation (Skinner, s. f.). Complementarily, Vygotsky's concept of the Zone of Proximal Development (ZPD) highlights the importance of guided learning, scaffolding, and peer collaboration in enabling learners to achieve outcomes beyond their independent capabilities (Vygotsky, 1978). This theoretical convergence ensures that gamified strategies are both motivational and pedagogically sound.

The use of mockups and emotionally engaging designs enhances the effectiveness of gamification by providing tangible representations of learning objectives. Mockups—whether as digital interfaces, 3D environments, or physical prototypes—

serve as scaffolds that mediate understanding and guide students toward incremental mastery. They also increase immersion and emotional connection to the learning material, allowing students to experience immediate progress, self-efficacy, and achievement, which strengthens both cognitive and affective engagement.

From a didactic perspective, gamification must be implemented intentionally to balance extrinsic and intrinsic motivation. While rewards and symbolic elements can reinforce desired behaviors, over-reliance on them risks diminishing intrinsic interest in learning and may negatively affect emotional well-being (Howard-Jones, 2014). Therefore, gamified activities must be carefully designed to ensure that external incentives complement internal motivation, allowing students to value the learning process itself rather than focusing solely on obtaining rewards.

Gamification aligns closely with global educational and sustainability objectives, particularly SDG 3 (Good Health and Well-being) and SDG 4 (Quality Education). By promoting emotional self-regulation, resilience, and cooperative behaviors, gamification supports the mental and emotional health of students, contributing to healthier learning experiences consistent with SDG 3. Furthermore, gamified learning strategies enhance inclusivity and equity in education, providing adaptive pathways, interactive feedback, and accessible tools that support students with diverse developmental needs, directly contributing to SDG 4's goal of inclusive and equitable quality education.

The integration of emerging technologies, such as e-learning, m-learning, and b-learning platforms, amplifies the potential of gamification. These technologies allow students to interact with content flexibly, receive immediate feedback, and engage in collaborative problem-solving activities across spatial and temporal boundaries. However, careful instructional planning is necessary to prevent cognitive overload, digital fatigue, or reduced attention spans, ensuring that technology serves as an enabler rather than a distraction.

Effective gamification requires that each symbolic and interactive element serves a clear educational purpose. Visual representations, game mechanics, and narrative components must be coherently aligned with curriculum goals, pedagogical frameworks, and developmental appropriateness. When designed thoughtfully, gamified environments can foster equity, empathy, and engagement, creating learning experiences that are meaningful, enjoyable, and impactful while respecting students' individual differences and promoting long-term academic and socio-emotional growth.

Gamification in education represents a transformative approach when integrated with theoretical grounding, intentional design, and alignment with global educational objectives. By combining behavioral reinforcement, social interaction, emotional engagement, and technological mediation, gamification supports holistic student development and prepares learners to thrive both academically and socially. When implemented in accordance with SDG 3 and SDG 4, gamification not only motivates and engages students but also contributes to the broader goals of well-being, inclusivity, and equitable quality education, demonstrating its potential as a scientifically and ethically grounded pedagogical tool.

REFERENCES

Birk, M. V., Mandryk, R. L., & Krolczyk, Z. (2020). The effects of avatar customization on player engagement in educational games [Conference session]. 2020 IEEE International Conference on Teaching, Assessment, and Learning for Engineering (TALE), Takamatsu, Japan (virtual). https://doi.org/DOI: 10.1109/TALE48869.2020.9368315

Gené, O. B. (n.d.). *Gamificación en educación* [Unpublished manuscript]. Universidad Politécnica de Madrid.

Gómez-Urquiza, J. L., Velando-Soriano, A., Membrive-Jiménez, M. J., Ramírez-Baena, L., Aguayo-Estremera, R., Ortega-Campos, E., & Cañadas-De la Fuente, G. A. (2023). Prevalence and levels of burnout in nursing students: A systematic review with meta-analysis. *Nurse Education in Practice*, *72*, 103753. Advance online publication. DOI: 10.1016/j.nepr.2023.103753 PMID: 37651959

Hamari, J., Koivisto, J., & Sarsa, H. (2014). Does gamification work? — A literature review of empirical studies on gamification. In *Proceedings of the 47th Hawaii International Conference on System Sciences* (pp. 3025–3034). IEEE. https://doi.org/DOI: 10.1109/HICSS.2014.377

Howard-Jones, P. A. (2014). Neuroscience and education: Myths and messages. *Nature Reviews. Neuroscience*, *15*(12), 817–824. DOI: 10.1038/nrn3817 PMID: 25315391

Huang, B., Hew, K. F., & Lo, C. K. (2019). Investigating the effects of gamification-enhanced flipped learning on undergraduate students' behavioral and cognitive engagement. *Interactive Learning Environments*, *27*(8), 1106–1126. DOI: 10.1080/10494820.2018.1495653

Koivisto, J., & Hamari, J. (2019). The rise of motivational information systems: A review of gamification research. *International Journal of Information Management*, *45*, 191–210. DOI: 10.1016/j.ijinfomgt.2018.10.013

Looyestyn, J., Kernot, J., Boshoff, K., Ryan, J., Edney, S., & Maher, C. (2017). Does gamification increase engagement with online programs? A systematic review. *PLoS One*, *12*(3), e0173403. Advance online publication. DOI: 10.1371/journal.pone.0173403 PMID: 28362821

Norman, D. A. (2004). *Emotional design: Why we love (or hate) everyday things*. Basic Books. DOI: 10.1145/985600.966013

Piaget, J. (1952). *The origins of intelligence in children* (Cook, M., Trans.). International Universities Press., DOI: 10.1037/11494-000

Ryan, R. M., & Deci, E. L. (2000). Self-determination theory and the facilitation of intrinsic motivation, social development, and well-being. *The American Psychologist, 55*(1), 68–78. DOI: 10.1037/0003-066X.55.1.68 PMID: 11392867

Seaborn, K., & Fels, D. I. (2015). Gamification in theory and action: A survey. *International Journal of Human-Computer Studies, 74*, 14–31. DOI: 10.1016/j.ijhcs.2014.09.006

Skinner, B. F. (1953). *Science and human behavior*. Macmillan.

Toda, A. M., Valle, P. H. D., Isotani, S., Cristea, A. I., Bittencourt, I. I., & Lima, F. (2018). The dark side of gamification: An overview of negative effects of gamification in education. In *Higher Education for All: From challenges to novel technology-enhanced solutions* (p. 14). Springer. DOI: 10.1007/978-3-319-97934-2_9

Usán Supervía, P., & Salavera Bordás, C. (Eds.). (2020). *Gamificación educativa: Innovación en el aula para potenciar el proceso de enseñanza-aprendizaje*. Pregunta Ediciones. https://dialnet.unirioja.es/servlet/libro?codigo=972682

Vygotsky, L. S. (1978). *Mind in society: The development of higher psychological processes* (Cole, M., John-Steiner, V., Scribner, S., & Souberman, E., Eds.). Harvard University Press., DOI: 10.2307/j.ctvjf9vz4

Chapter 8
Co-Designing a Serious Game for Early Literacy:
A Participatory Case Study from Mexico

Laura S. Gaytán-Lugo
https://orcid.org/0000-0002-7007-7500
Universidad de Colima, Mexico

Pedro C. Santana-Mancilla
https://orcid.org/0000-0002-4184-0116
Universidad de Colima, Mexico

Pablo A. Alcaraz-Valencia
https://orcid.org/0000-0003-2994-2395
Universidad de Colima, Mexico

Eduardo D. Jimenez Cisneros
Universidad de Colima, Mexico

Cristina Zéster Pelayo
Universidad de Colima, Mexico

ABSTRACT

Video games are increasingly recognized as engaging tools to enhance learning. In Mexico, where children's reading performance presents challenges, serious games offer innovative opportunities to foster early literacy. This study aimed to design and evaluate a serious game to support reading and writing skills in preschool children. Using a participatory design approach, teachers and children actively co-created the proposal to ensure relevance and acceptance. The game was developed with

DOI: 10.4018/979-8-3373-4657-1.ch008

the Unity platform and integrated three activities: completing words, matching letters with images, and a memory game. Evaluation sessions were carried out with children at a support school, complemented by teacher feedback. Results revealed strong acceptance of the technology, reflected in children's motivation, enjoyment, and sustained attention. Suggestions included increasing difficulty levels and incorporating phonetic feedback, providing insights for improving future iterations, and expanding educational impact.

INTRODUCTION

Knowing how to read is one of the fundamental pillars for acquiring and transmitting knowledge both in everyday life and in the academic world (Guzhñay Vélez, 2021). However, reading habits in Mexico continue to represent a significant educational challenge. Studies indicate that more than 70% of Mexicans do not read a single book per year (Camacho, 2013), and the country ranks second to last among 108 nations evaluated by UNESCO in terms of reading practices (Villamil, 2013). Data from INEGI's Reading Module (MOLEC) further reveal a downward trend: while 50.2% of adults reported reading at least one book in 2015, this proportion declined to 45.1% by 2018. Similarly, the OECD has documented decreasing reading performance among Mexican students, reflecting persistent difficulties with basic literacy skills (Schleicher, 2019).

Nowadays, one of the main challenges in education is the development of reading skills. When reading instruction relies exclusively on traditional methods and materials, students often display apathy and lack of motivation due to the monotony and limited variety of approaches used in the teaching–learning process (Vargas et al., 2023). These challenges underscore the need for innovative strategies to foster literacy from an early age. Research has consistently shown that promoting literacy at a young age has long-term positive effects on productivity and learning outcomes (Burns, Griffin, & Snows, 1999; Russo, Kosman, Ginsburg, Thompson-Hoffman, & Pederson, 1998; Slavin, Madden, Dolan, & Wasik, 1996; Swartz, Shook, & Klein, 2000; González & Delgado, 2009).

Given their motivational and engaging nature, video games represent a promising avenue for educational innovation. They have had a significant impact on young people (Gros Salvat, 2009) and are particularly relevant in Mexico, where the country is the leading consumer of video games in Latin America (Armendáriz Espadas & Sánchez Camargo, 2018; Endeavor & Santander, 2025). A video game is an interactive digital system in which players engage with rules, challenges, and feedback through input devices such as controllers, keyboards, mice, or touchscreens, with outcomes visualized on a screen (Juul, 2005; Entertainment Software Association

[ESA], 2023). Traditionally, their main purpose has been entertainment; however, video games encompass multiple branches, one of which is serious games. A serious game is a video game whose purpose goes beyond leisure; as its name suggests, it is designed with an explicit educational, health-related, or professional training objective. Educational serious games enhance learners' cognitive and motor skills (Evans et al., 2016).

Video games are now deeply embedded in people's daily lives. Worldwide, there are an estimated two billion players (Statista, 2018; Boyle et al., 2016). In Mexico alone, around 76 million people play video games (Endeavor & Santander, 2025), and according to Jiménez (2018), a large proportion of Mexican children spend at least one hour a day engaging with this type of technology. This widespread presence represents a valuable opportunity to leverage the appeal of video games for educational purposes. Recent evidence supports this perspective, showing that serious games are increasingly recognized for their role in education and training (Connolly et al., 2012; Fernández-Sánchez et al., 2023).

One of the main reasons for considering video games as tools to support literacy activities lies in their proven capacity to capture and sustain attention. Papert (1993) noted that many people learn from video games precisely because of the challenges they present: players actively seek strategies and information to overcome obstacles, much like students tackling an academic problem. Since completing a game usually requires multiple attempts, experiential learning is achieved through practice and iteration. These qualities position video games as a powerful medium for supporting literacy development in ways that are both entertaining and educational.

Furthermore, researchers have increasingly sought to harness the attention-grabbing power of video games by assigning them a serious purpose, as they offer multiple educational and socio-emotional benefits. For instance, Erickson (1977) argued that play contexts allow children to experience social interactions and explore alternative emotional outcomes. More recent studies have demonstrated that serious games can foster motivation, engagement, and socio-emotional learning in young learners, while also supporting the development of collaboration and problem-solving skills (Connolly et al., 2012; Fernández-Sánchez et al., 2023).

In this chapter, we present the design and development of a video game conceived as a technological support tool to foster reading and writing skills in preschool children.

LITERATURE REVIEW

Video Games and Education

Children increasingly use video games as their first means of accessing the digital world. Video games are attractive and entertaining because they use sounds, colors, and other features that capture attention; at the same time, they help develop skills that support early experiences in human–computer interaction (López Raventós, 2016). With the rapid advancement of technology and the growing presence of virtual environments in everyday life, it is common to see young children easily handling devices ranging from mobile phones to computers. This context suggests that video games can serve as valuable alternatives to support learning inside and outside the classroom (Moral Álvarez & Almazán Ruíz, 2017).

The video game industry has grown significantly in recent decades, becoming a significant element in the lives of children and adolescents. Its evolution has been remarkable: from the early 2D game OXO, considered one of the first video games, to more complex titles that gained popularity with consoles such as Nintendo's SNES (8 and 16 bits), and later with the emergence of 3D graphics on 32-bit systems like Sony's PlayStation. The creation of 3D accelerators on personal computers further enhanced visual quality (Belli & López Raventós, 2008). Over time, technological improvements have expanded the quality and popularity of games, making them accessible to audiences of all ages and opening possibilities for applications in education and training (Belli & López Raventós, 2008).

Video games also mirror pedagogical systems, in which learners are given increasingly challenging exercises. Incorporating these principles into interactive environments, such as games, provides powerful learning tools. A common approach is using pedagogical agents, avatars or characters that guide the player through assigned tasks, offering various supports to strengthen specific learning outcomes.

Although video games have long been associated primarily with leisure, their educational potential is often overlooked. During the 1980s, much scientific research focused on their adverse effects, shaping a critical public perception. However, later studies showed that negative consequences were minimal, while positive outcomes were significant (González González, 2011; López et al., 2023; Marinelli et al., 2023). The engaging nature of games has been harnessed to develop educational and serious games, which—though they may seem novel—have been studied for several decades. These games are designed to strengthen specific skills, such as reading comprehension or writing practice. By combining elements such as simulation with real-life contexts, educational video games generate greater interest among learners, as they can identify with the environment while pursuing well-defined learning goals (López Raventós, 2016).

Gee (2003) argues that video games allow players to consume knowledge and produce it, fostering feedback that requires the integration of previously acquired and new skills to solve problems. Similarly, Papert (1998) stated that learning is hard; it happens best when deeply engaging in complex and challenging activities. This author explained that children prefer difficult things if they are interesting. Unlike conventional study methods that rely on rote memorization and later assessment, video games evaluate learners instantly, as they overcome problems or challenges, promoting greater efficiency in knowledge retention.

While games have traditionally been seen as leisure activities, they can also function as tools for learning and personal development. Reported benefits include improvements in language and thought structuring; facilitation of meaningful learning; reduced anxiety about errors and failure; encouragement of active participation; and stimulation of creativity, intellectual competence, emotional resilience, and personal stability, all of which contribute to holistic development (Latorre, 2003; Marcano, 2008; López Raventós, 2016).

Educational Video Games for Literacy

The use of video games to support reading and writing processes is not new. There is a substantial background of projects that, in some cases, have yielded positive results across different age groups, particularly among preschool and elementary school students.

Lost in La Mancha is one of the many serious games currently available. It is an online educational video game for learning Spanish, designed for English-speaking learners. The player controls the protagonist, Collin, who must acquire enough knowledge of the Spanish language to survive in a fictional town called "La Mancha." The project is immersive, developed in 3D, and accessible from any mobile device via the internet. The learning activities are structured according to the curriculum of the Instituto Cervantes, following an active methodology that embodies the principle of learning by doing (Maniega, Yànez, & Lara, 2011).

It's a Deal! is another serious game, developed with technological support from the General Foundation of the University of Alicante using the Visionaire Studio 3.0 engine. This project provides a simulated experience for business English students, allowing them to discover the cultural rules underlying transactions in British contexts and practice their application in different negotiation stages. The game highlights the impact of intercultural exchanges and the role of linguistic behavior. Evaluations showed that students were enthusiastic about the game: among the positive responses, 31.3% considered it educational, 27.1% entertaining, and 27.1% instructive, as it helped users become familiar with business communication.

Additionally, 16.5% reported enjoying the learning experience through gameplay (Guillén & Aleson, 2011).

Another serious game was introduced by Gaytán-Lugo et al. (2015), aimed at strengthening reading comprehension skills among third-grade students. Dasha is a 2D video game developed with the Unity 3D engine under a user-centered design approach. It features a main character, an antagonist, secondary characters, interactive scenarios, and interfaces designed and tested with Balsamiq Mockups. A demo was presented to students, who were asked to complete in-game tasks and later respond to a questionnaire about their experience. Students described the game as fun and engaging, noting some challenges in completing tasks. Results showed that 90% of participants found the game efficient, immersive, and fluid; 85% considered it effective; 80% reported motivation and excitement in completing objectives; and 75% evaluated its learning curve positively.

Pipo is educational software aimed at children aged 0 to 12, offering various games designed by child psychologists and educators to promote learning through play while fostering intuition, reasoning, and creativity (CIBAL Multimedia, 2004).). The content is divided into five age groups (0–3 years, 4–6 years, 6–8 years, 8–10 years, and 10–12 years) and includes four subjects: mathematics, language, English, and environmental knowledge/music. The language subject supports literacy development explicitly, with exercises designed to help children recognize letters and words through images and sounds. Activities include completing words with missing letters, writing full words after hearing them, or, for younger children, reproducing the sound of a letter by clicking on it.

Among recent developments, an action-based video game developed by educational psychologists targets children's executive functions, such as attention, working memory, inhibition, and cognitive flexibility, which are foundational for reading. In a study with 150 Italian schoolchildren, those who played this specially designed action game experienced significant improvements in reading speed and accuracy, as well as a sevenfold gain in attention control compared to a control group (who played a programming game), with sustained performance benefits one year after the intervention (Pasqualotto et al., 2022).

Another recent initiative explores gamified puzzle games aimed at phonemic awareness, a critical early reading skill. In a study involving preschool children learning Malay (aged 5–6), puzzle-based blending games were shown to significantly improve letter-sound recognition, collaboration, readiness, and sustained interest in the learning process (Ungau et al., 2023).

These examples demonstrate how educational video games have been applied to support children's literacy development across different contexts and languages. From early projects to more recent initiatives that integrate executive function training and gamified phonemic awareness activities, these experiences highlight the potential of serious games to engage learners, foster motivation, and enhance reading and writing skills. While results vary depending on design and context, the evidence suggests that video games can be powerful tools when aligned with clear pedagogical objectives, offering opportunities for innovation and challenges for future research.

ANALYSIS AND DESIGN OF THE SERIOUS GAME

This section describes the analysis and design methodology of the proposed serious game, which served as the foundation for its subsequent evaluation. Since the project aims to support children through pedagogical activities, these activities needed to be integrated into the game design. Therefore, a preliminary study was carried out to delimit the proposal according to the needs identified through interactions with teachers and children. Based on this analysis, the necessary software and tools for development were selected.

This project emphasizes Human-Computer Interaction (HCI), or in this case, Child–Computer Interaction (CCI). These concepts are closely related, as Hourcade (2015) states that HCI and CCI are the study of the design, evaluation, and implementation of interactive computing systems. The main difference lies in the group of users involved: while HCI typically addresses young people and adults, CCI focuses on children, whose ways of perceiving and interacting with the world present unique challenges and opportunities for design.

The use of technology in such contexts can be fundamental, since, as noted by Wehmeyer et al. (2008), technology has the potential to be used effectively with children with disabilities to enhance their learning experiences. It is important to highlight, however, that although these concepts are similar, the main difference lies in how children perceive the world, which is markedly distinct from that of adolescents or adults. While the underlying model may be comparable, the techniques and approaches required to engage children involve unique challenges tied to the characteristics of this user group.

As Gee (2003) argues, video games embody learning principles that can be highly valuable for educational purposes in schools. He classifies these into three core pillars: student empowerment, problem-based learning, and deep understanding. Squire (2003) further emphasizes that video games can serve as dynamic learning environments where players actively construct knowledge through experimentation and feedback rather than passive reception. He argues that studying how games engage players can inform instructional design, encouraging educators to move beyond simple comparisons between games and traditional lectures toward understanding how interactive systems foster learning. In line with these ideas, Jackson

(2009) demonstrates how these principles can be operationalized in practice through game-based teaching, an instructional approach that integrates core features of video games into classroom design. Her findings indicate that applying such pedagogical techniques can increase motivation, engagement, and learning outcomes, even without relying directly on technology.

Participatory Design

This case study adopted a participatory design (PD) approach. PD is a creative methodology that seeks to engage and co-create with communities to address local problems (Participate in Design, 2019). It is also a design approach that invites all stakeholders (teachers, students, and others) into the design process to understand needs better and develop meaningful and satisfactory solutions (UX Magazine, 2017). Unlike traditional design approaches, PD recognizes all community members, from end users directly affected by the design to institutional stakeholders, as legitimate participants who can influence the project.

According to the consultancy Participate in Design (2019), five key principles of PD are: (1) reducing risk of failure and cost, (2) generating ownership of the outcome, (3) increasing confidence and self-efficacy, (4) creating realistic experiences while reducing resistance to change, and (5) fostering strong community bonds and greater engagement.

Figure 1. Representation of the stages of participatory design (Simonsen & Robertson, 2013)

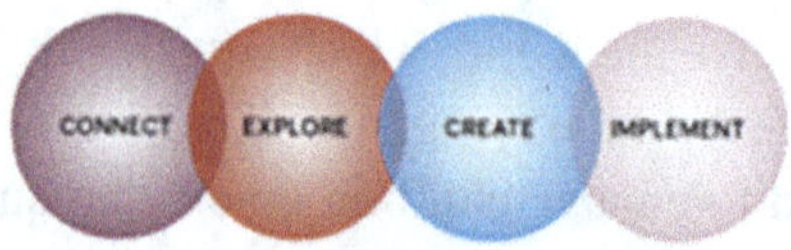

As shown in the Figure 1, participatory design unfolds across four fundamental stages:

- Connect. This stage begins by building a relationship with the target community. Together, opportunities for positive change are identified. The combined capacities of the community influence the creation, implementation, and sustainability of solutions. In this case, the process began with an initial visit to the collaborating school, which will be described in detail in the following section.

- Explore. This stage involves discovering and mapping collective knowledge about a place, its people, and available resources, in other words, understanding the context. By identifying the needs and assets of the community, more meaningful and innovative solutions can be achieved. Here, the focus was on the teacher and children who would ultimately use the game, considering both their current situation and the resources, didactic and technological, available to them.
- Create. At this stage, the information gathered is translated into possible solutions through brainstorming with the community. Proposals are tested and refined using prototypes, which should be low-cost and low-risk so that the community can actively contribute to concrete outcomes.
- Implement. This stage involves evaluation through the end users. When developing for children, it is particularly important that the product be easy to use, age-appropriate, attractive, and fun.

Contextual Analysis

In line with the participatory design approach, the contextual analysis encompassed two complementary stages: Connect and Explore.

Connect. During this stage, we established contact with a private school. An initial meeting was held with the lead teacher to discuss the study's objectives and to secure the teacher's and her students' participation. At this point, informed consent was obtained, and the necessary permissions were requested to interact with the children, ensuring the process was transparent and ethically conducted.

Explore. We proceeded to a formal visit to conduct the contextual analysis. The school employs two teachers trained in education and serves children between 4 and 7 years of age. Its facilities include a reception area and two classrooms, with curricular activities primarily focused on literacy and mathematics. We interviewed the teacher, who described the literacy practices typically used in the classroom. It is important to highlight that the school functions as a support center: not all children enrolled present learning difficulties, but many parents seek to provide their children with stronger tools and skills.

During this stage, we also reviewed the instructional materials and infrastructure available. The teacher shared the multimedia tools currently used for literacy activities and her experiences with traditional didactic strategies and digital resources. We also conducted informal conversations with three children (two girls and one boy), who described how they use the available digital tools. One research team member observed these interactions, identifying strengths and weaknesses in the multimedia resources. At the same time, the project advisor held discussions with the teacher regarding didactic strategies to be reinforced.

Finally, we agreed that the developer team would bring three prototype games in a subsequent visit. Progress in art design and game dynamics would be documented and shared with the teacher for feedback, closing the Explore stage with a clear roadmap for co-creation.

Requirements Analysis

The requirements analysis corresponds to the Create stage of participatory design. In this phase, the information gathered during the contextual exploration was translated into concrete proposals and possible solutions. Together with the teacher and children, ideas were refined and consolidated into a set of requirements that guided the development of the serious game.

According to Gómez Fuentes (2011), requirements analysis refers to the study of the elements necessary for software development and the determination of the features and limitations the system must have. Based on our visits and conversations with the teacher and some of the participating children, we identified the following requirements:

Functional Requirements

- The user must be able to select an activity from a menu.
- The user must be able to change activities without completing the current one.
- The system must provide immediate feedback (visual and/or auditory) for correct and incorrect actions.
- The game must include three difficulty levels that increase progressively.

User Requirements

- The system must allow interaction via both mouse and touchscreen.
- Visual elements (letters and images) must be large and clear enough for children aged 4–7.
- Instructions must be presented in short, age-appropriate sentences and/or through audio prompts.
- Completing words. The system must allow the user to complete words by dragging and dropping missing letters from a set displayed on the screen.

- Matching images. The system must allow the user to match images with their corresponding words through a series of exercises.
- Memory game. The system must allow the user to flip cards and find matching pairs until all pairs are completed.

Technical Requirements

- The system must run on a computer with Windows, or on a tablet/smartphone with Android.
- The game must be installable on devices with limited storage and processing capacity.

These requirements reflect the project's technical feasibility and emphasize a better interaction for children. The requirements ensure that children remain motivated and can interact effectively with the system, and guarantee that the game can be deployed on widely available devices in schools or at home.

System Design

The system design corresponds to the final phase of the Create stage and serves as the transition toward Implement within the participatory design process. At this point, the previously defined requirements were translated into structured representations, diagrams, and models that clarified how the serious game would function. This step ensured that developers and stakeholders—teachers and children—shared a common understanding of the proposed system.

Visual models are one of the most effective ways to communicate the game's logic to end users. Therefore, several diagrams and tables were created to illustrate use cases, system behavior, and activity flows. These representations served as technical documentation and communication tools during feedback sessions with the teacher.

Figures 2–4 illustrate the use cases for the three core game activities (Matching images, Completing words, and Memory). Tables 1–3 describe each activity's interaction sequences, preconditions, exceptions, and postconditions. These tables helped to define what the system should do in response to specific user actions, reinforcing the alignment between pedagogical objectives and interactive design.

Figure 2. Use case, video game: matching images

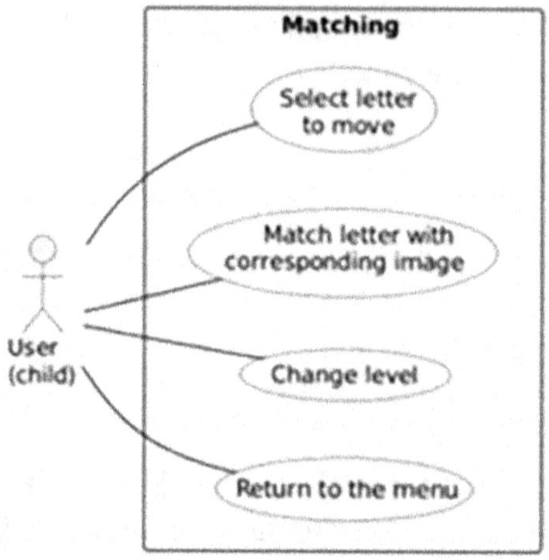

Figure 3. Use case, video game: completing words

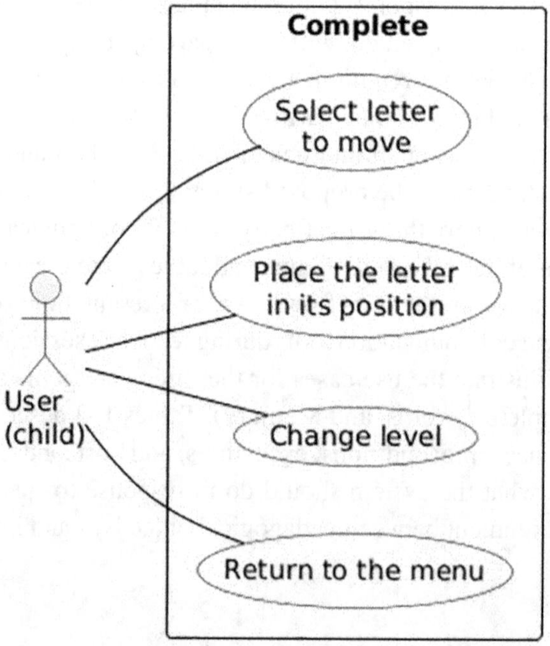

Figure 4. Use case, video game: memory game

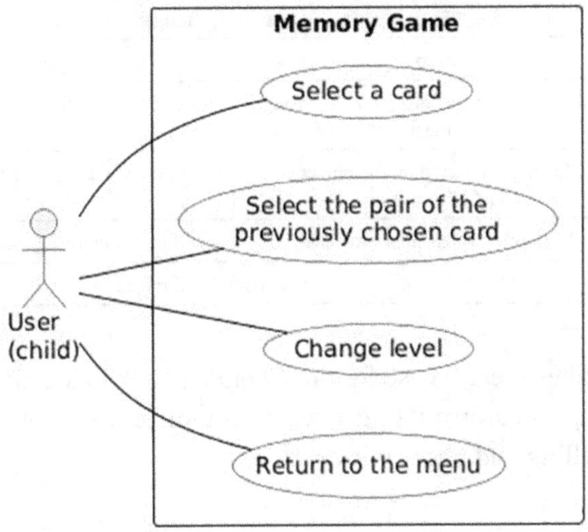

Table 1 presents the use case specification for the *Matching Images* activity. This game challenges children to associate letters with the corresponding images, reinforcing the relationship between sounds and symbols through immediate feedback.

Table 1. Matching Images

Name	**Matching Images**	
Actor	Child	
Description	The system must behave as described in this use case when the user starts the *Matching Images* game	
Precondition	The user selected the game from the menu.	
Normal Flow	Step	System Action
	Select the letter/card to move	System highlights the letter/card
	Place the letter/card on the corresponding object	System removes the matched pair and adds 1 point
	Select the button to change level	System loads a new level with higher difficulty
	Select the button to return to the menu	System returns to the main menu

continued on following page

Table 1. Continued

Name	Matching Images	
Exceptions	Step	System Action
	If the letter/card is placed on the wrong object	Player loses one life, and the letter/card returns to its initial position
	If the letter/card placed on the object is the last of the game	Button to change level is enabled
	If all three levels are completed	Button to return to the menu is enabled
Postcondition	The user completed the game	

Table 2 describes the use case for the *Completing Words* activity. In this game, children must drag and drop missing letters to complete words, an exercise designed to strengthen spelling and phonemic awareness.

Table 2. Completing words

Name	Completing words	
Actor	Child	
Description	The system must behave as described in this use case when the user starts the Completing Words game	
Precondition	The user selected the game from the menu.	
Normal Flow	Step	System Action
	Select the letter to move	System highlights the letter
	Place the letter in the target space	System locks the letter in place and adds 1 point
	Select the button to change level	System loads a new level with higher difficulty
	Select the button to return to the menu	System returns to the main menu
Exceptions	Step	System Action
	If the letter is moved to an incorrect space	Player loses one life, and the letter returns to its initial position
	If the letter placed correctly is the last needed to complete the word	Word is completed and button to change level is enabled
	If all three levels are completed	Button to return to the menu is enabled
Postcondition	The user completed the game	

Finally, Table 3 summarizes the use case for the *Memory Game*. Although not directly focused on reading or writing, this activity supports literacy indirectly by enhancing visual memory and concentration, while incorporating the same characters and letters used in the other activities.

Table 3. Memory Game

Name	**Memory game**	
Actor	Child	
Description	The system must behave as described in this use case when the user starts the Memory game	
Precondition	The user selected the game from the menu.	
Normal Flow	Step	System Action
	Select the cards to flip	System highlights the card
	Flip the card to check if it matches the previously flipped card	System removes the matched pair and adds 1 point
	Select the button to change level	System loads a new level with higher difficulty
	Select the button to return to the menu	System returns to the main menu
Exceptions	Step	System Action
	If the flipped card does not match the previous one	Player loses one life, and the card returns to its initial position
	If the flipped card is the last in the game	Button to change level is enabled
	If all three levels are completed	Button to return to the menu is enabled
Postcondition	The user completed the game	

To further clarify the flow and logic of the game, Figures 5–6 present two flowcharts: one outlining the general progression of the game, and another showing the logic of activity selection through the main menu. Together, these models provide a comprehensive overview of the game's architecture, ensuring consistency between learning objectives, user interactions, and technical implementation.

Figure 5. General flowchart of the game

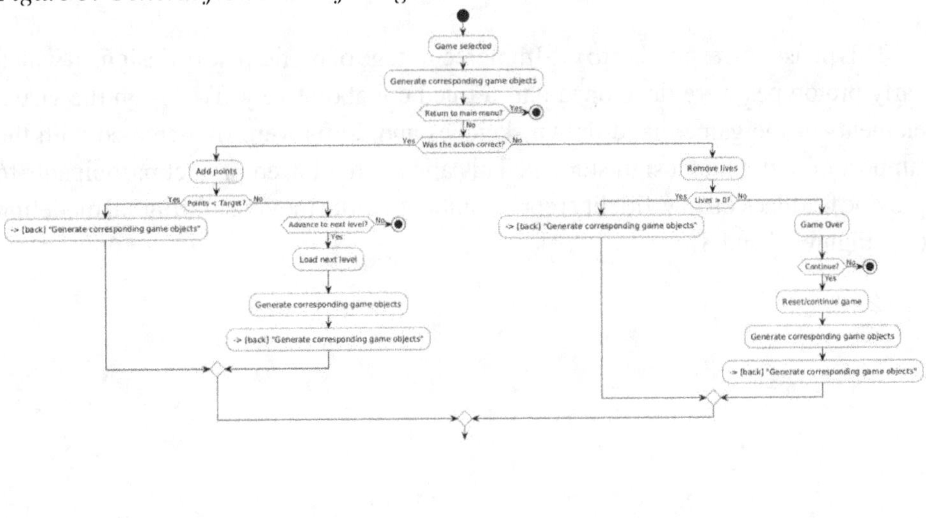

Figure 6. Flowchart of game selection using the menu

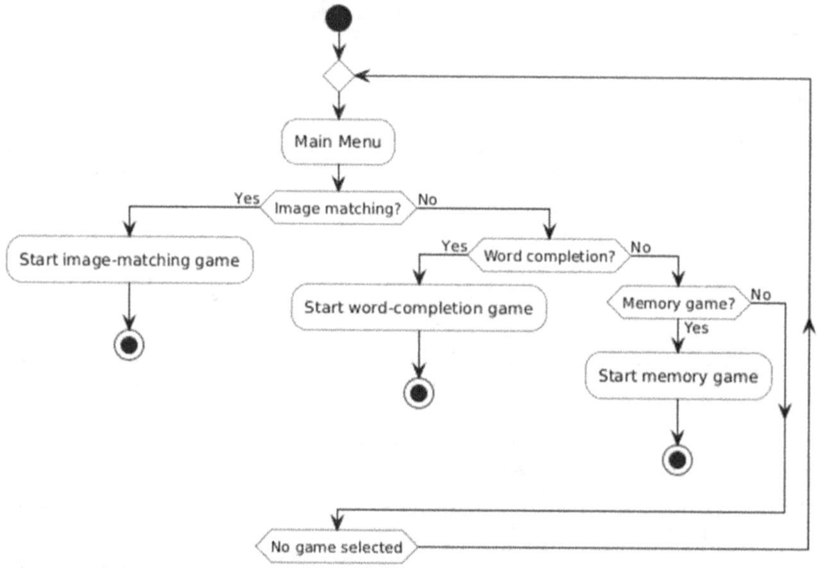

The requirements specifications provide a detailed blueprint of how each activity is expected to function and ensure that the pedagogical goals are consistently translated into interactive mechanics by outlining user interactions, system responses, exceptions, and postconditions. Likewise, they offer a framework for implementation, reduce ambiguity during development, and strengthen the alignment between instructional goals and technical design.

Art Design: Characters and Scenarios

This phase corresponded to the Implement stage of participatory design, in which early prototypes were developed and refined collaboratively. To design the visual elements of the game, hand-drawn sketches and drafts were first created with the support of a graphic design student. This approach allowed project participants to provide feedback on low-fidelity representations before moving into digital modeling (see Figures 7 and 8).

Figure 7. Sketch of the cards used in the game in general in its early versions

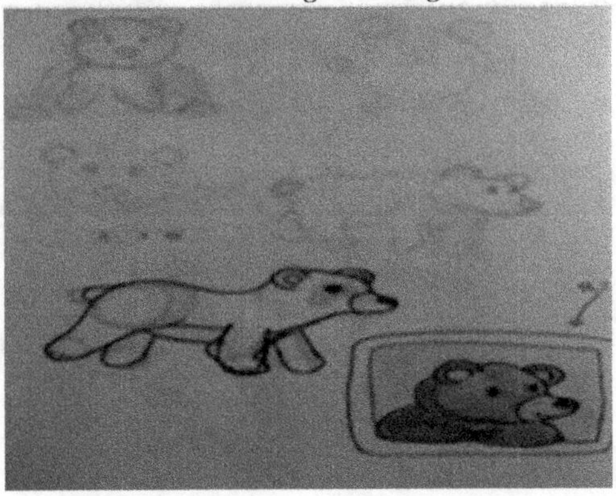

Figure 8. Sketch of the cards used in the game in general with different characters

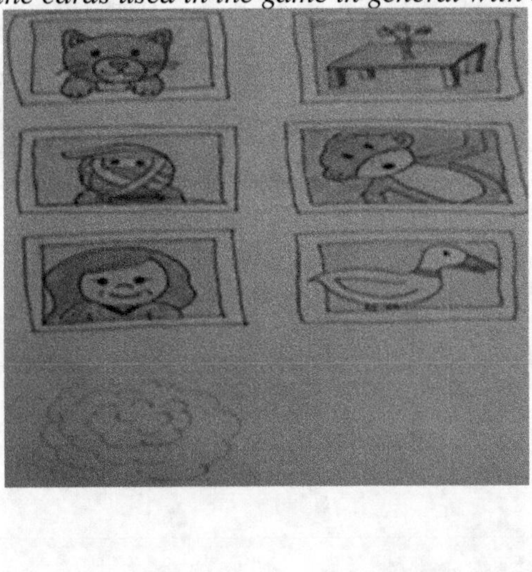

To validate the proposed visual style, children and the teacher were asked a simple question regarding their satisfaction with the images. Once the sketches were confirmed to appeal to the children and the teacher, the design team created the final digital models. These included avatars, buttons, markers, menus, and other interface components (see Figures 9–12).

Figure 9. Modeling the final version of the avatars

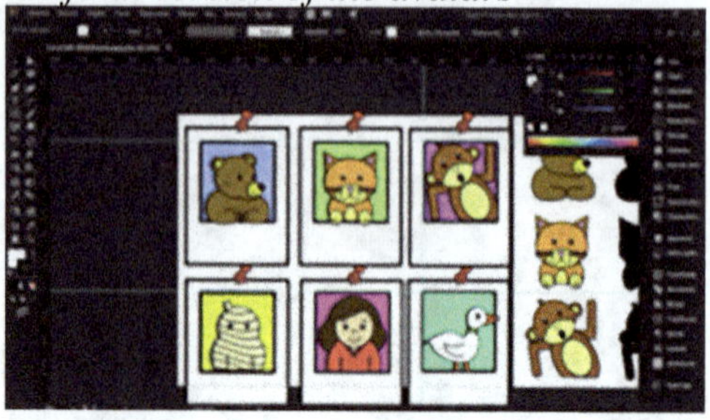

Figure 10. Buttons and markers in their final version

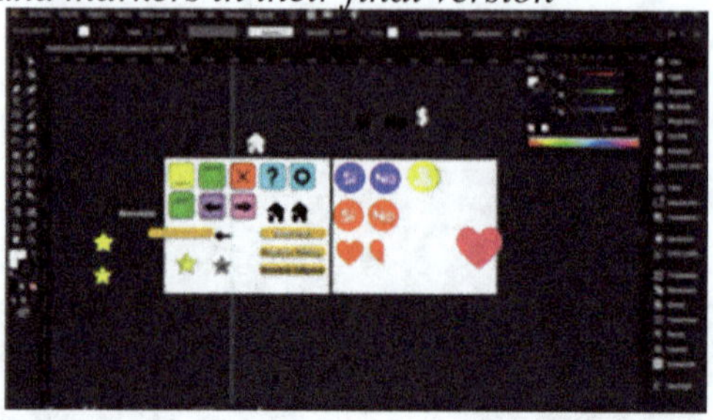

Figure 11. Modeling the room menu

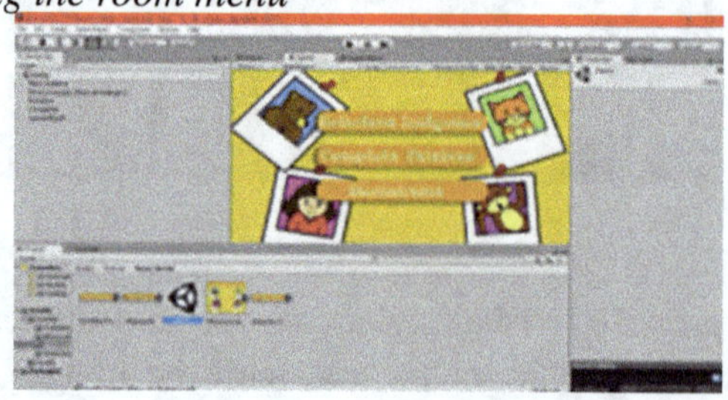

Figure 12. Design of the room menu, as well as the messages for each case

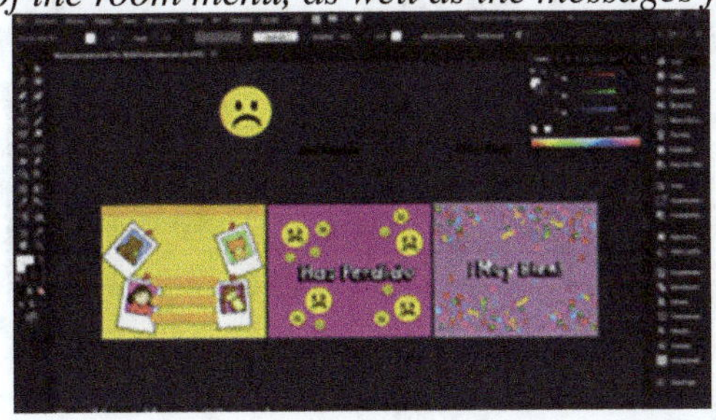

The project ensured that the prototypes were functional, engaging, and age-appropriate by incorporating children's and the teacher's perspectives into the visual design process. This iterative approach, which moved from sketches to finalized digital models, emphasized feedback and user-centered decision making, resulting in visual elements appealing to children and consistent with the game's pedagogical goals.

Game Dynamics Design and Development

This section shows the design of the dynamics based on the children's needs, following the advice of the teacher in charge of the school. The goal is to reinforce reading and writing skills by memorizing letters and sounds. These activities were created and presented through the video game and were part of the code generated when developing the dynamics using the Unity platform. The three dynamics presented are: completing words with corresponding letters, matching images to their corresponding letters, and the memory game.

Dynamic 1: Completing Words with Corresponding Letters

In this activity, children are shown incomplete words on the screen. They drag scattered letters to the correct positions to complete the word (see Figure 13). The game includes three levels of increasing difficulty, each requiring the completion of different words. For every correct placement, the child earns points; incorrect attempts reduce the number of lives. The activity ends when all words are completed or the player runs out of lives. The design emphasizes immediate feedback and progressive challenge, encouraging children to practice spelling interactively.

Figure 13. Example of the word completion module; the left shows an incomplete activity, while the right shows what happens once the activity is completed

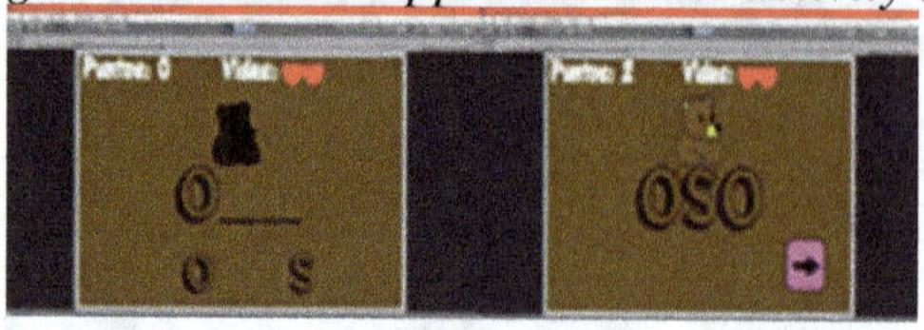

Dynamic 2: Matching Letters with Corresponding Images

This activity reinforces the connection between letters and phonemes through images. Children are presented with characters or objects alongside several letters. Their task is to drag each initial letter to the correct image (see Figure 14). As in the previous dynamic, three levels gradually increase the number of pairs to match. Correct answers are rewarded with points, while incorrect matches reduce lives. This design helps children strengthen phonemic awareness while engaging through simple, game-like interactions.

Figure 14. Final version of the word matching game

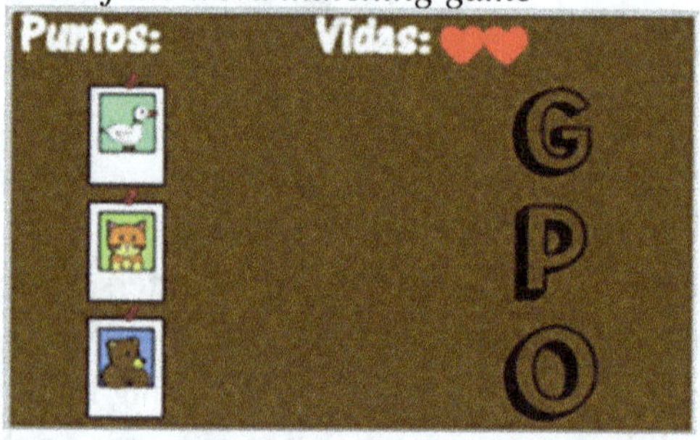

Dynamic 3: Memory Game

The memory game focuses on visual memory and concentration. Although not directly tied to reading and writing, it uses the same characters and letters introduced in the previous activities, reinforcing familiarity with phonemes (see Figure 15). Children flip pairs of hidden cards in search of matches. Correct pairs remain visible and add points, while incorrect attempts reduce lives. The game progresses across three levels, each with a larger grid and more cards to match. Including this dynamic supports cognitive processes such as attention, memory, and recall, which are fundamental for early literacy development.

Figure 15. Final version of the Memory Game

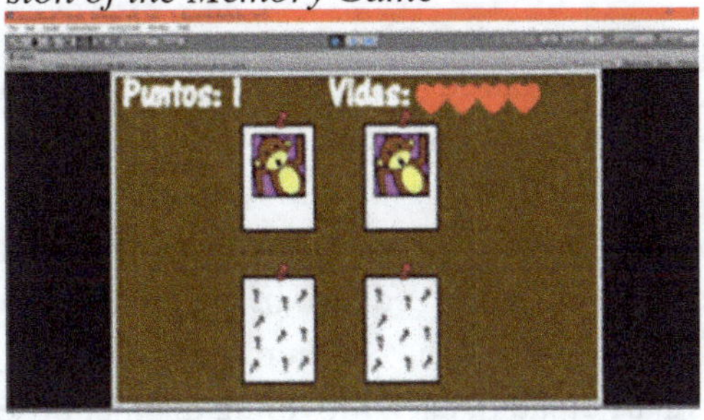

The three game dynamics were designed to integrate playfulness with pedagogical intent. The game promotes early literacy skills by combining word completion, letter–image association, and memory tasks while fostering motivation. These dynamics illustrate how interactive mechanics can be aligned with educational goals, creating learning opportunities through play.

EVALUATION OF THE SERIOUS GAME

Evaluation is one of the most important phases in developing interactive systems. Since the environments used to develop video games are not always perfect, it is essential to include evaluation in any system or application, as this activity ensures the design's quality, effectiveness, and efficiency (Schultz & Bryant, 2011). In this study, usability was chosen as the primary evaluation criterion to determine whether children found the design of each room simple and easy to use. According to Nielsen (2012), usability refers to the quality attribute that focuses on the ease with which a user can interact with an interface. In other words, it verifies that the product functions correctly and can be used without difficulty (García et al., 2017).

To conduct the evaluation, we returned to the support school previously described. First, we spoke with the lead teacher, who responded positively to our shared proposal. Once the days and times of our visits were agreed upon, we discussed with her the dynamics and teaching strategies usually applied with the children attending the school. This allowed us to understand the pedagogical context better and establish a foundation for the design and refinement of the game.

A total of three visits were made. The first visit was dedicated to gaining a more concrete understanding of the literacy activities carried out at the school and the specific skills targeted for improvement. The two subsequent visits focused on evaluating the serious game, during which the teacher and the children provided valuable feedback as participating evaluators.

First Evaluation

The prototype, designed based on initial visits and conversations with the participating teacher, was evaluated during two sessions at the support school. The evaluations consisted of inviting a child to interact with the prototype while systematically recording observations of errors and suggestions. It is important to note that the teacher also provided feedback based on her experience; however, in this phase, the focus was placed on the children's perspectives. During the first test, one boy and one girl participated, each providing distinct observations.

The first participant, a boy selected by the teacher, was asked to sit at a table where a laptop with the game preloaded was prepared. The laptop included a touchscreen, which the child preferred to use. He appeared curious about the activities, paid close attention to each, and commented about errors he noticed or exercises he did not understand. He completed each activity quickly and desired increased difficulty, considering the game too simple.

After his turn, the next participant, a girl, was invited to play. She also completed the activities quickly, though she experienced difficulties navigating the menu and moving objects in the image-matching activity. These aspects were noted for improvement in the prototype to prepare for a second test.

The teacher also had the opportunity to play the game and share her experience. She highlighted several issues, including navigation problems when selecting activities and errors in the life system. She also suggested adding feedback messages to indicate successful completion of activities and incorporating sounds that pronounced each letter and image used to facilitate and improve the overall experience.

Activity suggestions from the first test

Drawing on observations from both the teacher and the participating children, Table 4 organizes the activity suggestions according to their source and pedagogical purpose. This tabular format offers a clearer overview of how each recommendation contributes to refining the game.

Table 4. Activity suggestions from the first test

Suggestion	Source	Purpose
Add an Alphabet mode where words are formed with each letter of the alphabet	Children	Broaden practice opportunities and make activities more varied.
Include sounds (music, clicks, animal sounds, success/error cues), especially in Completing Words	Children	Increase engagement and provide auditory feedback.
Play a phonetic sound when tapping letters	Teacher & Children	Reinforce letter–sound association and phonemic awareness.

Suggestion	Source	Purpose
Add a representative image in each game	Teacher	Support comprehension and make tasks more intuitive.
Provide a clear instruction at the beginning of each game	Teacher	Guide children and reduce confusion at the start of activities.
Incorporate syllable reading practice	Teacher	Strengthen literacy through syllable recognition.
Add a difficulty level using syllables in Completing Words	Teacher	Introduce progression and adapt the challenge to children's literacy levels.

Errors found during the first evaluation

In this case, Table 5 presents the errors identified during the first evaluation, specifying their location within the game and the suggested fixes. This structure facilitates a more systematic analysis and supports future iterations of the development process.

Table 5. Errors found during the first evaluation and suggested fix

Issue	Location	Suggested Fix
Word "momia" auto-completes when restarting the game	Completing Words	Reset variables properly on restart to avoid preloaded text.
Change-level icon overlaps the bottom-right card	Memory game	Adjust interface layout and icon positioning.
The remaining lives from the previous session remain when restarting.	All games	Ensure variables reset correctly at the beginning of each session.
Score resets when changing level within the same game	All games	Modify scoring logic so points persist across levels.
Letters push other letters off-screen when dragged	Completing Words	Restrict draggable area or implement collision constraints.
Player cannot switch to another game until the current one ends	Main menu navigation	Enable game-switching from the menu at any point.

The first evaluation session provided valuable input from the teacher and the children. The activity suggestions highlighted opportunities to enrich the game with additional features such as sounds, syllable-based exercises, and more precise instructions. At the same time, the error reports identified technical issues requiring correction. Together, these insights informed the next iteration of the game, ensuring that subsequent versions were more functional and better aligned with the pedagogical needs of the users.

Second Evaluation

In the second evaluation, two children participated once again. Unlike the first test, only one error was identified in the Memory Game, which caused one card to remain flipped, showing the side that should have been hidden.

The participants used the game under the same conditions as in the first session (seated at a table with the game preloaded on a laptop). The first child initially had minor difficulties understanding the instructions, but after a short time, was able to complete the exercises without problem. When asked if he enjoyed the game, he responded affirmatively. The second participant, a girl, understood the instructions more easily and quickly completed each activity, stating that she enjoyed them, though she found them very easy. Both participants showed interest and enthusiasm before and during the test.

During this session, several aspects of the prototype that had been identified in the first evaluation were corrected and improved:

- The bug that caused the word momia to auto-complete in the Completing Words activity was fixed.
- In the Memory game, the "change level" button was repositioned to no longer overlap the bottom-right card (see Figure 16).
- All games added a button to allow users to return to the home screen at any time (see Figure 17).
- When restarting any game, the number of lives is reset to the default rather than being carried over from the previous session.
- The "change level" button was removed after completing the last level of each game.
- In levels 2 and 3 of the Memory game, the bug that caused the bottom-right card to appear flipped at the start was corrected.
- In the word completion dynamic, images were added from the beginning (see figure 18).

The second evaluation confirmed that the children perceived the game as enjoyable and easy to use, while the teacher recognized its potential as a classroom tool. The adjustments implemented not only resolved previous technical issues but also enhanced acceptance of the game as an effective learning aid.

Figure 16. The level change button is now next to the bottom right card and not overlapping it

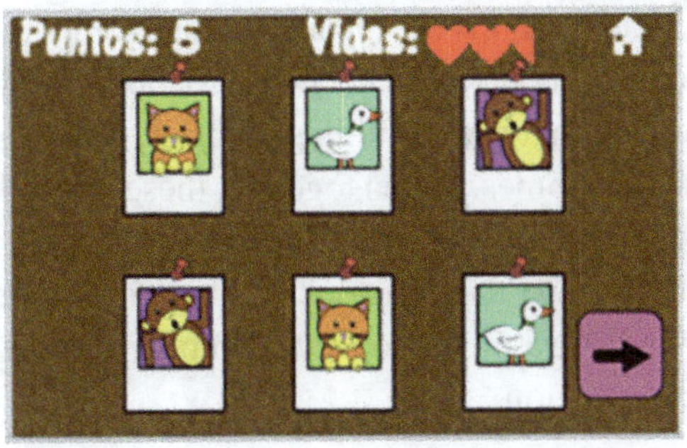

Figure 17. In the upper right corner is the house-shaped button which takes the user to the home screen

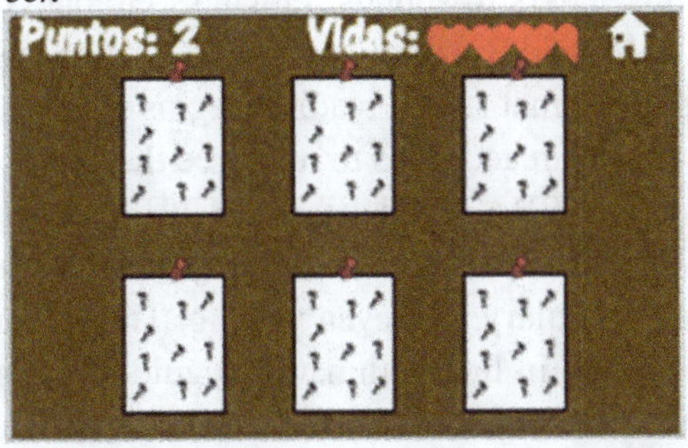

Figure 18. The image of the bear has been placed from the beginning instead of the silhouette. This is a suggestion because some children had difficulty recognizing the silhouette

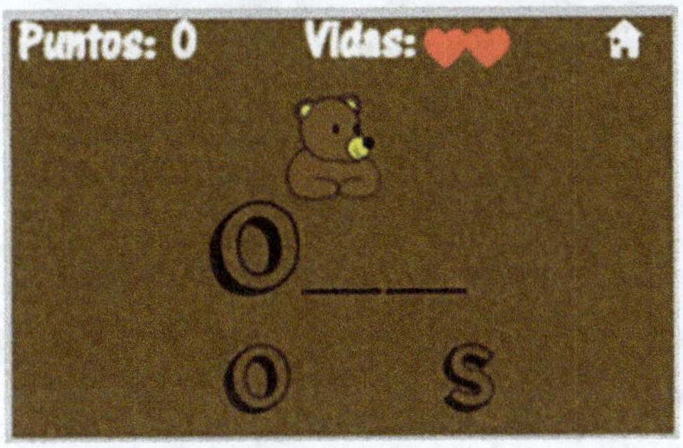

DISCUSSION

To complete our contribution, we compared serious games for early literacy across international and Mexican contexts. This comparison highlights both similarities and differences in educational goals, guiding theories, design strategies, evaluation methods, and reported outcomes. Taken together, these examples not only show the potential of serious games as tools to spark literacy development, but also reveal the broader conditions that shape their success. In this discussion, we interpret these findings in plain terms, share the lessons we can take away, and place our project within this global conversation.

Educational Objectives

One of the most notable differences among these international examples is their varied starting points. Some games are deeply rooted in phonics, a classic method that helps children link letters to sounds. Finland's GraphoGame (Borleffs et al., 2018; Ojanen et al., 2015) and Brazil's Escribo Play (Amorim et al., 2022) are clear examples. Both emphasize that strong reading begins with mastering these sound-letter relationships, using fun activities to reinforce the skill.

Canada's ABRACADABRA (Piquette et al., 2014) adopts a wider approach. Rather than zeroing in on just one aspect of literacy, it combines phonics with comprehension, fluency, vocabulary, and even writing. This balanced model provides children with a full toolkit, in line with national guidelines on effective learning. Malaysia's Mari Membaca (Abidin et al., 2024) takes a different route, inspired by brain-based learning from neuroscience. Its activities engage multiple senses, progressing gradually from letters to words, and are specifically designed for students who learn at a slower pace. An Italian case (Pasqualotto et al., 2022) pushes boundaries further. Instead of direct reading instruction, it uses an action video game to strengthen attention and executive functions like focus and self-control. The theory is that these improvements indirectly boost reading abilities, and research shows it can be effective.

Our participatory project draws from a constructivist perspective, focusing on enjoyment, challenges, and kids' active role in shaping the game. And, while all these cases harness the engaging power of games, their underlying theories vary widely, from behaviorist and phonics-based foundations to constructivist, cognitive, and neuroscience-driven models. This highlights the interdisciplinary appeal of serious games: effective literacy tools can stem from diverse ideas, as long as the gameplay supports clear learning goals.

Pedagogical depth

When it comes to educational tools, two approaches often stand in contrast: scientific precision and local relevance. Programs like GraphoGame and ABRACADABRA are built on deep expertise. They're carefully designed by specialists, grounded in the science of reading, and backed by thorough research studies. Their content is robust, but applying them in new cultural or linguistic settings often requires significant adjustments.

In contrast, tools like Escribo Play and Mari Membaca prioritize practical relevance. While still rooted in research, they were developed with local needs in mind. Escribo Play was created to support under-resourced schools in Brazil, while Mari Membaca was tailored to help slower learners in Malaysia.

Our project takes this a step further. By directly involving teachers and students from the start, we ensured the tool feels familiar and aligns with local culture and curricula. This makes it immediately usable in classrooms, though it has limitations: solutions designed this way may work wonderfully locally but often lack the extensive evidence needed to convince policymakers.

The trade-off is clear. Expert-driven designs deliver strong, measurable results but can feel out of place or hard to integrate in everyday classrooms. Community-driven designs connect deeply with users but may struggle to provide the large-scale evidence required for wider adoption. The challenge lies in finding ways to blend the strengths of both approaches.

Evaluation Strategies

The evaluation methods used for these projects highlight a balance between rigorous testing and practical feedback. Programs like ABRACADABRA, Escribo Play, and the Italian action game were assessed through large-scale studies involving many children. These studies used control groups, standardized tests, and even tracked progress over time. This thorough approach provides solid evidence that these games improve literacy skills, making them highly credible in academic and policy discussions.

In contrast, Mari Membaca and our project took a more hands-on, formative approach. They involved teachers and students in testing early versions, gathering feedback on usability and engagement. This process is crucial in the early stages, ensuring the games are enjoyable for kids and practical for teachers. However, these evaluations don't yet measure improvements in learning with the same level of rigor.

This difference reflects the stage of each project's development. New projects often start with smaller usability tests to refine the design before moving to more structured studies. This project, for example, is in its early phase, showing strong signs of classroom acceptance but lacking formal data on literacy gains. To move forward, the next step is clear: conducting more systematic trials to build a stronger case for its impact.

Reported Outcomes

The results from these projects show that serious games can effectively support children's reading skills, though each takes a unique approach. GraphoGame reliably improves children's ability to connect letters with sounds, especially in languages like Finnish and Spanish, where spelling is relatively simple. ABRACADABRA leads to broader progress in decoding and word reading, but its success relies on teachers actively incorporating it into their lessons. Escribo Play stands out with strong results, particularly in under-resourced schools, demonstrating that mobile games can help close educational gaps when challenges like access to technology are addressed. Mari Membaca shows that kids respond well to brain-based learning methods, and teachers value its focus on supporting slower learners, though its evidence is still small-scale. The Italian project offers a surprising finding: even action games not focused on reading can boost literacy by improving cognitive skills like attention.

Our approach, while lacking formal data on learning outcomes, achieves something equally important: cultural connection and engagement. Kids loved playing the games, teachers found them practical, and they blended seamlessly into the classroom. In places where imported or top-down solutions often fall short, this sense of belonging is a big win. However, to prove its educational value, future studies need to link this enthusiasm to clear improvements in reading skills.

Lessons Learned and Best Practices

Looking at these global experiences, several clear lessons stand out for creating effective literacy games. First, every game needs a strong educational foundation, whether it's focused on phonics (like GraphoGame), a mix of literacy skills (like ABRACADABRA), or cognitive training (like the Italian action game). Just as important, games must be fun, engagement isn't just a bonus; it's a core part of how kids learn. Involving teachers, and sometimes students, in the design process helps ensure the game feels right for the local culture and classroom, making it more likely to be used long-term. Evaluation should grow over time: start with small tests to check usability, then move to larger studies that measure actual learning gains. Finally, scalability is critical—without teacher training and reliable access to devices, even the best games can end up gathering dust.

These lessons explain why some projects, have grown from research ideas into widely used programs, while others, are still in early stages. The difference isn't just about how well the games are designed, it's also about how they're tested and supported with resources like technology and training.

The bigger picture is that no single approach has all the answers. The best literacy games combine strong teaching methods, fun design, input from teachers and students, careful testing, and practical support for scaling up. In the broader world of literacy games, the potential is exciting but complex. These tools can measurably improve children's reading skills, but their success depends on more than just the game itself. It requires bringing together solid teaching, motivation, thoughtful design, thorough evaluation, and a good fit with the local context. Our project illustrates that impact is not only about test scores—it also involves creating games that feel meaningful in the classroom and connect with both teachers and children. By blending global best practices with our participatory approach, this work opens up the possibility of developing literacy games that are effective, sustainable, and genuinely embraced by the communities they are meant to serve.

CONCLUSIONS AND FUTURE WORK

Video games can be a valuable tool for learning. In this project, prototype testing yielded positive responses from the children, particularly regarding their attention to completing the activities. This level of engagement demonstrated the educational potential of video games: the fact that children remained focused on overcoming challenges suggested that their learning process became more effective. Another key finding was the role of challenge as a motivating factor. During the evaluations, children completed the activities relatively quickly, and one participant explicitly stated that he would prefer higher difficulty levels. Increasing challenge levels, therefore, could enhance children's interest and lead to more effective learning outcomes in the future.

The study also provided concrete insights into how children's attention can be captured through playful activities, while identifying opportunities for improvement in future iterations of educational games. Nonetheless, certain limitations must be acknowledged. First, the evaluation involved a small sample size, limited to a few children from a single support school, which prevents generalization. Second, the short-term sessions captured only immediate reactions, without assessing long-term learning outcomes or retention. Third, the prototype was restricted to three activities with limited difficulty levels, constraining the range of literacy skills addressed. Finally, the study relied primarily on qualitative observations and informal feedback, which, while suitable for the context, limit comparability with other studies.

Future development should address these areas. For instance, difficulty levels could be refined by sequencing the introduction of letters and allowing practice at the letter or syllable level. Incorporating phonetic feedback that reproduces the sound of a word once completed could also strengthen literacy practice. For the Memory Game, improvements include moving beyond character-based cards to integrate letters with sound effects, embedded in progressively complex levels where children connect letters, images, and sounds simultaneously. Another important opportunity is enabling teachers to act as active users who can create and add activities, making the game more adaptable and expanding its classroom value. Although such features require significant development, they represent promising avenues for increasing the tool's educational impact.

As a final remark, this study contributes to understanding how serious games can be integrated into early literacy development by combining playful interaction with pedagogical goals. The prototype's design, evaluation, and refinement demonstrated that video games can capture children's attention, foster motivation, and provide meaningful opportunities for practicing reading and writing skills. While the project had limitations in scale and scope, it highlights the potential of technology-based interventions to complement traditional educational practices. By addressing the challenges identified and pursuing the future work proposed, this line of research can advance toward scalable and adaptive digital tools that meaningfully support literacy learning in early childhood education.

REFERENCES

Abidin, S. R. Z., Noor, S. F. M., Ashaari, N. S., & Yadegaridehkordi, E. (2024). Improving literacy skills using the serious game model compatible with brain-based learning. *Multimedia Tools and Applications*, *84*(1), 95–129. DOI: 10.1007/s11042-024-20305-9

Amorim, A. N., Jeon, L., Abel, Y., Albuquerque, E. X. S., Soares, M., Silva, V. C., & Oliveira Neto, J. R. (2022). Escribo play learning games can foster early reading and writing for low-income kindergarten children. *Computers & Education*, *177*, 104364. DOI: 10.1016/j.compedu.2021.104364

Armendáriz Espadas, P. (2018). *Los videojuegos educativos en México* (Universidad de las Américas Puebla). Retrieved from http://catarina.udlap.mx/u_dl_a/tales/documentos/lnd/armendariz_espadas_p/etd_3021084549481.pdf

Belli, S., & López Raventós, C. (2008). Breve historia de los videojuegos. *Athenea Digital*, *179*(14), 159–179. DOI: 10.5565/rev/athenead/v0n14.570

Borleffs, E., Glatz, T. K., Daulay, D. A., Richardson, U., Zwarts, F., & Maassen, B. A. M. (2018). GraphoGame SI: The development of a technology-enhanced literacy learning tool for Standard Indonesian. *European Journal of Psychology of Education*, *33*(4), 595–613. DOI: 10.1007/s10212-017-0354-9

Boyle, E. A., Hainey, T., Connolly, T. M., Gray, G., Earp, J., Ott, M., Lim, T., Ninaus, M., Ribeiro, C., & Pereira, J. (2016). An update to the systematic literature review of empirical evidence of the impacts and outcomes of computer games and serious games. *Computers & Education*, *94*, 178–192. DOI: 10.1016/j.compedu.2015.11.003

Burns, M. S., Griffin, J., & Snows, C. E. (1999). *Starting out right. A guide promoting children s reading success*. National Academic Press.

Camacho-Quiroz, R. (2013). La lectura en México, un problema multifactorial. *Contribuciones Desde Coatepec*, (25), 153–156.

Connolly, T. M., Boyle, E. A., MacArthur, E., Hainey, T., & Boyle, J. M. (2012). A systematic literature review of empirical evidence on computer games and serious games. *Computers & Education*, *59*(2), 661–686. DOI: 10.1016/j.compedu.2012.03.004

Endeavor & Santander. (2025). Game On: El auge del Gaming en México. Retrieved from https://mexico.endeavor.org/gaming/

Entertainment Software Association. (2023). *Essential facts about the computer and video game industry*. Entertainment Software Association. Retrieved from https://www.theesa.com/resources/essential-facts-about-the-us-video-game-industry/

Erickson, F. (1977). Some Approaches to Inquiry in School-Community Ethnography. *Anthropology & Education Quarterly*, *8*(2), 58–69. https://www.jstor.org/stable/3216407. DOI: 10.1525/aeq.1977.8.2.05x1396r

Evans, F., Spinelli, A., Zapirain, E., Soriano, F., & Massa, S. M. (2016). Proceso de desarrollo de serious games. Diseño centrado en el usuario, jugabilidad e inmersión. *III Congreso Argentino De Ingeniería (Cadi) - IX Congreso Argentino De Enseñanza de la Ingeniería (Caedi)*.

Fernández-Sánchez, M. R., González-Fernández, A., & Acevedo-Borrega, J. (2023). Conceptual Approach to the Pedagogy of Serious Games. *Information (Basel)*, *14*(2), 132. Advance online publication. DOI: 10.3390/info14020132

García, L., Pernett, A., & Cano, J. (2017). Estudio exploratorio de usabilidad para niños de Colombia. *Zona Próxima, 9444*(26), 12–30. Retrieved from https://www.redalyc.org/pdf/853/85352029002.pdf

Gee, J. P. (2003). What video games have to teach us about learning and literacy. *Computers in Entertainment*, *1*(1), 20. DOI: 10.1145/950566.950595

Gómez Fuentes, M. (2011). *Notas del Curso: Análisis de Requerimientos*. Retrieved from https://www.cua.uam.mx/pdfs/conoce/libroselec/Notas_Analisis_Requerimiento.pdf

González, M. J., & Delgado, M. (2009). Rendimiento académico y enseñanza-aprendizaje de la lectoescritura en Educación Infantil y Primaria: Un estudio longitudinal. *Infancia y Aprendizaje*, *32*(3), 265–276. DOI: 10.1174/021037009788964114

González González, C. S., & Blanco Izquierdo, F. (2011). Videojuegos educativos sociales en el aula. *Revista ICONO14. Revista Científica de Comunicación y Tecnologías Emergentes*, *9*(2), 59. DOI: 10.7195/ri14.v9i2.46

Gros Salvat, B. (2009). Certezas e interrogantes acerca del uso de los videojuegos para el aprendizaje. *Comunicación: Revista Internacional de Comunicación Audiovisual. Publicidad y Estudios Culturales*, *1*(7), 251–264.

Guzhñay Vélez, K. J. (2021). Aprendizaje de lengua y literatura mediante rúbricas de evaluación. *Sociedad & Tecnología*, *4*(2), 174–190. DOI: 10.51247/st.v4i2.103

Hourcade, J. P. (2015). *Child-Computer Interaction. University of Iowa's Department of Computer Science*. Editorial Board of Interacting with Computers.

INEGI. (2018). Disminuye la Población Lectoraern México: Módulo de Lectura (MOLEC) 2018. Instituto Nacional de Estadística y Geografía. Retrieved from https://www.inegi.org.mx/contenidos/saladeprensa/boletines/2018/EstSociodemo/MOLEC2018_04.pdf

Jackson, J. (2009). Game-based teaching: What educators can learn from videogames. *Teaching Education*, *20*(3), 291–304. DOI: 10.1080/10476210902912533

Jiménez, D. (2018). Niños ya no juegan en la calle, nuevos entretenimientos causan obesidad. Retrieved from https://www.excelsior.com.mx/comunidad/2018/01/08/1211772

Juul, J. (2005). *Half-real: Video games between real rules and fictional worlds.* MIT Press.

Latorre, A. (2003). *La investigación-Acción: Conocer y cambiar la práctica educativa.* Editorial Graó.

López, J. Y. A., Nuñoncca Huaycho, R. N., Yallercco Santos, F. I., Talavera-Mendoza, F., & Rucano Paucar, F. H. (2023). The impact of serious games on learning in primary education: A systematic literature review. *International Journal of Learning. Teaching and Educational Research*, *22*(3), 379–395. DOI: 10.26803/ijlter.22.3.23

López Raventós, C. (2016). El videojuego como herramienta educativa. Posibilidades y problemáticas acerca de los serious games. *Apertura, Revista de Innovación Educativa, 8*(1), 1–51. Retreived from http://www.udgvirtual.udg.mx/apertura//index.php/apertura/article/view/825

Magazine, U. X. (2017). Participatory Design in Practice. Retrieved from https://uxmag.com/articles/participatory-design-in-practice

Marcano, B. (2008). Juegos Serios Y Entrenamiento En La Sociedad Digital. *Teoría de La Educación Educación y Cultura En La Sociedad de La Información, 9*, 5. Retrieved from https://dialnet.unirioja.es/servlet/articulo?codigo=2778746&info=resumen

Marinelli, C. V., Nardacchione, G., Trotta, E., Di Fuccio, R., Palladino, P., Traetta, L., & Limone, P. (2023). The Effectiveness of Serious Games for Enhancing Literacy Skills in Children with Learning Disabilities or Difficulties: A Systematic Review. *Applied Sciences (Basel, Switzerland)*, *13*(7), 4512. DOI: 10.3390/app13074512

Moral Álvarez, J., & Almazán Ruíz, E. (2017). El uso de los videojuegos como recurso didáctico para el aprendizaje de inglés (Tesis para licenciatura). Universidad de Jaén, Andalucía, España. Retrieved from http://tauja.ujaen.es/bitstream/10953.1/5745/1/Moral_lvarez_Jess_TFG_Educacin_Primaria.pdf

Multimedia, C. I. B. A. L. (2004). Ven a jugar con Pipo. CIBAL Multimedia S.L. Retrieved from http://www.pipoclub.com/webonline/guia/catalogo.pdf

Nielsen, J. (2012). Usability 101: Introduction to Usability. Nielsen Norman Group. Retrieved from https://www.nngroup.com/articles/usability-101-introduction-to-usability/

Ojanen, E., Ronimus, M., Ahonen, T., Chansa-Kabali, T., February, P., Jere-Folotiya, J., Kauppinen, K.-P., Ketonen, R., Ngorosho, D., & Pitk, Ã¤nen, M., Puhakka, S., Sampa, F., Walubita, G., Yalukanda, C., Pugh, K., Richardson, U., Serpell, R., & Lyytinen, H. (. (2015). GraphoGame â€“ a catalyst for multi-level promotion of literacy in diverse contexts. *Frontiers in Psychology, 6*. Advance online publication. DOI: 10.3389/fpsyg.2015.00671

Papert, S. (1993). The children's machine. Perseus Book Group. Retrieved from https://pdfs.semanticscholar.org/e744/f03a3586f8e79dee595a3dbdef2e327b28cd.pdf

Papert, S. (1998). Does Easy Do It? Children, Games, and Learning. Retrieved from http://www.papert.org/articles/Doeseasydoit.html

Participate in Design. (2019). Our Design Philosophy. Retrieved from https://participateindesign.org/approach/what

Pasqualotto, A., Altarelli, I., de Angeli, A., Menestrina, Z., Bavelier, D., & Venuti, P. (2022). Enhancing reading skills through a video game mixing action mechanics and cognitive training. *Nature Human Behaviour*, *6*(4), 545–554. DOI: 10.1038/s41562-021-01254-x

Piquette, N. A., Savage, R. S., & Abrami, P. C. (2014). A cluster randomized control field trial of the ABRACADABRA web-based reading technology: Replication and extension of basic findings. *Frontiers in Psychology*, *5*, 1413. DOI: 10.3389/fpsyg.2014.01413

Russo, M., Kosman, G., Ginsburg, A., Thompson-Hoffman, S., & Pederson, J. (1998). *A compact for reading and School-home Links*. Department of Education.

Schleicher, A. (2019). PISA 2018: Insights and Interpretations. Retrieved from https://www.oecd.org/pisa/PISA%202018%20Insights%20and%20Interpretations%20FINAL%20PDF.pdf

Schultz, C., & Bryant, R. (2011). *Game Testing All in One*. Mercury Learning & Information, Herndon.

Simonsen, J., & Robertson, T. (Eds.). (2013). *Routledge international handbook of participatory design* (Vol. 711). Routledge.

Slavin, R. E., Madden, N. A., Dolan, L., & Wasik, B. A. (1996). *Every child, every school: Success for all.* Corwin Press, Inc.

Squire, K. (2003). Video games in education. *Int. J. Intell. Games & Simulation*, *2*(1), 49–62. https://www.biblioteken.fi/sites/default/files/content/10.1.1.100.8500.pdf

Statista. (2018). Number of active video gamers worldwide from 2014 to 2021. Retrieved from https://www.statista.com/statistics/748072/number-pc-gamers-world-platform

Swartz, S. L., Shook, R. E., & Klein, A. F. (2000). California Early Literacy Learning. Redlaus, CA: Foundation for California early literacy learning.

Ungau, S., Nasip, F., Linyaw, K., & Yusop, Y.Tang Tien Mee. (2023). Gamification in Improving Reading Skills of Preschool Children: Blending Through Puzzle Game. *Journal of Cognitive Sciences and Human Development*, *9*(1), 193–220. DOI: 10.33736/jcshd.5479.2023

Vargas, F., Restrepo, S., & Tapia, M. (2023). Fomento al hábito por la lectura en estudiantes de educación básica primaria en el Estado de México. (2023). *Revista de Ciencias Sociales*, *3*(3), 282–291. https://www.cienciaysociedaduatf.com/index.php/ciesocieuatf/article/view/97

Villamil, J. (2013). Entre 108 países, México es penúltimo lugar en lectura. Revista Proceso. Retrieved from_https://www.proceso.com.mx/339874/entre-108-paises-mexico-es-penultimo-lugar-en-lectura

Wehmeyer, M. L., Palmer, S. B., Smith, S. J., Davies, D. K., & Stock, S. (2008). The efficacy of technology use by people with intellectual disability: A single-subject design meta-analysis. *Journal of Special Education Technology*, *23*(3), 21–30. DOI: 10.1177/016264340802300303

ADDITIONAL READING

Biancarosa, G., & Griffiths, G. G. (2012). Technology Tools to Support Reading in the Digital Age. *The Future of Children*, *22*(2), 139–160. https://www.jstor.org/stable/23317415. DOI: 10.1353/foc.2012.0014

Gaytan-Lugo, L. S., Prietch, S. S., Santana-Mancilla, P. C., Rodriguez-Ortiz, M. A., Bautista-Flores, P. M., Fajardo-Flores, S. B., & Sanchez, J. A. (2023). Codesigning a Spanish literacy platform for deaf children. *Proceedings of the XI Latin American Conference on Human Computer Interaction*, 1–8. https://doi.org/DOI: 10.1145/3630970.3631064

Godinez, K. D., Gaytán-Lugo, L. S., Alcaraz-Valencia, P. A., & Arellano, R. M. (2017). Evaluation of a Low Fidelity Prototype of a Serious Game to Encourage Reading in Elementary School Children. *Proceedings of the 8th Latin American Conference on Human-Computer Interaction*, 1–4. https://doi.org/DOI: 10.1145/3151470.3156640

Papert, S. (1980). *Mindstorms: children, computers, and powerful ideas*. Basic Books, Inc.

Read, J. C., & Gilutz, S. (2016). Research Methods for Child Computer Interaction. *Proceedings of the 2016 CHI Conference Extended Abstracts on Human Factors in Computing Systems - CHI EA '16*, 927–930. https://doi.org/DOI: 10.1145/2851581.2856678

Read, J. C., & MacFarlane, S. (2006). Using the fun toolkit and other survey methods to gather opinions in child computer interaction. *Proceeding of the 2006 Conference on Interaction Design and Children - IDC '06*, 81. https://doi.org/DOI: 10.1145/1139073.1139096

Sørensen, B. H., & Meyer, B. (2007). Serious Games in language learning and teaching – a theoretical perspective. *Situated Play, Proceedings of DiGRA 2007 Conference*, 559–566. http://www.digra.org/dl/db/07312.23426.pdf

Zapušek, M., Cerar, Š., & Rugelj, J. (2011). Serious computer games as instructional technology. 1056–1058. 2011 *Proceedings of the 34th International Convention MIPRO*, 1056–1058. https://ieeexplore.ieee.org/abstract/document/5967211

KEY TERMS AND DEFINITIONS

Engagement: The level of attention, focus, and active participation demonstrated by learners while interacting with educational content.

Learning Outcomes: Specific skills, or attitudes that learners are expected to achieve as a result of an educational activity or intervention, serving as measurable indicators of the effectiveness of the learning process.

Motivation in Learning: An internal process that drives learners to initiate, persist, and complete educational activities, significantly influenced by elements such as challenge, feedback, and interactivity.

Participatory Design: A design approach that involves end-users and stakeholders in the development process, ensuring that their needs, experiences, and perspectives directly shape the design of technologies.

Playful Learning: An educational approach that integrates play elements into structured learning activities, fostering curiosity, creativity, and enjoyment while achieving educational goals.

Serious Games: Interactive digital games designed with the primary goal of promoting learning and knowledge acquisition through engaging and playful activities.

Technology Acceptance: The degree to which users are willing to adopt and use a technological system, often influenced by factors such as perceived usefulness and ease of use.

Chapter 9

Analog and Digital Gameplay in the Human Brain:

A Cognitive Neuroscience Perspective on Board and Video Gaming

Sergio Rivera-Tello
https://orcid.org/0000-0002-7183-7452
Departamento de Bioingeniería Traslacional, Universidad de Guadalajara, Mexico & Instituto de Neurociencias, CUCBA, Mexico

Julio Cesar Llamas-Alonso
Universidad Autónoma del Estado de Hidalgo, Mexico

Luis Angel Llamas-Alonso
https://orcid.org/0000-0002-4736-769X
Universidad Autónoma de Baja California, Mexico

ABSTRACT

This chapter explores board and video games from a cognitive neuroscience perspective, emphasizing their growing relevance in education and healthcare. It outlines the core elements of games—mechanics, narratives, and feedback systems—central to game-based learning and gamification, and presents key mechanics as practical resources for designers in both analog and digital formats. Empirical findings are reviewed on cognitive, behavioral, and neural outcomes: video games engage dopaminergic reward pathways to enhance attention, flexibility, and multitasking, while board games foster social reasoning, executive control, and long-term plan-

DOI: 10.4018/979-8-3373-4657-1.ch009

ning. Neuroimaging and behavioral evidence shows both benefits and risks, from motivational gains to addictive patterns. The chapter concludes with real-world applications and methodological challenges, underscoring the need for ecologically valid designs, interdisciplinary collaboration, and serious games for cognitive, educational, and mental health purposes.

INTRODUCTION

Games are among the oldest cultural artifacts of human civilization, serving both as entertainment and as tools for teaching, ritual, and socialization. Across cultures, games have functioned as instruments for transmitting knowledge, reinforcing social hierarchies, fostering cooperation, and even simulating conflict in safe environments. In recent years, there has been a surge of interest in understanding how games, both analog (such as board games, card games and tabletop role-playing games) and digital (including video games and virtual reality experiences) affect the human brain and cognition. This interest in games lies in their capacity to simulate complex real-world challenges within a control and structured environment. This is relevant because it makes the games a well-suited tool for studying how the brain learns, adapts, and changes through experience, which is relevant in the field of cognitive neuroscience. At the same time, the growing integration of gamified strategies into educational programs, therapeutic interventions, and cognitive training platforms reflects a shift in how society understands and leverages the power of gaming.

Globally, the video game industry is valued at approximately $230 billion USD, with projections reaching $400 billion by 2027 (Statista, 2025). In parallel, the board game industry has experienced remarkable growth since the COVID-19 pandemic. Valued at $14.37 billion USD in 2024, it is expected to reach $32 billion by 2032 (Fortune Business Insights, n.d.), reflecting a renewed global interest in analog forms of play. The continued rise of both industries highlights their expanding relevance not only in entertainment but also in education, healthcare, and cognitive development. This widespread popularity has also sparked increasing academic interest in understanding how digital and analog gameplay influence human behavior and cognition (Martinez et al., 2023).

Over the past 25 years, there has been a steady increase in research studies exploring the impact of games on cognition and behavior. Figure 1.A shows the number of publications indexed in PubMed for each type of game. As expected, video games have a clear lead in terms of publication volume. However, Figure 1.B presents the relative frequency of publications over time, revealing a noticeable spike in board game research around 2020, likely influenced by the global COVID-19 quarantine. These trends suggest that while video game research remains dominant, interest in board games is experiencing a resurgence, with a growing number of studies being published. At the same time, research on video games seems to be leveling off or showing a modest decline in recent years.

Figure 1. **A.** *Histogram with the number of publications in PubMed related to video (blue) and board games (red).* **B.** *Relative frequency of publications. Data was retrieved from PubMed using the search terms "Video Games" and "Board Games".*

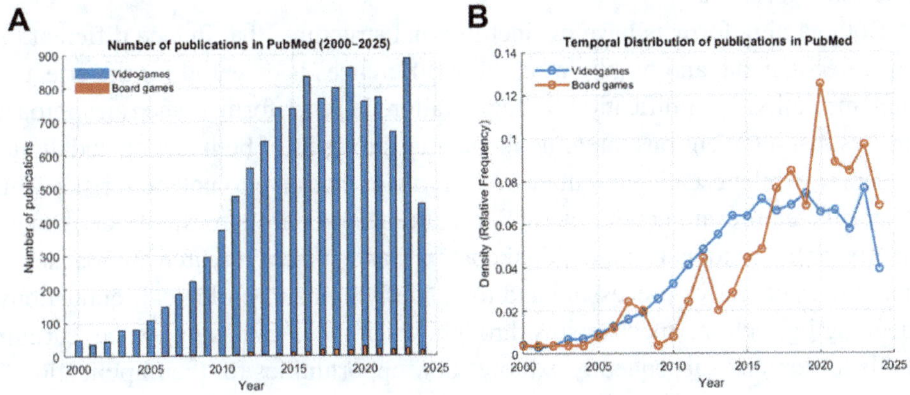

Board games, once considered primarily as casual family entertainment, have experienced a significant resurgence in recent years, probably due to a combination of several factors. These include accessible pricing, the appeal of screen-free social interaction, and the increasing desire for novel experiences that contrast with digital entertainment. Modern board game design has evolved dramatically, incorporating sophisticated mechanics such as card drafting, deck building, tile placement, and worker placement. These systems could engage players in strategic thinking, collaboration, emotional regulation, and social negotiation (Menon et al., 2019; Türkoğlu, 2019). Moreover, modern board games are emerging as valuable tools for cognitive intervention and for the development of emotional and social skills across various populations, including school-age children and older adults (Ammar et al., 2024; Cès et al., 2024; Vita-Barrull et al., 2024).

At the same time, the video game industry has continued to grow and innovate, delivering increasingly immersive experiences. Advances in technology have led to the development of virtual reality (VR), augmented reality (AR), and spatial audio formats that heighten sensory engagement and presence. These innovations allow players to explore richly detailed environments, interact in real time with dynamic systems, and even experience emotionally resonant narratives. Research on video games has identified beneficial effects on cognitive performance, such as enhanced attention, problem-solving, and visuospatial skills (Bavelier & Green, 2019). However, these outcomes are not universal, as they depend on the cognitive processes engaged by each game, player characteristics, and contextual factors (Choi et al., 2020). Alongside potential benefits, studies also point to risks, including excessive play or the reinforcement of maladaptive behaviors (Demuyakor, 2021). Video games should therefore be understood as complex tools whose impact on cognition arises from dynamic interactions between game features, individual profiles, and situational variables.

Both gaming formats have distinct internal structures that induce different effects. Recognizing and highlighting these differences is essential for the effective implementation of gamification strategies tailored to each format. Such an approach ensures that interventions integrate the unique strengths of both analog and digital gameplay, while research simultaneously remains attentive to potential risks. This chapter therefore examines the internal structure of both board games and video games, their potential as tools in educational contexts, and current research approaches. It emphasizes cognitive processing and the underlying neurobiological foundations, shedding light on the mechanisms through which these games influence learning and behavior, and subsequently explores new opportunities for their application.

INTERNAL STRUCTURE OF BOARD AND VIDEO GAMES

Games, whether analog or digital, are constructed from a series of interconnected systems known as mechanics, which function as the essential architecture of the play experience. These mechanics form the internal structure of games—the underlying rules and systems that influence player behavior, progression, interaction, and feedback. These mechanics define not only the possible actions available to players but also the constraints, rewards, and challenges that shape how play unfolds. In both, board games and video games, understanding this structure is crucial for leveraging their pedagogical potential and gamification strategies.

Cognitive and Neurofunctional Outcomes of Gaming

At the heart of every game lies a set of core mechanics that define how a game is played and how challenges are presented. In board games, these might include *area control* (e.g., *Risk, Ankh*), which involves players competing for dominance over specific regions of the board. *Set collection* (e.g., *Ticket to Ride*) rewards players for gathering specific groups of items to earn points. *Tile placement* (e.g., *Carcassonne*, *Dorfromantik*) challenges players to strategically arrange pieces, earning points based on how well tiles align or create patterns. Meanwhile, *worker placement* (e.g., *Everdell*) tasks players with assigning limited workers to various actions or locations to gather resources and build their strategy. Table 1 presents a synthesis of the most influential mechanics found in modern and classic board games, with its associated cognitive processes and titles.

Table 1. List of the most important board game mechanics, cognitive processes involved and popular reference games

Mechanic	Cognitive processes	Reference games
Area Control	Long-term planning, dominance estimation, spatial control	*Chinese Checkers, Ankh, Blood Rage, War of the Ring*
Bluffing	Theory of mind, emotional control, deception detection	*Clue, Blood on the Clocktower, Coup, The Resistance*
Deck Building	Working memory, probabilistic reasoning, strategy updating	*Pokémon Trading Card Game (TCG), Magic: The Gathering, Dominion, Dune: Imperium, Star Realms*
Drafting	Anticipation, strategic filtering, decision inhibition	*7 Wonders, Sushi Go!, Between Two Cities*
Negotiation	Empathy, perspective-taking, verbal reasoning	*Monopoly, Catan, Chinatown*
Push Your Luck	Risk assessment, impulsivity control, reward prediction	*UNO, Quacks, Heat Pedal to the Metal*
Roll and Move	Probabilistic reasoning, tactical adjustment, multiple scenarios evaluation	*Snakes and Ladders, Monopoly, Backgammon*
Set Collection	Category learning, short-term memory, goal evaluation	*Ark Nova, Concordia, Ticket to Ride,*
Storytelling	Narrative reasoning, imagination, episodic memory, empathy	*Dixit, Dungeons and Dragons, Once Upon a Time*
Strategy (General)	Abstraction, long-term planning, error monitoring	*Chess,* Go, *Twilight Struggle, Brass: Birmingham*
Tile Placement	Visual-spatial reasoning, pattern completion	*Scrabble, Carcassonne, Cascadia, Dorfromantik*
Trick-Taking	Pattern recognition, rule-based reasoning, memory updating	*The Crew, Fox in the Forest, Skull King*
Worker Placement	Strategic planning, inhibition, multitasking	*Agricola, Everdell, Viticulture*

From a cognitive perspective, board games can serve as effective tools for stimulating Executive Functions (EF) — a set of higher-order cognitive processes that enable individuals to plan, focus attention, remember instructions, regulate behavior, and adapt flexibly to new situations. These sets of processes make possible mentally playing with ideas, thinking before acting, meeting novel unanticipated challenges and resisting temptations (Diamond, 2012). Executive Functions include key components such as updating working memory, or the ability to hold and manipulate information. Inhibition which is the capacity to suppress automatic or impulsive responses and cognitive flexibility, the ability to shift perspectives or strategies in response to changing demands.

By requiring players to follow complex rules, anticipate opponents' moves, and adjust strategies dynamically, board games provide a rich and motivating context for exercising these abilities, thereby supporting learning, emotional regulation, and autonomy in both children and adults (Cristofori et al., 2019). One study found strong effects on verbal short-term memory, with board game–based cognitive interventions producing greater improvements than those observed in control groups of children (Estrada-Plana et al., 2024).

Similarly, Ammar et al. (2024) demonstrated that regular participation in board games (*Snakes and Ladders, Ludo, Chess*) can benefit older adults, improving both cognitive performance and physical balance. Over an eight-week intervention, older participants who engaged in board-game sessions showed significant gains in the Mini–Mental State Examination (MMSE), Berg Balance Scale, and Dynamic Gait Index, along with a reduced risk of falls compared to a control group. These results suggest that board games that are strategic with visuospatial elements can serve as an effective strategy to maintain cognitive vitality, physical stability, and overall well-being in later life.

Each game mechanic involves different cognitive strategies that could activate distinct brain regions or circuits—for instance, area control and tile placement relies on long-term planning and spatial reasoning, engaging possibly in regions such as the hippocampal formation (McNaughton et al., 2006) and the parietal cortex (Gunia et al., 2021). Bluffing activates theory of mind and emotional regulation, supported by the supramarginal gyrus as a key component for the sociocognitive process of deception (Meier et al., 2021). Mechanics like deck building and drafting require working memory and strategic updating, possibly recruiting brain areas such as the dorsolateral prefrontal cortex (dlPFC) and frontostriatal updating mechanisms driven by dopaminergic pathways (Nyberg & Eriksson, 2016). Meanwhile, push your luck games emphasize reward anticipation and impulsivity control, engaging brain circuitry like the "reward system" comprising the medial and orbital prefrontal cortex, ventral striatum (VS), dopaminergic midbrain, amygdala and insula (Haber & Knutson, 2010; Murch & Clark, 2016). The study of this brain circuit could be important to better understand how games influence the brain to better design strategies applied in education and healthcare.

Building on the idea of the brain's reward system, it is plausible that mesolimbic–cortical dopaminergic circuits underlie the intrinsic enjoyment and sustained engagement many individuals experience while playing games. Midbrain dopamine neurons in the ventral tegmental area (VTA) project to the ventral striatum, dorsal striatum, and prefrontal cortex, where they encode *reward prediction errors*—phasic signals indicating whether outcomes are better or worse than expected (Schultz, 2016). This computational role explains why outcomes that are contingent, surprising, and informative—features central to most games—evoke motivational and learning signals.

A seminal neuroimaging study using positron emission tomography (PET) demonstrated that video game play produces real-time dopamine release in the striatum, and the degree of release correlated with task performance (Koepp et al., 1998). Subsequent magnetic resonance imaging (MRI) work revealed structural and functional plasticity in reward circuits, including gray matter increases and altered ventral striatal responsiveness after regular gaming practice (Kühn et al., 2011; Lorenz et al., 2015). These findings highlight that games engage the very circuits that drive motivation, reward-based learning, and behavioral persistence.

Dopamine's role extends beyond motivation: it gates synaptic plasticity. In animal models, pairing sensory stimulation with dopaminergic activity alters cortical representations. Bao et al. (2001), for example, showed that concurrent stimulation of the VTA with auditory tones reorganized the auditory cortex, facilitating neuroplasticity. Such results provide a mechanistic bridge between dopamine release during rewarding events and long-term changes in cortical processing.

These mechanisms resonate with the cognitive benefits attributed to video games. Bavelier and Green (2019) report that action video games can enhance attentional control and perceptual discrimination. Green and Bavelier, (2012) demonstrated improvements in cognitive flexibility, while Stockdale et al. (2017) observed enhanced inhibitory control among players. Training studies have further shown gains in multitasking and task-switching abilities (Llamas-Alonso et al., 2019). Extending beyond these executive and attentional domains, evidence also indicates that video game experience enhances probabilistic learning, with gamers showing superior categorization performance under uncertainty and greater reliance on hippocampal and declarative memory systems (Schenk et al., 2017). This suggests that gaming not only sharpens cognitive control but also fosters more effective learning strategies when outcomes are ambiguous. Taken together, these findings support the idea that dopamine-mediated plasticity provides a plausible substrate for the transfer of gaming-related experience to a broad set of core cognitive functions.

The same dopaminergic mechanisms that support learning and motivation can also underlie maladaptive use. The World Health Organization's ICD-11 includes "gaming disorder," characterized by impaired control, prioritization of gaming over other activities, and functional impairment (World Health Organization, 2021). Reviews suggest that problematic gaming shares neurobiological features with behavioral addictions, including altered striatal activation patterns (Weinstein & Lejoyeux, 2020). While most players do not develop addiction, excessive use can result in withdrawal-like symptoms and disruptions in academic, social, and emotional functioning. This underscores the importance of promoting responsible gaming practices, particularly among children and adolescents, whose developing brains may be more vulnerable to the reinforcing properties of games and the potential impact on academic and psychosocial development.

In the context of board games, several factors may contribute to the players' motivation. For example, social interaction provides emotional connection, cooperation or competition. Strategic thinking and cognitive challenges may also be rewarding. These game attributes are present in some board games genres, for example, *Eurogames*, which is characterized by low randomness and high complexity. Titles such as *Catan*, *Carcassonne*, or *Agricola* reward careful long-term planning, resource management, and optimization strategies rather than luck-based outcomes. This reduction of chance increases the salience of decision-making and encourages players to rely on analytical thinking, foresight, and adaptive planning. For instance, one study found that preschoolers enjoyed cooperative board games such as *Granny's House*, *Secret Door*, and *Mr. Troll* more than competitive ones, suggesting that these formats provide a more engaging and rewarding context for fostering the early development of social interaction skills (Eriksson et al., 2021).

More narrative-driven mechanics, such as storytelling, could stimulate imagination and episodic memory, as well as activate regions related to reading stories, like visual and premotor areas (Speer et al., 2009). Games like *Gloomhaven* or *Dungeons & Dragons* (D&D) exemplify how narrative can become central to gameplay. In *Dungeons & Dragons* there is a range of cognitive, social, and psychological benefits that extend beyond entertainment. A Rapid Evidence Assessment conducted by Henrich and Worthington (2023) highlights that while no single personality type defines D&D players, participation in the game is consistently associated with positive outcomes, including enhanced social skills, creativity, and emotional regulation.

The board game *Go*—a centuries-old, highly strategic game that requires players to capture territory by surrounding their opponent's tokens on a grid—offers a compelling case study. The fundamental goal in this game is to occupy the largest area of the board, which encourages long-term spatial planning and dominance estimation. Neuroimaging research has shown that expert *Go* players exhibit increased gray matter volume in regions involved in reward evaluation and decision-making, most notably the bilateral nucleus accumbens (Kim, 2025). This region is a central component of the mesolimbic reward system, which mediates pleasure, motivation, and reinforcement learning. The observed structural changes in these areas suggests a form of neural adaptation driven by the cognitive demands of sustained strategic training and long-term engagement with the game. Recent functional imaging work further expands this view. Lee et al. (2025) demonstrated that expert Go players rely not only on cortical reward and decision-making circuits but also on cerebellar networks when making intuitive, rapid estimations of territory size—an ability linked to the Approximate Number System (ANS). Their study revealed heightened activation in the right cerebellum during difficult estimation tasks, rather than in the traditional parietal regions typically associated with numerical reasoning. This finding suggests that intuitive quantitative reasoning in expert players is supported by automatized cerebellar processes, reflecting neural efficiency developed through extensive practice.

Board games promote slower-paced, embodied interactions, narrative reasoning, and face-to-face negotiation, strategic thinking, patience, supporting cognitive functions such as working memory, inhibitory control, complex collaboration, strategy and theory of mind (Moya-Higueras et al., 2023; Romero et al., 2015). In addition, these games provide opportunities for learning, accomplishment, excitement (D'Astous & Gagnon, 2007) and motivation (Klein, 1992). They can improve learning rate in students of elementary schools (Asemani Barekat, 2023) and even prevent cognitive decline in aging populations (Pozzi et al., 2023).

In summary, games (digital and analog) offer a unique intersection of motivation and learning by engaging reward-driven processes in the mesolimbic–cortical dopaminergic system. During play, well-timed feedback, uncertainty, and goal progress elicit dopamine signals that sustain intrinsic enjoyment and gate cortical reorganization, creating opportunities for cognitive enhancement. Board/analog formats also contribute distinctive affordances—face-to-face social cues, turn-based planning, and tangible components—that can scaffold executive control and metacognitive reflection. Yet the same reward processes can become maladaptive when unbounded, fostering compulsive patterns or crowding out other activities. To isolate causal mechanisms, future research should deploy preregistered randomized designs, address selection effects, and experimentally manipulate mechanics (e.g., feedback timing, reward schedules, social interaction) across digital and analog media to test their impact on prediction-error signaling and learning. Ultimately, harnessing games for education and well-being—whether on a screen or around a table—requires pairing their motivational power with safeguards that promote balanced, prosocial, and reflective engagement.

Cognitive Specificity of Gaming Effects

Even though numerous video game genres have been described in scholarly taxonomies. For example, Wolf identified approximately 42 categories, which a 2024 systematic review later condensed into 25 popular genres for comparability (Starosta et al., 2024). However, not all genres share equal prevalence or cognitive impact. Shooter games (e.g., *Fortnite*, *Call of Duty*, *Halo*), which belong to the broader action category, consistently emerge as the most widely played worldwide

(Bavelier & Green, 2019; Statista, 2023). Their fast-paced gameplay and demand for rapid responses highlight their relevance for research on cognitive processes such as attention, processing speed, and executive control. More broadly, many video games are built around core loops such as combat systems (e.g., *NieR: Automata*), exploration (e.g., *The Legend of Zelda*), or role-playing progression (e.g., *Skyrim*). These mechanics create highly dynamic, real-time experiences that involve motor coordination, reaction time, goal setting, and adaptation. Within educational contexts, such systems can be leveraged to train decision-making under pressure, systems thinking, and iterative problem-solving. Given that the classification of video game genres remains a research challenge—and that many games combine three or more genres simultaneously—we have chosen instead to describe popular core video game mechanics in Table 2.

Table 2. List of the most important video game mechanics, cognitive processes involved and popular reference games

Mechanic	Cognitive processes	Reference games
Action Timing / Reflexes	Processing speed, motor control, reaction inhibition	*Fortnite, Call of Duty, Super Meat Boy, Cuphead*
Branching Dialogue	Social cognition, moral reasoning, theory of mind	*Mass Effect, The Walking Dead, Disco Elysium*
Combat Systems	Visual-motor integration, working memory, task-switching	*Dark Souls, Devil May Cry, Bayonetta, Street Fighter*
Crafting / Building	Sequential reasoning, planning, visual-spatial mapping	*Minecraft, Terraria, Valheim*
Exploration	Spatial navigation, curiosity, environmental memory	*The Legend of Zelda: Breath of the Wild (BOTW), Subnautica, Journey*
Loot Upgrade Systems	Reward anticipation, decision-making under uncertainty	*Diablo III, Borderlands, Destiny 2*
Platforming	Motor coordination, timing, spatial attention	*Celeste, Super Mario Odyssey, Hollow Knight*
Puzzle Solving	Logical reasoning, pattern recognition, cognitive flexibility	*Portal, The Witness, Baba Is You*
Resource Management	Executive function, prioritization, working memory	*StarCraft II, Factorio, Cities: Skylines*
Role-Playing Progression	Goal setting, feedback processing, identity projection	*Skyrim, Final Fantasy VII, Persona 5*
Sandbox / Open World	Self-directed goals, exploration, system thinking	*Grand Theft Auto V, Red Dead Redemption 2*
Stealth Mechanics	Planning, risk prediction, inhibition of dominant responses	*Metal Gear Solid, Hitman, Dishonored*

Video games—particularly action video games, the most popular genre—typically engage users through audiovisual stimulation, rapid decision-making, hand-eye coordination, multitasking, and reward-based feedback, all of which activate motivational and dopaminergic pathways (Bavelier & Green, 2019; Palaus et al., 2017). However, the neurobiological effects of gaming extend beyond dopaminergic reward pathways. Action and strategy video games activate several neural networks supporting multiple executive functions such as working memory, attentional and spatial navigation, including the prefrontal cortex, anterior cingulate, parietal areas, and hippocampus. These regions coordinate planning, error monitoring, and updating of goals in real time (Bavelier & Green, 2019; Kühn & Gallinat, 2014). Functional imaging studies show increased frontoparietal connectivity and hippocampal plasticity following sustained gaming, suggesting that video games engage both motivational and executive-memory circuits, thereby supporting goal-directed learning and cognitive flexibility. Action games include mechanics that involve the execution of combos that rely on selective attention, rapid error correction and timing, which are processed in the cerebellum and premotor areas. These brain regions allow players to anticipate trajectories, compensate for latency and execute with accurate timing, within the mili-second range (O'Reilly et al., 2008).

Moreover, exploration mechanics, navigating in open worlds, reading maps, or using landmarks, are abilities that involve spatial cognition. This spatial navigation is processed in the hippocampus and the retrosplenial complex, evidenced by theta brain rhythm during navigation tasks (Do et al., 2021).

To wrap up the discussion on cognitive specificity, the following argument provides useful insight: Although popular discourse often frames video games as either beneficial or harmful, such generalizations are misleading. Green and Bavelier (2015) emphasize that different genres elicit distinct, often non-overlapping cognitive effects: some commercial video games induce large-scale improvements in attentional control and probabilistic reasoning, whereas others show little or no transfer beyond the gaming context. For example, *action shooters* like *Doom* or *Call of Duty* have been repeatedly associated with enhancements in visuospatial attention, visual acuity, and rapid decision-making (Bavelier & Green, 2019; Green & Bavelier, 2012). In contrast, *life simulation* games such as *The Sims* may foster resource management and social decision-making but are unlikely to train visuospatial attention, nor do they typically sensitize players to violent content. This contrast illustrates why it is dangerous to generalize game effects as universally "good" or "bad": the relationship between a game's mechanics, the cognitive processes it stimulates, and the behavioral outcomes it produces is complex and domain-specific. Furthermore, cross-cultural perspectives are essential to avoid a Western-centric view of gaming and cognition. The cultural meanings of play, competition, and cooperation differ markedly across societies, influencing both how games are designed and how players interpret their experiences. For example, studies comparing Eastern and Western players suggest variations in preferred genres, motivational drivers, and social play styles, which can moderate cognitive and emotional outcomes (Nuyens et al., 2023). Recognizing these cultural dimensions allows for more inclusive research frameworks and prevents overgeneralizing findings derived primarily from Western samples.

Narrative Structures and Engagement

Beyond mechanics, both board and video games use narrative elements to enhance immersion and emotional investment. In analog games, storytelling is often emergent—arising through player interaction (e.g., *Dixit* or tabletop role-playing such as the popular *Dungeons & Dragons*), while in digital games, narratives are more explicitly scripted or branching (e.g., *Death Stranding, The Last of Us*).

These stories support narrative identity, enabling players to reflect on choices, consequences, and ethical dilemmas—key aspects in educational contexts such as history, ethics, and social-emotional learning. Narrative design also shapes pacing, goal structures, and player motivation; in educational gamification, this can help sustain engagement across long-term learning processes by embedding goals within a meaningful fictional context. When combined with role-playing elements, narrative design supports identity exploration and collaborative learning, making the educational process more immersive, memorable, and socially engaging.

Beyond cognitive and educational benefits, narrative-driven video games have been shown to support health and well-being (Baranowski et al., 2008). For example, immersive storylines can enhance psychological outcomes such as adherence to nutritional regimens to prevent obesity (Hwang & Lu, 2018), increase physical activity through active gameplay (Hwang & Lu, 2018) and generally mental health (Kowal et al., 2021) probably explained by the emotional engagement and the sense of purpose. By providing context, emotional resonance, and branching choices that model ethical reasoning and judgment, narratives not only enrich learning experiences but also foster motivation, deeper immersion, and potential health-related benefits.

Interactive Systems and Feedback

A critical component of game design is the feedback system—how the game responds to player actions. Whether through scoring in a board game or visual/audio effects in video games, feedback supports self-regulation and metacognition (Checa-Romero & Gimenez-Lozano, 2024). Well-designed feedback loops help players assess their progress, adjust strategies, and develop growth mindsets through iterative failure and success.

One compelling example of a feedback system in board games is narrative progression—a dynamic in which the board state and its components evolve visibly throughout the game, providing continuous visual and spatial feedback to the player. In *Dorfromantik*, a tile-placement game, players take turns placing hexagonal tiles to construct a harmonious landscape by aligning elements such as train tracks, rivers, and clusters of houses. With each tile placed, the board expands and transforms, offering an immediate and tangible representation of the player's progress. This unfolding visual narrative not only reinforces engagement but also fosters a sense of accomplishment and immersion.

In video games, particularly in the cognitively demanding action genre, feedback systems are central to player engagement and performance. Real-time visual, auditory, and haptic cues—such as health bars, damage indicators, and cooldown timers—provide continuous information about the player's actions and their consequences. Games like *Overwatch* or *Call of Duty* require rapid decision-making and precise coordination, and the immediate feedback these systems provide allows players to adjust strategies, refine motor responses, and optimize cognitive resources. By reinforcing successful behaviors and signaling errors, these interactive systems not only sustain engagement but also promote learning, attention, and executive function under high-pressure conditions (Bavelier & Green, 2019).

In gamification, feedback systems are often abstracted into forms such as Points, Badges, and Leaderboards (PBL). While these elements can drive short-term motivation, when implemented without meaningful interaction or cognitive challenge, they may lead to superficial engagement. In contrast, when feedback is closely linked to core mechanics—such as completing quests, crafting functional tools, or solving contextual logic puzzles—it encourages deep cognitive involvement and sustained learning (Liu et al., 2021).

VIDEO GAMES AS TOOLS FOR HEALTH AND EDUCATION

Before describing how video games contribute to health and educational outcomes, it is important to clarify the distinctions among *gamification*, *serious games*, and *game-based learning*. While these terms are sometimes used interchangeably, their content has different levels of game integration and intentionality. For instance, *Gamification* refers to the use of game elements (e.g., points, badges, leaderboards) in non-game contexts to increase motivation and engagement. *Serious games*, in contrast, are video games that have been designed with specific non-entertainment purposes such as explicit educational, therapeutic, or cognitive training goals. Finally, *Game-based learning* lies between these two, describing the pedagogical use of commercial or serious video games as tools to achieve specific learning objectives. Clarifying these distinctions helps prevent conceptual misusage and ensures accurate interpretation of cognitive and behavioral outcomes when applying game principles in educational or health interventions.

Understanding the internal structure of games enables educators, healthcare professionals, and designers to extract pedagogically and behaviorally valuable mechanics and adapt them to real-world learning and service environments in non-game context. In this regard, gamification—the application of game design elements in non-game settings—is an innovative strategy that effectively fosters motivation and sustained participation. For example, incorporating progress bars or rewarding patients for engaging in desired health behaviors, such as increasing daily step counts or adhering to medication schedules, transforms routine tasks into engaging challenges. This transformation turns ordinary events into exciting, goal-oriented experiences that promote active participation and facilitate learning (Buheji, 2019).

Beyond individual motivation, gamification also supports social dynamics by encouraging collaboration, cooperation, and social connection among participants. As McGonigal (2011) highlights, well-designed game elements can build meaningful communities, foster teamwork, and strengthen social bonds, which are essential for both educational and healthcare settings. By leveraging these principles, gamification can create more dynamic, interactive environments that improve outcomes and enrich user experiences.

Several gamification techniques, originally developed in video games and mobile applications, are now being increasingly adopted in hospitals, psychological clinics, and educational settings. Among the most widely used game design elements are points, storyline, and feedback, which have been shown to be particularly effective in medical education (Aster et al., 2024). Key techniques include:

- **Progress Bars / Tracking**: Visual indicators of progress toward a goal to encourage persistence.
- **Points / Scores:** Rewarding users with points for completing tasks or behaviors.
- **Badges / Achievements:** Visual symbols or certificates earned for reaching milestones.
- **Leaderboards:** Ranking participants to introduce friendly competition.
- **Challenges / Quests / Missions:** Structured tasks or goals to complete, often with increasing difficulty.
- **Levels / Experience Points (XP):** Systems where users "level up" as they accumulate experience.
- **Rewards / Incentives:** Tangible or intangible prizes given for desired actions.

- **Feedback / Immediate Response:** Instant reactions to user actions to reinforce learning and behavior.
- **Unlockable Content / Features:** Rewards that become available only after certain achievements.
- **Storytelling / Narrative:** Embedding tasks in a meaningful story to boost immersion.
- **Social Interaction:** Incorporating collaboration, competition, or sharing with peers.
- **Timers / Time Limits:** Adding urgency or pacing to encourage action.
- **Random Rewards / Loot Boxes:** Introducing unpredictability to increase excitement.
- **Card set collection:** Card-based challenges where patients collect cards to track and reinforce healthy behaviors or treatment adherence.
- **Tile placement:** Tiles representing completed exercises to build a visual "path" toward recovery.
- **Storyline:** Give meaning to the user's actions and transform isolated tasks into a coherent adventure.

Apps like *MyFitnessPal* and *Fitbit* use points, goals, and stats to encourage healthy habits such as exercise, proper nutrition, and sleep. These systems turn wellness into a game-like experience, promoting sustained behavior change through visible progress and achievable milestones. Similarly, platforms like *Pill Reminder Medisafe* gamify medication adherence by sending encouraging messages and rewards when users take their prescriptions on time. In the field of mental health, apps like *Happify* and *SuperBetter* use game-based challenges and interactive activities to help users build emotional resilience, practice mindfulness, and cope with stress or depression. Another interesting app is Lumosity, a brain training platform that uses gamification to support cognitive health. It offers short, game-like tasks that target memory, attention, flexibility, problem-solving, and processing speed.

In real-life educational settings, gamification techniques have shown tangible benefits. For example, platforms like *Kahoot!* and *Quizizz* use competitive quizzes with points and leaderboards, turning review sessions into fun, dynamic games that increase student participation. Similarly, *ClassDojo* employs a reward system that gives students badges and positive feedback for good behavior and effort, helping to build a positive classroom culture. Project-based learning platforms such as *Duolingo* apply levels, streaks, and immediate feedback to language learning, motivating students to practice regularly and track their improvement. In more formal environments, teachers create "*quest*" or "*mission*"-based curriculums where students complete tasks in sequence, encouraging mastery and self-paced progression.

Overall, gamification empowers individuals—whether patients or students—to take an active, engaged role in their personal development. In healthcare and mental health, gamification transforms therapeutic and preventive activities into interactive, goal-oriented experiences that improve consistency, build healthy habits, and support long-term well-being. Similarly, in educational settings, gamification goes beyond mere entertainment. It leverages core psychological motivators such as achievement, competition, and social connection to make learning more meaningful, enjoyable, and motivating.

Previously, we described how gamification elements are implemented in health and educational contexts. We now turn to how games can, either unintentionally or intentionally, promote learning opportunities in these domains through game-based-learning. To this matter, it is important to differentiate between traditional games and serious games. Although this distinction has been described previously, it is necessary to revisit it here for conceptual clarity. Games can be broadly classified into two main categories based on their primary purpose. On one hand, traditional video games—such as *Super Mario Bros*, *Call of Duty*, or *Fortnite*—are designed primarily for entertainment and enjoyment, without an explicit educational objective, so related to unintentional learning or effects related to education or health settings (Llamas-Alonso & Llamas-Alonso, 2025). On the other hand, serious games are intended to educate, train, or raise awareness among users, incorporating pedagogical or skill-development goals (Krath et al., 2021; Laamarti et al., 2014). These intentional games are structured to promote cognitive and social competencies, including critical thinking, problem-solving, strategic decision-making, and teamwork, fostering active and contextualized learning (Gee, 2003). Moreover, the use of serious games in educational settings allows for the assessment and reinforcement of skills interactively, providing immediate feedback and realistic simulations that can enhance teaching and learning processes.

Board games differ from video game gamification in mechanics that are more tangible and social. *Monopoly, Catan* and *Scrabble* are some traditional board games that primarily were designed for entertainment purposes without an explicit educational objective. Nevertheless, they often result in incidental learning: players practice negotiation, probability assessment, and memory updating without being consciously aware of the educational value. However, there are many serious educational board games that were designed for this purpose. For instance, *Timeline* encourage historical learning of scientific inventions and political events. This game promotes memorization of historical dates. Another notable example is *The Color Monster*, a children's emotional education game. Its purpose is to help children identify, label, and regulate emotions by associating colors with different feelings (e.g., yellow for happiness, blue for sadness, red for anger). The game mechanic requires players to work together to sort emotional tokens into jars, fostering emotional intelligence, empathy, and communication skills. In therapeutic and educational contexts this game demonstrates how serious board games can be tailored to early childhood, promoting socio-emotional learning in a playful, accessible manner.

Coming back to the intentionality of promoting beneficial effects, debate remains over whether serious or traditional (commercial) games yield greater benefits. In this regard, Silva et al., (2021) conducted a systematic review of 53 studies on Autism Spectrum Disorder (ASD) interventions using both game types and reported measurable benefits for autistic participants, most often in social-communication, emotion recognition, executive attention, and behavioral regulation. However, the evidence base is methodologically mixed (few randomized designs and limited blinding), and many improvements are confined to proximal, task-specific measures rather than clearly demonstrated generalization to everyday functioning. On balance, the review does not support a clear superiority of serious over commercial games; rather, it concludes that both categories can be useful, while emphasizing the need for better-controlled trials and outcome measures that capture naturalistic social behavior and broader transfer.

Regarding traditional games specifically, benefits were most consistent for exergames (movement-based titles), which were associated with reductions in repetitive/stereotyped behaviors and modest gains in engagement (e.g., initiative, eye contact, peer conversation), alongside lower stress/anxiety in several reports. Serious games, for their part, showed targeted gains (e.g., emotion recognition and attentional control), but affective resilience remains underexplored across both categories. In short: commercial games can produce meaningful, domain-relevant improvements, and current data do not justify prioritizing serious games categorically—what matters most is fit to goals, intensity/structure of use, and assessing change with ecologically valid outcomes.

Even though transfer benefits to everyday activities remain a challenge, some promising findings support positive effects on reading in developmental dyslexia for example. In Italian-speaking children with dyslexia, a randomized comparison of action versus non-action games—using mini-games drawn from the commercial title *Rayman Raving Rabbids* (Nintendo Wii)—showed that just 12 hours of action-game play, without any phonics content, sped up reading with no loss of accuracy and also improved attention; the reading gains were larger than those expected from a full year of spontaneous development, indicating meaningful transfer to everyday literacy demands (Franceschini et al., 2013).

These benefits generalize beyond transparent writing systems. In English-speaking children with dyslexia, action-oriented mini-games from *Rayman Raving Rabbids* again increased word recognition and pseudoword decoding, boosted focused visual attention, and accelerated shifting from vision to audition—a skill that supports letter-to-sound mapping during reading. The same training improved phonological short-term memory and phoneme blending, and changes in attention and working memory together explained over 30% of the improvement in reading speed, consistent with an attention-based pathway to better reading (Franceschini et al., 2017; Franceschini & Bertoni, 2019).

Finally, there is early dose–response evidence: in a clinical program using two off-the-shelf action titles—*Plants vs. Zombies: Garden Warfare* (*PlayStation 3*) and *Nanostray 2* (*Nintendo DS*)—over twelve one-hour sessions, only the children who measurably improved their in-game performance showed faster phonological decoding and better phonological short-term memory; in these high-learners, decoding gains were comparable to a year of natural reading development. This pattern supports the idea that commercial action games exercise a multisensory attentional system whose plasticity can yield practical, day-to-day reading benefits (Franceschini & Bertoni, 2019).

It is important to emphasize that as these technologies become increasingly integrated into healthcare and education environments, ethical considerations must also be addressed and considered. For instance, gamified health applications collect sensitive personal and biometric data that could raise privacy and data-protection concerns (Mavroeidi et al 2019). Moreover, the inclusion of reward mechanics such as loot boxes—often resembling gambling—poses psychological and regulatory challenges, particularly for younger users (Zendle & Cairns, 2019). Overall, ethical design requires transparency, informed consent, age regulations, trained monitors for underage players as well as safeguards to prevent addictive patterns or exploitative monetization, ensuring that the motivational affordances of games serve users' well-being rather than commercial manipulation.

BOARD AND VIDEO GAMES RESEARCH APPROACHES AND OPPORTUNITIES

The scientific study of board and video games in cognitive neuroscience, health, and education presents substantial opportunities for growth. One promising direction involves developing novel experimental designs in which cognitive paradigms are embedded in ecologically valid contexts that closely resemble real gameplay. This includes not only adapting existing tasks to game-like formats but also designing original games, ensuring they incorporate all the critical characteristics of paradigms used to evaluate specific cognitive processes.

Although video games have received extensive exploration within neurosciences, analog board games remain an underexplored field. The lack of neuroimaging studies investigating board games limits our understanding of how social, motivational and strategic aspects of analog gaming contribute to cognitive development and brain plasticity. Future research should aim to bridge this gap by employing neuroimaging techniques to capture the neural dynamics underlying board gaming.

Research should also move beyond isolated case studies to encompass the full spectrum of the gaming population. This includes casual players, highly engaged hobbyists, and the rapidly expanding professional gaming sector, which spans competitive video games, esports, such as *League of Legends*, and board games from the traditionally *Chess* and *Go* to Trading Card Games (TCGs) like *Pokémon, Lorcana, Yu-Gi-Oh!* and *Magic: The Gathering*. Also, longitudinal studies are particularly important for capturing the sustained cognitive, social, and emotional effects of gaming over time and the neuroplastic changes involved.

One of the most debated topics in game research is the transfer of skills from play to other domains. A growing body of evidence suggests that games can enhance cognitive abilities closely aligned with in-game demands. Future research should also focus on this topic. Meta-analytic evidence indicates that transfer is strongest for domains overlapping with gaming demands, such as selective attention and visuospatial processing, but weaker for unrelated domains (Bediou et al., 2018). Concerns about selection bias persist, as individuals with higher baseline abilities may self-select into cognitively demanding genres. Moreover, publication bias and underpowered samples complicate the interpretation of findings (Sala et al., 2018). Thus, while the evidence for cognitive enhancement is compelling, generalizability is constrained by methodological limitations.

Other future opportunities could include the design of AI-driven adaptive games, which adjust difficulty and feedback in real time within a laboratory, creating highly individualized training environments. Clinical interventions, where games are designed as diagnostic and therapeutic tools, rehabilitation or preventive strategies for Attention Deficit Hyperactivity Disorder (ADHD), depression or anxiety. Moreover, games designed to teach specific topics in universities.

These emerging opportunities also call for adapting neuroimaging and psychophysiological methods to authentic gaming environments. Advances in mobile, wireless Electroencephalographic (EEG) technology—such as *Emotiv* and *Muse* systems—make it feasible to record neural activity in settings optimized for play, including game rooms, esports arenas, and community tournaments. This wireless technology has been proven to capture accurate EEG activity within psychophysiological paradigms (Balart-Sánchez et al., 2019). Conducting research in these environments preserves the naturalistic qualities of gameplay while enabling high-quality neuroscientific data.

Building on these methodological innovations and perspectives, the future of game research lies in interdisciplinary collaboration and the design of innovative methodologies. Neuroscientists, educators, psychologists, and game designers should work together to develop "serious games" as research instruments and commercial assets that are both engaging to play and useful in specific educational and healthcare contexts.

Moreover, a persistent challenge—and opportunity—in this field is demonstrating transfer from game-based training to everyday activities. We therefore propose a mechanism-first approach: start from a disorder, health, or educational problem that is clearly characterized by a specific cognitive bottleneck (e.g., focused visuospatial attention, cross-modal attentional shifting, response inhibition, working memory), then select traditional commercial games whose core mechanics intensively exercise that process (e.g., fast target selection and temporal precision for visuospatial attention; visual-auditory cue switching for cross-modal shifting; stealth/puzzle play with stop-go demands for inhibition). Crucially, evaluate success with ecologically valid outcomes that matter in daily life—such as natural-text reading speed/accuracy, teacher-rated on-task classroom behavior, or parent-logged functional gains—rather than relying only on laboratory proxies. The dyslexia literature provides a proof of principle: brief, structured action-video-game training improves attention and transfers to everyday reading (Franceschini et al., 2013, 2017; Franceschini & Bertoni, 2019), while evidence from autism interventions underscores that measuring real-world generalization should be a design priority whether one uses serious or commercial titles (Silva et al., 2021).

Finally, recent findings highlight the urgent need to better define thresholds of gameplay that are beneficial versus harmful, yet the current evidence base remains insufficient. For instance, in a large sample of highly engaged gamers ($N = 14{,}740$), those at risk of Gaming Disorder reported playing an average of about 42 hours per week ($M = 42.1$, $SD = 19.0$ under the APA framework; $M = 42.6$, $SD = 19.3$ under the WHO framework), whereas gamers not at risk reported approximately 27 hours per week (Katz et al., 2024), while pediatric guidance for young children (ages 2–5) recommends limiting screen use to ≤1 hour per day of high-quality programming, with co-viewing encouraged and screens avoided during meals and in the hour before bedtime (AAP, policy reaffirmed 2022) (American Academy of Pediatrics, 2016), these stricter limits reflect the fact that the developing brain is more vulnerable to negative outcomes from excessive media exposure; therefore, further research is needed to establish clearer age-specific thresholds and covariables to guide safer gaming practices across the transitions from school age to adolescence and adulthood.

Similarly, sociodemographic factors such as gender, family structure, and extracurricular physical activity have been identified as predictors of gaming addiction risk in school children (Rodríguez-Fernández et al., 2024), but we still lack longitudinal evidence to explain how these variables interact with psychological vulnerabilities over time. Collectively, these findings suggest not only those games can have diverse effects depending on multiple interacting factors, but also that much more research is needed—particularly longitudinal and mechanistic studies—to translate these insights into reliable guidelines and interventions.

CONCLUSIONS

Board and video games differ in mechanics and context. Fast-paced mechanics in video games stimulate dopaminergic circuits that reinforce rapid learning, motor control and attention. In contrast, board games rely on slower, socially embedded mechanics—such as negotiation, storytelling, and long-term strategic planning. Despite these differences, both forms of play converge on a common pathway: the brain's reward system. By triggering dopamine release in mesolimbic–cortical circuits, games could promote neuroplasticity, reinforcing the behaviors and cognitive strategies practiced repeatedly during gameplay. Describing these neurobiological foundations is critical for understanding why gamification holds so much promise in education and healthcare. When integrated into learning environments or therapeutic interventions, game-based elements recruit the same reward-driven mechanisms that sustain motivation and learning in natural play. This makes gamification a uniquely powerful tool to foster adherence, resilience, and engagement in contexts where maintaining long-term effort is essential. Looking into the near future, emerging technologies are rapidly transforming the boundaries of what constitutes a "game." Artificial intelligence now enables adaptive games that adjust difficulty and feedback dynamically based on a player's performance, cognitive state, or emotional cues, offering unprecedented personalization in both learning and therapy (Fisher & Kulshreshth, 2024). Meanwhile, advances in brain–computer interfaces (BCIs) allow direct neural input and output, opening possibilities for rehabilitation, attention training, and assistive communication (Elashmawi et al., 2024). These innovations blur the line between game, tool, and neural prosthesis, suggesting a future in which interactive systems are not merely entertaining but integrative components of cognitive and emotional enhancement.

The growing sector of both, analog and digital games, underscores the importance of advancing experimental research. Future studies should prioritize ecologically valid designs that capture the complexity of real-world gameplay, ensuring that findings translate into practical applications for cognitive development, education, and health.

REFERENCES

Ammar, M., Amjad, I., Nisar, M., & Ghoneim, O. S. (2024). Effects of board games on balance in association with cognition in community-dwelling older adults. *Journal of Musculoskeletal Surgery and Research : Official Publication of Saudi Orthopaedic Association*, *8*(3), 256–263. DOI: 10.25259/JMSR_122_2024

Asemani Barekat, N. (2023). The Effect of Board Games on the Academic Achievement and Learning Motivation of Fourth-Grade Elementary Student. *International Journal of Elementary Education*, *12*(3), 68–75. DOI: 10.11648/j.ijeedu.20231203.13

Aster, A., Laupichler, M. C., Zimmer, S., & Raupach, T. (2024). Game design elements of serious games in the education of medical and healthcare professions: A mixed-methods systematic review of underlying theories and teaching effectiveness. *Advances in Health Sciences Education : Theory and Practice*, *29*(5), 1825–1848. DOI: 10.1007/s10459-024-10327-1 PMID: 38563873

Balart-Sánchez, S. A., Vélez-Pérez, H., Rivera-Tello, S., Gómez Velázquez, F. R., González-Garrido, A. A., & Romo-Vázquez, R. (2019). A step forward in the quest for a mobile EEG-designed epoch for psychophysiological studies. *Biomedizinische Technik*, *64*(6), 655–667. DOI: 10.1515/bmt-2017-0189 PMID: 31322998

Bao, S., Chan, V. T., & Merzenich, M. M. (2001). Cortical remodelling induced by activity of ventral tegmental dopamine neurons. *Nature*, *412*(6842), 79–83. DOI: 10.1038/35083586 PMID: 11452310

Baranowski, T., Buday, R., Thompson, D. I., & Baranowski, J. (2008). Playing for real: Video games and stories for health-related behavior change. *American Journal of Preventive Medicine*, *34*(1), 74–82. DOI: 10.1016/j.amepre.2007.09.027 PMID: 18083454

Bavelier, D., & Green, C. S. (2019). Enhancing attentional control: Lessons from action video games. *Neuron*, *104*(1), 147–163. DOI: 10.1016/j.neuron.2019.09.031 PMID: 31600511

Bediou, B., Adams, D. M., Mayer, R. E., Tipton, E., Green, C. S., & Bavelier, D. (2018). Meta-analysis of action video game impact on perceptual, attentional, and cognitive skills. *Psychological Bulletin*, *144*(1), 77–110. DOI: 10.1037/bul0000130 PMID: 29172564

Buheji, M. (2019). Gamification techniques to re-invent public healthcare services: A case study. *International Journal of Human Resource Studies*, *9*(2), 339. DOI: 10.5296/ijhrs.v9i2.14888

Cès, P., Duflos, M., Tricard, E., Jhean-Larose, S., & Giraudeau, C. (2024). Playing board games to increase emotional competencies in school-age children and older people: A systematic review. *Leisure Sciences*, *•••*, 1–24. DOI: 10.1080/01490400.2024.2373415

Checa-Romero, M., & Gimenez-Lozano, J. M. (2024). Video games and metacognition in the classroom for the development of 21st century skills: A systematic review. *Frontiers in Education*, *9*, 1485098. Advance online publication. DOI: 10.3389/feduc.2024.1485098

Choi, E., Shin, S. H., Ryu, J. K., Jung, K. I., Kim, S. Y., & Park, M. H. (2020). Commercial video games and cognitive functions: Video game genres and modulating factors of cognitive enhancement. *Behavioral and Brain Functions : BBF*, *16*(1), 2. DOI: 10.1186/s12993-020-0165-z PMID: 32014027

Cristofori, I., Shalom, D., & Grafman, J. (2019). Executive functions. In D'Esposito, M., & Byrne, J. H. (Eds.), *Encyclopedia of the cognitive neurosciences* (2nd ed.). Elsevier., DOI: 10.1016/B978-0-12-804281-6.00011-2

D'Astous, A., & Gagnon, K. (2007). An inquiry into the factors that impact on consumer appreciation of a board game. *Journal of Consumer Marketing*, *24*(2), 80–89. DOI: 10.1108/07363760710737085

Demuyakor, J. (2021). Battling Underaged Online Video Gamers: Probing the Negative Effects of Online Video Gaming Addictions on Young Adolescents. *Asian Journal of Media and Communication*, *5*(2). Advance online publication. DOI: 10.20885/asjmc.vol5.iss2.art3

Diamond, A. (2012). Activities and programs that improve children's executive functions. *Current Directions in Psychological Science*, *21*(5), 335–341. DOI: 10.1177/0963721412453722 PMID: 25328287

Do, T. T. N., Lin, C. T., & Gramann, K. (2021). Human brain dynamics in active spatial navigation. *Scientific Reports*, *11*(1), 13036. Advance online publication. DOI: 10.1038/s41598-021-92246-4 PMID: 34158525

Elashmawi, W. H., Ayman, A., Antoun, M., Mohamed, H., Mohamed, S. E., Amr, H., Talaat, Y., & Ali, A. (2024). A Comprehensive Review on Brain–Computer Interface (BCI)-Based Machine and Deep Learning Algorithms for Stroke Rehabilitation. *Applied Sciences (Basel, Switzerland)*, *14*(14), 6347. DOI: 10.3390/app14146347

Eriksson, M., Kenward, B., Poom, L., & Stenberg, G. (2021). The behavioral effects of cooperative and competitive board games in preschoolers. *Scandinavian Journal of Psychology*, *62*(3), 355–364. DOI: 10.1111/sjop.12708 PMID: 33543787

Estrada-Plana, V., Martínez-Escribano, A., Ros-Morente, A., Mayoral, M., Castro-Quintas, Á., Vita-Barrull, N., Terés-Lleida, N., March-Llanes, J., Badia-Bafalluy, A., & Moya-Higueras, J. (2024). Benefits of playing at school: Filler board games improve visuospatial memory and mathematical skills. *Brain Sciences*, *14*(7), 642. DOI: 10.3390/brainsci14070642 PMID: 39061383

Fisher, N., & Kulshreshth, A. K. (2024). Exploring Dynamic Difficulty Adjustment Methods for Video Games. *Virtual Worlds*, *3*(2), 230–255. DOI: 10.3390/virtualworlds3020012

Fortune Business Insights. (n.d.). *Board games market size, share & trends analysis [2032]*. Retrieved September 3, 2025, from https://www.fortunebusinessinsights.com/board-games-market-104972

Franceschini, S., & Bertoni, S. (2019). Improving action video games abilities increases the phonological decoding speed and phonological short-term memory in children with developmental dyslexia. *Neuropsychologia*, *130*, 100–106. DOI: 10.1016/j.neuropsychologia.2018.10.023 PMID: 30395809

Franceschini, S., Gori, S., Ruffino, M., Viola, S., Molteni, M., & Facoetti, A. (2013). Action video games make dyslexic children read better. *Current Biology*, *23*(6), 462–466. DOI: 10.1016/j.cub.2013.01.044 PMID: 23453956

Franceschini, S., Trevisan, P., Ronconi, L., Bertoni, S., Colmar, S., Double, K., Facoetti, A., & Gori, S. (2017). Action video games improve reading abilities and visual-to-auditory attentional shifting in English-speaking children with dyslexia. *Scientific Reports*, *7*(1), 5863. Advance online publication. DOI: 10.1038/s41598-017-05826-8 PMID: 28725022

Gee, J. P. (2003). What video games have to teach us about learning and literacy. [CIE]. *Computers in Entertainment*, *1*(1), 20. DOI: 10.1145/950566.950595

Green, C. S., & Bavelier, D. (2012). Learning, attentional control, and action video games. *Current Biology*, *22*(6), R197–R206. DOI: 10.1016/j.cub.2012.02.012 PMID: 22440805

Green, C. S., & Bavelier, D. (2015). Action video game training for cognitive enhancement. *Current Opinion in Behavioral Sciences*, *4*, 103–108. DOI: 10.1016/j.cobeha.2015.04.012

Gunia, A., Moraresku, S., & Vlček, K. (2021). Brain mechanisms of visuospatial perspective-taking in relation to object mental rotation and the theory of mind. *Behavioural Brain Research*, *407*, 113247. DOI: 10.1016/j.bbr.2021.113247 PMID: 33745982

Haber, S. N., & Knutson, B. (2010). The reward circuit: Linking primate anatomy and human imaging. *Neuropsychopharmacology : Official Publication of the American College of Neuropsychopharmacology, 35*(1), 4–26. DOI: 10.1038/npp.2009.129 PMID: 19812543

Henrich, S., & Worthington, R. (2023). Let your clients fight dragons: A rapid evidence assessment regarding the therapeutic utility of 'Dungeons & Dragons.'. *Journal of Creativity in Mental Health, 18*(3), 383–401. DOI: 10.1080/15401383.2021.1987367

Hwang, J., & Lu, A. S. (2018). Narrative and active video game in separate and additive effects of physical activity and cognitive function among young adults. *Scientific Reports, 8*(1), 11020. Advance online publication. DOI: 10.1038/s41598-018-29274-0 PMID: 30030456

Katz, D., Horváth, Z., Pontes, H. M., Koncz, P., Demetrovics, Z., & Király, O. (2024). How much gaming is too much? An analysis based on psychological distress. *Journal of Behavioral Addictions, 13*(3), 716–728. DOI: 10.1556/2006.2024.00036 PMID: 39024045

Kim, K. W. (2025). Go and the brain: Cognitive and neural impacts of training. *Psychiatry Investigation, 22*(4), 357–364. DOI: 10.30773/pi.2024.0387 PMID: 40262784

Klein, J. D. (1992). Effect of instructional gaming and reentry status on performance and motivation. *Contemporary Educational Psychology, 17*(4), 364–370. DOI: 10.1016/0361-476X(92)90074-9

Koepp, M. J., Gunn, R. N., Lawrence, A. D., Cunningham, V. J., Dagher, A., Jones, T., Brooks, D. J., Bench, C. J., & Grasby, P. M. (1998). Evidence for striatal dopamine release during a video game. *Nature, 393*(6682), 266–268. DOI: 10.1038/30498 PMID: 9607763

Kowal, M., Conroy, E., Ramsbottom, N., Smithies, T., Toth, A., & Campbell, M. (2021). Gaming Your Mental Health: A Narrative Review on Mitigating Symptoms of Depression and Anxiety Using Commercial Video Games. *JMIR Serious Games, 9*(2), e26575. DOI: 10.2196/26575 PMID: 34132648

Krath, J., Schürmann, L., & Von Korflesch, H. F. O. (2021). Revealing the theoretical basis of gamification: A systematic review and analysis of theory in research on gamification, serious games and game-based learning. *Computers in Human Behavior, 125*, 106963. DOI: 10.1016/j.chb.2021.106963

Kühn, S., Romanowski, A., Schilling, C., Lorenz, R., Mörsen, C., Seiferth, N., Banaschewski, T., Barbot, A., Barker, G. J., Büchel, C., Conrod, P. J., Dalley, J. W., Flor, H., Garavan, H., Ittermann, B., Mann, K., Martinot, J.-L., Paus, T., Rietschel, M., & Gallinat, J. (2011). The neural basis of video gaming. *Translational Psychiatry, 1*(11), e53–e53. DOI: 10.1038/tp.2011.53 PMID: 22833208

Laamarti, F., Eid, M., & El Saddik, A. (2014). An overview of serious games. *International Journal of Computer Games Technology, 2014*(1), 358152. DOI: 10.1155/2014/358152

Lee, T., Jo, H. J., Kim, M., & Kwon, J. S. (2025). The neural basis of intuitive approximate number system in board game Go (Baduk) experts. *Scientific Reports, 15*(1), 16400. DOI: 10.1038/s41598-025-98605-9 PMID: 40355626

Liu, Y. C., Wang, W. T., & Lee, T. L. (2021). An Integrated View of Information Feedback, Game Quality, and Autonomous Motivation for Evaluating Game-Based Learning Effectiveness. *Journal of Educational Computing Research, 59*(1), 3–40. DOI: 10.1177/0735633120952044

Llamas-Alonso, J., Guevara, M. A., Hernández-González, M., Hevia-Orozco, J. C., & Almanza-Sepúlveda, M. L. (2019). Action video game players require greater EEG coupling between prefrontal cortices to adequately perform a dual task. *Entertainment Computing, 30*, 100302. Advance online publication. DOI: 10.1016/j.entcom.2019.100302

Llamas-Alonso, J. C., & Llamas-Alonso, L. A. (2025). Videojuegos y aprendizaje: Impacto cognitivo, neurobiológico y aplicaciones educativas. Video Games and Learning: Cognitive, Neurobiological Impact, and Educational Applications. *Humanus Nexus, 9*(16), nueva época. ISSN 3061-7235.

Lorenz, R. C., Gleich, T., Gallinat, J., & Kühn, S. (2015). Video game training and the reward system. *Frontiers in Human Neuroscience, 9*, 40. DOI: 10.3389/fnhum.2015.00040 PMID: 25698962

Martinez, L., Gimenes, M., & Lambert, E. (2023). Video games and board games: Effects of playing practice on cognition. *PLoS One, 18*(3), e0283654. Advance online publication. DOI: 10.1371/journal.pone.0283654 PMID: 36972271

Mavroeidi, A.-G., Kitsiou, A., Kalloniatis, C., & Gritzalis, S. (2019). Gamification vs. Privacy: Identifying and Analysing the Major Concerns. *Future Internet, 11*(3), 67. DOI: 10.3390/fi11030067

McGonigal, J. (2011). *Reality is broken: Why games make us better and how they can change the world*. Penguin Press.

McNaughton, B. L., Battaglia, F. P., Jensen, O., Moser, E. I., & Moser, M. B. (2006). Path integration and the neural basis of the "cognitive map.". *Nature Reviews. Neuroscience*, *7*(8), 663–678. DOI: 10.1038/nrn1932 PMID: 16858394

Meier, S. K., Ray, K. L., Mastan, J. C., Salvage, S. R., & Robin, D. A. (2021). Meta-analytic connectivity modelling of deception-related brain regions. *PLoS One*, *16*(8), e0248909. Advance online publication. DOI: 10.1371/journal.pone.0248909 PMID: 34432808

Menon, D., Romero, M., & Viéville, T. (2019). Computational thinking development and assessment through tabletop escape games. *International Journal of Serious Games*, *6*(4), 3–18. DOI: 10.17083/ijsg.v6i4.319

Moya-Higueras, J., Solé-Puiggené, M., Vita-Barrull, N., Estrada-Plana, V., Guzmán, N., Arias, S., Garcia, X., Ayesa-Arriola, R., & March-Llanes, J. (2023). Just Play Cognitive Modern Board and Card Games, It's Going to Be Good for Your Executive Functions: A Randomized Controlled Trial with Children at Risk of Social Exclusion. *Children (Basel, Switzerland)*, *10*(9), 1492. Advance online publication. DOI: 10.3390/children10091492 PMID: 37761453

Murch, W. S., & Clark, L. (2016). Games in the brain: Neural substrates of gambling addiction. *The Neuroscientist*, *22*(5), 534–545. DOI: 10.1177/1073858415591474 PMID: 26116634

Nyberg, L., & Eriksson, J. (2016). Working memory: Maintenance, updating, and the realization of intentions. *Cold Spring Harbor Perspectives in Biology*, *8*(2), a021816. Advance online publication. DOI: 10.1101/cshperspect.a021816 PMID: 26637287

O'Reilly, J. X., Mesulam, M. M., & Nobre, A. C. (2008). The cerebellum predicts the timing of perceptual events. *The Journal of Neuroscience : The Official Journal of the Society for Neuroscience*, *28*(9), 2252–2260. DOI: 10.1523/JNEUROSCI.2742-07.2008 PMID: 18305258

Palaus, M., Marron, E. M., Viejo-Sobera, R., & Redolar-Ripoll, D. (2017). Neural basis of video gaming: A systematic review. *Frontiers in Human Neuroscience*, *11*, 248. DOI: 10.3389/fnhum.2017.00248 PMID: 28588464

Pozzi, F. E., Appollonio, I., Ferrarese, C., & Tremolizzo, L. (2023). Can traditional board games prevent or slow down cognitive impairment? A systematic review and meta-analysis. *Journal of Alzheimer's Disease*, *95*(3), 829–845. DOI: 10.3233/JAD-230473 PMID: 37638443

Rodríguez-Fernández, A., Ruíz-De la Fuente, M., Maury-Sintjago, E., Petersen, S., Paredes, V., & Montero, B. (2024). Sociodemographic Factors Associated with Video Game Addiction in Schoolchildren from the South-Central Region of Chile. *Children (Basel, Switzerland), 11*(10), 1156. DOI: 10.3390/children11101156 PMID: 39457120

Romero, M., Usart, M., & Ott, M. (2015). Can serious games contribute to developing and sustaining 21st century skills? *Games and Culture, 10*(2), 148–177. DOI: 10.1177/1555412014548919

Sala, G., Tatlidil, K. S., & Gobet, F. (2018). Video game training does not enhance cognitive ability: A comprehensive meta-analytic investigation. *Psychological Bulletin, 144*(2), 111–139. DOI: 10.1037/bul0000139 PMID: 29239631

Schenk, S., Lech, R. K., & Suchan, B. (2017). Games people play: How video games improve probabilistic learning. *Behavioural Brain Research, 335*, 208–214. DOI: 10.1016/j.bbr.2017.08.027 PMID: 28842270

Schultz, W. (2016). Dopamine reward prediction error coding. *Dialogues in Clinical Neuroscience, 18*(1), 23–32. DOI: 10.31887/DCNS.2016.18.1/wschultz PMID: 27069377

Silva, G. M., Souto, J. J. de S., Fernandes, T. P., Bolis, I., & Santos, N. A. (2021). Interventions with serious games and entertainment games in autism spectrum disorder: A systematic review. *Developmental Neuropsychology, 46*(7), 463–485. DOI: 10.1080/87565641.2021.1981905 PMID: 34595981

Speer, N. K., Reynolds, J. R., Swallow, K. M., & Zacks, J. M. (2009). Reading stories activates neural representations of visual and motor experiences. *Psychological Science, 20*(8), 989–999. DOI: 10.1111/j.1467-9280.2009.02397.x PMID: 19572969

Starosta, J., Kiszka, P., Szyszka, P. D., Starzec, S., & Strojny, P. (2024). The tangled ways to classify games: A systematic review of how games are classified in psychological research. *PLoS One, 19*(6), e0299819. Advance online publication. DOI: 10.1371/journal.pone.0299819 PMID: 38913664

Statista. (2023, January 10). *Video game industry - Statistics & Facts*. Video Gaming & ESports. https://www.statista.com/topics/868/video-game-industry/

Statista. (2025, July 4). *Industria del videojuego: valor de mercado global*. https://es.statista.com/estadisticas/598622/valor-de-mercado-del-videojuego-en-el-mundo/

Stockdale, L., Morrison, R. G., Palumbo, R., Garbarino, J., & Silton, R. L. (2017). Cool, callous and in control: Superior inhibitory control in frequent players of video games with violent content. *Social Cognitive and Affective Neuroscience*, *12*(12), 1869–1880. DOI: 10.1093/scan/nsx115 PMID: 29040750

Türkoğlu, B. (2019). The effect of educational board games training programme on the social skill development of the fourth graders. *Elementary Education Online*, *18*(3), 1326–1344. DOI: 10.17051/ilkonline.2019.612180

Vita-Barrull, N., Estrada-Plana, V., March-Llanes, J., Sotoca-Orgaz, P., Guzmán, N., Ayesa, R., & Moya-Higueras, J. (2024). Do you play in class? Board games to promote cognitive and educational development in primary school: A cluster randomized controlled trial. *Learning and Instruction*, *93*, 101946. DOI: 10.1016/j.learninstruc.2024.101946

Weinstein, A., & Lejoyeux, M. (2020). Neurobiological mechanisms underlying internet gaming disorder. *Dialogues in Clinical Neuroscience*, *22*(2), 113–126. DOI: 10.31887/DCNS.2020.22.2/aweinstein PMID: 32699511

World Health Organization. (2021). *International statistical classification of diseases and related health problems* (5th ed.). https://icd.who.int

Zendle, D., & Cairns, P. (2019). Loot boxes are again linked to problem gambling: Results of a replication study. *PLoS One*, *14*(3), e0213194. DOI: 10.1371/journal.pone.0213194 PMID: 30845155

Chapter 10
Collaborative Training Design in a Simulation System Integrating Virtual Reality in Residents

Madeleine Gabriela Contreras Davito
https://orcid.org/0009-0005-2528-098X
Universidad de Guadalajara, Mexico

José Martínez-Chávez
Instituto Mexicano del Seguro Social, Mexico

Jesús Cabral-Araiza
https://orcid.org/0009-0006-9078-6044
Universidad de Guadalajara, Mexico

Sonia Martínez-Solís
https://orcid.org/0009-0003-1205-9923
Instituto Tecnológico Superior de Jalisco, Mexico

Armando Ariel Gutierrez-Lopez
https://orcid.org/0009-0001-1301-3789
Universidad de Guadalajara, Mexico

ABSTRACT

Virtual reality is increasingly being incorporated into the field of medical training. The Mexican Social Security Institute is recognized for training personnel in various

DOI: 10.4018/979-8-3373-4657-1.ch010

specialties; in this case, the focus is on the development of surgical clinical skills that medical residents at Regional Hospital 45 must acquire. Within this context, attending physicians have shown interest in incorporating virtual reality into the residents' learning process. On a daily basis, residents often share how their own motivation drives them to integrate information they have encountered across different technology-mediated platforms. Virtual reality is examined here as a tool which, from a collaborative perspective, contributes to surgical clinical training. The emphasis is placed on integrating three equally important components: the pedagogical, the technological, and the patient-centered orientation.

INTRODUCTION

The Mexican Institute of Social Security (IMSS) is a public institution in Mexico that provides health coverage in the different states of the Mexican Republic. Its network ranges from family clinics to highly specialized hospitals.

It should be noted that, as of August 31, 2022, the Official Gazette of the Federation published the decree that creates the decentralized public body called *Health Services of the Mexican Institute of Social Security for Welfare* (IMSS-Bienestar). The most significant change lies in its transformation from a program that primarily served the needs of rural communities to a decentralized public institution responsible for providing health services to people without social security throughout the country.

For the purposes of this proposal, it is important to clarify that the Regional Hospital of Specialties No. 45 in Guadalajara, Jalisco, Mexico, belongs exclusively to the ordinary regime of the IMSS, that is, it serves only the insured.

With regard to the medical-surgical specialty, this area of health care has become increasingly widespread in hospitals which, fortunately, are equipped not only with the necessary human resources, but also with the infrastructure, equipment and facilities necessary to incorporate procedures aimed at guaranteeing quality standards. This, of course, includes the training of healthcare professionals.

Such interest has attracted the attention of the divisions responsible for the teaching processes. A notable example, which serves as a useful reference for this proposal, is the Simulation Center for Clinical and Surgical Excellence of the IMSS Jalisco. This center teaches courses with a clinical-surgical approach, aimed at strengthening competencies to improve the quality and safety of medical care. The interest of this hospital is to contribute to the training of resident doctors through the integration of a collaborative system that allows the use of virtual reality technology in their education.

The Simulation Centers for Clinical and Surgical Excellence are pioneers and a key component of health education within the Mexican Institute of Social Security.

They were created to strengthen training and continuing education processes for both internal and external users, through the clinical simulation strategy applied by a multidisciplinary health team.

Specialized medical training is a rigorous process aimed at ensuring the acquisition of the knowledge and clinical skills necessary for professional practice in various areas of medicine. In Mexico, this process begins with the approval of the **National Examination for Medical Residency Applicants (ENARM),** a standardized assessment that selects general practitioners to enter specialized programs in hospitals accredited by the Ministry of Health and other educational institutions (CIFRHS, 2023).

Among the candidates who pass the ENARM, those who opt for the specialty of general surgery face challenges during their training both in the acquisition of knowledge and in its practical application in real clinical situations. Specifically, first-year residents in the specialty must develop complex surgical skills in a high-demand healthcare environment, with limited time for self-directed learning.

At the **Regional General Hospital No. 45** of the Mexican Institute of Social Security in Guadalajara, Jalisco, Mexico, specialists in various medical fields are trained. In general surgery, approximately ten residents enter each year, completing the first year of their specialty in this hospital unit before continuing their training in the **High Specialty Unit of Western National Medical Center**. During this first year, residents perform clinical and academic functions, including outpatient care, emergency services, inpatient follow-up, communicating clinical updates about patients, reviewing scientific papers, and preparing conferences, all under the supervision of a staff specialist physician.

In this context, there has been a growing interest among residents in using digital resources to complement their training; This phenomenon is not exclusive to this disciplinary area.

It is a reality that students are learning in an increasingly digitized world. The challenge lies in finding a balance and ensuring that personal and human interaction, which should be prioritized by the academic instructor or teacher, whether in classrooms or other training spaces, does not diminish. To some extent, it is also the instructor's responsibility to take an active interest in the methods, modes, and spaces in which students currently learn.

Increasingly, spaces that connect in a tangible way with social networks are being integrated, not only as individual activities, but also in groups where it is increasingly common to exchange information about TikTok creators, YouTubers, Instagram channels or Facebook profiles, as well as the use of downloadable applications on mobile devices that facilitate access to information and the development of various skills. Examples include physical activity, language practice, crafts, cooking, landscaping, and countless other possibilities, including, as discussed herein, access to skill approaches related to surgical practice.

This reinforces the notion that the paradigm in education has changed with respect to access to information and sources. While the teacher used to occupy a central role in the transmission of knowledge, students now make content preferences and select resources based on user characteristics on different social platforms (Bingyan et al., 2024). For example, assessing the quality of resources such as short videos related to health sciences illustrates how virtual resources can provide a foundation for academic learning without compromising scientific rigor, transcending the boundaries of classrooms and institutions, and supporting the professional exchange of information in fields such as hospitals.

In the following sections, we will develop how the integration of resources, specifically those that involve virtual reality, is conceptualized within a training activity. The objective is to establish academic bases where information and communication technologies converge with the scientific-academic knowledge of the educational process, both in the classroom and in the clinical field, and extending beyond to specific professional environments such as hospitals.

TRAINING PROCESSES FOR RESIDENT DOCTORS IN SURGICAL CLINICS: FROM TRADITIONAL TEACHING TO THE USE OF VIRTUAL REALITY AND SIMULATION

In the formative training of medical graduates, it is commonly recognized that learning must be spread over time, and scientific advances often determine the pace, methods, pathways, and even direction of continuing professional development.

Historical examples illustrate this, such as the demands derived from wars, famines, public health needs, epidemics or even pandemics that have marked the 21st century. While it might be assumed that barriers to incorporating technology and scientific knowledge have been resolved, the continued preparation of human resources has been shown to be essential, and even vital, to address these urgent health and social challenges.

Being connected and transmitting information to build support networks within communities and across various domains has become a reality. Each effort contributes to collecting experiences and providing them with a more structured foundation based on lived experiences. This constitutes a form of learning, through which current and future professionals can take advantage of the tangible contributions of digital technology.

It is therefore not surprising that traditional methods of instruction, knowledge sharing, and skill development are now mediated by information and communication technologies, including social media, and increasingly shaped by trends such as virtual reality and artificial intelligence.

It should be noted that within the broad field of virtual reality, there are multiple alternatives that facilitate learning. The possible integration of these approaches will be discussed in the relevant sections of this model.

A study by Acevedo-Osorio, et. Al. (2025) on the impact of virtual reality on the strengthening of psychomotor skills in Surgical Instrumentation students in Pereira, Colombia, took a sample of 50 students enrolled in the third or fourth semester Surgical Instrumentation program who were 18 years of age or older, without medical conditions that affect their motor skills and without previous experience in the use of simulators for medical practice, This study consisted of training the selected students in the use of medical simulators, for which the pre- and post-training participants were evaluated in the areas of precision, execution time, economy of movements, technical quality and safety, as a result they found significant improvements in these areas in contrast to those students who were not participants in the training. This highlights the effectiveness of using virtual reality as a pedagogical tool to break down the barriers found in traditional methods.

For their part, Tokuno et al. (2025) in their study "Immersive Virtual Reality Simulation for Medical Student Procedural Training: Assessment of Cognitive Load and Usability" conducted an additional analysis to a previous study published in 2023 involving 30 medical students with no or limited experience in the use of virtual reality and who had no experience in chest tube placement, This study made a comparison between a group of students who learned with an online system, and another group that also added the virtual reality experience, in this study the students who had a virtual reality training showed greater technical skills when evaluated in simulations based on mannequin, compared to the group that only had online learning.

The study by Tokuno et al. (2025) raised the question of whether using immersive virtual reality tools on students with no experience in this field could, instead of bringing benefits to their learning, cause an increase in cognitive load by decreasing their ability to do so, contrary to what was thought, the results showed that the load was not significant and also the students adapted easily and quickly to the reality tools virtual, allowing them to feel comfortable after a few rehearsals.

In addition, Issleib et al. (2025) conducted a comparative study of basic life support (BLS) learning based on virtual reality, in contrast to training with mannequins, whose data from January 2023 to July 2023 were obtained from the Department of Anesthesiology of the University Medical Center Hamburg-Eppendorf where 110 participants were made up of medical and nursing staff from the hospital. This study mentions BLS training with virtual reality as an attractive alternative to traditional teaching with mannequins, since its immersive nature allows it to simulate realistic scenarios of medical action, however, it is also mentioned that they failed to demonstrate non-inferiority statistically, although clinical non-inferiority is observed, that is, although the study does not reach the statistical threshold to demonstrate that BLS learning with virtual reality does not is inferior or worse than learning with mannequins, the clinical and practical evidence does indicate that such training is comparable to traditional training.

Finally, a meta-analysis carried out by Sung et al. (2024), 45 studies involving 3329 people, published between 2017 and 2024 with a variation between 13 and 164 participants per study, were selected at the end of the exclusion criteria, of these 45 studies 38 implemented virtual reality and 5 augmented reality and mixed reality that includes augmented reality, All studies belong to the training area of medical sciences, mainly being the degrees of Medicine, Nursing and Dentistry. The meta-analysis showed that students who participated in the use of virtual reality obtained a higher knowledge score than those who followed traditional models in medicine, nursing and dentistry careers, they also obtained greater effectiveness in the acquisition and improvement of skills in medicine and nursing careers, but with negative results in dentistry, as well as demonstrating a positive effect on the learning attitude, improving satisfaction and confidence levels.

Overall, simulation allows participants to explore a virtual universe, pursue goals, and foster accurate understanding. It begins with a scenario that, through effects and variations, approximates interactive reality within a 3D environment (Asad et al., 2021).

In medical settings, simulated and immersive devices promote cognitive engagement while incorporating pragmatic components, allowing critical thinking to bridge the gap between existing knowledge and direct experiential learning. The meta-analysis carried out by Sung et al. (2024), also showed that most of the studies reviewed were done in Asia, followed by Europe and North America, which highlights the lack of Latin American representativeness in the analysis, mentioning a group of low-income countries which have few studies carried out due to high costs and technical limitations.

The studies analyzed show that implementing virtual reality tools in the teaching-learning process in medical sciences not only increases learning levels, but also helps to generate and reinforce the skills required for professional practice by allowing them to practice in realistic simulated environments and with 3D models, this learning model encourages students to generate a positive attitude in the educational process. increasing their satisfaction and confidence levels, because contrary to the belief that involving students without prior knowledge of spaces simulated by virtual reality could generate a great mental load that hinders the acquisition of knowledge, studies show that the mental load is minimal and does not affect in a negative way, but allows students to adapt and learn effectively in these environments.

MODEL TPACK

Virtual reality has been increasingly incorporated into medical education. The Mexican Social Security Institute stands out for its commitment to the training of specialized personnel; in this case, the interest is focused on the development of clinical surgical skills among the resident physicians of the Regional Hospital 45. Given the need to strengthen surgical competencies, treating physicians have shown interest in using virtual reality as an innovative resource within the learning process. Residents frequently report how their own motivation drives them to use information from various technology platforms. This article examines virtual reality as a tool that, from a collaborative approach, can favor clinical surgical development through the integration of three equally relevant dimensions: pedagogical, technological and disciplinary, according to the TPACK model.

The surgical training of resident physicians requires a combination of theoretical knowledge, technical skills and clinical decision-making in highly complex scenarios. Today, virtual reality (VR) has become relevant as a support tool to simulate medical procedures, reduce risks, and improve skill acquisition in controlled environments.

The Regional Hospital 45 of the Mexican Institute of Social Security has been characterized by promoting innovations that strengthen medical education. In this context, the insertion of immersive technologies such as virtual reality has aroused interest

In the educational context and also increasingly in health research, the TCPACK model is used to analyze how technology is integrated into teaching and professional practices

To be able to show how technology, content (medical systems) and methodology (research, virtuality, intervention) are integrated in an articulated way. The following text is developed:

As a subject of study, there is the difficulty that the practitioner presents to have trial and error before arriving at the operating room and not being able to face their areas of opportunity in advance. Likewise, some virtual tools were considered as support for the situation, case analysis is used as a methodology for the support of the document. If the three previous positions are worked on the fly, the TCPACK can be consolidated.

The medical system needs artificial assistants to be able to rely on them and does not take lives because it does not know how to do it, how to care for them, how to treat them, etc. It is considered a rubric to be able to evaluate the interaction between the tool, the use and the results of the experience.

The data that is collected is the experience of the professional in the area and their results in the tool they use, the process is validated, but the final goal will always be their result, the best thing about it is that they can try as many times as necessary until they achieve what they need, without damaging any lives.

Several tools are considered for different areas of surgery, with a 6-month trial for the duration of the course of the course, where the results of error reduction in face-to-face operations will be evaluated.

Table 1. Evaluation scale

Criterion	Excellent (10)	Good (8)	Satisfactory (6)	Insufficient (4 or less)
1. Technical implementation of AI	AI is robustly integrated, with accurate and adaptive algorithms.	It works properly, with minimal errors or limitations.	It has minor errors that partially affect its performance.	AI fails at key tasks or doesn't adapt to the surgical environment.
2. Recognition and analysis of the clinical case	Correctly identifies the type of surgery, risks and needs of the patient.	He acknowledges the case with acceptable accuracy, though he omits minor details.	Recognizes the case partially, with errors in diagnosis or approach.	Fails to identify the clinical case or interprets it incorrectly.
3. Virtual Patient Interaction	Clear, empathetic communication adapted to the patient's profile.	Functional interaction, although with limitations in empathy or language.	Basic interaction, with generic or insensitive responses.	Poor, confusing, or inappropriate communication for the clinical context.
4. Surgical Procedure Proposal	It suggests an appropriate, safe and well-founded procedure.	It proposes a valid option, although with technical details that could be improved.	The proposal is functional but incomplete or not very precise.	The proposal is incorrect, risky or not applicable.
5. Decision-making during simulation	It responds with clinical logic, adapting to changes and complications.	Make acceptable decisions, even if slowly or hesitantly.	Make basic decisions, with minor mistakes.	Makes wrong decisions or doesn't respond to complications.
6. Ethics and safety in the use of AI	Respect ethical principles, privacy and safety of the virtual patient.	Comply with basic ethical and safety standards.	It has minor omissions in ethical or safety aspects.	It ignores ethical principles or puts the patient's integrity at risk.
7. Evaluation of the simulated surgical outcome	Successful result, with minimal human intervention and high accuracy.	Acceptable result, with moderate intervention.	Functional result, but with obvious errors.	Failed result or with serious consequences for the virtual patient.
8. Critical reflection and improvement of the system	Analyze strengths and weaknesses, propose viable improvements.	It recognizes areas for improvement, although without depth.	Limited or poorly structured reflection.	There is no reflection or proposal for improvement.

- 80–100 points: Outstanding mastery of the use of AI in surgery.
- 60–79 points: Good management, with areas of technical or ethical improvement.
- 40–59 points: Basic performance, requires reinforcing clinical and technological foundations.
- Less than 40 points: Inappropriate or risky use of AI in a surgical context.

COLLABORATIVE MODEL AT THE IMSS REGIONAL HOSPITAL: PROPOSAL FOR TRAINING IN SURGICAL CLINIC INTEGRATING VIRTUAL REALITY AND SIMULATION THROUGH THE ANALYSIS OF THREE MAIN COMPONENTS: TECHNOLOGICAL, PEDAGOGICAL AND HOLISTIC ORIENTATION

For many decades, the use of reality simulation systems has been common to train a variety of human skills. In the field of engineering, it is widely used in air travel and spacecraft, among other applications. Similarly, it is used in motor racing, as well as in commercial and combat aviation.

Its use has spread to less expected areas, but with equally successful results. It was only a matter of time before concrete actions in the health sector benefited from mannequins, prosthetics or other devices that simulate the conditions and reactions of the human body. Today, its widespread use is not surprising and has allowed "technological miracles", such as performing remote operations in real time, among many other medical-surgical or interventional procedures.

The **SimOne** is considered the first large-scale human simulator controlled by a computer. It was developed at the University of California by Abrahamson and Denson for the training of anesthesiologists in the late 1960s. She had heart and lung sounds, thoracic ventilatory movements, blinking, and pupillary dilation or contraction. However, it did not gain popularity (only one unit was built) and was eventually abandoned due to its high cost. […] It was a high-fidelity simulator for cardiological examination that allowed blood pressure to be measured using the auscultatory method, it presented pulses and heart sounds at four points synchronized with the pulse and modulated with breathing. […] In this context, we will discuss certain aspects of human psychological conditions, as well as some pedagogical and holistic aspects of intervention, in order to understand and maximize the benefits of simulators in medical practice (Salas, 2017, p. 6).

It is no longer surprising that virtual teaching and pedagogical simulation elements are a reality in both virtual and face-to-face classrooms, and that they are here to stay. In fact, its use continues to grow daily, and the trend is unlikely to slow down. While not yet completely universal, usage rates are much higher than they were in 2019.

The pandemic accelerated the adoption of virtual teaching, artificial intelligence, and simulators. As with other paradigms, the urgency to adapt is imperative in the various domains of daily human activity, not to mention professional practice.

It is a reality that students are learning in an increasingly digitized world. The challenge lies in finding a balance and ensuring that personal and human interaction, which should be prioritized by the academic instructor or teacher, whether in classrooms or other training spaces, does not diminish.

To some extent, it is also the instructor's responsibility to take an active interest in the methods, modes, and spaces in which students currently learn.

Increasingly, spaces that connect tangibly with social networks are being incorporated, not only as individual activities, but also within groups where it is increasingly common to exchange information about TikTok creators, YouTubers, Instagram channels or Facebook profiles.

Attention should be paid to what vocational training entails, for example in terms of surgical skills, but also in areas such as patient safety (HC) and communication, as these are cross-cutting competencies that medical students must acquire. International guidelines and consensus define communication and patient safety competencies (Martínez-García et al., 2025) as essential; therefore, they must be integrated into the development of academic training and specialized skills.

An important aspect that motivated this research project is the observation in daily professional activity, hospital training and the validation of the importance of interdisciplinarity in these health sciences. This confirms that learning opportunities in clinical settings are much more diverse and realistic than those found in textbooks, classrooms, or digital tools.

In addition, it is important to note that nothing compares to the real clinical learning experience: interviewing a patient for the first time, entering operating rooms and accompanying them on a post-surgical visit.

Thus, the virtual reality and simulation approach proposed in this chapter represents, above all, an opportunity to incorporate and evaluate which devices can be integrated. This project seeks to take advantage of the resources that the Institute itself provides to its resident doctors and explore external tools available through expanded digital information and communication technologies, without neglecting the collaborative process of the relationship between the doctor and the objective of contributing to the training of future specialists.

The proposed collaborative model emphasizes the interaction of three components for the integration of virtual reality and simulation in the surgical clinic:

a) **The pedagogical component**, which contributes to the systematization of shared knowledge, attitudes, skills and competencies with a methodological approach.
b) **The technological component**, which aims to generate interest in exploring virtual reality platforms, tools and devices applied to strengthen, practice, expand, compare and critically examine the theoretical and practical knowledge required.
c) **The holistic orientation component**, aimed at the patient from a humanistic perspective, focusing on patient safety and effective communication.

For the resident in training, the fundamental aspects arise from the collaboration with the doctor who incorporates these technologies, encouraging the development of self-confidence, critical thinking, self-management and continuous improvement of skills.

The general process proposed in this project is as follows:

1. **Selection and definition of simulation requirements**: It consists of choosing and defining the requirements for the different levels of simulations, including the type of objectives, to finally suggest a basic tool within the existing virtual reality resources. This option is submitted for evaluation by the faculty trainer. If non-free tools are considered, institutional support can be sought if budgetary viability allows it, although it is not mandatory. The aim is to open up a range of possibilities, where, as indicated in the next point, the professional trainer can also propose their own tools.
2. **Clearly define the teacher's role and type of feedback**: This should be approached from a self-management and collaboration perspective.
3. **Develop a model that considers both practical-clinical and theoretical aspects**: This includes communication with the patient, the needs of the student and the teaching planning derived from the model. Strategies must go beyond the mere integration of the devices chosen for virtual reality simulation.
4. **Inclusion of an assessment stage as a requirement**: This stage should integrate self-assessment, peer assessment, and instructor assessment within each learning activity.

a) Pedagogical component

Undoubtedly, one of the psycho-emotional burdens of teaching medicine, directly or indirectly, to students who begin their professional practice in this field involves pedagogical elements that must consider the respect and moral and academic authority that an instructor with more hours of experience and professional practice inspires. In addition, it is important to remember that the emotional well-being of the student plays an important role in the progress of the designed practice. It is not simply a matter of preparing real or simulated environments; It is also about the tools and preparation of the student who performs the intervention, which, by the way, shows how prepared the student is for this professional challenge.

> *The learning process for novice surgeons can be lengthy and demanding, as it requires acquiring specific skills to carry out procedures safely and effectively. In this context, educational innovation refers to significant changes in teaching-learning processes, including new methodologies and technologies, with the aim of improving educational quality and adapting to the needs of general surgeons in training (Romero, 2025, p. 6).*

When teaching begins, the teacher-student dyad begins a dynamic shaped by the personal elements of each individual. Many of these elements are unconscious, the needs or impulses, as some would call them, that arise without the learner being fully aware of them, making the pedagogical experience of teaching unique in each class. Therefore, although the didactic elements remain the same, the individuals are not identical, since they are constantly evolving.

What specific factors related to psychomotor and emotional aspects can benefit from the use of simulators? Ramírez-Sánchez et al. (2018) highlight the following:

A. Mental training (TM) creates a clear mental environment and, depending on the student, promotes better safety conditions with respect to the procedure they intend to perform.
B. Similarly, MT generally promotes an appropriate controlled relaxation environment, allowing most participants to handle the procedures they are performing with greater awareness and composure.
C. AT also facilitates muscle memory, which is essential in any psychomotor activity to master or gain experience in fine and gross motor skills.

Figure 1. Usefulness of Mental Training in Surgery

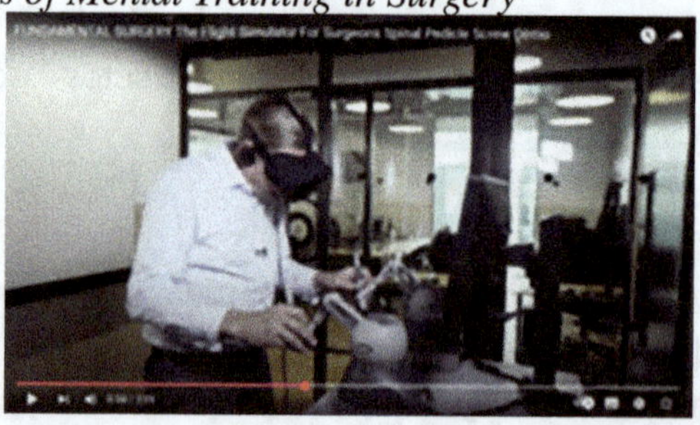

[In the mental imagination of the step-by-step surgical procedure

In non-physical mental training
What effects does it produce?

- A controlled environment allows for appropriate decision-making
- Identifies critical moments and how to resolve them
- Creates nearly involuntary movement sequences

Combined with physical skills, academic knowledge, and emotional intelligence INCREASES SURGICAL COMPETENCIES]
Source: Ramírez-Sánchez et al. (2018, p. 184).

It is necessary to take into account that in simulated training, the individual personality of the student plays a fundamental role in the success or failure of the achievement of the objectives set. Likewise, the role of the instructor or mediator between the desired skills and the student is fundamental.

As for the skills that should prevail in the educator, the following stand out:

A. **Empathy and passion for teaching**: Favorable results will not be achieved if, despite having valid knowledge, the instructor does not teach with the required motivation, empathy and care. It is hoped that this attitude will be reflected, at least ideally, in the future physician in his or her interactions with patients.
B. **Seek recognition of teaching knowledge or authority**: It is known that educators in the health sector are not always well regarded as accepting criticism or opposing opinions when expressing an idea. However, the mindset must prevail that everyone can learn something at any time, including their students' own instructors.
C. **Building a good relationship with students**: Exploring the benefits of establishing a positive relationship with students before introducing new content, often for the first time, facilitates well-rounded teaching and learning. Asking casual questions about the environment, the individual, or previous experience in simulation environments can greatly support effective pedagogy, and instructors should never overlook this.
D. **Ongoing professional development**: Undoubtedly, a crucial aspect of the professional responsibility of instructors is their continuous training. To teach cutting-edge techniques and use simulation systems effectively, instructors must engage in lifelong learning. Unlike a decade ago, investment is no longer necessarily on the books; today, it involves online resources and various ICT tools that instructors must use.

The pedagogical component is the essential link aimed at promoting collaborative learning, while ensuring, as mentioned above, that the integration of virtual reality or simulation is supported by academic foundations. The objective is to guide these resources, following criteria agreed upon within the scientific community, so that they can serve as a kind of guarantee among residents. By serving as a means of comparison, dialogue, and exchange (Guerrero-Martínez & Martínez-Castillo, 2022), these tools can foster assertiveness, responsibility, and even creativity within the group, ultimately strengthening their professional achievements.

In summary, particularly with regard to the use of technology such as virtual reality, which can be understood as an important aspect of the use of digital platforms, and based on the existing literature, it is crucial to establish a connection between technological use and the principles that contribute to the expansion of learning. This approach represents an active and collaborative pedagogical approach. Access to information freely and autonomously is, to a certain extent, inevitable. As Salas-Flores et al. (2024) point out, this approach aims to develop competencies that respond actively and dynamically, fostering interest in collaborative work, decision-making, and strengthening communication.

b) Technological component

Regarding the interest that gave rise to this proposal, it is considered relevant to integrate virtual reality as a system, that is, the knowledge or resources generated autonomously by the professional in training can be incorporated into an organized whole, where the elements are interrelated to support learning according to what is expected for residents.

The following elements are considered to expand this system in terms of technology:

| Pedagogical relevance | Interactivity & Immersive Experience | Technological accessibility and usability | Integrated Assessment & Feedback |

It is also considered useful, for practical purposes, to make a division to analyze virtual reality options. Ultimately, the goal is to have a rubric-like guide that supports self-directed learning and allows useful conclusions to be drawn for continued use.

a) VR in downloadable mobile apps

Here are some options that are interesting to consider to ensure that professional practice does not encounter conflict and that the maximum benefits are obtained from mobile technology. These benefits include easy access, portability, and intuitive interfaces that simplify functionality.

Firstly, **tactile surgery** was identified as a strong and widely recognised application.

It is a free mobile application developed to support the training of medical students and residents through interactive 3D surgical simulations. It includes more than 150 to 400 surgical procedures in approximately 17 specialties, including orthopedics, ophthalmology, neurosurgery, general surgery, among others.

The app works as a guide, taking users step-by-step through the procedures. It offers visual instructions, realistic charts, and assessments to track progress at the end of practice. It also provides a community for sharing results and monitoring individual progress, as well as reference libraries for performing procedures. The application has been evaluated in more than 100 surgical residency programs.

Touch Surgery is available free of charge, allowing access to more than 150 basic procedures. The **Premium version** requires payment and provides an institutional license for residency programs.

It can be used on a smartphone, tablet, or PC. As an app, its minimum requirements may vary depending on the user's needs.

Figure 2. Images taken from Medtronic Digital Surgery

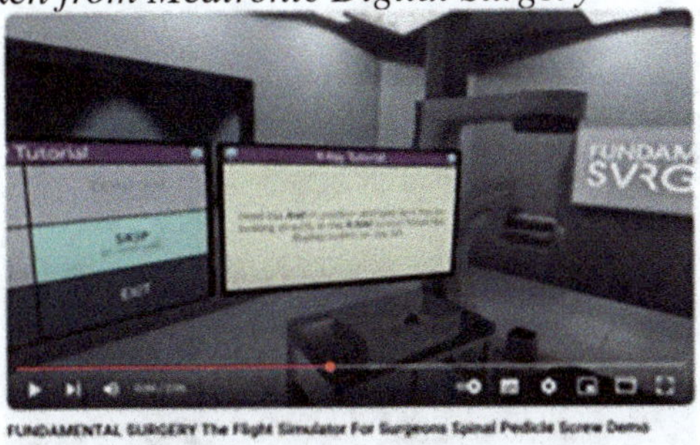

(https://www.youtube.com/watch?v=_Fhqd070FBw).

An interesting aspect regarding feedback is that it is integrated with progress statistics and activity reports, using solutions that provide real-time feedback through algorithms, allowing information to be extracted from video recordings stored on a device. Another key feature is that it is based on scientific research evidence gathered from global experiences. Therefore, it is a comprehensive application in terms of the aforementioned criteria: pedagogical relevance, interactivity and immersive experience, technological accessibility and usability, as well as integrated evaluation and feedback.

Can this be extended to the other two components, both pedagogical and holistic patient-oriented? Yes, it requires that this self-directed activity, enabled by access to a personal device such as a mobile phone, serve as a bridge for collaborative work with other residents and for sharing experiences. However, this also involves constantly considering who the end user is and translating that knowledge into real-life situations with case studies.

Next up is **ARCollab**, an app that simulates and specializes in the heart, helping users study and manipulate it without the need for a physical organ.

This application has similar requirements to the previous one, with the advantages of low-cost interaction, accessibility, usability, and the ability to organize surgical planning.

In addition, 3D models allow for realistic interaction, which until now has focused only on the heart. These cardiac models are manipulated using gestures.

A major advantage is that it eliminates the need to manufacture physical cardiac models, while allowing collaboration with other users. The premise is collaboration, as it was designed for interaction between cardiologists and surgeons, who can perform interventions within this 3D environment with their patient.

Although not strictly a feedback mechanism, it allows you to save the current properties of the model and reload them later.

Figure 3. ARCollab

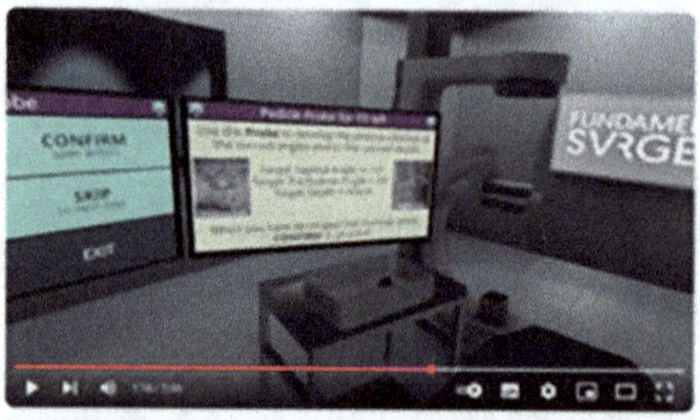

FUNDAMENTAL SURGERY The Flight Simulator For Surgeons Spinal Pedicle Screw Demo

Tomado de: https://github.com/poloclub/arcollab?tab=readme-ov-file#readme

Table 2. Application comparison table

Application	Platform	Specialties Covered	Access model	Key features
Tactile surgery	iOS / Android	17 (up to ~400 procedures)	Free basic, premium, or institutional modules	Step-by-step guidance, testing, progress tracking, community
ARCollab	iOS (AR)	Cardiovascular planning	Experimental/Academic	Team interaction with 3D models

These two examples allow users to become familiar with more focused aspects of collaborative learning. They serve as a starting point for guiding and sharing knowledge; Both from the role of the trainer and from the perspective of the resident, they allow self-directed learning and subsequently facilitate collaboration in relation to the knowledge acquired.

b) VR as systems

Osso VR

This system consists of a virtual reality headset, an internet station, and an optional PC (required for some functions). Its cost ranges from approximately 37,000 to 93,000 Mexican pesos. It is clinically validated and has undergone robust analysis, which means it requires a dedicated space for its operation. The interaction between the device and the user occurs through the headset and connected tools. External accessories are needed for optimal use, and institutions could cover the cost of equipment to support practice, which would help make medical training more organic (MedicalExpo, 2024).

Its interface is handy because it provides a list of cases, allowing the user to select the case they want to practice multiple times. However, integrated interaction is limited; Simulation does not begin with the admission of patients, but jumps directly to cases.

Considering the points raised above, one potential area for improvement is to incorporate interaction or preparation before surgery, taking full advantage of the device's capabilities.

Figure 4. Images taken from Osso VR (https://www.youtube.com/watch?v=bqra7wslwCM).

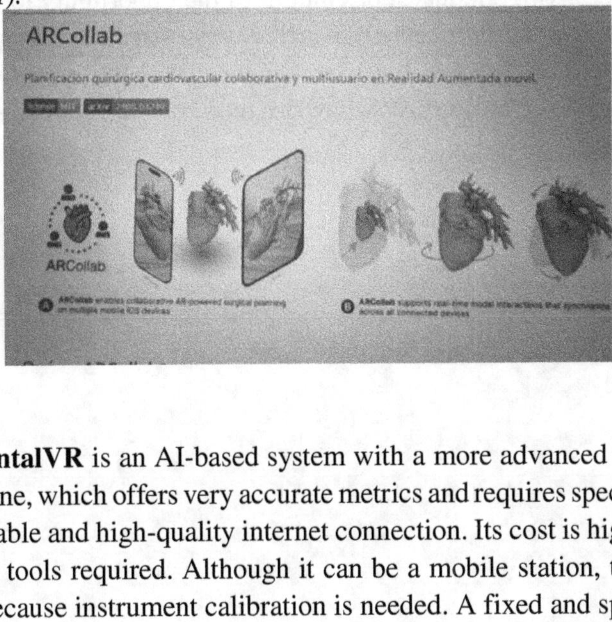

FundamentalVR is an AI-based system with a more advanced approach than the previous one, which offers very accurate metrics and requires specific hardware. You need a stable and high-quality internet connection. Its cost is higher due to the hardware and tools required. Although it can be a mobile station, this is not recommended because instrument calibration is needed. A fixed and spacious area is necessary for comfortable use. As the practice progresses, performance improves, errors decrease, and execution time is reduced. It is reported that a resident may need around 20 virtual reality simulations to master a basic laparoscopic technique (Fundamental XR, n.d., https://www.youtube.com/watch?v=0NtCRXOuLto).

Figure 5. Images taken from Fundamental XR (https://www.youtube.com/watch?v=0NtCRXOuLto).

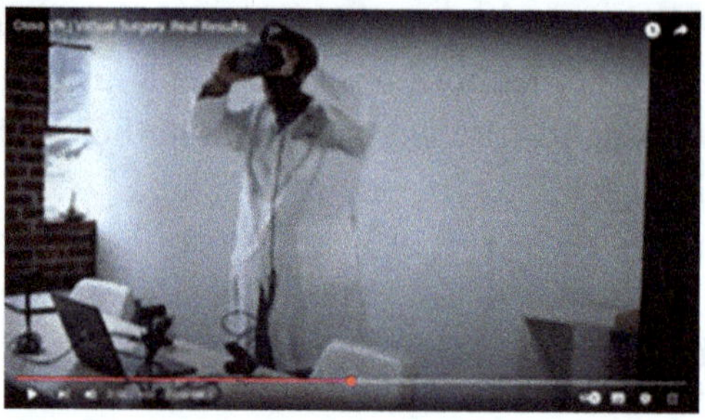

VirtaMed is a fixed station that, depending on the user's needs, allows the manipulation of extremity procedures. It's expensive, but it provides very realistic simulations. It is not portable, but includes curricular support and the use of real instruments integrated into the simulation. This is where universities or workplaces should consider giving graduates or employees the opportunity to make minimal mistakes in actual practice. The system includes assessments or minimum requirements to complete the exercises, but does not interact with the patient, only addresses the procedure (VirtaMed, https://www.virtamed.com/en/products-and-solutions/simulators/arthros)

Figure 6. Images taken from VirtaMed (https://www.youtube.com/watch?v=psXNC2XrLS0).

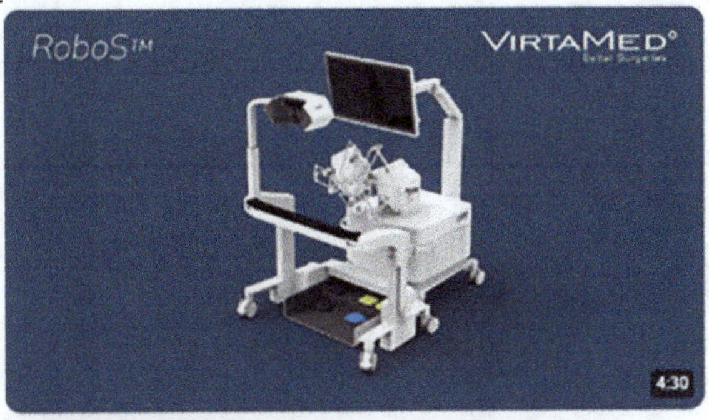

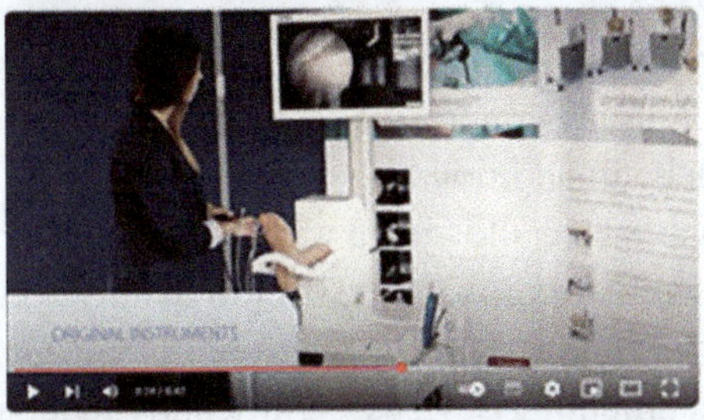

VirtaMed ArthroS™ Ankle

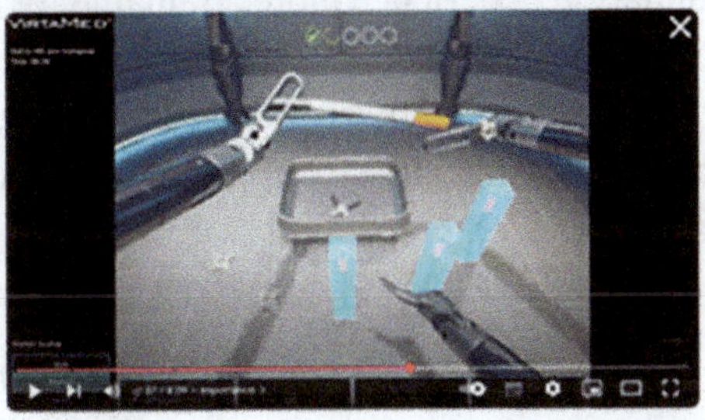

VirtaMed RoboS™

Sim Surgery is a virtual reality and artificial intelligence application developed by **Smart Surgery Technology**, where both medical students and experienced surgeons can practice and refine the skills needed to operate robotic surgical systems (Dana, 2023), such as the **Da Vinci** Surgical System. This system consists of a slave robot controlled by the surgeon, which improves precision and dexterity during surgical procedures, reduces tremors, and provides an exceptionally clear view of the patient's anatomy (CEMTRO Clinic, 2019).

According to Dana (2023), the application allows the transmission of high-quality 3D anatomical models to virtual reality headsets, with the support of artificial intelligence. This allows medical students or doctors in training to more accurately identify the anatomical components of the area being operated on. Some of the advantages of using this system include:

- Residents can effectively learn minimally invasive surgery and improve their surgical skills.
- The intraoperative image recognition system helps clinicians identify critical organ structures.
- Reduced operation time and improved surgical efficiency.
- Prevention of infections and operational errors.
- It helps hospitals reduce medical disputes.
- Improves trust between doctors and patients.

The integration of **artificial intelligence** within **Sim Surgery** also allows medical students to gain a highly immersive visual and tactile experience using 3D anatomical organ models. In addition, the system is deployed on personal and relatively affordable VR platforms, allowing a wider range of users to access these advanced training tools, thereby improving the overall quality and effectiveness of their surgical practice. By leveraging **Ubitus' technology**, the application does not require high-performance computing devices, significantly reducing technological barriers and making the simulation experience more attainable for both educational institutions and individual students (Ubitus, 2022). This combination of AI-powered guidance and accessible virtual reality hardware represents an important step forward in democratizing surgical training and expanding hands-on opportunities for medical students in basic and advanced procedural skills.

Figure 7. Image taken from Dana, 2023: "The immersive simulation application allows doctors to practice robotic surgery with virtual reality streaming."

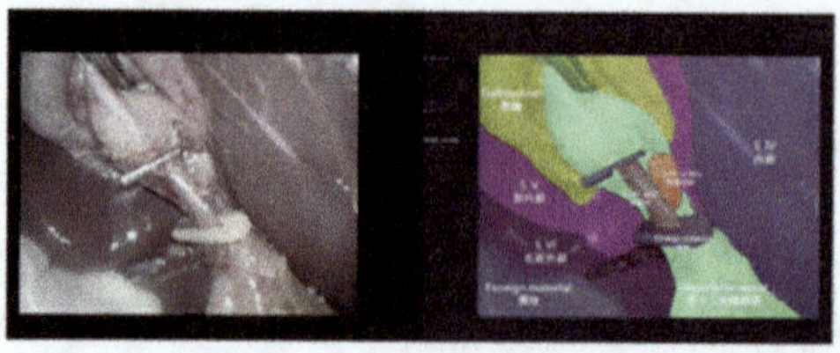

Cirugía de vesícula, a través de Realidad Aumentada e Inteligencia Artificial.

Table 3. Virtual Reality Systems Comparison Table

Platform	Minimum requirements	Estimated cost (MXN/year)	Advantages	Disadvantages	Pedagogic	Patient-Oriented Component/ Interaction
Osso VR	VR headset, Internet, PC optional	37,000–93,000	Robust, clinically validated, multi-user analysis	Requires hardware, institutional cost	Yes	No
FundamentalVR	VR headsets, haptic hardware, stable internet	28,000–74,000	Advanced Haptics, Accurate Metrics	Costly and heavy learning curve	Yes	No
VirtaMed Laboratory	Fixed station with dedicated hardware	930,000–2,790,000	Full realism, real instruments, curricular support	Very expensive, not portable	Yes	Some cases
Sim Surgery	VR headset, PC, broadband network	No data available	Less invasive surgeries, reduces operation time, improves efficiency	Lack of Cost Transparency, Technological Accessibility, Virtual Reality Learning Curve	Yes	Some cases

The review of these virtual reality examples provides a perspective, as mentioned at the beginning of this section, aimed at analyzing the components that adhere to a collaborative model for the use of virtual reality in the surgical training of residents. While the applications or systems themselves address aspects of feedback, it is important to extend this to what will be discovered or shared within a group, consistent with the learning objectives set by the supervising physician. It is true that self-directed learning is encouraged, especially when mobile devices facilitate its implementation.

Another interesting aspect to consider regarding the use of this technology is that it recreates characters and interactions, which requires an integrated approach. This approach, discussed below, not only emphasizes practice in a safe environment, but also promotes placing the patient at the center, with a more human-centered perspective.

c) Comprehensive patient-oriented component in simulation

Based on the above discussion, it is possible to expand on the idea that this model aims to place the person at the forefront of collaboration, directly oriented towards the patient, from a humanizing perspective, focusing on patient safety and effective communication.

Without a doubt, the most important component in this process lies with the end user: the patient. At the end of the day, they will experience the benefits and improvements in treatments and interventions, which will be reflected in their overall health. In the case of cancer patients supported by Virtual Reality (VR), promising results have been observed. For example: *"Based on the review carried out and the ongoing experience, it can be proposed that ICTs are useful to promote higher levels of well-being and lower levels of discomfort in different groups of cancer patients (children, adolescents and adults) and in various contexts (outpatients and hospitalized)"* (Espinoza et al., 2013, p. 258).

Some of the basics to consider in virtual interventions that apply to real patients should include the following elements:

1. Remember that human dignity must be the guiding principle in all procedures, whether virtual or face-to-face.
2. Humane treatment and warmth in interactions with patients should be prioritized in any type of treatment or intervention.
3. Explanations and details of the procedures should be provided regardless of whether the patient requests them.
4. The patient may be advised to keep a family member or mental health professional in mind if any medical information may be too distressing.
5. If necessary, the clinician should consult with a mental health professional to review their practices or methods of comprehensive communication and assess their impact on the patient's overall well-being.
6. Medical staff must have or develop social skills to ensure the best possible patient disposition and maximize the likelihood of achieving comprehensive health goals.
7. Part of explaining the virtual procedure to the patient may include highlighting cost savings related to travel and safety, which helps the patient feel confident in the procedure.
8. Interdisciplinary collaboration with colleagues and other professionals can provide significant benefits both before and after a medical intervention, whether surgical or pharmacological.
9. Depending on the patient's psychosociocultural context, family support is invaluable, not only because they are often the first point of contact or source of motivation, but also because they are natural allies in the patient's comprehensive care. The clinician should be prepared to communicate effectively with the family and form the necessary alliances to make unconventional interventions more effective, involving as many family members as possible.

It is also important to clarify that this collaborative proposal, described above in previous sections, aims not only to promote the ability of professionals to operate freely and autonomously in a respectful environment, but also to bring them closer to real-life experiences.

Some models have already been implemented in medical training settings that, for the purposes of this research, have been carefully selected based on the daily experiences of interaction, observation and feedback of the residents. For example, the OSCE (Objective Structured Clinical Examination) station model promotes the interactive development of an exam composed of a predetermined number of stations (12 to 18) through which all students rotate. At each station, competencies are assessed, either with a real or simulated patient (taking a history, physical examination, diagnosis, or management) or without a patient (radiographic interpretation, database research, or analysis of research papers). Some universities implement this model, for example, the Faculty of Medicine of the National Autonomous University of Mexico, which has applied it since 1996 and incorporated it into the Practical Phase of the Professional Exam since 2002.

From these experiences, it is evident that it is possible, on the one hand, to connect with learning closer to real life in a virtual way, providing favorable aspects in the construction of knowledge, as well as in know-how, considering a more comprehensive approach that prioritizes surgical training from a humanistic perspective.

Another example that may be useful to incorporate into this collaborative model, specifically within the patient-oriented component, is the Boston Children's Hospital Simulator Program, which developed the SimZones system (Roussin & Weinstock, 2017). This methodological innovation provides a conceptual framework to adapt the simulation to the needs and profiles of the participants. One of its most valuable methodologies is the debriefing process, which essentially consists of simple feedback and a complete conversation. Its elements include an "emotional decompression" phase, where aspects of the simulation experience are shared; a description phase, narrating what the group wishes to communicate; an analysis phase, guided by the facilitator, where participants reflect and share their experience without judgment and develop a plan for improvement; and finally, a summary phase, aimed at transferring learning to professional practice.

The SimZones model has been expanded and even combined with other approaches. It starts with elements that allow for self-guided induction and experimentation, building trust. In the literature, this is known as Sim0 or Zone 0, with the possibility of progressing through different zones to Zone 5. Some authors classify the zones by skill level, starting from an intuitive phase and progressing to more complex cognitive processes that integrate combined cognitive and motor reflection.

A constructive aspect of these simulation options is that, by interacting with resources such as simulated patients, communication skills can be actively developed. This, as mentioned above, fosters a key element: the therapeutic relationship between patient and physician, all within a clinical simulation environment.

For example, when considering the surgical scenario, performing a simulation involves recreating everyday scenes while paying attention to the details that make a difference. Of course, the main actors participate on stage, and there is a pre-learning phase, similar to the distribution of roles in a theatrical performance: scripts are reviewed, possible questions are posed, and then participation takes place on stage. Once the action has occurred, the experience is reviewed through the report, but it does not end there. There is a post-learning phase, which in the case of simulation allows us to review possible areas for improvement without the risk of fatal consequences.

In fact, a theoretical-methodological model of learning and training based on simulation has been developed, which especially reinforces this collaborative component. For residents, this promotes processes that involve an analytical perspective, since, as noted above, differences in the variations experienced and changes in conditions can be observed. In addition, it encourages a deductive perspective, used by the person performing the simulation, since the conclusions are drawn based on the role assumed (Eliosa, 2022).

As mentioned in previous paragraphs, in the health sector there are specific spaces and roles that allow attention to be focused on the integration of simulation tools and access to new ways of dealing with a condition. This applies to healthcare personnel, such as doctors and nurses. Below is an example:

> *Nursing staff play a crucial role in the monitoring and prevention of obesity from Primary Care along with other disciplines. However, teens spend little time in healthcare settings. Therefore, nurses acquire among their competencies the ability to create an optimal environment in schools for the conduct of nutrition education sessions so that adolescents acquire knowledge and skills, monitor obese patients, propose activities and alternatives, etc. (Diego-Cordero et al., 2017, p. 89).*

CONCLUSIONS

Undoubtedly, virtual environments are here to stay. What was once considered science fiction is now commonplace. There are several factors to consider when talking about current education and the use of simulators within it.

Increasingly, we will be forced to optimize our time, partly due to the greater distances over which humans interact and the associated costs of travel, and partly due to the need to interact with remote people who help solve various situations. It is therefore essential to understand that human activity and its availability will become increasingly important. Virtual interaction is no longer a luxury; it is a necessity. In the case of simulation systems for medical training, they are an invaluable help in most cases.

For this proposal, it is evident that, as with technology in general, what is developed today continues to evolve and expand to include options arising from everyday practice. Consequently, the focus has been placed on prioritizing relationships between professionals, promoting collaboration, strengthening work teams and guiding leaders, in this case, those who contribute to the training of resident physicians, to continuously improve, with an emphasis on a more human contact with patients. Each health professional has, as seen, a range of possibilities, which is part of what in this historical moment of the digital era, is observed as personalization in training, use of available technology, curiosity that comes from academic background and as has been seen individual, even from the context in the praxis that is found.

Although, in everyday terms, when talking about the human dimension, something that affects each individual is receiving positive comments. The role of the instructor, especially in the training of residents at the graduate level, is crucial, since these are professionals who, as mentioned above, are already on a trajectory that involves facing real-life challenges. Through their clinical rotations and practice in various healthcare contexts, they have already been exposed to the reality of addressing specific medical issues and, more importantly, direct patient care.

There are different guidelines to ensure that patient-centered counseling is as effective as possible. Beyond the technological and pedagogical aspects already discussed, communication between the members of the health team that provides such care is essential. Therefore, the recommendation is to employ direct methods such as the **MIMO feedback model** for residents, which reflects the essence of this chapter: a collaborative approach, a type of learning in which experiences based on simulation and virtual reality are integrated to reinforce the knowledge and skills already acquired.

The acronym **MIMO,** as described by Mendoza (2023), refers to a set of recommended actions in communication with the purpose of providing constructive feedback to residents:

- **M – Keep**: Emphasize what needs to be preserved, making clear what was done correctly and therefore should continue.
- **I – Incorporate**: Rather than framing feedback in terms of error, this step focuses on highlighting what needs to be incorporated or added to improve performance.
- **M – Improve**: Reinforcing the widely recognized idea that "practice makes perfect," this action emphasizes that human beings are capable of continuous improvement. Even when technical mastery is achieved, skills and competencies can always be refined. This perspective fosters professional growth and patient confidence, not by creating perceptions of incompetence or rejection, but by encouraging constant improvement.
- **O – Omit:** Particularly in healthcare contexts where accuracy is critical, this action highlights the importance of understanding and rationalizing the consequences of adverse events. In medicine, such events are recognized as a public health problem. The patient safety culture, therefore, aims to omit

these situations through effective communication and structured feedback, which encourage reflection and action aligned with error prevention.

In summary, therefore, the integration of this chapter necessarily emphasizes both collaborative training through technologies such as virtual reality and simulation, and the development of a strong patient safety culture. The goal is to promote higher standards of care while advancing the comprehensive education and professional development of medical residents.

The development of the necessary points to bring about a change in the culture of training resident doctors in the institutional setting also involves revisiting relevant topics as points of reflection, which are presented below.

A. The pandemic has established as a norm the need to look for virtual alternatives in various fields of teaching and learning.
B. Pedagogical analyses derived from virtual environments are necessary and often differ from previous analyses of traditional in-person educational practices.
C. Students, although they are the main recipients of education, also require the development and consideration of so-called soft skills (empathy, integral communication, assertiveness, among others) to fully benefit from virtual environments, particularly when using simulation systems.
D. Teachers must understand that their role as mediators requires them to stay at the forefront of technology for educational purposes, especially in virtual environments or in those that mainly use simulators.
E. It is always desirable to carry out a comprehensive evaluation of the designed virtual environment, the strategies used for the specific teaching of the contents and the characteristics, at least general, of both the students and the teachers involved in a virtual simulation project, since not everyone starts with the same skills, abilities, motivations or personality.
F. Likewise, when creating a virtual environment or using simulators, the necessary didactic tools should never be improvised, as objectives may be compromised and final goals may not be achieved.
G. One of the main advantages of simulation is that data, outcomes, and procedures are recorded, quantified, and analyzed, and then serve multiple purposes in teaching and learning, not only for students but also for practicing physicians and, in specific respects, for patients.
H. Simulation as a didactic pedagogical tool facilitates the repetition and variations of conditions appropriate to each student, increasing the level of difficulty in the planned interventions.
I. The ideal technology is one that, in a collaborative environment adapted to contextual situations, allows participants to enjoy the experience, deepen their

knowledge and stay motivated, recognizing learning as a continuous and progressively refined process.

J. Whether in real or simulated conditions, the patient must be the central focus, expanding the perspective to their needs; Beyond providing solutions through scientific procedures, which is valid, it is essential to always guarantee a human approach that prioritizes safety.
K. The paradox of our time is that while technology is widely accessible and each learner determines the pace and depth of learning, technology cannot yet replace what is achieved through personal contact: addressing genuine human needs, such as feeling safe in times of vulnerability and the desire to solve health-related problems in the best way possible.

REFERENCES

Acevedo-Osorio, G. O., Cortes-Benítez, P. L., Blanco-Vanegas, A. M., & Montero-Caicedo, L. L. (2025). Impact of virtual reality on the strengthening of psychomotor skills in Surgical Instrumentation students in Pereira, Colombia. *Medical Education*, *26*(5), 101083. DOI: 10.1016/j.edumed.2025.101083

Asad, M., Naz, A., Churi, P., & Tahanzadeh, M. (2021). Virtual reality as a pedagogical tool to improve experiential learning: a systematic review of the literature. *International Research in Education*, 1–17. https://doi.org/DOI: 10.1155/2021/7061623

CEMTRO Clinic. (2019). *Da Vinci robotic surgery*. Robotic Surgery. Retrieved September 6, 2025, from http://www.icirugiarobotica.com/cirugia-robotica-da-vinci/

Dana. (2023). *The immersive simulation application allows physicians to practice robotic surgery with virtual reality transmission*. Health Simulation Network. Retrieved September 6, 2025, from https://reddesimulacionensalud.com/tecnologia/la-aplicacion-de-simulacion-inmersiva-permite-a-los-medicos-practicar-cirugia-robotica-con-transmision-de-realidad-virtual/

de Diego-Cordero, R., Fernández-García, E., & Badanta Romero, B. (2017). Use of ICT to promote healthy lifestyles in children and adolescents: The case of overweight. *Spanish Journal of Health Communication*, *8*(1), 79–91. DOI: 10.20318/recs.2017.3607

Eliosa, V. (2022). 6 types of learning that can be reinforced through simulation. https://blog.pearsonlatam.com/columna-de-opinion/6-tipos-de-aprendizaje-que-pueden-reforzarse-mediante-la-simulacion

Espinoza, M., Baños, R. M., García-Palacios, A., & Botella, C. (2013). Virtual reality in psychological interventions with cancer patients. *Psycho-Oncology*, *10*(2-3), 247–261. DOI: 10.5209/rev_PSIC.2013.v10.n2-3.43447

Fundamental, X. R. (n.d.). FUNDAMENTAL SURGERY. The flight simulator for surgeons [Video]. YouTube. https://www.youtube.com/watch?v=0NtCRXOuLto

Guerrero-Martínez, S. F. & Martínez-Castillo, M. F. (2022). YouTube, Instagram, emerging educational environments in times of remote teaching and collaborative learning. INNOVA Research Journal, 7(3.1), 1-12. DOI: 10.33890/innova.v7.n3.1.2022.2146

Inter-institutional Commission for the Training of Human Resources for Health (CIFRHS). (2023). National Exam for Medical Residency Applicants. https://cifrhs.salud.gob.mx/site1/enarm/2023/index.html

Issleib, M., Geiger, A., Pinnschmidt, H. O., Hilz, P., Zöllner, C., & Moll-Khosrawi, P. (2025). Virtual reality as a training method for basic life support of the medical staff on general wards: A randomized controlled non-inferiority trial. *Virtual Reality (Waltham Cross)*, *29*(3), 141. Advance online publication. DOI: 10.1007/s10055-025-01216-y

Martínez-García, M., González-Caminal, G., & Gomar-Sancho, C. (2025). Quantitative analysis of communication and patient safety competencies included in a clinical simulation program for the degree in Medicine. *Medical Education*, *26*(4), 101041. DOI: 10.1016/j.edumed.2025.101041

MedicalExpo. (2024). Osso VR surgical training simulator. https://www.medicalexpo.com/prod/osso-vr/product-301294-1007883.html

Medtronic Digital Surgery. (2021, September 28). Tactile surgery. Medtronic Enterprise [Video]. YouTube. Retrieved September 4, 2025, https://www.youtube.com/watch?v=_Fhqd070FBw [REMOVED HYPERLINK FIELD]

Mendoza, L. (2023, August 11). *Unraveling the MIMO method and its importance in feedback.* Health Simulation Network. https://reddesimulacionensalud.com/desarrollo-profesional/desentranando-el-metodo-mimo-y-su-importancia-en-el-feedback/

Osso, V. R. (2017, August 23). Osso VR virtual surgery. Real results [Video]. YouTube. https://www.youtube.com/watch?v=bqra7wslwCM

Osso, V. R. (2023). Guide to using virtual reality in medical education programs. Osso's virtual reality blog. https://www.ossovr.com/post/guide-to-using-vr-in-medical-education-programs

Ramírez-Sánchez, N. A., Vega-Peña, N. V., Domínguez-Torres, L. C., & Sanabria-Quiroga, Á. E. (2018). Mental training and surgeons: A strategy for improvement. *Iatreia*, *31*(2), 180–190. DOI: 10.17533/udea.iatreia.v31n2a06

Romero Castillo, J. S. (2025). Educational Innovations in Laparoscopy: A Comparative Meta-Analysis Between Mechanical Simulation and Traditional Training [Undergraduate Thesis, Universidad Veracruzana. "Dr. Rafael Lucio" High Specialty Center]. Veracruz. https://cdigital.uv.mx/handle/1944/53563

Roussin, C. J., & Weinstock, P. (2017). SimZones: An organizational innovation for simulation programs and centers. *Academic Medicine*, *92*(8), 1114–1120. DOI: 10.1097/ACM.0000000000001746 PMID: 28562455

Salas, M. A. (2017). The use of simulation in medical education. Mini physiological checks, 4 (1), 3-10. http://sedici.unlp.edu.ar/handle/10915/126449

Salas-Flores, L. O., Rojas Espinoza, B. I., Pinedo Paz, M. A., & Vega Vilca, C. S. (2024). ICT and collaborative learning in higher education: A systematic review. Court. *Journal of Education Sciences and Legal Sciences*, *4*(9), 579–591. DOI: 10.59659/revistatribunal.v4i9.94

Simulation Center for Clinical and Surgical Excellence. Jalisco (CeSiECQ Jalisco). https://sites.google.com/view/cesiecq/p%C3%A1gina-principal

Sung, H., Kim, M., Park, J., Shin, N., & Han, Y. (2024). Effectiveness of Virtual Reality in Healthcare Education: Systematic Review and Meta-Analysis. *Sustainability (Basel)*, *16*(19), 8520. DOI: 10.3390/su16198520

Tokuno, J., Knobovitch, R. M., Botelho, F., Fried, H. B., Carver, T. E., & Fried, G. M. (2025). Immersive Virtual Reality Simulation for Medical Student Procedural Training: Assessment of Cognitive Load and Usability. *Surgical Innovation*, *32*(4), 378–384. DOI: 10.1177/15533506251339920 PMID: 40298260

Ubitus. (2022). *Empowering Surgeons! HuiShu Technology's AI-assisted system and virtual reality platform boost hands-on training for medical students.* Retrieved September 6, 2025 from https://smartsurgerytek.com/empowering-surgeons-huishu-technologys-ai-assisted-system-and-vr-platform-boost-practical-training-for-medical-students/ [REMOVED HYPERLINK FIELD]

VirtaMed. (n.d.). ArthroSTM. Retrieved September 6, 2025, from https://www.virtamed.com/en/products-and-solutions/simulators/arthros

VirtaMed. (s.f.). VirtaMed ArthroSTM Tobillo [Video]. YouTube. https://www.youtube.com/watch?v=psXNC2XrLS0

Chapter 11
Evaluation of Dissolution Profiles With BioSimuLab Simulator Based on NOM-177-SSA1 Mexican Standard

Martín Hernández-Rivera
https://orcid.org/0009-0001-4793-8835
Universidad de Guadalajara, Mexico

Nelson Bruno de Almeida-Cunha
https://orcid.org/0000-0002-9276-159X
Universidad de Guadalajara, Mexico

César Ricardo Cortez-Álvarez
https://orcid.org/0000-0002-3763-7115
Universidad de Guadalajara, Mexico

ABSTRACT

The predominance of expository teaching in pharmaceutical sciences, focused on theoretical and lecture-based methods, limits practical application and hinders understanding of biopharmaceutical processes such as bioavailability, bioequivalence, and dissolution—essential for ensuring drug efficacy, quality and safety. To address this challenge, BioSimuLab was developed as a pedagogical simulator that reproduces dissolution processes in accordance with NOM-177-SSA1, generating simulated data for reference and test drugs. This tool enables the analysis of dissolution profiles, application of statistical reasoning, and evaluation of bioequiv-

DOI: 10.4018/979-8-3373-4657-1.ch011

alence through parameters such as the similarity factor (f_2) and linear regression. By promoting discovery-based learning and evidence-driven decision-making, BioSimuLab enhances analytical, technical, and interpretive skills, strengthens understanding of pharmacokinetic principles, and bridges the gap between theory and professional practice in pharmaceutical sciences, aligning educational outcomes with professional competencies.

INTRODUCTION

Traditional approaches in pharmaceutical sciences face significant challenges stemming from the predominance of expository methods focused on the transmission of theoretical knowledge and the limited inclusion of practical experiences that place students in contexts closer to professional reality. The development of BioSimuLab promotes discovery-based learning and the development of statistical reasoning by enabling students to interact with simulated (near-real) data, formulate hypotheses, conduct analyses, and make evidence-based decisions supported by technology while fostering teamwork (Cabero-Almenara & Costas, 2016; Sánchez et al., 2019). This tool is designed to address the gaps between theory and practice for applied contexts such as pharmaceutical quality control, bioequivalence studies, and risk assessment. More specifically, the structure of BioSimuLab allows the simulation of drug dissolution profiles in accordance with the guidelines established in NOM-177-SSA1, which specifies the criteria for demonstrating drug interchangeability and establishing bioequivalence tests (Secretaría de Salud, 2013).

One of the main experimental studies related to pharmaceutical sciences is biopharmaceutical assays, which seek to optimize drug therapy, reducing adverse effects and generating the maximum benefit from the drug. The therapeutic activity generated by a drug is the result of several physicochemical processes, which are closely related to the chemical properties of the drug and the organism (Darlami & Sharma, 2024). This complexity of factors is the reason why a drug can reach the site of action in sufficient quantity and speed to be able to develop its effect; in other words, for the drug to exhibit good bioavailability.

Some pharmaceutical alternatives may differ in the rate of absorption of the drug they contain, and despite these differences, they may still be considered bioequivalent because such differences are intentional, are established in the medical information, and do not influence the achievement of the necessary plasma concentrations during multi-dose pharmacological treatment, or such differences in absorption rate are considered medically irrelevant in the particular case. In this way, biopharmaceutical studies aim to externally control the formulation of the drug (e.g., release, dissolution, route of administration, among others) and modulate the pharmacological response as desired (Nguyen et al., 2023).

Establishing with certainty the veracity and proper interpretation of bioavailability, pharmacological effect, and clinical response studies is complex due to ethical factors, limitations in experimental design, analytical considerations, and multiple sources of variation, such as pathophysiological ones (Wu et al., 2024). Therefore, bioequivalence should not be assumed to be synonymous with therapeutic equivalence. Although it represents a fundamental starting point for the comprehensive evaluation of a drug, this type of study does not directly analyze clinical effectiveness.

A comparative assessment of clinical efficacy involves comparing the therapeutic effects between products, which requires the use of advanced techniques, increasing the cost and complexity of the study. Furthermore, these effects are not always easily measurable and may be subject to external influences, such as psychological and environmental factors (Cárdenas-Rodríguez et al., 1996). In this context, bioequivalence studies provide scientific evidence that two formulations do not differ significantly in the rate and extent to which the drug reaches the systemic circulation, and, therefore, are unlikely to exhibit clinically relevant differences in therapeutic efficacy or clinical performance

In this sense, the use of simulators bridges the theory-to-practice gaps and facilitates immediate feedback, promoting reflection and the integration of new competencies, while also fostering self-directed learning, critical thinking, and evidence-based decision-making, making it an essential tool in pharmaceutical education. The objective of this chapter is to present and explain the use of BioSimuLab to promote the development of statistical reasoning and decision-making within a pharmaceutical sciences context, specifically related to dissolution testing as established by NOM-177-SSA1, in the classroom setting.

THEORETICAL FRAMEWORK

Pedagogical Foundations for the Use of Simulators in Health Sciences Teaching

The teaching of pharmaceutical sciences presents several challenges that hinder the holistic education of students (Hidalgo et al., 2017). Tutorial sessions are designed to strengthen both theoretical understanding and practical skills through highly interactive learning experiences, while simulation offers a dynamic environment where learners engage in lifelike scenarios that promote critical thinking and the practical application of knowledge (Kaddoura et al., 2024). The integration of high-fidelity technologies, whether virtual (software-based) or physical (manikins with physiological responses), is therefore essential to foster active learning, problem-solving, safe experimentation, and data-driven decision-making in subjects that are currently taught exclusively through theoretical instruction(Kaddoura et al., 2024).

In this context, several theoretical frameworks have been developed to explain the adoption and use of technology in education. One of the most influential is the Unified Theory of Acceptance and Use of Technology (UTAUT), which seeks to explain users' intention to adopt technology and their actual usage behavior (Venkatesh et al., 2012). Compared to earlier theories—such as the Technology Acceptance Model (TAM), the Theory of Planned Behavior (TPB), and Kolb's Experiential Learning Theory—the UTAUT provides a more comprehensive perspective by incorporating additional factors such as system usability, facilitating conditions, experience, and social context (Neves et al., 2025). According to Casallas-Hernández et al. (2025), the UTAUT comprises four main constructs: performance expectancy (the perception that the system enhances job performance), effort expectancy (the perceived ease of use), social influence (the perceived pressure or support from others), and facilitating conditions (the availability of resources and technical support). These relationships are moderated by four factors: gender, age, experience, voluntariness of use, hedonic motivation, price value, and habit, which influence how strongly each construct affects the intention or behavior to use technology (Venkatesh et al., 2012).

Recent findings align with previous studies that identify perceived usefulness and technological integration as key predictors of students' intention to adopt high-fidelity simulations to develop competencies and gain clinical experience (Granić, 2023). Since habit and facilitating conditions are the most significant predictors of behavioral intention and technology use, this will allow the user to increase familiarity and resources to solve real-life situations (Neves et al., 2025). Since habit and facilitating condition are the most significant predictor of behavioral intention and use of technology, it will allow the user to increase familiarity and resources to solve real-life situations (Neves et al., 2025). Therefore, the use of simulation in the teaching context improves students' clinical skills and comprehensive abilities by allowing them to navigate complex situations, experience consequences in a controlled environment, and engage in repeated practice and experimentation (Casallas-Hernández et al., 2025; Huon et al., 2024; Lei et al., 2022).

A growing number of professional councils encourage the incorporation of emerging technologies into the education of future healthcare professionals. Among these, the Accreditation Council for Pharmacy Education (ACPE), the Health and Care Professions Council (HCPC), and the Center for the Advancement of Pharmacy Education (CAPE) stand out for promoting pedagogical strategies that connect didactic learning with clinical practice while maintaining a safe and controlled environment (Lei et al., 2022; Serag-Bolos et al., 2018). Healthcare and pharmaceutical sciences require the development of both technical and clinical expertise, as well as solid scientific knowledge. Simulation has proven to be an effective method for teaching and assessment in clinical education. According to Miller's Pyramid of Assessment, students who demonstrate clinical competence in a simulated environment are more likely to maintain this competency when transitioning from the didactic curriculum to clinical rotations (Miller, 1990).

Abdulhussain et al. (2022) reviewed the use of high-fidelity simulation (HFS) in biomedical courses for health professions students, comparing it with traditional teaching methods. Their analysis included both students and residents and revealed that HFS is more commonly applied in advanced clinical training than in preclinical education. Overall, HFS was found to be more effective than traditional methods in enhancing the understanding of core biomedical concepts. Similarly, a meta-analysis conducted (Lei et al., 2022) examined the impact of HFS on nursing students' knowledge, professional skills, and clinical abilities. Results indicated significant improvements in knowledge acquisition, professional skills, and key clinical competencies—including critical thinking, clinical judgment, and communication—demonstrating the strong educational benefits of HFS in nursing education.

In the field of pharmaceutical sciences, Ledbetter et al. (2020) evaluated the impact of an interactive oncology simulation on third-year pharmacy students' confidence and perceptions of pharmacists' roles. Across two cohorts (2016–2017), 66 students participated in a two-hour, four-station activity simulating different oncology practice settings. Post-activity surveys showed significant improvements in students' confidence and understanding of pharmacists' roles, demonstrating the effectiveness of simulation. Likewise, Serag-Bolos et al. (2018) reported significant knowledge gains in post-simulation assessments and improved perceptions of pharmacists' roles, as well as increased confidence in preparing patient-specific regimens among 109 pharmacy students. Overall, these studies highlight the capacity of simulation to enhance both knowledge and understanding of oncology pharmacy practice.

Although Kaddoura et al. (2024) found no significant difference in knowledge retention between high-fidelity simulation and case-based tutorials in a 16-week pharmacology course, students preferred simulation, describing it as more engaging, realistic, and effective for reinforcing learning. While HFS proved equally effective for knowledge retention, its interactive and immersive qualities made it the favored approach among students.

Despite the demonstrated value of simulators in pharmaceutical education and related health sciences, several subject areas remain underexplored. Particularly, in terms of competencies and skills related to technical and clinical management, this includes analytical and regulatory activities that ensure the quality, efficacy, and safety of medicines, such as dissolution profiling, period-based coefficient of variation (CV%), similarity factor (f_2), and linear regression, which are essential for solving drug-related problems (Morais et al., 2021). It is essential to leverage the didactic potential of simulation technologies in new contexts, such as bioequivalence studies.

Addressing this gap, BioSimuLab was developed—a simulator designed to replicate experimental drug dissolution processes in the classroom. Its purpose is to teach students to evaluate drug quality, efficacy, and safety in accordance with the Mexican Official Standard NOM-177-SSA1, through data-driven decision-making, effective oral and written communication of ideas, and the development of research skills. It also aims to foster the ability to argue, explain, and interpret solutions to interchangeability problems using the verbal and mathematical language of descriptive statistics, connecting statistical concepts to support interpretations, which facilitates the selection of the medication that ensures quality, efficacy, and safety. This process is called statistical reasoning, a concept presented below.

Statistical Reasoning to Facilitate Learning and Interpret Results

According to Garfield et al. (2008), statistical reasoning involves the way people reason with statistical ideas and make sense of statistical information; it can involve connections from one concept to another (for example, measure of central tendency and dispersions) or combining ideas about data and chance. Statistical reasoning also means understanding and being able to explain statistical processes and interpret statistical results.

In this context, Biggs and Collis (1982) developed a useful method to analyze statistical reasoning in task solving: the SOLO taxonomy (Structure of the Observed Learning Outcome), which assesses the quality of students' responses and allows the identification of progress in their reasoning, classifying reasoning into five levels: pre-structural, uni-structural, multi-structural, relational, and extended abstract.

According to Orta and Sánchez (2018), a response is classified as pre-structural when it does not contain relevant elements; if it presents a single element, it corresponds to the uni-structural level; if it shows two or more elements without establishing clear relationships between them, it is placed at the multi-structural level. When the elements are integrated coherently, the response is at the relational level. Finally, the extended abstract level is reached by expanding a relational response and applying it to other situations or problems, which often requires posing additional tasks to identify this level. Table 4 presents the description of the levels of understanding in the SOLO taxonomy for the proposed teaching sequence aimed at learning mathematical concepts related to the development of statistical reasoning applied to the dissolution profile testing of medication.

Table 1. Description of the Levels of Understanding in the SOLO Taxonomy.

Level	Capability	Related Operation	Consistency and Closure
Pre-structural	Superficial responses without statistical reasoning. Relevant statistical ideas and concepts are not addressed. Variables are described qualitatively.	No statistical operations are used. Justifications are circular or lack a statistical basis (for example, "because they are similar").	There is no consistency in the reasoning; the process concludes without analyzing or understanding the problem.
Uni-structural	An estimator (mean, mode, median, maximum, or minimum) is selected to compare samples without considering measures of dispersion. Variables are described quantitatively.	Only one aspect of the sample is compared without integrating other statistical measures. Limited generalization.	Reasoning is inconsistent, as it is based on a single measure. The process concludes with incomplete responses.
Multi-structural	Central tendency and dispersion measures are used, but without relating them. Variables are described quantitatively	Multiple statistical measures are employed independently, without establishing connections between them. Comparisons are incomplete.	There is some sense of consistency, but inconsistencies may arise due to the lack of integration between measures.
Relational	Measures of central tendency and dispersion are related to support comparisons, considering the risk when making decisions. Variables are described quantitatively.	Multiple statistical measures are integrated to justify comparisons. Aspects such as variability and the risk of making decisions are considered.	Relationships between elements are well established within the given context. Reasoning is concluded with an appropriate justification.
Extended abstract	Statistical measures and their relationships are extrapolated to new contexts. Inference is used to generate hypotheses or predictions.	Deduction and induction are combined to generalize to untested situations. Solutions are formulated in new contexts.	Inconsistencies are resolved through statistical reasoning. Multiple alternatives are considered, and critical reflection is encouraged.

Regarding the teaching of statistics, Garfield et al. (2008) highlight several key considerations to ensure the effectiveness of a technology-enhanced didactic sequence:

- **Encouraging discussion of students' results and findings:** Each proposed activity is followed by a collaborative analysis session, promoting reflection and deeper understanding.
- **Teaching students to explain and justify their conclusions:** Students learn to communicate their interpretations clearly and effectively, supporting the development of critical reasoning.
- **Providing immediate feedback through box-and-whisker plots:** These visual tools present information in an accessible format, reducing the need for students to make complex inferences from numerical data they may not yet fully master.
- **Promoting collaborative learning:** This approach is especially valuable in technology-supported statistics education, such as when using simula-

tors. These tools facilitate joint exploration and inquiry, enabling students to actively construct their own knowledge and comprehension of statistical concepts.

For this reason, the simulator design focused on examining statistical reasoning related to variability, taking into account estimators such as measures of dispersion and central tendency, as well as graphical representations (dot plots and box-and-whisker plots) and the raw data. This aims to generate connections between the concepts, the parameters involved in dissolution profile tests, and their correct interpretation.

Bioequivalence Studies

When bioavailability studies are designed for comparative purposes, as in the case of bioequivalence studies, the goal is to demonstrate that a drug exhibits similar biopharmaceutical characteristics to another and, therefore, can be substituted without loss of therapeutic efficacy. This type of study is conducted to determine bioequivalence between reference (patented) drugs and generic drugs, which fosters economic competitiveness within the pharmaceutical industry and makes these products more financially accessible and affordable to the population (Gozzo et al., 2022).

In comparative bioavailability studies, the aim is to determine whether two or more formulations show no significant differences in the rate and extent of absorption at the drug's site of action when the same molar dose is administered under similar conditions; that is, whether they are bioequivalent. The main regulatory authorities worldwide indicate that various *in vivo* and *in vitro* methods can be used to establish bioequivalence, in order of preference: pharmacokinetic studies, pharmacodynamic studies, clinical studies, and *in vitro* studies (Polli, 2008). Although pharmacokinetic studies are generally preferred over pharmacodynamic studies as an alternative to comparative clinical studies, both *in vivo* and *in vitro* methods are acceptable for establishing bioequivalence.

In vitro can replace *in vivo* testing in certain cases, offering cost reduction, a more direct assessment of product performance, and ethical advantages. They allow avoiding human testing when bioequivalence is evident or predictable, reduce expenses for highly variable drugs, and focus directly on drug dissolution and permeability, without the physiological factors that complicate *in vivo* studies (Polli, 2008). Additionally, they comply with the ethical principle of avoiding unnecessary human experimentation and accelerate drug development. Despite the obvious benefits that *in vitro* studies offer as a replacement for *in vivo* testing to demonstrate bioequivalence, Mitra & Wu (2012) highlighted important limitations: *in vitro* results do not always reflect actual behavior in the body, as they do not replicate physiological conditions such as variable pH, intestinal motility, or metabolism. They are less suitable for complex or unconventional formulations, only evaluate drug release (not actual absorption or bioavailability), and can be affected by variability in methods and equipment between laboratories, which limits their reproducibility and comparability.

When differences in key bioavailability parameters are small, they can be detected using traditional statistical methods, such as hypothesis testing through analysis of variance (Cárdenas-Rodríguez et al., 1996). However, when variability in the results is high, a clinically relevant difference may be masked and not detected as statistically significant. In such cases, rather than focusing solely on differences, the analysis should emphasize the degree of similarity between the products being evaluated (U.S. Food and Drug Administration [FDA], 1997).

One of the first criteria applied to determine bioequivalence was to examine the difference between the Cmax and AUC obtained with the products under study. Differences of up to 20% between the mean values of the aforementioned bioavailability parameters were, and still are, considered acceptable to assume bioequivalence (Cárdenas-Rodríguez et al., 1996). This parameter is based on the consensus that, for most drugs, this magnitude would not cause therapeutic failure or an increase in toxic effects. The exception to this generalization, of course, is drugs with a narrow therapeutic index.

The current trend at the FDA and other regulatory authorities worldwide is to adopt the bioequivalence criterion based on the 90% confidence interval (CI) for Cmax and AUC ratios, within a range of 80% to 125% (Gozzo et al., 2022). Currently, the FDA and the Mexican Pharmacopoeia (FEUM) recommend that the main aspects to consider for determining significant differences due to treatments are: plasma concentration–time profiles, Cmax, Tmax, and AUC to infinity (Secretaría de Salud, 2013; FDA, 1997). Whenever feasible, other pharmacokinetic parameters such as absorption rate, elimination half-life, plasma clearance, and others, should be subjected to statistical comparisons with respect to their mean values and variances.

According to NOM-177-SSA1, to establish interchangeability between generic and reference drugs, it is necessary to conduct, in a scientific, technical, and high-quality manner, and in compliance with regulations, tests that demonstrate that they are equivalent within a defined interval (Secretaría de Salud, 2013). The main tests include bioavailability, bioequivalence, and the comparison of dissolution profiles. The dissolution profile test is used as an important tool to determine *in vitro* bioequivalence between a testing (target) drug and a reference drug. This test is used particularly to determine or support bioequivalence in specific cases where *in vivo* studies may not be necessary, or to complement information, such as: Class I drugs (high solubility and high permeability) and some Class III drugs (high solubility and low permeability) of the Biopharmaceutics Classification System; comparison of final formulations and previous versions of a drug; when formulation changes are made; and studies to replace clinical trials for certain drugs, among others (FDA, 1997).

Depending on the characteristics of the drug, a slow dissolution can ensure that the drug's bioavailability is limited by factors such as the absorption coefficient and gastric emptying, in addition to the dissolution process itself. Since the response to absorption and gastric emptying is relatively consistent in humans, biopharmaceutical characteristics are usually the most important aspects for determining the product's bioavailability. In these cases, the rate-limiting step for drug absorption is gastric emptying (FDA, 1997). In the case of low-solubility/high-permeability drugs (Class II of the BCS), drug dissolution can be the rate-limiting step for drug absorption, and an *in vivo–in vitro* correlation can be expected. The FDA (1997) recommends a dissolution profile in multiple media for medicinal products in this category. In the case of high-solubility/low-permeability drugs (Class III of the BCS), permeability is the rate-controlling step, and only a limited *in vivo–in vitro* correlation is possible, depending on the relative rates of dissolution and intestinal transit. Class IV drugs (low solubility/low permeability) present significant challenges for oral drug delivery. Therefore, it is important to understand some fundamental aspects of dissolution theories to establish the best methods for identifying mathematical models to determine drug interchangeability.

Theories of Dissolution

The dissolution of drugs in a solvent is considered a molecular dispersion of the drug in the dissolution medium, determined by the affinity of both molecular species (Abrami et al., 2022). Dissolution can become the limiting factor for absorption when it exhibits slow dissolution kinetics compared to the faster kinetics of disintegration or absorption of the active ingredient. The intrinsic dissolution rate is influenced by the solid-state properties of the drug, such as crystallinity, polymorphism, amorphism, hydration, solvation, particle size, shape, and surface area (Gopal Rangarao et al., 2022).

Mathematical models provide quantitative data on the dissolution process, including the dissolution rate constant. The main theories that describe the solid–liquid dissolution phenomenon are based on several assumptions: that the dissolving particle is spherical in shape, that mass transfer occurs through diffusion processes, and that a sink condition (non-saturation of the solution) is maintained, meaning that the volume is 5 to 10 times greater than the saturation volume (Cárdenas-Rodríguez et al., 1996). According to Gopal Rangarao et al. (2022), two major theories explain how solid particles dissolve in a liquid. The first and most widely accepted is the diffusion layer theory. Under sink conditions, this theory proposes that the dissolution rate is determined by a rate constant with zero-order kinetics, indicating that the dissolution process is independent of drug concentration. However, under non-sink conditions or near saturation of the medium, the dissolution rate follows first-order kinetics, and the process becomes dependent on the drug concentration. The second theory, known as the surface renewal theory, explains dissolution differently by assuming that the medium is in motion, thereby simulating the dynamic conditions of gastric fluids.

The determination of the in vitro dissolution rate is carried out under apparent sink conditions, but as the drug concentration in the medium increases, it approaches the solubility limit. For most poorly water-soluble drugs, the dissolution rate constitutes the rate-limiting step in the absorption process.

Criteria and Requirements for Evaluating Dissolution Profiles, According to NOM-177-SSA1

NOM-177-SSA1 establishes the main criteria and general requirements for evaluating dissolution profiles as an interchangeability test for immediate-release pharmaceutical dosage forms. One of the main aspects to consider before performing this test is ensuring the quality of the manufactured drug, that the expiration date has not been reached, proper registration with the health authority (for example, COFEPRIS in Mexico), and the assay percentage of the test drug, which must be within pharmacopeia limits (not differing by more than 5% from that of the reference). Once these aspects have been considered, the dissolution profile test is carried out under the main conditions considered by the Official Standard:

1. Perform dissolution profiles with at least 12 units of both the test drug and the reference drug in three dissolution media. Dissolution should be carried out using Apparatus I (basket) at 100 rpm or Apparatus II (paddle) at 50 rpm, employing 900 mL of the following dissolution media: 0.1 N hydrochloric acid solution pH 1.2 or simulated gastric fluid without enzyme; pH 4.5 buffer solution; pH 6.8 buffer solution or simulated intestinal fluid without enzyme. The mean values of the profiles should be used for comparison.
2. These mean values can only be used if the coefficient of variation (CV) at the first sampling time (up to 15 minutes) is below 20% and does not exceed 10% at the remaining sampling times.
3. To perform the dissolution profile, at least five sampling times should be selected to appropriately characterize the ascending curve and the plateau phase. Only two points should be on the plateau of the curve, and the other three distributed between the ascending and inflection phases. The sampling times must be the same for the profiles being compared

4. If both the target drug and the reference drug dissolve 85% or more within 15 minutes or less in at least one dissolution medium, it is not necessary to use the similarity factor (f_2), and the products are classified as very rapidly dissolving.
5. The withdrawn volume may or may not be replaced; when the volume is not replaced, no more than 10% of the dissolution medium should be withdrawn. In any case, the aliquot volume taken at each sampling must be considered when calculating the percentage dissolved
6. If the %CV of the dissolved percentage exceeds the limit established in point 4 of this section, the comparison should be performed using an independent multivariate confidence region procedure, a model-dependent approach, or a time-series model.

These points are fundamental for understanding the relevance of the dissolution profile as a test to determine the interchangeability of reference and generic drugs. This is based on evaluating that the drug release, dissolution, and absorption process, as projected according to the drug formulation, is not the rate-limiting step of bioavailability. For example, NOM-177-SSA1(Secretaría de Salud, 2013) and other health authorities consider certain conditions sufficient and necessary for the exemption of *in vivo* studies: high solubility and permeability of the active pharmaceutical ingredient (Class I according to the BCS), immediate-release solid oral dosage form, similar pharmaceutical composition, and very rapid dissolution (85% in less than 15 minutes). The dissolution profile test simulates physiological conditions using buffer solutions, temperature, and agitation. Therefore, the FDA (1997) advocates a conservative conclusion that, if the mean gastric residence (emptying) time T50% is 15–20 minutes under fasting conditions, a medicinal product that achieves 85% dissolution in 15 minutes under mild dissolution test conditions in 0.1 N HCl is expected to behave like a solution and generally should not have any bioavailability issues.

Evaluation and Interpretation of Dissolution Profiles, According to NOM-177-SSA1

The interpretation of the dissolution test, on the other hand, allows the use of mathematical tools to determine the absence of differences (f_1 factor) or similarity (f_2 factor) in the drug release and dissolution processes, as well as predictions of the active ingredient's absorption, thereby determining interchangeability (Rivas et al., 2023). While the difference factor (f_1) calculates the percent difference (%) between the two curves at each time point and serves as a measure of the relative error between the two curves, the similarity factor (f_2) is a logarithmic reciprocal square root transformation of the sum of squared errors and corresponds to a measure of the similarity in percent dissolution between the two curves, not allowing a difference greater than 10% between the mean dissolved amount of the reference drug and that of the test drug (FDA, 1997). Regarding the evaluation and interpretation of the dissolution profile, the standard establishes several key points:

1. The percentage dissolved should be calculated with respect to the nominal dose of the drug.
2. The percentages dissolved at each sampling time for each dosage unit should be reported, as well as the mean percentages dissolved, the coefficients of variation, and the maximum and minimum values in each of the dissolution media.
3. If the %CV of the dissolved percentage is less than or equal to 20% for the first sampling time (up to 15 minutes) and less than or equal to 10% for subsequent times (over 15 minutes), the dissolution profiles are compared using f_2 as defined in the following equation:

$$f_2 = 50 \cdot Log\left(\frac{1}{\sqrt{1+\frac{\sum_{i=1}^{n}|R_i - T_i|^2}{n}}} \cdot 100\right)$$

Where:
n = number of sampling times.
R_i= Average percentage of the reference drug dissolved at the i-th sampling time.
T_i= Average percentage of the target drug dissolved at the i-th sampling time

4. Calculate the f_2 value in each of the dissolution media, compare the mean values from the first sampling time up to at most one sampling time after the reference drug has reached 85% dissolved, with a minimum of three points. If the f_2 value is greater than or equal to 50 in at least one of the three dissolution media, the dissolution profiles are considered similar
5. If both the target drug and the reference drug dissolve 85% or more within 15 minutes or less in a dissolution medium, it is not necessary to use the f_2 factor, and the products are classified as very rapidly dissolving.
6. If the %CV of the dissolved percentage exceeds the limit established in point 3 of this section, the comparison should be made using an independent multivariate confidence region procedure, a model-dependent approach, or a time-series model.

In theory, both factor f_1 and factor f_2 can be used to analyze equivalence in the dissolution profile test. However, factor f_1, being limited to measuring the average percentage difference point by point between profiles, without using a logarithmic scale or considering the overall shape of the dissolution profile, may overlook relevant differences in the dissolution rate (Costa & Sousa Lobo, 2001). Therefore, it is not considered sufficient to declare equivalence, and its use is restricted to a complementary analysis. In contrast, factor f_2 proves to be more robust and useful in practice, since it employs a logarithmic scale that smooths out minor differences while assigning greater weight to large discrepancies between profiles (Costa & Sousa Lobo, 2001). For these reasons, it has been established as the main criterion of similarity by regulatory agencies such as the FDA, the EMA, and NOM-177-SSA1-2013 (Gozzo et al., 2022).

As mentioned above, if both the reference and test drugs dissolve 85% or more in less than 15 minutes, it is not necessary to use factor f_2, since the drugs are classified as very rapidly dissolving and may potentially be exempt from more extensive bioequivalence studies (for example, if they belong to BCS Class I, if they are immediate-release oral solid dosage forms, if they have a similar pharmaceutical composition, among other factors). Likewise, if they do not meet the previously mentioned condition and the coefficient of variation of the percentage dissolved for both drugs (reference and test) is less than or equal to 20% for the initial sampling times (up to 15 minutes) and less than or equal to 10% for the subsequent times (beyond 15 minutes), it is reasonable to compare the dissolution profiles using f_2 (Secretaría de Salud, 2013).

The calculation of f_2 is performed using the percentage of drug dissolved at each time point, and once 85% of the dose has been dissolved, only one additional data point should be taken for the reference drug (Secretaría de Salud, 2013). When f_2 takes values between 50 and 100, the profiles are considered similar (FDA, 1997). In cases where the drugs present a CV different from that mentioned above, another model must be used, and here we will focus on the first-order regression model, which is often compatible with dissolution profiles.

To better understand the aspects mentioned in NOM-177-SSA1-2013, we will take an example to analyze how the main points are applied. Let us suppose that a dissolution profile is being carried out between a reference drug and a target drug, and all the technical aspects outlined in the Official Standard have been followed. The results of the percentage of drug dissolved for the reference and target drugs over time, along with the corresponding CVs, are presented in Table 2.

Table 2. Average of the percentage of drug dissolved for the reference and target drugs over time.

Time (min)	Dissolution of the Reference Drug (%)	Dissolution of the Target Drug (%)	Coefficient of Variation
5,0	5,5	3,5	18,3
10,0	41,5	27,5	7,3
15,0	65,5	43,5	6,3
20,0	82,5	59,5	5,4
25,0	90,0	70,0	3,6
30,0	94,5	78,5	2.1

It is observed that the drugs do not reach a dissolution greater than 85% within 15 minutes, and that the coefficients of variation (CV%) of the percentage dissolved in the dissolution media are less than 20% at the first sampling time and less than 10% at subsequent times. Therefore, the use of the similarity factor f_2 formula is indicated to evaluate the interchangeability of these drugs. The NOM-177-SSA1-2013 states that drugs show similarity in the dissolution profile if the f_2 value is greater than or equal to 50 in at least one of the three dissolution media. To this end, the f_2 value is calculated in each of the dissolution media, and the mean values are compared from the first sampling time up to, at most, one sampling time after the reference drug has reached 85% dissolved drug, with a minimum of 3 points. The data in Table 1 do not allow establishing the exact experimental time at which 85% dissolution of the reference drug occurs; it is between 20–25 minutes. For calculation purposes, it is assumed that the desired percentage occurs at 25 minutes for the reference drug (90% dissolved). Therefore, one subsequent sampling time is taken, the data of the percentage of reference drug dissolution, corresponding to 30 minutes (where 94.5% is dissolved). Based on the data in Table 1, the correct way to perform the similarity factor calculation is to include all experimental time points. The calculation of the similarity factor yields the following value:

$$f_2 = 50 \cdot Log\left(\frac{1}{\sqrt{1+\frac{1869}{6}}} \cdot 100\right) = 37.62.$$

This value is not within the acceptable similarity range (50–100), and therefore these drugs cannot be considered interchangeable, at least based on the data from this dissolution medium.

On the other hand, we will now analyze how to determine the interchangeability of drugs in a hypothetical case where the values shown in Table 3 were obtained.

Table 3. Average of the percentage of drug dissolved for the reference and target drugs over time.

Time (min)	Dissolution of the Reference Drug (%)	Dissolution of the Target Drug (%)	Coefficient of Variation
10,00	67,76	67,89	21.3
20,00	75,12	74,98	10,32
30,00	80,74	80,33	6,39
35,00	86,81	86,07	5,46
40,00	99,29	93,36	3,60

It is observed, in Table 2, that the drugs do not reach more than 85% dissolution in less than 15 minutes, and that the coefficients of variation (CV%) of the dissolved percentage in the dissolution media exceed 20% at the first sampling time and 10% at least at one of the subsequent times, in accordance with the Official Standard. Therefore, it is not possible to apply the similarity factor f_2 formula to evaluate the interchangeability of these drugs, and an alternative approach is required (for example, Hixson-Crowell, Higuchi, Baker–Lonsdale, Korsmeyer-Peppas, quadratic, regression, logistic, Gompertz, Hopfenberg, etc.).

In this case, a model-dependent approach is chosen, specifically the first-order linear regression model. This choice is justified because the data show a good fit to this model ($r^2 > 0.93$), and it is assumed that the dissolution profile of the hypothetical drugs meets the criteria for surface change across the dissolution process, which causes disintegration and fragmentation (Pineda, 2017). According to Costa & Sousa Lobo (2001), the first-order regression model is suitable when the dosage form contains water-soluble active pharmaceutical ingredients incorporated in porous matrices, releasing proportionally to the amount of remaining drug, which implies that the release rate decreases over time.

Pineda (2017) establishes some basic principles for using a regression model to fit the kinetic model between the arithmetic mean of the percentage dissolved (y) versus time (x). The author states that the first-order model ($y = \beta_0 e^{\beta_1 x}$) is applied when the surface area of the dosage form changes during the dissolution process and belongs to the classification model based on physicochemical properties. For this, the least squares method is applied to estimate the representative parameters (β_0, β_1), via a 90% confidence interval (LCI (β_i), UCI (β_i)), in addition to the goodness-of-fit indicator (r^2), its prediction error or regression standard deviation ($S_{y/x}$), the Akaike criterion, in addition to supporting at least one significant effect of the model ($F < 0.05$).

According to Pineda (2017), since the similarity criterion allows for a difference of ±10% between the arithmetic mean of the percentage dissolved at each time for the test drug compared to the reference drug, two regression models are proposed for the reference drug: $(\bar{y}_i - 10\%, x_i)$y $(\bar{y}_i + 10\%, x_i)$. To determine the similarity of the kinetic models of the reference and test drugs, it is necessary to use the 90% confidence intervals for their parameters (intercept or the amount of drug immediately dissolved at time zero (β_0) and slope or dissolution constant for the first-order kinetic model (β_1) in both models of the reference drug: $LCI_{R-10\%}(\beta_i), UCI_{R-10\%}(\beta_i)$ y $LCI_{R+10\%}(\beta_i), UCI_{R+10\%}(\beta_i)$.

In this way, a broader general model is obtained that assumes ±10% values of the LCI and UCI of the reference drug, using the 90% confidence interval. That is, a general model will be proposed that ranges from $LCI_{R-10\%}(\beta_0), UCI_{R-10\%}(\beta_0)$ to $LCI_{R+10\%}(\beta_0)$and $UCI_{R+10\%}(\beta_0)$ for the confidence interval of the intercept of the reference drug, and from $LCI_{R-10\%}(\beta_1), UCI_{R-10\%}(\beta_1)$ to $LCI_{R+10\%}(\beta_1)$and $UCI_{R+10\%}$ (β_1) for the confidence interval of the reference drug slope. If in the general model $[LCI_{R-10\%}(\beta_0) - UCI_{R+10\%}(\beta_0)]$ y $[LCI_{R-10\%}(\beta_0) - UCI_{R+10\%}(\beta_0)]$ includes $LCI_T(\beta_0) - UCI_T(\beta_0)$ and $LCI_T(\beta_1) - UCI_T(\beta_1)$, then similarity is observed in the intercept and slope, and the kinetic models of both drugs are concluded to be similar, and therefore, they are considered interchangeable (Pineda, 2017).

To better understand the aspects mentioned above, we will take an example to analyze how the main points are applied. Assuming the coefficients of variation from Table 2, we will use the model-dependent approach (regression) to determine interchangeability. Suppose that the values in Table 4 represent the percentage of drug dissolved for the reference and target drugs, their respective values transformed into the natural logarithmic scale, as well as the value of the percentage dissolved -10% $(\bar{y}_i - 10\%, x_i)$and +10% $(\bar{y}_i + 10\%, x_i)$.

Table 4. Average dissolution percentages of reference and target drugs, including 10% variability for the reference, with corresponding natural logarithms over time.

Time (min)	Dissolution of R (%)	Dissolution of T (%)	LN Dissolution of R*	LN Dissolution of T*	LN Dissolution of R +10%*	LN Dissolution of R -10%*
10,00	67,76	67,89	4,22	4,22	4,31	4,11
20,00	75,12	74,98	4,32	4,32	4,41	4,21
30,00	80,74	80,33	4,39	4,39	4,49	4,29
35,00	86,81	86,07	4,46	4,46	4,56	4,36
40,00	99,29	93,36	4,60	4,54	4,69	4,49

* Note: The percentage dissolved values were transformed into the natural logarithmic scale to facilitate calculations.

Dissolution R: Percentage of dissolution for the reference drug; Dissolution T: Percentage of dissolution for the target drug; LN Dissolution R: Natural logarithm of the percentage of dissolution for the reference drug; LN Dissolution T: Natural logarithm of the percentage of dissolution for the target drug; LN Dissolution R +10%:

Natural logarithm of the percentage of dissolution for the reference drug + 10%; LN Dissolution R -10%: Natural logarithm of the percentage of dissolution for the reference drug - 10%.

Based on these values, the regression model is constructed, and the general model is established, formed from the ±10% values of the LCI and UCI (with a 90% confidence interval) of the reference drug. It is then analyzed whether the confidence interval of the test drug is included within the general model. Using the previous table, we obtain:

Model for the reference drug -10%: [0.008 – 0.015], which corresponds to $LCI_{R-10\%}(\beta_1)$, $UCI_{R-10\%}(\beta_1)$ and [3.867 – 4.085], which corresponds to $LCI_{R-10\%}(\beta_0)$, $UCI_{R-10\%}(\beta_0)$; $r^2 = 0.95$, $F = 53.743$, $p = 0.005$, $S = 0.04$.

Model for the reference drug +10%: [0.008–0.015], which corresponds to $LCI_{R+10\%}(\beta_1)$, $UCI_{R+10\%}(\beta_1)$ and [4.067 – 4.285], which corresponds to $LCI_{R+10\%}(\beta_0)$, $UCI_{R+10\%}(\beta_0)$; $r^2 = 0.93$, $F = 53.743$, $p = 0.005$, $S = 0.04$.

General Model: [0.008 – 0.015], which corresponds to $LCI_{R-10\%}(\beta_1)$, $UCI_{R+10\%}(\beta_1)$ and [3.867 – 4.285], which corresponds to $LCI_{R-10\%}(\beta_0)$ and $UCI_{R+10\%}(\beta_0)$.

Model for the target drug: [0.008 – 0.012], which corresponds to $LCI_T(\beta_1)$, $UCI_T(\beta_1)$ and [4.053 – 4.171], which corresponds to $LCI_T(\beta_0)$ and $UCI_T(\beta_0)$; $r^2 = 0.98$, $F = 137.394$, $p = 0.001$, $S = 0.02$.

Therefore, we see that the confidence interval of the broader general model, formed from the ±10% values of the LCI and UCI (with a 90% confidence interval) of the reference drug [0.008–0.015] for the slope and [3.867 – 4.285] for the intercept – includes the confidence interval of the slope and intercept of the target drug, [0.008 – 0.012] and [4.053 – 4.171], respectively. This leads to the conclusion that the drugs are interchangeable.

SIMULATOR DESIGN

Contribution of the SOLO Taxonomy and Technology Educational Theory

The study of drug interchangeability testing represents a real-world problem that enables students to develop statistical reasoning and learn through problem-solving, while simultaneously acquiring knowledge and concepts specific to pharmaceutics sciences. This approach aligns with the characteristics of problem-based learning (PBL) described by Vera Velázquez et al. (2021), an active methodology which enhances meaningful learning. Likewise, the use of active methodologies in the pharmaceutical field, as noted by Limberger (2013), encourages students to construct their own knowledge with greater autonomy and motivation, develop a deeper understanding of the subject, retain content more effectively, and strengthen interdisciplinary connections.

Since the objective of the teaching sequence is to analyze how statistical reasoning develops in students who complete a didactic sequence designed based on the SOLO Taxonomy, focused on descriptive statistics concepts and supported by technology, the next step is to characterize the levels of statistical reasoning. This taxonomy describes the progression of learning from basic levels to more complex levels of understanding. In this way, BioSimuLab promotes progressive comprehension and the development of statistical reasoning, while also fostering the transfer of knowledge to real situations in professional pharmaceutical practice.

The first two stages of the medication dissolution profile test (analysis of the time required for 85% dissolution and calculation of the CV) are designed to facilitate students' understanding of statistical reasoning. Based on the SOLO taxonomy, two worksheets are proposed (see the "User Guide" section), where students must answer questions related to the topic that promote the progression of reasoning levels. For example, when comparing measures of central tendency and dispersion, greater variability is identified in Target Drug 2 compared to the Reference Drug and Target Drug 1.

This scenario is presented so that students perceive the variability of the data and understand its significance in terms of risk. With greater dispersion, students are expected to use different measures of central tendency and dispersion, as well as graphical representations such as scatter plots and box-and-whisker plots (Figure 1 and Figure 2, respectively).

Figure 1. Scatter plot of the percentage of drug dissolved over time, created in the worksheet 1.

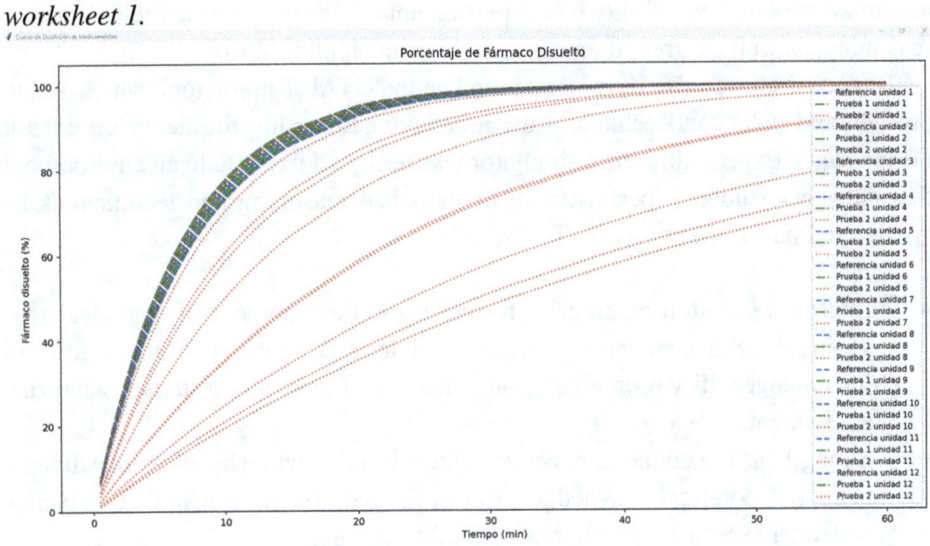

Figure 2. Box-and-whisker plot created in Worksheet 2.

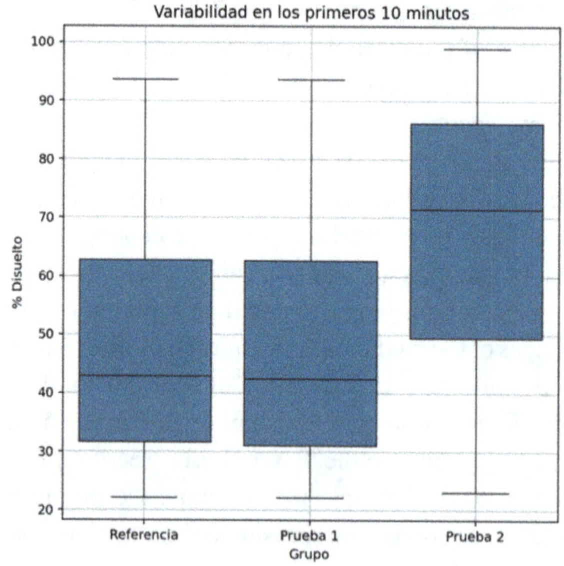

It is intended that they begin to differentiate between estimators and relate them to each other in order to make sense of variability, which supports data-driven decision-making and gives meaning to the various statistics that may be considered (Garfield et al., 2008; Orta y Sánchez, 2018). This strategy promotes the emergence of different levels of understanding according to the SOLO taxonomy and, based on this, allows for analyzing the development of statistical reasoning in students who participated in the activity designed under this approach. This will lead to better assimilation of data variability by the participants, thereby fostering their statistical reasoning, as well as strengthening analytical and applied skills.

BioSimuLab was also developed based on the UTAUT predictors, which aim to promote and understand technology usage behavior. Regarding the theory´s predictor Performance Expectations, the simulator was designed to emulate an environment that enhances students' performance in statistical reasoning and technical skills applied to Pharmacology. Specifically, it:

- Improves decision-making by fostering the development of statistical reasoning, teaching students to argue, explain, and interpret solutions to drug interchangeability problems through the use of descriptive statistics and risk assessment.
- Strengthens the connection between theory and practice by allowing students to apply theoretical knowledge within a simulated environment that replicates real-world scenarios of interchangeability testing.

- Facilitates data visualization and interpretation by enabling the export of dissolution data from three drugs (one reference and two target drugs) to an Excel file, thus providing interoperability and making data analysis and interpretation easier.

Concerning Effort Expectation (perceived ease of use), BioSimuLab was designed with an intuitive and user-friendly interface, featuring visual cues for running simulations and exporting results. When users hover over the "Run" and "Export" buttons, immediate guidance is provided, and an integrated help option is available. Additionally, a comprehensive instructional manual is included, covering key considerations, potential export errors, usage instructions, and a general overview of the simulator's functions.

In relation to Facilitating Conditions (availability of resources): The simulator is accessible and functional on computers with Microsoft operating systems, requiring no specialized infrastructure. Its ability to export data to Excel enhances interoperability with other analysis tools. Moreover, BioSimuLab is cost-effective, as it eliminates the need for laboratory materials and is available as free software. In the future, it will be hosted in the repository of the Master's Program in Mathematics Teaching at the University of Guadalajara.

With respect to Social Influence: BioSimuLab adheres to the Mexican Official Standard NOM-177-SSA1, reinforcing its academic and professional validity for both individual and group data analysis. Its design supports the learning of statistical concepts and facilitates the teaching of drug interchangeability testing from a regulatory perspective, using graphical and visual information suitable for classroom discussion. Consequently, it can be integrated into various courses—such as Regulatory and Health Legislation or Biopharmaceutics and Pharmacokinetics—within the Bachelor's program in Pharmaceutical Chemistry and Biology, promoting acceptance and recommendation among faculty and students in the pharmaceutical field.

In this sense, the simulator was proposed to develop statistical reasoning, by adopting a didactic sequence based on SOLO Taxonomy and some predictors of the UTUAT to increase intention to use, acceptance, and usage behavior of emerging technology to foster professional competences among students, especially on those related to the quality, efficacy, and safety of medicines.

Contribution of NOM-177-SSA1

BioSimuLab was designed to serve as an educational resource for teaching dissolution profile testing in the experimental design course at a public university in Mexico. This simulator is developed in the Python programming language, using packages such as Tkinter, Pandas, and Matplotlib, and consists of two main modules:

the administrator interface and the user interface. Its implementation is designed to be intuitive and efficient for use in the classroom or in self-learning contexts. The simulator generates data following an exponential dissolution model, defined by the equation:

$$f(t) = 400e^{-0.1400463423698196(t)},$$

where t represents time in minutes, and 0.1400463423698196is the dissolution constant, established so that the reference drug complies with the dissolution profile proposed in NOM-177-SSA1. In other words, the reference drug must dissolve at least 85% within a maximum of 15 minutes, and in this way, these parameters serve as an alternative for analyzing bioequivalence studies.

BioSimuLab generates an Excel file named **BioSimuLab.xlsx**, which contains three spreadsheets with dissolution data corresponding to three types of hypothetical drug brands (using 400 mg ibuprofen as the example drug for the simulation). Each type of drug is evaluated in 12 units, with 60 measurement time points. This structure follows the requirements established in NOM-177-SSA1, which mandates at least five sampling points and evaluation of 12 units for each type of drug. In addition, a higher data density is included during the first 20 minutes in order to analyze in greater detail the variations in drug dissolution. This interval corresponds to a critical phase of the dissolution process that closely reflects real conditions, since the mean gastric emptying time (T50%) is approximately 15 to 20 minutes under fasting conditions (FDA, 1997).

The sheets contain the following information:

- **Sheet 1:** Dissolution data for the reference drug.
- **Sheet 2:** Dissolution data for Target Drug 1 (bioequivalent profile).
- **Sheet 3:** Dissolution data for Target Drug 2 (non-bioequivalent profile).

The following considerations were made to simulate Test Drugs 1 and 2:

- **Target Drug 1:** A controlled variability variable, denoted as ε, is introduced. This variable modifies the dissolution constant of the reference drug while ensuring compliance with NOM-177-SSA1. Since Test Drug 1 dissolves more than 85% within 15 minutes or less, calculating the similarity factor f_2, mentioned in NOM-177-SSA1 is not necessary.
- **Target Drug 2:** Two variability variables were incorporated, and the dissolution constant was modified to 0.11904634236968196, making it significantly different from the reference drug. The variability variables denoted as $\varepsilon_1$and ε_2,increase the variability such that Target Drug 2 does not meet the range

of dissolved drug coefficient of variation established by NOM-177-SSA1. Therefore, additional statistical tests are required to determine similarity in the dissolution profiles.

According to NOM-177-SSA1, for Test Drug 2, the %CV (coefficient of variation) of the dissolved drug must be ≤20% for the first sampling time and ≤10% for subsequent times in order to be accepted. Target Drug 2 does not meet this criterion; therefore, NOM-177-SSA1 recommends performing the comparison using a model-independent multivariate confidence region procedure, a model-dependent approach, or a time-series model (Secretaría de Salud, 2013).

In addition to the two worksheets mentioned before, BioSimuLab includes two more, which propose the estimation of f_2 similarity factor, and allows the use a model-dependent approach, in this case, linear regression, which will be carried out to compare the "*y*"-intercept and the slope of the fitted line with those of the reference drug. For both the interception and the slope, upper and lower limits will be established corresponding to a ±10% variability. Figure 3 show the worksheet generated for the determination of interchangeability according to the calculation of the similarity factor (f_2). Figure 4 provide a diagram that the students could create from the Worksheet 4 for comparison of the linear regression of the drugs to determine bioequivalence.

Figure 3. Worksheet 3 for the calculation and interpretation of the similarity factor (f_2).

Actividad 2: BioSimuLab

Alumno:

Lea cuidadosamente la siguiente información.

En esta actividad, eres encargado de evaluar y seleccionar un medicamento que cumpla con los criterios para ser considerado genérico intercambiable. Para ello, utilizarás el simulador **BioSimuLab**, una herramienta que genera datos de disolución para analizar la equivalencia entre medicamentos.

El simulador generará un archivo en formato Excel con los perfiles de disolución de tres medicamentos de **400 mg**:

- **Medicamento de referencia:** Producto original con el cual se comparan los demás.
- **Medicamento de prueba 1 y 2:** Alternativas genéricas cuya equivalencia será evaluada.

Utiliza los datos del simulador y conocimientos previos de Biofarmacia y Farmacocinética para contestar las preguntas indicadas. Anota tus respuestas en un documento de Word y guarda el archivo en la misma carpeta del simulador, con el nombre de "BioSimuLabact2_#*n*", donde *n* es el número del equipo asignado por el aplicador. Incluye al inicio los nombres de todos los integrantes del equipo. Asegúrate de fundamentar cada respuesta con la justificación correspondiente.

Preguntas:

1. Con base en la NOM-177-SSA1, ¿cuáles son los pasos que se siguen para realizar la prueba del coeficiente de variación (CV %) por periodos?
2. Con base en la NOM-177-SSA1, ¿se cumple el criterio del CV % en cada periodo del perfil de disolución?
3. ¿Qué procedimiento se sigue en caso de que los valores de CV % excedan los límites de aceptación establecidos en la NOM-177-SSA1?
4. ¿Cuál de los dos medicamentos de prueba se adquiere? Argumenta tu respuesta con datos estadísticos. Usa un informe estadístico que contenga variables independientes y dependientes del experimento, medidas de tendencia central y de dispersión, y un diagrama de caja y bigote, el cual te servirá para justificar tu respuesta.

Al terminar la actividad, adjunta el archivo Word con tus respuestas, el archivo de Excel generado por el simulador, y la hoja de trabajo de Excel al apartado correspondiente a Actividad 2 BioSimuLab en Classroom.

1

Figure 4. Analysis and Interpretation of Linear Regression data created in Worksheet 4.

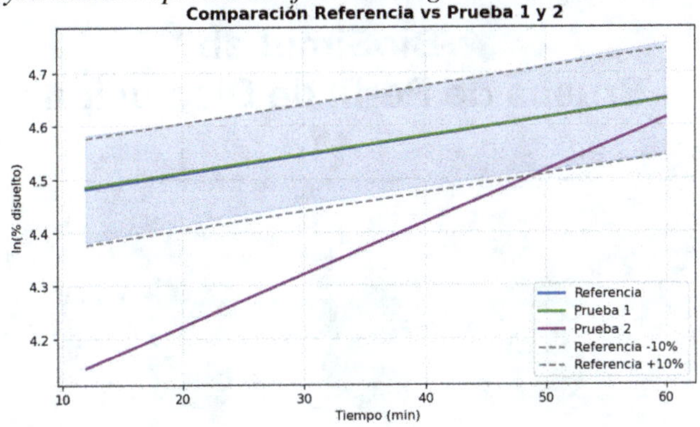

In this sense, BioSimuLab facilitates the understanding of technical aspects of pharmacokinetics and has significant educational value. As noted by Orozco-Rodríguez et al. (2023) simulators and digital laboratories allow the recreation of realistic environments that promote active student participation in all stages of the statistical process: from problem formulation, data generation and collection to data analysis, interpretation, and decision-making. This directly contributes to meeting the graduation profile for the Bachelor's degree in Pharmaceutical-Biology Chemistry, since the graduation profile establishes that:

> *"The Pharmaceutical-Biology Chemistry professional is one who applies their knowledge, skills, and attitudes in the production of goods and services aimed at the prevention, diagnosis, treatment support, and monitoring of diseases. This is achieved through the performance and interpretation of chemical, microbiological, food, clinical biochemical, toxicological, and pharmaceutical analyses and procedures, following quality standards and sanitary regulations, thereby promoting public health and social well-being to meet societal needs" (Universidad de Guadalajara, 2025).*

USER GUIDE

The student will have access to a folder containing the following materials: BioSimuLab.exe (simulator), User Guide.pdf and Worksheet.xlsm, which includes the four worksheets that will be used throughout the teaching sequence.

The BioSimuLab simulator has the interface shown in Figure 5. When the "run button" is clicked, a message appears confirming that the simulation has been performed correctly. At this point, the dissolution data for three drugs are generated: the reference drug, target 1 and target 2.

Figure 5. BioSimuLab simulator interface.

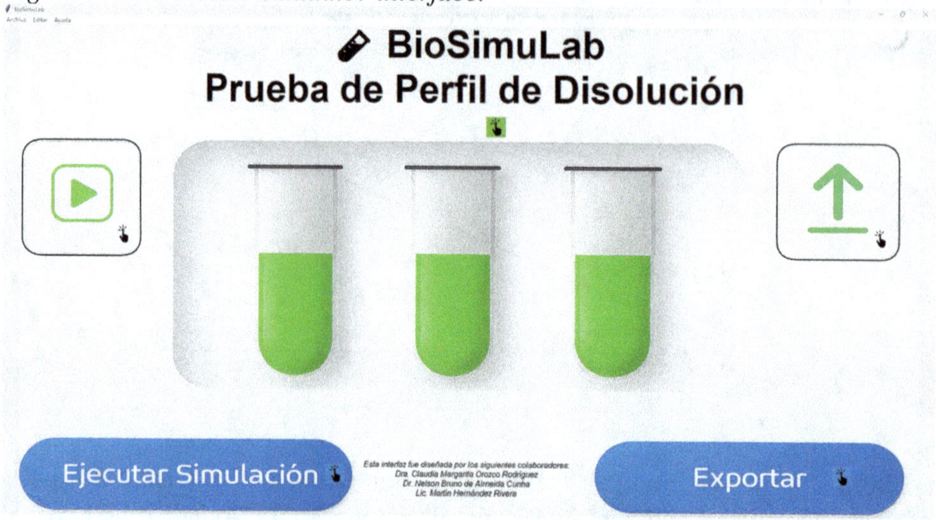

After selecting the export button, the system displays a window with the message **"Data exported to the BioSimuLab.xlsx file"**. This file is automatically saved in the same folder where the simulator is located. This document contains three spreadsheets with the dissolution results expressed in milligrams dissolved and in percentage dissolved, organized according to the type of drug (reference, target 1 and target 2), as shown in Figure 6.

Figure 6. File generated after exporting results.

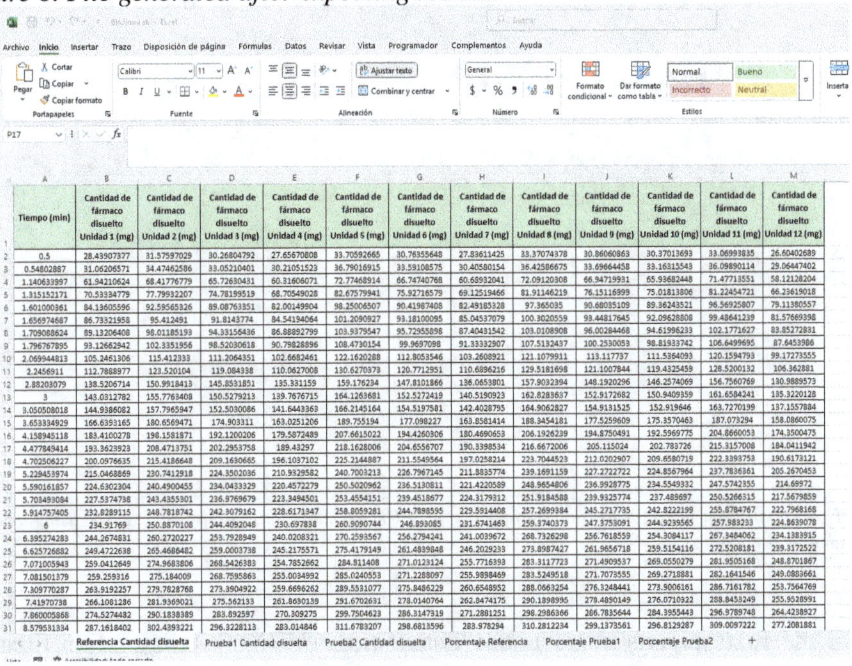

Tiempo (min)	Cantidad de fármaco disuelto Unidad 1 (mg)	Cantidad de fármaco disuelto Unidad 2 (mg)	Cantidad de fármaco disuelto Unidad 3 (mg)	Cantidad de fármaco disuelto Unidad 4 (mg)	Cantidad de fármaco disuelto Unidad 5 (mg)	Cantidad de fármaco disuelto Unidad 6 (mg)	Cantidad de fármaco disuelto Unidad 7 (mg)	Cantidad de fármaco disuelto Unidad 8 (mg)	Cantidad de fármaco disuelto Unidad 9 (mg)	Cantidad de fármaco disuelto Unidad 10 (mg)	Cantidad de fármaco disuelto Unidad 11 (mg)	Cantidad de fármaco disuelto Unidad 12 (mg)
0.5	28.43907377	31.57597029	30.26804792	27.65670808	33.70592665	30.76355648	27.83611425	33.37074378	30.86060863	30.37013693	33.06993835	26.60402689
0.54802887	31.06206571	34.47462586	33.05210401	30.21051523	36.79016915	33.59108575	30.40580154	36.42586675	33.69664458	33.16315543	36.09890114	29.06447402
1.140633997	61.94210624	68.41776779	65.72630431	60.31606071	72.77468914	66.74740768	60.68932041	72.09120308	66.94719931	65.93682448	71.47713551	58.12128204
1.315152171	70.53334779	77.79932207	74.78199519	68.70549028	82.67579941	75.92716579	69.12519466	81.91146219	76.15116999	75.01813806	81.22454721	66.23619018
1.601000361	84.13605596	92.59565326	89.08763351	82.00149904	98.25006507	90.41987408	82.49185328	97.365035	90.68035109	89.36243521	96.56925807	79.11380557
1.656974687	86.73321958	95.412491	91.8143774	84.54194064	101.2090927	93.18100095	85.04537079	100.3020559	93.44817645	92.09628808	99.48641239	81.57669398
1.709088624	89.13206408	98.01185193	94.33156436	86.88892799	103.9379547	95.72955898	87.40431542	103.0108908	96.00284468	94.61996233	102.1771627	83.85272831
1.796767895	93.12662942	102.3351956	98.52030618	90.79828896	108.4730154	99.9697098	91.33332907	107.5132437	100.2530053	98.81933742	106.6499695	87.6453986
2.069944813	105.2461306	115.412333	111.2064351	102.6682461	122.1620288	112.8053546	103.2608921	121.1079911	113.117737	111.5364093	120.1594793	99.17273555
2.2456911	112.7888977	123.520104	119.084338	110.0627008	130.6270373	120.7712951	110.6896216	129.5181698	121.1007844	119.4325459	128.5200132	106.362881
2.88203079	138.5206714	150.9918413	145.8531851	135.331159	159.176234	147.8101866	136.0653801	157.9032394	148.1920296	146.2574069	156.7560769	130.9889573
3	143.0312782	155.7763408	150.5279213	139.7676715	164.1263681	152.5272419	140.5190923	162.8283637	152.9172682	150.9409359	161.6584241	135.3220128
3.050508018	144.9386082	157.7965947	152.5030086	141.6443363	166.2145164	154.5197581	142.4028795	164.9062827	154.9131525	152.919646	163.7270199	137.1557884
3.653334929	166.6393165	180.6569471	174.903311	163.0251206	189.755194	177.098227	163.8581414	188.3454181	177.5259609	175.3570463	187.073294	158.0860075
4.158945118	183.4100278	198.1581871	192.1200206	179.5872489	207.6615022	194.4260306	180.4690653	206.1926239	194.8750491	192.5969775	204.8660053	174.3500475
4.477849414	193.3623923	208.4713751	202.2953758	189.43297	218.1628006	204.6556707	190.3398534	216.6672006	205.115024	202.783726	215.3157008	184.0411942
4.702506227	200.0976635	215.4186648	209.1630665	196.1037102	225.2144887	211.5549564	197.0258214	223.7044523	212.0202907	209.6580719	222.3393753	190.6173121
5.229453974	215.0468869	230.7412918	224.3502036	210.9329582	240.7003213	226.7967145	211.8835774	239.1691159	227.2722722	224.8567964	237.7836361	205.2670453
5.590161857	224.6302304	240.4900455	234.0433329	220.4572279	250.5020962	236.5130811	221.4220589	248.9654806	236.9928775	234.5549332	247.5742355	214.69972
5.703493084	227.5374738	243.4355301	236.9769679	223.3494501	253.4554151	239.4518677	224.3179312	251.9184588	239.9325774	237.489697	250.5266315	217.5679859
5.914757405	232.8289115	248.7818742	242.3079162	228.6171347	258.8059281	244.7898595	229.5914408	257.2699384	245.2717735	242.8222199	255.8784767	222.7968168
6	234.91769	250.8870108	244.4092048	230.697838	260.9090744	246.893085	231.6741463	259.3740373	247.3753091	244.9239565	257.983233	224.8639078
6.395274283	244.2674831	260.2720227	253.7928949	240.0208321	270.2593567	256.2794241	241.0039672	268.7326298	256.7618559	254.3084117	267.3484062	234.1383915
6.625726882	249.4722638	265.4686482	259.0003738	245.2175571	275.4179149	261.4839848	246.2029233	273.8987427	261.9656718	259.5154116	272.5208181	239.3172522
7.071005943	259.0412649	274.9683806	268.5426383	254.7852662	284.811408	271.0123124	255.7716393	283.3117723	271.4909537	269.0550279	281.9505168	248.8701867
7.081501379	259.259316	275.184009	268.7595863	255.0034992	285.0240553	271.2288097	255.9898469	283.5249518	271.7073555	269.2718881	282.1641546	249.0883661
7.309770287	263.9192257	279.7828768	273.3904922	259.6696262	289.5531077	275.8486229	260.6548952	288.0663254	276.3248441	273.9006161	286.7161782	253.7564769
7.41970738	266.1081286	281.9369021	275.562133	261.8630139	291.6702631	278.0140764	262.8474175	290.1898995	278.4890149	276.0710322	288.8458249	255.9528991
7.860005868	274.5274482	290.1838389	283.892597	270.309275	299.7504623	286.3147319	271.2881251	298.2986366	286.7835644	284.3955443	296.9789748	264.4238927
8.579531334	287.1618402	302.4393221	296.3228113	283.014846	311.6783207	298.6813596	283.978294	310.2812234	299.1373561	296.8129287	309.0097222	277.2081881

Each drug is evaluated using 12 units, with a total of 60 measurements. This design complies with NOM-177-SSA1, which requires at least five sampling points and the evaluation of 12 units per drug. The resulting data will be used to complete the worksheets.

Some considerations for the correct use of the simulator must be taken into account:

- Before exporting the data, students must ensure that they have previously run the simulation.
- Data should not be exported if an Excel file with the same name is open, as this could cause errors.

Figure 7 describes the process of drug interchangeability evaluation, step by step. This flowchart outlines the decision-making process for proceeding with the assessment of drug dissolution profiles. Students will work on the specific worksheets, following the procedure outlined in the document Worksheet.xlsm.

Figure 7. Flowchart for the determination of drug interchangeability.

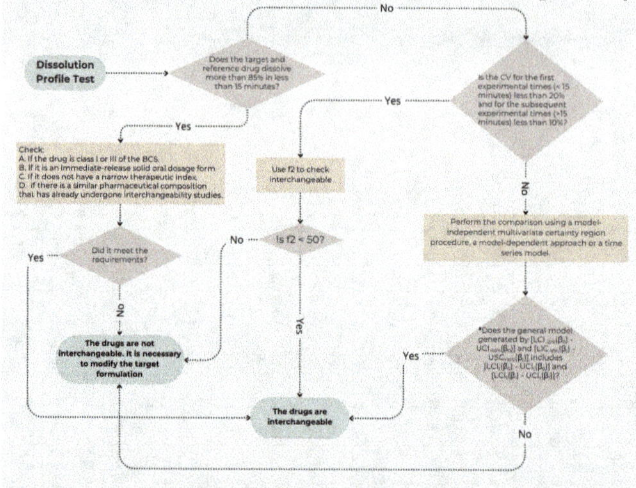

**Note: First-order linear regression parameters (90% CI) for interchangeability comparison using a model-dependent approach.*

In the first spreadsheet, named "Estadísticas 85%", the dissolution times at which each of the 12 units of the three drugs reach 85% are calculated. As shown in Figure 8, the spreadsheet includes a table for recording these calculations and a macro button that clears the data (a feature included in all spreadsheets). For clarity, the worksheets corresponding to the different activities can be hidden.

Figure 8. Spreadsheet "Estadísticas 85%."

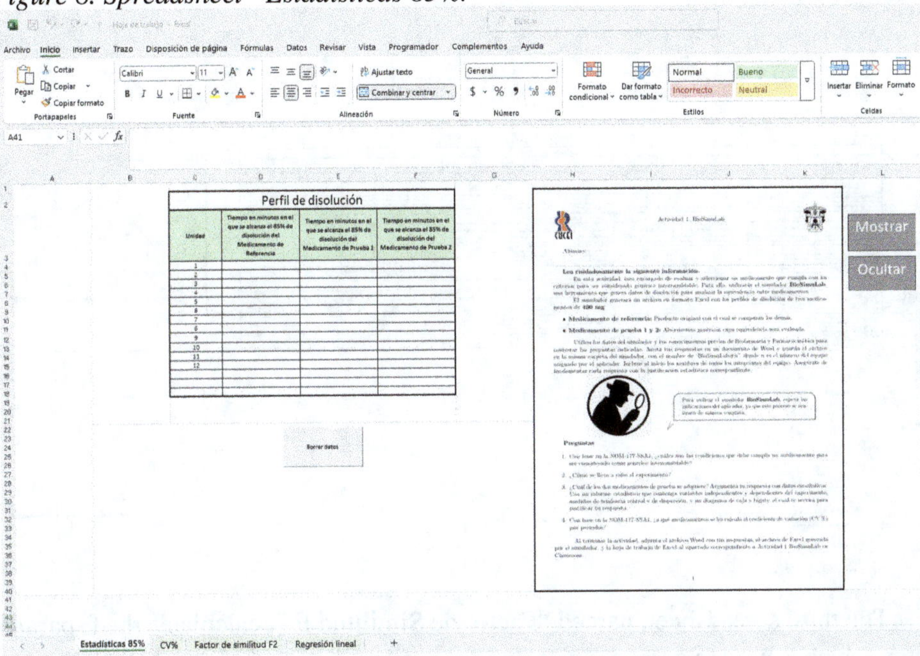

The second spreadsheet, named *CV%*, evaluates the coefficient of variation (CV). According to NOM-177-SSA1, the CV for the first period (≤15 minutes), must be less than or equal to 20%, while for subsequent periods (>15 minutes), it must be less than or equal to 10%. The spreadsheet includes a predefined table with analysis times of 12 and 15 minutes for the first period, and 20, 25, 30, 40, 45, 50, and 60 minutes for the second period. The layout of this sheet is illustrated in Figure 9.

Figure 9. Spreadsheet "CV%".

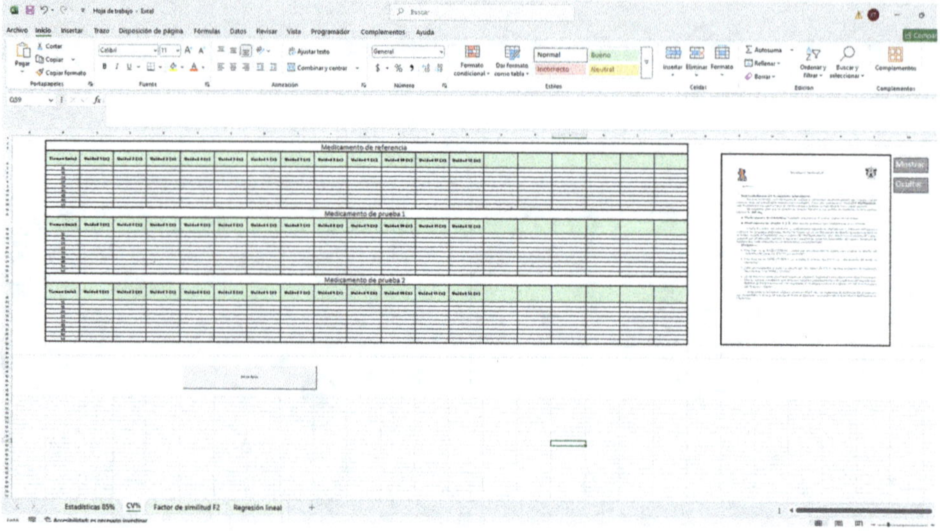

The third spreadsheet, named "Factor de Similitud F_2", calculates the f_2 parameter, which is used to compare dissolution profiles. A value greater than or equal to 50 indicates that the profiles are similar; otherwise, they do not meet the similarity criterion. The layout of this spreadsheet is shown in Figure 10.

Figure 10. Spreadsheet "Factor de Similitud F_2".

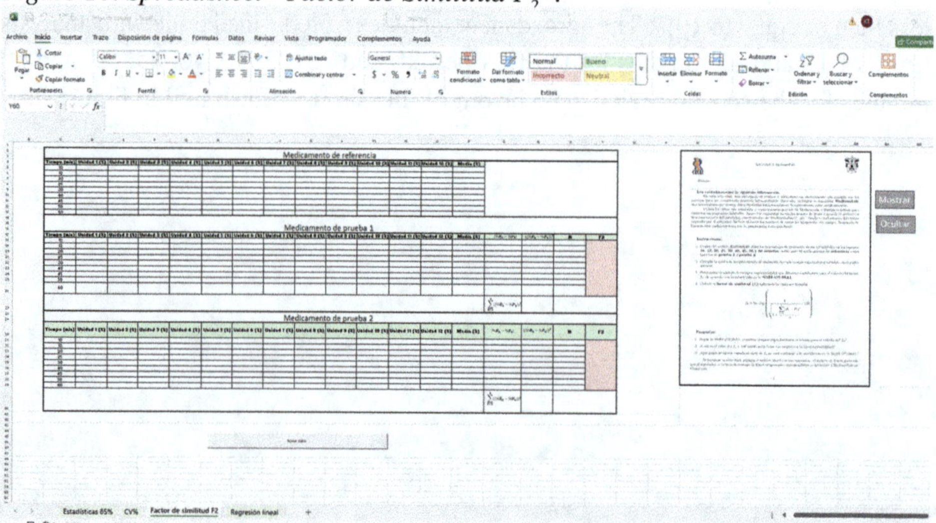

Finally, the fourth spreadsheet, named "Regresión Lineal", use the average percentage of the 12 units of the three types of drugs at the specified times to perform a linear regression to compare the dissolution profiles. It also includes the values of the reference drug ±10% of the average percentage of dissolution. Using a statistical software (e.g., Statgraphics, SPSS, or similar), the student must determine the values of R^2, F, P, and S, as well as the confidence intervals of the slope and intercept. Based on this information, a general model is constructed and then compared with the models of the test drugs. The spreadsheet of this activity is shown in Figure 11.

Figure 11. Spreadsheet "Regresión Lineal".

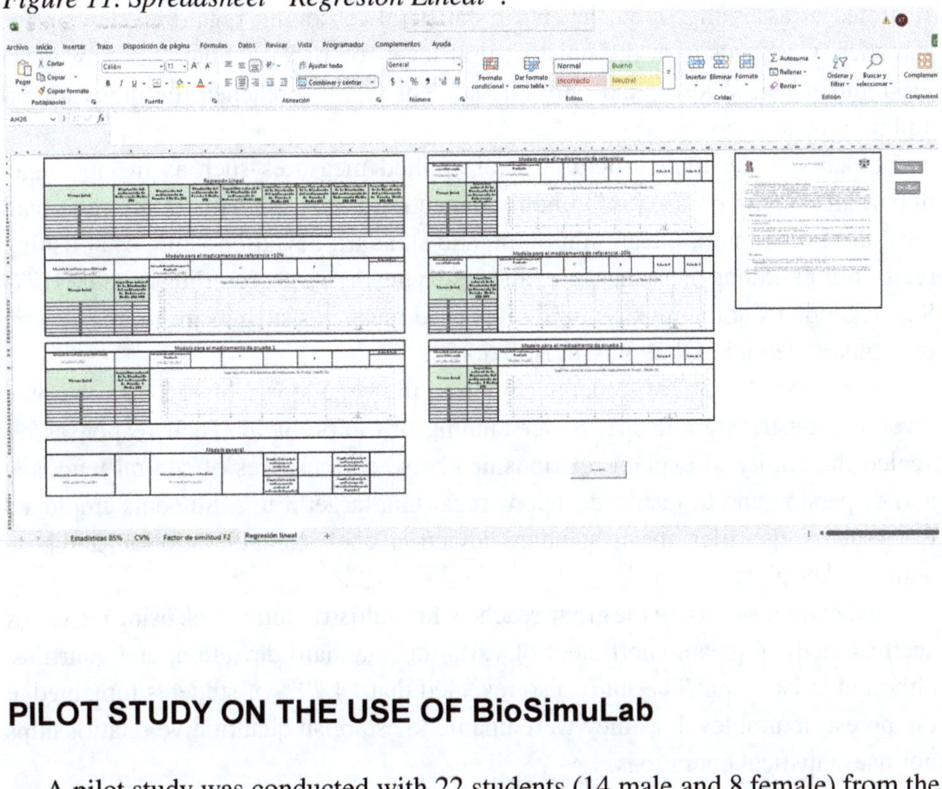

PILOT STUDY ON THE USE OF BioSimuLab

A pilot study was conducted with 22 students (14 male and 8 female) from the Bachelor's degree in Pharmaceutical-Biology Chemistry and in Chemical Engineering at a public university in Mexico, during the period from August to September 2025. The purpose of the study was to evaluate the clarity of the activities and the interpretation of results in the first BioSimuLab worksheet.

In this pilot study, an activity was designed to compare the effectiveness of using the simulator versus the traditional teaching method. Following a phase of concept formalization, the activities were implemented. Activity 1 followed the traditional teaching approach, in which students analyzed static data corresponding to the dissolution times of reference and test drugs (as established in worksheets 1 and 2 of this chapter). The objective was for students to analyze data behavior and determine the interchangeability of test drugs with the reference drug through dissolution profile analysis according to NOM-177-SSA1, while also identifying optimal statistical measures of central tendency and dispersion (mean, standard deviation, interquartile range, coefficient of variation, among others). Activity 2 followed the same procedure but used randomly generated data from the simulator. In both activities, students' statistical reasoning was assessed through questions designed to promote interpretation and critical reflection.

According to the SOLO Taxonomy (Table 4), students who completed Activity 1, aimed at assessing initial levels of statistical reasoning regarding descriptive statistics, were mostly at the unistructural level (63.64%), while 27.27% were at the multistructural level, and only one student (4.55%) reached the prestructural and relational levels.

Students at the multistructural level applied measures such as mean, range, maximum, or minimum, but without connecting them. Students at the relational level used maximum, mean, minimum, and standard deviation while establishing relationships among these measures and justifying their use according to NOM-177-SSA1. Students at the unistructural level used measures such as mean, maximum, or standard deviation, but only in isolation.

In contrast, 71.43% of students who used the simulator achieved the relational level, demonstrating a deeper understanding of the problem. Their responses revealed the ability to explain relationships between measures of central tendency and dispersion and to justify decisions regarding target drugs. Students employed tools such as quartiles, mean, standard deviation, coefficient of variation, and box-and-whisker plots.

Meanwhile, 14.29% of the group reached the multistructural level, using measures such as median, mean, coefficient of variation, standard deviation, and quartiles, although in isolation. The study also revealed that 14.29% of students remained at the preestructural level, as they were unable to establish quantitative relationships nor use statistical operations.

Although this is a pilot study, the results indicate that the use of BioSimuLab facilitated students' progression from unistructural and multistructural levels to the relational level (Figure 12).

Figure 12. Sankey diagram of Activity 1 (a) and Activity 2 (b)

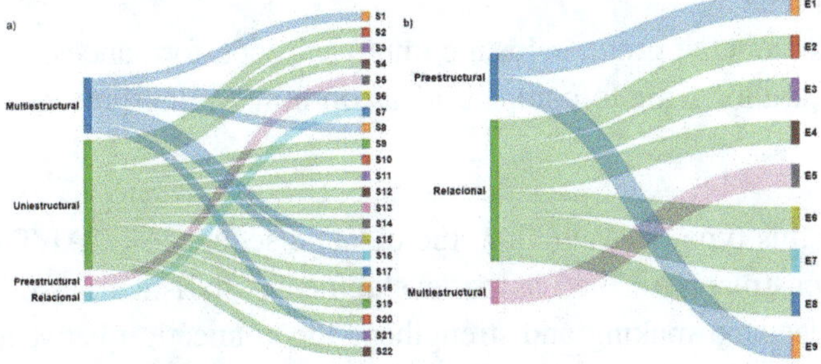

Additionally, once Activity 2 is complete, a questionnaire will be completed to evaluate the students' experience with the didactic sequence and their attitude toward the use of technology (specifically, BioSimuLab), in which students describe their experience in each situation, according to the following options: Strongly Disagree, Disagree, I Don't Know, Agree, and Strongly Agree. These questions will be reviewed by experts to determine content, construct and criterion validity, aiming to establish a more accurate assessment of the aspects mentioned earlier; some propositions for perceiving student's experience would be:

1. I identify the estimators or statistics used to describe the variability of a data set.
2. I correctly explain the data variability.
3. In decision-making, I associate greater variability with greater risk.
4. I reflect on how variability affects decision-making in the problems posed in the activities.
5. When analyzing data, I incorporate interpretations of data variability and context, not just statistical summaries or graphs.
6. I consider estimators or statistics that differ from the mean, when context requires it.
7. I consider the context of the problem to describe data
8. I explain in my own words what the estimators used in solving the activities mean.
9. I justify my interpretations with estimators or statistics.
10. Working with simulated data in the BioSimuLab activity improved my understanding of variability.
11. The graphical representations created in the simulator activity facilitated my understanding of data variability.
12. The simulator helped me connect theory with practice in bioequivalence testing.

13. Collaborating with my colleagues makes it easier for me to interpret the variability of the data.
14. Feedback from the group helps me improve my performances.
15. Teamwork allows me to compare ideas on how to interpret variability in the data.

Based on this type of evaluation, the didactic sequence UTAUT performance expectancy construct is fulfilled, as the development of statistical reasoning improves data-driven decision-making and strengthens the connection between theory and practice. The use of simulated data allowed students to visualize trends and patterns of variability, providing a more realistic learning experience aligned with professional practice. This was made possible by BioSimuLab's interoperability, which enables students to work with, analyze, and interpret data directly from an Excel file. Furthermore, working with dynamic data rather than predefined datasets promoted the development of statistical reasoning and strengthened students' analytical skills.

CONCLUSION

The objective of this chapter was to present and explain the use of BioSimuLab to promote the development of statistical reasoning and decision-making within a pharmaceutical sciences context, specifically related to dissolution testing as established by NOM-177-SSA1, in the classroom setting. Given that pharmaceutical sciences education faces significant challenges stemming from the predominance of expository methods and limited inclusion of practical experiences, the use of BioSimuLab can bridge the gaps between theory and practice, specially in the field of bioequivalence. In this regard, understanding the processes of bioavailability, bioequivalence, and dissolution profiles is a fundamental aspect in the training of professionals capable of ensuring the quality, efficacy, and safety of medicines. However, the complexity inherent to these studies, influenced by multiple biological, pharmacokinetic, and methodological variables, requires the development of statistical and analytical competencies that enable the rigorous interpretation of experimental data and grounded decision-making.

The use of simulations, including oral absorption modeling and *in vitro–in vivo* correlation, have become essential tools for guiding formulation development. The application of computational modeling in drug development offers several benefits. It integrates all available *in vitro* and *in vivo* data to provide a comprehensive understanding of formulation bioperformance, offers a mechanistic insight into both *in vitro* formulation behavior and *in vivo* outcomes, and enables the exploration of multiple scenarios in a shorter timeframe with fewer experiments, thereby accelerating product development. In addition, modeling and simulation methods are increasingly employed in regulatory review and align with current trends in the pharmaceutical industry, which aims to. When used complementarily to guide formulation development, these tools can significantly increase the likelihood of achieving bioequivalent endpoints.

Furthermore, simulators promote data-driven learning and informed decision-making, which are key skills in the modern pharmaceutical industry, where digitalization, computational modeling, and predictive analysis are growing trends. By interacting with simulators, students develop the ability to design experiments, evaluate results, and optimize processes, reflecting real-world pharmaceutical research and development practices.

In this context, BioSimuLab is presented as an innovative educational resource that integrates computational simulation with the regulatory criteria established in NOM-177-SSA1. Its design fosters active learning based on inquiry and experimentation with simulated data, enabling students to practice hypothesis formulation, apply statistical methods, critically interpret results according to data variability, and prepare students to perform effectively in an industrial environment that increasingly relies on technology and computational simulation. The tool also contributes to the strengthening of statistical reasoning while simultaneously promoting the meaningful acquisition of technical concepts inherent to bioequivalence studies and dissolution profiles.

Consequently, the implementation of BioSimuLab in the university context represents a pedagogically valuable strategy that, in addition to addressing the curricular requirements of student training, responds to the current demands of higher education oriented toward professional practice. By fostering the integration of theory, simulated experimentation, and current regulations, this proposal contributes to the training of professionals with the competencies required to ensure drug quality, promote public health, and responsibly address the needs of society.

REFERENCES

Abdulhussain, Y., Ghelani, H., Henderson, H., Sudhir, M., Mascarenhas, S., Radhakrishnan, R., & Jan, R. K. (2022). The use and effectiveness of high-fidelity simulation in health professions education: Current update. *Simulation, 98*(12), 1085–1095. Advance online publication. DOI: 10.1177/00375497221101066

Alcántara Pineda, A. (2017). *Métodos estadísticos para comparar perfiles de disolución requeridos por la NOM-177.* https://farmazine.mx/articulos/metodos-estadisticos-para-comparar-perfiles-de-disolucion-requeridos-por-la-nom-177

Biggs, J. B., & Collis, K. F. (1982). *Evaluating the Quality of Learning: The SOLO Taxonomy (structure of the Observed Learning Outcome).* Academic Press. https://books.google.com.mx/books?id=x4qcAAAAMAAJ

Cabero-Almenara, J., & Costas, J. (2016). La utilización de simuladores para la formación de los alumnos. *Revista Prisma Social, 17*, 343–372.

Cárdenas Rodríguez, H. Lilia., Cortés Arroyo, A. Rosa., & Universidad Autónoma Metropolitana (México). Unidad Xochimilco. (1996). *Aspectos biofarmacéuticos de la evaluación de medicamentos / Hilda Lilia Cárdenas Rodríguez, Alma Rosa Cortés Arroyo.* Casa abierta al tiempo, Universidad Autónoma Metropolitana.

Casallas-Hernández, N., Castillo-Daza, C. A., & González-Guzmán, V. A. (2025). Acceptance and effectiveness of high-fidelity simulation in nursing education: Application of the Technology Acceptance Model (TAM). *Clinical Simulation in Nursing, 105*, 101765. DOI: 10.1016/j.ecns.2025.101765

Costa, P., & Sousa Lobo, J. M. (2001). Modeling and comparison of dissolution profiles. *European Journal of Pharmaceutical Sciences, 13*(2), 123–133. DOI: 10.1016/S0928-0987(01)00095-1

Darlami, J., & Sharma, S. (2024). The role of physicochemical and topological parameters in drug design. *Frontiers in Drug Discovery, Volume 4-2024.* DOI: 10.3389/fddsv.2024.1424402

Garfield, J. B., Ben-Zvi, D., Chance, B., Medina, E., Roseth, C., & Zieffler, A. (2008). *Developing students' statistical reasoning* (SCOPUS:84891388863). Springer Netherlands. DOI: 10.1007/978-1-4020-8383-9

Gozzo, L., Caraci, F., & Drago, F. (2022). Bioequivalence, Drugs with Narrow Therapeutic Index and The Phenomenon of Biocreep: A Critical Analysis of the System for Generic Substitution. *Healthcare (Basel), 10*(8), 1392. Advance online publication. DOI: 10.3390/healthcare10081392

Granić, A. (2023). Technology Acceptance and Adoption in Education. In *Handbook of Open, Distance and Digital Education* (pp. 183–197). Springer., DOI: 10.1007/978-981-19-2080-6_11

Hidalgo Cajo, B. G., Mayacela Alulema, Á. G., & Hidalgo Cajo, I. M. (2017). Estrategias didácticas para potenciar el aprendizaje de Farmacología clínica. *Revista Habanera de Ciencias Médicas*, *16*(3), 439–453.

Huon, J.-F., Nizet, P., Tollec, S., Vene, E., Fronteau, C., Leichnam, A., Tching-Sin, M., Michelet-Barbotin, V., Foucault-Fruchard, L., & Nativel, F. (2024). A systematic review of the impact of simulation on students' confidence in performing clinical pharmacy activities. *International Journal of Clinical Pharmacy*, *46*(4), 795–810. DOI: 10.1007/s11096-024-01715-z

Kaddoura, R., Faraji, H., Otaki, F., Radhakrishnan, R., Stanley, A., Paulus, A., Jackson, L., Jayyousi, R. A., Mascarenhas, S., Sudhir, M., Alfroukh, J., Ghelani, H., Azar, A. J., Khamis, A. H., & Jan, R. K. (2024). High-fidelity simulation versus case-based tutorial sessions for teaching pharmacology: Convergent mixed methods research investigating undergraduate medical students' performance and perception. *PLoS One*, *19*(8), e0302609. DOI: 10.1371/journal.pone.0302609

Ledbetter, E., Lau, S., Enterline, A., Sibbitt, B., & Chen, A. M. H. (2020). A Simulation Activity to Assess Student Pharmacists' Knowledge and Perceptions of Oncology Pharmacy. *American Journal of Pharmaceutical Education*, *84*(5), 7474. DOI: 10.5688/ajpe7474

Lei, Y.-Y., Zhu, L., Sa, Y. T. R., & Cui, X.-S. (2022). Effects of high-fidelity simulation teaching on nursing students' knowledge, professional skills and clinical ability: A meta-analysis and systematic review. *Nurse Education in Practice*, *60*, 103306. DOI: 10.1016/j.nepr.2022.103306

Limberger, J. B. (2013). Metodologias ativas de ensino-aprendizagem para educação farmacêutica: Um relato de experiência. *Interface: Comunicacao, Saude, Educacao*, *17*(47), 969–975. DOI: 10.1590/1807-57622013.3683

Miller, G. E. (1990). The assessment of clinical skills/competence/performance. *Academic Medicine*, *65*(9), S63–S67. DOI: 10.1097/00001888-199009000-00045

Mitra, A., & Wu, Y. (2012). Challenges and Opportunities in Achieving Bioequivalence for Fixed-Dose Combination Products. *The AAPS Journal*, *14*(3), 646–655. DOI: 10.1208/s12248-012-9378-x

Morais, Y. de J., dos Santos, V. R. C., & Soler, O. (2021). Simulação realística como mediadora do processo ensino-aprendizagem na graduação em Farmácia: Revisão sistemática. *Research. Social Development, 10*(10), e241101018783–e241101018783. DOI: 10.33448/rsd-v10i10.18783

Neves, C., Oliveira, T., Cruz-Jesus, F., & Venkatesh, V. (2025). Extending the unified theory of acceptance and use of technology for sustainable technologies context. *International Journal of Information Management, 80*, 102838. DOI: 10.1016/j.ijinfomgt.2024.102838

Nguyen, V. T. T., Darville, N., & Vermeulen, A. (2023). Pharmacokinetics of Long-Acting Aqueous Nano-/Microsuspensions After Intramuscular Administration in Different Animal Species and Humans—A Review. *The AAPS Journal, 25*(4), 4. Advance online publication. DOI: 10.1208/s12248-022-00771-5

Orozco-Rodriguez, C., Palafox González, A., & Valenzuela García, C. (2023). A realistic situation, proposed from data generated within the GeOrder Simulator to elicit the statistical reasoning. *Heliyon, 9*(9), e19330. DOI: 10.1016/j.heliyon.2023.e19330

Orta, J., & Sánchez Sánchez, E. (2018). Niveles de razonamiento sobre variación estadística de estudiantes de nivel medio superior al resolver problemas en un contexto de riesgo. *Educación Matemática, 30*(1), 47–71. DOI: 10.24844/EM3001.02

Polli, J. E. (2008). In Vitro Studies are Sometimes Better than Conventional Human Pharmacokinetic In Vivo Studies in Assessing Bioequivalence of Immediate-Release Solid Oral Dosage Forms. *The AAPS Journal, 10*(2), 289–299. DOI: 10.1208/s12248-008-9027-6

Rivas, K. A., Lemus García, C. R., Montelong, M. V., Cortez Álvarez, C. R., Barajas Menzoza, M. A., Avalos, A. V., & Garduño, A. C. (2023). Estudio Comparativo de Perfiles de Disolución de Tabletas de 500 mg de Paracetamol para Determinar su Intercambiabilidad. *Artículos del Congreso Internacional de Investigación Academia Journals Chetumal, 15*(5), 2.1-2.6.

Sánchez Sánchez, E., Silvestre Castro, E., & García Ríos, V. N. (2019). Patrones de razonamiento sobre pruebas de significación de estudiantes de bachillerato. *Patterns of reasoning on signification tests of high school students.* http://hdl.handle.net/10481/55045

Secretaría de Salud. (2013). *NORMA Oficial Mexicana NOM-177-SSA1-2013, Que establece las pruebas y procedimientos para demostrar que un medicamento es intercambiable. Requisitos a que deben sujetarse los Terceros Autorizados que realicen las pruebas de intercambiabilidad. Requisitos para realizar los estudios de biocomparabilidad. Requisitos a que deben sujetarse los Terceros Autorizados, Centros de Investigación o Instituciones Hospitalarias que realicen las pruebas de biocomparabilidad.* https://www.dof.gob.mx/

Serag-Bolos, E. S., Chudow, M., Perkins, J., & Patel, R. V. (2018). Enhancing Student Knowledge Through a Comprehensive Oncology Simulation. *American Journal of Pharmaceutical Education, 82*(3), 6245. DOI: 10.5688/ajpe6245

Universidad de Guadalajara. Centro Universitario de Ciencias Exactas e Ingenierías (CUCEI) & Coordinación Licenciatura en Químico Farmacéutico Biólogo. (2025). *Perfil de Ingreso y Egreso.* https://www.cucei.udg.mx/carreras/farmaceutica/es/perfil-de-ingreso-y-egreso

U.S. Department of Health and Human Services, Food and Drug Administration, Center for Drug Evaluation and Research. (1997, agosto). *Guía para la industria: Pruebas de disolución de formas de dosificación oral sólidas de liberación inmediata.* https://www.fda.gov/

Venkatesh, V., Thong, J. Y. L., & Xu, X. (2012). Consumer Acceptance and Use of Information Technology: Extending the Unified Theory of Acceptance and Use of Technology. *Management Information Systems Quarterly, 36*(1), 157–178. DOI: 10.2307/41410412

Vera Velázquez, R., Maldonado Zúñiga, K., Castro Piguave, C., & Batista Garcet, Y. (2021). Metodología del aprendizaje basado en problemas como una herramienta para el logro del proceso de enseñanza- aprendizaje: Metodología del aprendizaje basado en problemas. *Sinapsis: La revista científica del ITSUP, 1*(19), 15. DOI: 10.37117/s.v19i1.465

Wu, K., Kwon, S. H., Zhou, X., Fuller, C., Wang, X., Vadgama, J., & Wu, Y. (2024). Overcoming Challenges in Small-Molecule Drug Bioavailability: A Review of Key Factors and Approaches. *International Journal of Molecular Sciences, 25*(23), 13121. Advance online publication. DOI: 10.3390/ijms252313121

KEY TERMS AND DEFINITIONS

Pharmaceutical Equivalents: These are identical dosage forms that contain the same amount of the identical active ingredient, but not necessarily the same excipients, and which comply with all current pharmacopeial specifications.

Pharmaceutical Alternatives: Products administered by the same route, containing the same molar dose of the drug(s) or active substance(s), which may differ in dosage form (tablets or capsules), in the chemical form of the drug or active substance (different salts, different esters), or in both, and which comply with pharmacopeial specifications.

Bioequivalence: Relationship between two pharmaceutical equivalents or pharmaceutical alternatives when, under similar conditions, they obtain comparable bioavailability.

Bioavailability: It is the measure of the rate and extent to which a therapeutically active molecule reaches the systemic circulation (blood that will be distributed throughout the body) from the drug product originally administered.

Interchangeability: It refers to the possibility of replacing a drug with an equivalent one without significant clinical changes in efficacy or safety.

Therapeutic Equivalents: Drugs that are pharmaceutically equivalent and expected to have the same clinical effect and safety profile when administered to patients under the same conditions.

Cmax: It is a pharmacokinetic term that refers to the maximum concentration a drug reaches in plasma after its administration.

AUC (Area Under the Curve): It represents the total exposure of the body to a drug over time after its administration.

Chapter 12
Immersive Maze-Based Memory Tasks in Virtual Reality: Bridging Game Design and Neuroscience

David Fernández-Quezada
https://orcid.org/0000-0002-6943-7492
Centro Universitario de Ciencias de la Salud, Universidad de Guadalajara, Mexico

Diana Emilia Martínez-Fernández
Centro Universitario de Ciencias de la Salud, Universidad de Guadalajara, Mexico

ABSTRACT

Immersive maze-based memory tasks in virtual reality represent a novel intersection between game design and neuroscience, providing controlled yet ecologically valid environments for investigating spatial memory, navigation strategies, and executive functions. This chapter explores how VR-based adaptations of classical paradigms (radial arm, Morris water, and floor mazes) enable dynamic manipulation of environmental complexity, multisensory cues, and cognitive load. By integrating principles of serious game design, these immersive tasks enhance engagement and motivation while preserving experimental rigor, allowing researchers to evaluate hippocampal-dependent learning and memory consolidation. Evidence from experimental and clinical studies demonstrates VR's potential for early detection of cognitive decline, rehabilitation of spatial deficits, and personalized cognitive

DOI: 10.4018/979-8-3373-4657-1.ch012

training. Bridging interactive game mechanics with neuroscientific inquiry, this work highlights VR as a transformative platform for translational research and next-generation neurorehabilitation.

INTRODUCTION

Memory represents a fundamental cognitive function essential to the survival of many living organisms, enabling them to retain information derived from past experiences, including previous interactions with the environment and the outcomes associated with them. Because the external world is dynamic and constantly changing, humans, like many other animals, possess a remarkable capacity to regulate and adapt their memories with great flexibility. As new experiences occur, the brain continuously forms and updates memory traces, selectively determining which events should be stored, which previously encoded memories have become outdated and require modification, and which are no longer relevant and should be forgotten. This adaptive process not only allows for efficient information management but also contributes to the construction of a coherent sense of self and temporal continuity. Memory therefore acts as a critical framework for guiding learning, decision-making, and problem-solving, shaping both individual behavior and collective human experience (Josselyn et al., 2017).

Numerous studies have shown that memory formation involves the activation of small, specialized groups of neurons distributed across multiple brain regions. Following the initial encoding phase, many of these neurons are reactivated during offline periods, such as sleep, a process that contributes to the stabilization and consolidation of the neural networks representing the memory. During retrieval, a significant portion of these same neurons becomes reactivated, supporting the formation of a stable memory representation commonly referred to as the memory engram. This complex network-level phenomenon enables the storage of distinct memories by engaging separate ensembles of neurons and generating unique patterns of neural activity, thus allowing for efficient differentiation, integration, and retrieval of stored information (Eichenbaum, 1999; Merlo et al., 2024). Moreover, converging evidence highlights the central role of medial temporal lobe structures, particularly the hippocampus and entorhinal cortex, in the formation, maintenance, updating, and retrieval of memories. These brain regions operate as highly interactive hubs, integrating multimodal sensory inputs and transforming them into long-lasting representations, further supporting the idea that distinct neural ensembles and activity patterns within these structures are essential for encoding and preserving stable memory representations (Rolls, 2022).

The development of a memory instigates during the initial experience, when specific subpopulations of neurons across the brain become selectively activated in response to relevant stimuli. This heightened activity leads to elevated intracellular calcium levels within these neurons, which in turn trigger a cascade of downstream signaling mediated by calcium-dependent proteins. These molecular pathways promote both short-term natural plasticity and long-term mechanical modifications at the synaptic level, leading to strengthened connectivity between neurons involved in the same representation. Increased neuronal activation also induces the transcription of plasticity-related genes, including a class known as immediate early genes (IEGs), whose expression is essential for the acquisition and consolidation of new information. These genes serve as molecular switches, initiating a series of protein synthesis events that remodel synapses and establish persistent changes in synaptic strength. Among these, genes such as c-Fos, Arc, and Egr1 have been widely studied as key markers of neuronal plasticity and memory formation, as their expression directly correlates with the recruitment of neurons into memory-encoding ensembles. Studies have proved that a fundamental aspect of learning involves these gene-driven signaling mechanisms, which facilitate long-term potentiation (LTP) and long-term depression (LTD), thereby enabling the adaptive reorganization of neural circuits specifically within the networks of presynaptic and postsynaptic neurons engaged during the learning process (Kandel, 2012; Tischmeyer & Grimm, 1999).

Following the initial neuronal activation that drives the construction of a memory, a process of memory consolidation takes place during the subsequent hours, allowing the experience to be stabilized and stored for future retrieval. Research on memory consolidation has demonstrated that de novo protein synthesis within this period is essential for the successful formation of long-lasting memories, as it provides the structural and functional substrates necessary to sustain plasticity-related changes in synaptic connectivity. Protein synthesis-dependent consolidation occurs predominantly within the first six hours after learning, suggesting the existence of a sensitive window during which newly acquired information must be integrated into memory; disruption of this critical period leads to significant memory impairments. On a broader timescale, consolidation also occurs over weeks to years through a distinct process known as systems consolidation. In this mechanism, memories are initially encoded in the hippocampus through rapid synaptic plasticity and are gradually transferred to distributed cortical regions for long-term storage, ensuring robustness against hippocampal damage and enabling retrieval through neocortical pathways (Flexner et al., 1963; McGaugh, 2000).

Interestingly, when an animal retrieves a previously formed and consolidated memory, the same neural network originally engaged during its creation is reactivated, a process referred to as pattern completion. Research has shown that neurons in the amygdala, which were highly active during the original learning experience, are also strongly reactivated when the memory is retrieved. Moreover, the greater the reactivation of these neurons, the stronger the animal's ability to remember and express the learned behavior, showing a direct link between neuronal activity and memory strength (Reijmers et al., 2007). This process illustrates that memory retrieval is not a passive replay of stored representations but rather a dynamic reconstruction that integrates past information with ongoing contextual cues, allowing memories to be continuously updated to remain adaptive and relevant.

Despite significant advances in our understanding of memory mechanisms, traditional methods for assessing memory, ranging from paper-based neuropsychological tests to standard computerized paradigms, often fall short in capturing the dynamic, multimodal, and context-rich nature of real-world memory use. Spatial navigation and episodic memory, for instance, rely heavily on contextual cues, multisensory integration, and executive control processes that are rarely activated in artificial laboratory settings. These limitations have motivated the development of novel approaches capable of simulating real-life cognitive demands within controlled experimental frameworks. Recent advances in immersive technologies have opened unprecedented opportunities for understanding, evaluating, and enhancing human cognition. Among these, virtual reality (VR) has emerged as a particularly powerful tool, offering controlled yet ecologically valid environments in which users can engage in complex cognitive tasks that closely mirror real-world challenges (Cimadevilla et al., 2023).

VR technologies provide a unique opportunity to replicate naturalistic conditions while retaining experimental control, thus combining ecological validity with precise manipulation of sensory and cognitive variables. Through head-mounted displays and advanced rendering systems, VR allows researchers to construct three-dimensional environments enriched with visual, auditory, and even haptic cues that engage multiple cognitive systems simultaneously. Among the various applications of VR in cognitive neuroscience, maze-based paradigms stand out as particularly promising for studying memory processes, as they closely resemble classic spatial navigation tasks traditionally used in animal research while introducing innovations that make them suitable for human participants (Chitale et al., 2022).

Historically, maze-based tasks have played a central role in experimental memory research, beginning with classic rodent paradigms such as the Morris Water Maze, Radial 8-Arm Maze, and T-Maze. These paradigms have been instrumental in understanding the contributions of hippocampal and cortical circuits to spatial learning, navigation strategies, and long-term memory formation. In the Morris water maze, for example, rodents must locate a hidden platform using distal visual cues, providing robust measures of spatial memory accuracy, learning rates, and flexible navigation strategies. Similarly, the radial arm maze has been used to assess working memory and reference memory simultaneously, as animals learn to distinguish between previously visited and unexplored arms within a fixed spatial configuration. Translating these paradigms into human research has historically been challenging due to differences in sensory modalities, task demands, and ecological relevance; however, VR-based adaptations have successfully overcome many of these obstacles (Cimadevilla et al., 2023; Dale, 1986; Mei et al., 2020).

In virtual maze paradigms, researchers can systematically manipulate environmental complexity, cognitive load, and sensory inputs while recording fine-grained behavioral metrics such as decision times, error patterns, and exploration strategies. Unlike traditional paper-and-pencil or computer-based tasks, VR enables participants to navigate immersive environments using naturalistic cues and bodily movements, enhancing engagement and ecological validity. Importantly, VR-based mazes allow integration of multimodal sensory information, including visual landmarks, auditory signals, olfactory cues, and even dynamic social interactions, that modulate memory performance and strategy selection in ways that closely resemble real-world navigation. This technological flexibility makes VR-based paradigms highly suitable for probing both hippocampal-dependent spatial memory and executive functions, as well as for dissociating between egocentric and allocentric navigation strategies (Hořejší et al., 2025).

VIRTUAL REALITY TECHNOLOGIES IN NEUROSCIENCE RESEARCH

Virtual reality has traditionally been described as an "interactive visual system enhanced by specialized processing and complemented with multisensory modalities designed to create the perception of immersion within a simulated environment." Over the past two decades, VR has evolved from being considered an experimental technological innovation into a powerful scientific and clinical tool with significant applications in neuroscience, psychology, education, and rehabilitation. Today, VR is recognized as a promising technological resource that enables researchers and clinicians to simulate controlled, multisensory environments where the body, environment, and brain are closely interconnected. Through these interactive environments, VR facilitates the study of cognitive processes and supports both the enhancement and rehabilitation of spatial cognitive functions, providing significant benefits for diagnosing and treating spatial memory impairments (Chirico et al., 2016, 2020; Hofmann et al., 2003).

One of the key advantages of VR lies in its ability to replicate real-world conditions while preserving high ecological validity. Traditional laboratory-based cognitive assessments often rely on highly simplified and artificial tasks, which can fail to capture the complexity of real-life cognitive demands. In contrast, VR provides fully interactive environments where spatial orientation, decision-making, and navigation can be evaluated under realistic yet controlled conditions. This ability to balance experimental control with ecological fidelity makes VR particularly valuable in the study of spatial memory, as it allows researchers to evaluate participants' abilities to acquire, retain, and manipulate spatial information in scenarios that closely resemble everyday environments. Importantly, several studies have demonstrated a strong correlation between performance in VR-based tasks and performance in equivalent real-world tasks, highlighting the translational value of VR as a diagnostic and training tool for cognitive functions associated with navigation and memory formation (Hořejší et al., 2025; Krajčovič et al., 2024).

Furthermore, VR environments can be easily manipulated to design experimental tasks that would otherwise be difficult, unsafe, or impossible to implement in real-world contexts. For example, researchers can simulate complex city-like layouts, multilevel structures, or hazardous environments without exposing participants to actual risk. This flexibility enables the study of spatial learning, orientation strategies, and problem-solving behaviors in dynamic settings that challenge cognitive processing. Similarly, VR allows the creation of scenarios where controlled stressors can be introduced, such as unexpected obstacles, reduced visibility, or time constraints, to explore how cognitive performance is modulated under pressure. Such designs are invaluable in clinical contexts, where subtle deficits in spatial memory or executive functioning can be detected earlier than through standard neuropsychological testing (Jonson et al., 2021; Montana et al., 2019).

Beyond research, VR has been increasingly applied in rehabilitation to restore or strengthen spatial functions in patients with cognitive-spatial deficits arising from neurological injury, neurodegenerative disease, or developmental disorders. Clinical studies have provided strong evidence that VR-based interventions can serve as an effective complement to traditional rehabilitation methods, enhancing patient motivation, engagement, and adherence to treatment protocols. For instance, stroke patients undergoing VR-based training show significant improvements in navigation skills and visuospatial integration compared to conventional therapies. Similarly, VR tasks designed for individuals with mild cognitive impairment (MCI) or early-stage Alzheimer's disease have demonstrated high sensitivity in detecting subtle deficits in hippocampal-dependent spatial memory while simultaneously providing targeted training to preserve cognitive abilities for longer periods. These findings underscore the potential of VR not only as an assessment tool but also as an innovative therapeutic resource capable of promoting neuroplasticity and functional recovery (Cogné et al., 2017; Jonson et al., 2021; Sagaspe et al., 2023).

However, the rapid technological evolution of VR hardware and software has introduced new challenges for researchers and clinicians. The diversity of available devices, ranging from basic computer-based systems to fully immersive head-mounted displays, requires careful methodological standardization to ensure the comparability of findings across studies. Likewise, software frameworks must be optimized to accurately measure spatial abilities while avoiding confounding factors such as motion sickness, sensory mismatches, or unrealistic interaction constraints. Consequently, a growing body of research emphasizes the need to refine VR-based protocols, calibrate device performance, and integrate advanced metrics such as eye-tracking, body kinematics, and physiological monitoring to enhance the precision and interpretability of results (van der Ham et al., 2015).

The sense of immersion in VR, defined as the degree to which individuals feel "present" in a simulated environment, depends largely on the technological capabilities of the system to replicate realistic interactions and stimuli. Scientific literature commonly distinguishes three main types of VR systems, each offering different levels of immersion and interactivity. Nonimmersive VR systems involve the use of two-dimensional virtual environments displayed on a computer monitor, where participants interact using keyboards, joysticks, or gamepads. These setups are common in early VR applications and serious games; however, they provide limited depth perception and reduced embodiment, leading to a weaker sense of presence. In contrast, immersive VR systems integrate multiple components, such as high-resolution head-mounted displays, surround audio, motion sensors, and haptic feedback, to deliver fully simulated, three-dimensional environments. By continuously tracking users' head movements and providing stereoscopic visualization, these systems generate a natural sense of spatial presence and agency. Finally, semi-immersive VR systems combine features of both approaches; participants view stereoscopic images on large monitors or projection screens, while head-tracking or partial haptic feedback enhances interactivity, resulting in an intermediate level of immersion between the two extremes (Cipresso et al., 2018; D'Cunha et al., 2019).

An equally important feature of VR is its ability to generate a strong sense of presence, the subjective experience of being physically situated within a simulated space. Presence is closely associated with the level of engagement and realism perceived by the user, and it has a direct influence on the effectiveness of VR-based tasks. When participants feel fully immersed, their cognitive and emotional responses to virtual stimuli closely resemble those elicited in real-world contexts. This enhanced embodiment enables researchers to study spatial cognition under naturalistic conditions while retaining full control over the experimental variables. For example, in maze-based paradigms designed to evaluate spatial memory, a high sense of presence promotes the use of allocentric strategies, relying on external landmarks and spatial maps, rather than purely egocentric strategies based on body-centered cues. This distinction is particularly relevant in clinical settings, as disruptions in allocentric navigation have been linked to hippocampal dysfunction and early cognitive decline (Minderer et al., 2016).

In recent years, VR has emerged as a widely adopted tool in neuroscience, offering a broad spectrum of applications for both research and clinical practice. Its ability to create immersive and interactive environments has proven particularly valuable for enhancing spatial memory across diverse contexts. By simulating complex, realistic scenarios, VR enables the study, assessment, and rehabilitation of spatial cognitive functions with a level of precision and ecological validity that traditional methods cannot easily achieve (Cogné et al., 2017). Within cognitive neuroscience, VR has been successfully integrated with multimodal neuroimaging techniques such as fMRI, EEG, and fNIRS to investigate the neural mechanisms underlying spatial navigation, episodic memory retrieval, and decision-making in three-dimensional contexts. These combined approaches allow researchers to link behavioral performance with dynamic patterns of neural activity, providing insights into hippocampal-cortical interactions and network-level plasticity during learning (Ma et al., 2023; Parmar et al., 2023).

Moreover, virtual reality facilitates immersive and interactive learning environments in which users can actively manipulate, navigate, and engage with spatially complex concepts, thereby enhancing comprehension and promoting better retention of spatial information. By combining immersive environments with engaging tasks, VR strengthens spatial memory and enhances the ability to form accurate mental maps of surroundings. This makes VR particularly valuable as both an educational and rehabilitative tool. For example, in children with specific learning disabilities, VR-based serious games have been shown to enhance visuospatial reasoning and cognitive flexibility while maintaining a playful, motivating, and safe environment (Fernández-Batanero et al., 2022). Similarly, architectural training programs have adopted VR simulations to help professionals visualize large-scale spatial layouts, improving design planning and navigation skills in real-world contexts.

Another major advantage of VR lies in its cross-disciplinary applicability. In healthcare, VR-based tools are used to evaluate orientation strategies and diagnose spatial deficits in patients with traumatic brain injuries, neurodegenerative conditions, and psychiatric disorders. In rehabilitation sciences, adaptive VR environments facilitate motor and cognitive retraining by gradually adjusting task difficulty to match individual progress, leveraging reward-based feedback to sustain motivation. In education, immersive VR lessons allow students to interactively explore three-dimensional environments, such as navigating anatomical models, complex urban structures, or molecular landscapes, promoting deeper cognitive engagement compared to traditional didactic approaches. In architecture and engineering, VR simulations facilitate spatial planning, hazard training, and environmental design, enabling professionals to anticipate navigation challenges before real-world implementation. Finally, in entertainment and gaming industries, VR enhances experiential learning by integrating cognitive, motor, and social processes in highly interactive environments (Wiebe et al., 2022).

Overall, the use of VR for studying and enhancing spatial memory provides significant benefits across multiple disciplines, creating new opportunities to understand the neural mechanisms of navigation and orientation while offering powerful diagnostic and therapeutic applications. By immersing users in realistic, interactive environments, VR facilitates the development of spatial memory and strengthens cognitive abilities related to orientation, decision-making, and problem-solving. This technology enhances users' capacity to learn, adapt, and interact effectively with their surroundings, ultimately supporting better performance in both real-world and simulated contexts (Kellems et al., 2020; Weiss et al., 2003). As VR hardware becomes more accessible and software frameworks continue to evolve, future research will benefit from increasingly sophisticated experimental paradigms that combine ecological validity with advanced computational analyses. Integrating VR with machine learning models, behavioral tracking, and neuroimaging promises to transform the study of human cognition, enabling the development of personalized cognitive interventions and next-generation rehabilitation strategies grounded in precise neuroscientific evidence.

DIFFERENT VIRTUAL MAZE SCENARIOS FOR MEMORY EVALUATION

The neuroscience underpinning maze-based memory tasks is deeply rooted in the functional role of the hippocampus and its integration within broader neural circuits responsible for spatial cognition and episodic memory. The hippocampus, specifically the CA1 and CA3 subfields and the dentate gyrus, plays a critical role in encoding spatial representations, integrating sensory information, and supporting path planning through mechanisms such as place cells, grid cells, and head-direction cells (Cimadevilla et al., 2023).

Historically, paradigms like the Morris Water Maze and the Radial Arm Maze in rodent studies have served as gold standards for investigating spatial learning and memory consolidation. The Morris Water Maze rapidly became a gold-standard paradigm for studying spatial learning and memory in rodents. In this task, animals are placed in a circular pool filled with opaque water and must locate a hidden platform using distal visual cues. Performance is measured through variables such as escape latency, path efficiency, and search strategies. The radial arm maze is another widely used paradigm to assess working memory, reference memory, and decision-making strategies. Typically consisting of eight to twelve arms radiating from a central platform, RAM evaluates the subject's ability to remember which arms contain rewards and which have been previously visited. Beyond the Morris Water Maze and radial arm maze, several other paradigms have been developed to assess different aspects of spatial memory and executive function. The Barnes Maze, a dry-land alternative, evaluates allocentric navigation using distal cues and reduces stress-related confounds, making it suitable for studies involving stress-sensitive populations. The T-Maze and Y-Maze are widely used to measure spontaneous alternation behavior, working memory, and cognitive flexibility, relying on hippocampal-prefrontal and striatal interactions. Additionally, complex virtual mazes have emerged as powerful tools for exploring real-world navigation within ecologically valid settings, enabling the integration of multisensory cues and monitoring decision-making strategies. These paradigms complement each other by targeting distinct neural circuits and cognitive processes, providing a multidimensional framework for studying learning, memory, and executive control across both animal and human research (Cimadevilla et al., 2023; Dale, 1986; Mei et al., 2020).

These tasks provide researchers with valuable tools to investigate hippocampal-dependent processes, mechanisms of synaptic plasticity such as long-term potentiation, and the interactions between the hippocampus and prefrontal and parietal cortical regions implicated in executive control and decision-making. When adapted to virtual reality environments for human studies, these paradigms preserve their scientific rigor while enabling unprecedented manipulation and control over diverse environmental and cognitive variables. In this context, we present a series of experiments employing maze-based paradigms in VR to assess spatial memory and learning

Radial Maze Paradigms in Virtual Reality for Memory Research

The development of VR systems for spatial memory research has progressed significantly over the past decade, and one of the pioneering studies in this field was conducted by Xu and colleagues. Their work represents one of the first successful adaptations of the classical radial arm maze, widely used in rodent experiments, into a fully immersive VR paradigm suitable for human participants. By integrating this well-established behavioral task within a virtual environment, the study opened new possibilities for translational research, enabling direct comparisons between animal and human memory systems (Xu et al., 2012).

In this study, the researchers created a virtual environment composed of an eight-arm radial maze surrounded by a naturalistic landscape featuring mountains, grasslands, and trees under a simulated late-afternoon sky. A short brick rampart enclosed the maze, and several distinctive external landmarks served as extra-maze cues, allowing participants to use environmental references to guide spatial navigation strategies, figure 1.

Figure 1. The virtual maze consists of eight arms radiating from a central hub and is divided into three distinct regions for internal coding: the central area (green), the arm passage (light blue), and the baiting area (dark blue). The right panel shows a representative immersive view experienced by participants through MR-compatible goggles during control sessions. At the start of each trial, a red arrow is displayed, randomly pointing to one of the maze arms, which may or may not contain a reward. This randomized cue introduces potential misleading information, requiring participants to rely on their spatial memory and navigational strategies rather than following the directional hint. Image modified and adapted from Xu et al., 2012.

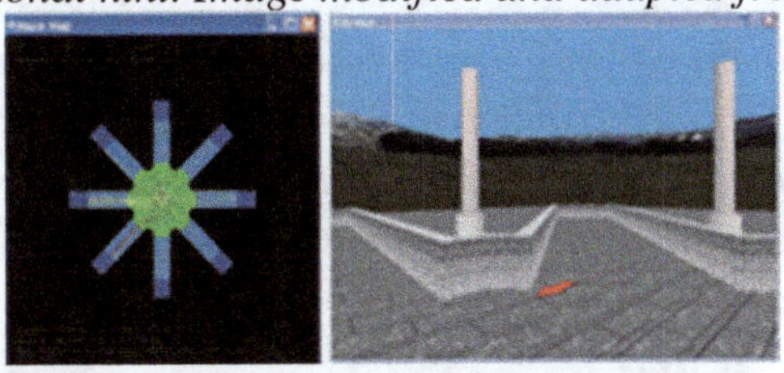

To adapt the task to humans, the original food-pellet rewards used in rodent experiments were replaced by visual reward icons represented by large U.S. dollar ($) symbols placed at the ends of selected arms. The VR system was developed using Microsoft Visual C/C++ to build the software architecture and OpenGL to render high-quality, interactive visualizations. The experimental setup included MR-compatible video goggles and input devices, such as joysticks or button boxes, which allowed participants to navigate within the maze while undergoing functional magnetic resonance imaging (fMRI) scanning (Xu et al., 2012).

Xu et al. demonstrated that this VR-based adaptation could effectively reproduce the behavioral dynamics of rodent radial arm maze tasks in human participants. By testing the system with 54 volunteers, the study confirmed its feasibility within MRI environments and highlighted its potential for investigating multiple memory systems, including spatial, working, and episodic memory (Xu et al., 2012).

In a study of 2017, a VR experiment was designed to investigate how environmental context modulates human recognition memory. In this study, thirty-three healthy young adults navigated through a four-arm VR maze (figure 2) to locate and memorize discrete items presented at specific locations within the environment. The experiment consisted of three sequential phases: learning, encoding, and retrieval. During all phases, participants performed a navigation task that required reaching a target room and either memorizing or recognizing the displayed stimulus. The VR environment, developed using the Unity3D game engine, was presented on a 32-inch computer screen, and participants interacted with the system using a keyboard and mouse. The learning phase aimed to familiarize participants with the maze layout and the user interface. In the encoding phase, participants memorized 80 images encountered during navigation, while in the retrieval phase, they explored the maze again and evaluated recognition performance using a new set of 80 images (20 per room), half of which had been previously presented and half of which were novel. Upon entering each target room, an image was displayed for one second, after which participants indicated whether they had seen it before, using a six-point confidence scale ranging from 1 ("sure unfamiliar") to 6 ("sure familiar"), following traditional recognition memory paradigms (Pacheco et al., 2017).

Figure 2. Overview of the virtual maze environment. The design consists of a central chamber connected to four surrounding rooms. In each room, twenty visual items are placed on a single wall. During each trial, the user interface highlights the corresponding target room in the upper-right corner by displaying a representative texture. Based on Pacheco D, et al. (2017).

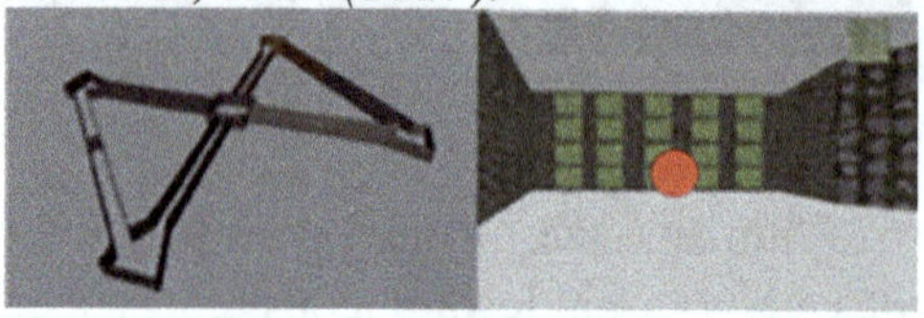

All images contain 360 objects across eight semantic categories: food, furniture, human body, musical instruments, buildings, tools, clothes, and animals. For each participant, 80 images were randomly selected from this dataset and assigned to three experimental conditions: congruent items, presented in the same room and position during both encoding and retrieval (20 images); incongruent items, presented in a different room and position (20 images); and novel items, introduced only during retrieval (40 images). This design enabled a direct comparison of recognition performance under different contextual conditions (Pacheco et al., 2017).

The results revealed that spatial context exerted a significant influence on recognition memory performance, as accuracy was notably higher when the contextual information during retrieval was congruent with that present during encoding compared to trials with incongruent contexts. These findings extend the current evidence by demonstrating these effects under ecologically valid experimental conditions achieved through the use of immersive VR technology (Pacheco et al., 2017).

Building upon previous advances in the use of VR for spatial memory research, a head-mounted display radial arm maze (HMD-RAM) was developed as a novel tool for assessing visuospatial learning and memory in humans, figure 3. This system adapts the classical radial arm maze paradigm, widely used in animal studies, into an immersive environment designed to enhance ecological validity and translational relevance. The program was built using a 3D development platform and operated on a high-performance workstation running Windows 7 and equipped with an Nvidia GeForce graphics card. The virtual environment consisted of an eight-arm maze radiating from a central hub, with chests placed at the ends of each arm containing either rewards or non-rewards (Kim et al., 2018).

Figure 3. View of the Head-Mounted Display Radial Arm Maze (HMD-RAM). The virtual environment features an eight-arm maze designed to evaluate spatial navigation and memory performance using immersive virtual reality, adapted from Kim et al. (2018).

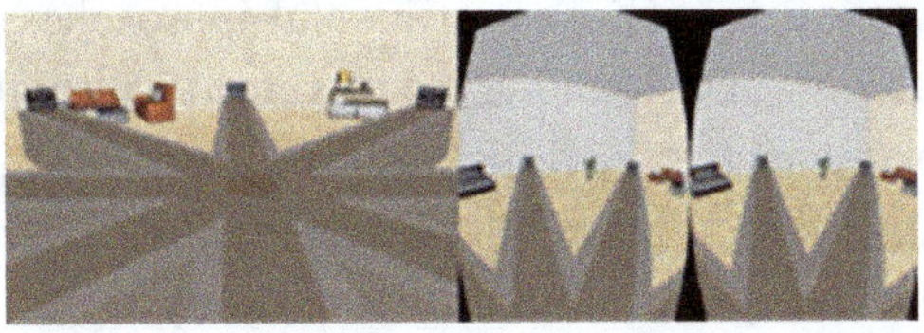

The immersive setup used an Oculus DK2 head-mounted display, providing a 100° field of view and a resolution of 960 × 1,080 pixels per eye, while tracking head movements across three degrees of freedom (yaw, pitch, and roll). Navigation was performed using a one-handed joystick, and stereo auditory feedback was presented whenever participants successfully located a reward. To facilitate spatial orientation, the virtual room contained landmark cues, including colored wallpaper and pieces of furniture, which participants could use to encode spatial relationships and navigate more effectively. The viewpoint dynamically adjusted according to head movements, simulating naturalistic exploration and increasing ecological validity (Kim et al., 2018).

Two studies were conducted to evaluate the system. Study 1 involved 20 participants completing the task with HMD, while Study 2 included another 20 participants performing the same task on a flat monitor for comparative purposes. In both studies, participants navigated the maze from a first-person perspective to locate four hidden treasures as quickly as possible within five blocks of trials, each lasting up to five minutes. The configuration of the environment and reward locations remained constant across blocks, allowing participants to consolidate spatial memory progressively (Kim et al., 2018).

The primary dependent measures included working memory errors, reference memory errors, detection time, travel distance, and head movement patterns. Results from Study 1 revealed a progressive decrease in behavioral errors across blocks, demonstrating effective spatial learning. Additionally, visuospatial memory was strongly correlated with performance outcomes, whereas verbal memory showed no association, consistent with findings from traditional rodent models. When comparing device types, results indicated that the HMD condition elicited greater presence and immersion compared to the flat monitor but also induced slightly higher levels of simulator sickness. Post-experiment questionnaires revealed that participants in the HMD condition relied more heavily on landmark-based navigation strategies, suggesting that immersive cues facilitate spatial orientation and memory encoding more effectively than standard screen-based approaches (Kim et al., 2018).

Virtual Reality Adaptation of the Morris Water Maze Paradigm

To further expand the diversity of experimental approaches using immersive VR for spatial cognition, Ben-Zeev et al. (2020) introduced a Virtual Morris Water Maze paradigm that complements the previous studies by Xu et al. (2012), Pacheco et al. (2017), and Kim et al. (2018). While earlier research primarily focused on short-term spatial navigation and recognition memory, this study significantly advances the field by integrating long-term spatial learning and memory assessment within large-scale virtual environments enriched with extra-maze cues (Ben-Zeev et al., 2020).

In this work, the authors developed spatial cognition tasks specifically adapted for VR goggles to evaluate participants' ability to accurately return to the precise location of a hidden target after multiple days of training. The tasks were programmed using Vizard 5 Virtual Reality software and executed with the Oculus Rift DK2 headset, which provided an immersive first-person perspective and real-time head tracking to dynamically adjust the viewpoint. Navigation was performed via an Xbox controller, allowing smooth interaction with the environment and fine control of orientation (Ben-Zeev et al., 2020).

Two main paradigms were introduced: the Virtual Morris Water Maze (VMWM) and the Virtual Radial Arm Water Maze (VRAWM). Unlike previous VR studies that tested short-term encoding and retrieval, this experiment systematically explored multi-day learning effects by training healthy participants (n = 40) across several sessions. In the VMWM, participants navigated a 51 × 51 × 27 m arena containing three distinct extra-maze cues and a circular pool (diameter = 25 m), searching for a hidden platform within 25 seconds per trial. The VRAWM introduced a more complex environment with eight enclosed arms, allowing researchers to examine the contribution of cue quantity by comparing groups exposed to either two or four extra-maze cues (Ben-Zeev et al., 2020).

The findings revealed optimal performance when participants completed three trials per day with three spatial cues in the VMWM and two trials per day with two cues in the VRAWM. These results underscore the importance of external cue availability and training intensity for effective spatial learning. Notably, the study extended the methodological scope of VR-based paradigms by demonstrating their suitability for long-term spatial memory evaluation, an aspect less addressed by previous VR-based maze tasks (Ben-Zeev et al., 2020).

By integrating dynamic head-tracking, large-scale environments, and ecologically valid extra-maze landmarks, this work provides a powerful tool for studying spatial cognition across extended timescales.

Remaining this progressive exploration of VR-based spatial memory paradigms, Eileen H. J. Wang et al. (2025) introduced a recently published adaptation of the classic Morris Water Maze for assessing flexible, rapid one-trial working memory in both young and older adults, figure 4. This study notably extends VR methodology into the domain of aging, offering new insights and immediate relevance to current research needs.

Figure 4. Schematic representation of the virtual environment. Left inset: participant's view from the center of the arena facing north. Right view: participants navigated a circular arena (green circle), starting from four possible positions (yellow arrows), with eight target locations (small circles) and external landmarks serving as spatial cues. Adapted from Wang et al. (2025).

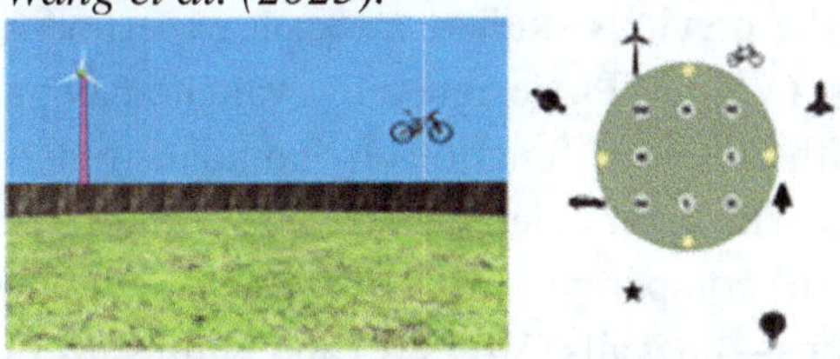

In this investigation, participants across three age brackets, Young Adults (18–44 years), Young Elderly (60–69 years), and Older Elderly (≥ 70 years), were immersed in a three-dimensional VR environment implementing a delayed-matching-to-place (DMTP) protocol. The virtual maze, designed in MazeMaker v3.0.5, presented a circular arena with allocentric cues (external landmarks) displayed on a 14-inch portable PC running Windows 10. Navigation operated in first-person, with participants issuing movement and rotation commands via arrow keys while their view updated dynamically, mirroring real-world orientation (Wang et al., 2025).

Each participant completed eight distinct DMTP problems, each requiring them to locate a hidden $100 bill in the maze. During sample visits, subjects searched for the goal and either received confirmation upon success or were guided to the correct location after a timeout. In the test visits, participants attempted to retrieve the goal from the learned location. A 5-second undistracted delay was contrasted with a 15-second distracted delay (involving reading a silent four-frame comic) to assess impacts of interference on working memory. Trials began from four randomized starting points (N, E, S, W), enhancing the demand for cognitive flexibility. Critically, probe trials (on the 4th and 8th DMTP problems) withheld the target location, allowing for analysis of pure search strategies devoid of goal feedback (Wang et al., 2025).

Key behavioral metrics included latency to target, frequency of unsuccessful trials, freezing time (periods of immobility), and the convex hull area of the search path (as a percentage of arena size). Notably, while younger participants and young-elderly maintain consistent performance levels, decline emerged more clearly in the older-elderly group, especially during probe trials requiring allocentric navigation. Moreover, performance on these trials correlated significantly with Montreal Cognitive Assessment (MoCA) scores, accounting for up to 17 percent of variance beyond age effects, suggesting high sensitivity to broader cognitive integrity (Wang et al., 2025).

Complex Maze Paradigm in Virtual Reality for Spatial Navigation and Memory Research

To complement the previous studies, a recent experiment introduced the Virtual Floor Maze Test (VR-FMT), designed to evaluate navigational strategies and their relationship with executive functions by comparing performance in real and virtual environments. The main objectives were to: (i) develop a VR adaptation of the floor maze test, (ii) compare performance between the real environment (RE) and two VR conditions—no walls (VE-NW) and with walls (VE-W), (iii) examine the contribution of distal visual cues by manipulating wall height, and (iv) explore associations between navigation performance and cognitive test outcomes (Martelli et al., 2019), figure 5.

Figure 5. view of the virtual maze entrance under the VE-NW and VE-W conditions, alongside a top-down schematic of the maze layout generated in Unity 3D. Adapted from Martelli et al. (2019).

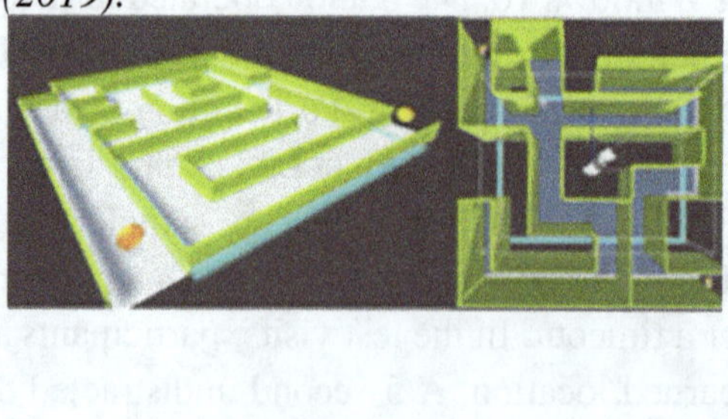

A total of 55 healthy adults participated in the experiment. The maze was built using a Matlab interface that allowed flexible block-based design, saving multiple configurations, and customizing features such as block size and maze dimensions. The virtual environment was rendered using Unity3D and displayed via an HTC VIVE headset, allowing precise tracking of head position at 90 Hz and recording behavioral metrics, including completion time, path length, and number of re-routings (Martelli et al., 2019).

Participants completed the FMT under three conditions: RE, VE-NW, and VE-W. For the VR conditions, the virtual maze was designed to match the real maze's dimensions exactly (3.22 m × 3.68 m), using a 7 × 8 block grid aligned one-to-one with the physical maze. In VE-NW, walls were nearly invisible (0.02 m height), allowing full visibility of the floor plan, whereas in VE-W, walls were set at 2 m height, obstructing distal cues. The order of conditions was counterbalanced across participants to control for learning effects, and performance was measured using both automated recordings and a stopwatch (Martelli et al., 2019).

The findings from the VR-FMT experiment revealed significant differences between real and virtual navigation performance. Completion times in the virtual environment were significantly longer than in the real environment, regardless of wall height. This discrepancy may be attributed to participants' reduced ability to effectively plan their exit during the initial planning phase and/or differences in gait patterns between real and virtual navigation contexts. In the VE-NW condition (no walls), despite longer completion times, only one participant re-routed while exiting, suggesting that participants acquired and used spatial information effectively, similar to performance in the RE. However, introducing high walls in the VE (VE-W) substantially affected performance. The VE-W condition led to increased completion times, a greater number of re-routes, and longer path lengths, indicating that blocking distal visual cues reduced spatial awareness and forced participants to rely on less efficient navigation strategies. Furthermore, correlational analyses showed that only the time to exit the maze in the VE-W condition was significantly associated with cognitive test performance (Martelli et al., 2019).

Extending the application of VR-based maze paradigms into clinical contexts, a novel and innovative approach was proposed through the development of a serious game designed for cognitive stimulation and memory training. Unlike traditional cognitive rehabilitation methods, which rely on printed exercises or specialist-led sessions, this system leverages immersive VR environments to increase engagement, reduce treatment-related stress, and enable personalized assessment of memory performance (Varela-Aldás et al., 2020).

This solution combines maze-based navigation tasks with pattern memorization exercises, incorporating two operational modes: an autonomous mode, where users focus on memorizing geometric shapes and colors while the system guides them to the exit, and a manual mode, where participants actively navigate the maze, adding an executive function component to the task. Performance data are automatically stored and transmitted securely to a server for specialist analysis, enabling remote monitoring and individualized feedback (Varela-Aldás et al., 2020).

The innovation lies in integrating VR immersion, real-time data collection, and interactive memory training into a single cost-effective, portable platform. By merging engaging cognitive tasks with automated performance tracking, this system represents a significant advancement in digital neurorehabilitation, expanding VR maze paradigms from experimental research into practical clinical applications (Varela-Aldás et al., 2020).

Pushing the boundaries of VR-based cognitive assessment, this study introduced an innovative memory training and evaluation system developed using the Unity 3D game engine. Unlike earlier experimental paradigms focused solely on maze navigation or recognition performance, this platform integrates immersive gamification, real-time interaction, and automated data management to provide a comprehensive digital tool for cognitive stimulation and memory monitoring (Varela-Aldás et al., 2020).

The application was designed as a serious game combining maze exploration with pattern memorization tasks of geometric shapes and colors, offering two distinct modes: an autonomous mode for guided navigation and focused memorization, and a manual mode where participants control their movement to reach the maze exit, figure 6. Technically, the system leverages Unity's PhysX physics engine, Mechanism animation system, and C# scripting to create dynamic interactions, including rotating objects, adaptive colliders, and visual effects for enhanced realism. Navigation integrates Smooth Artificial Locomotion techniques, while Unity's NavMesh system allows for seamless autonomous pathfinding (Varela-Aldás et al., 2020).

Figure 6. Difficulty levels and main components of the immersive virtual reality application. The images illustrate scene views at the basic level and at the advanced level. Adapted from Varela-Aldás et al. (2020).

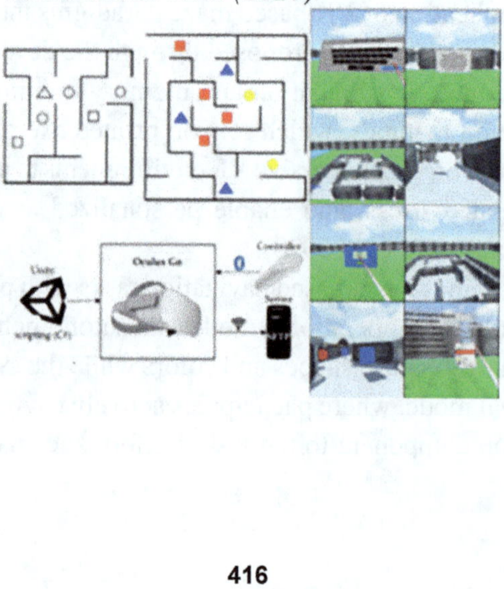

A key innovation lies in its automated data collection and remote analysis. Performance data, including completion times, correct responses, and interaction metrics, are securely transferred to a university-managed SFTP server using SSH. NET protocols, enabling specialists to review results remotely and track longitudinal progress. The system's design prioritizes portability, cost-effectiveness, and accessibility, using Oculus Go HMDs with integrated controllers and lightweight hardware requirements, making it suitable for both clinical and home environments (Varela-Aldás et al., 2020).

Results from 29 participants demonstrated a significant correlation between performance in the VR-based maze task and standardized assessments, such as the face–pair test, validating the system's reliability for objective memory evaluation. Moreover, repeated sessions revealed improvements in memory retention, particularly in the autonomous mode, underscoring its potential as both a training tool and an assessment platform (Varela-Aldás et al., 2020).

Moving beyond traditional navigation tasks, a new immersive VR paradigm was designed to investigate spatial learning and wayfinding under real-time environmental changes and cognitive stressors. In this study, 48 participants (24 female; ages 17–32) explored a 7.5 m × 7.5 m virtual maze (figure 7) using an HTC VIVE Pro Eye head-mounted display within an environment created in Unity. The maze contained 12 distinctive landmarks (paintings) strategically positioned to support spatial orientation, and the task design was adapted from previously validated dual-solution navigation studies (Varshney et al., 2024).

Figure 7. Map of the virtual environment. Landmarks are indicated by orange boxes, while black boxes represent walls. The difference between control and stress trials is illustrated, with stress trials showing a blocked path on the right side. Adapted from Apurv Varshney et al. (2024).

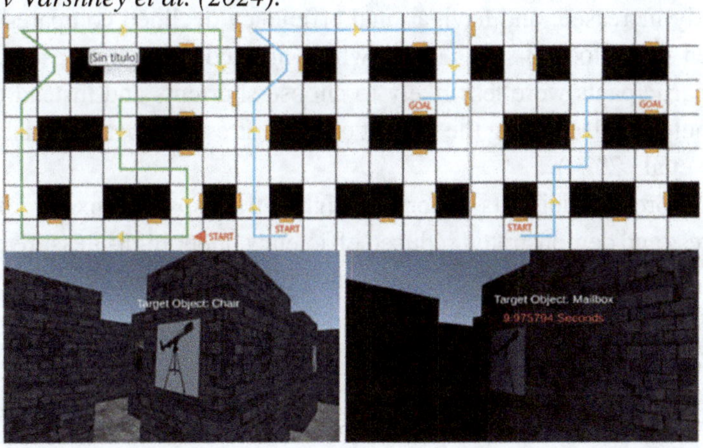

The experiment consisted of three phases. During the learning phase, participants followed a guided route passing all landmarks while naming them aloud on the first trial, repeating the route five times to consolidate spatial memory before retracing it independently. In the testing phase, participants performed 24 wayfinding trials, divided evenly between control and stress conditions. Stress trials introduced dynamic manipulations designed to simulate unpredictable environments, including sudden path obstructions accompanied by loud crashing sounds, time pressure with a 20-second limit and countdown beeps, threat-inducing auditory cues replacing neutral background sounds, and reduced visibility through fog and dim lighting that limited sightlines to 2.5 meters. After each trial, participants rated their perceived stress levels on a 1–7 scale (Varshney et al., 2024).

The findings of this immersive VR study demonstrate that acute stress significantly alters navigation strategies, leading participants to favor habit-based, learned-route strategies over more flexible, cognitive shortcuts, even when the latter were available. Under high-stress conditions, participants navigated less efficiently, exhibiting longer travel distances, lower trial completion rates, and increased reliance on previously learned paths. These behavioral changes suggest that stress induces a shift from goal-directed navigation to automatized spatial responses (Varshney et al., 2024).

Notably, the immersive virtual reality approach used here differs from traditional desktop-based studies by incorporating proprioceptive cues and the physical cost of navigation, providing a more ecologically valid assessment of wayfinding under stress. The inclusion of blocked paths as a stressor closely mirrors real-world navigation challenges, such as those encountered by firefighters facing obstructed corridors, enhancing the study's realism and translational relevance (Varshney et al., 2024).

In trials where participants' initial paths were blocked and additional stressors were introduced, darkened environments, threatening auditory cues, fog-induced visibility reduction, and strict 20-second time limits, self-reported stress levels significantly increased, and navigational efficiency declined compared to control trials. Even in unblocked stress trials, where all navigation options remained accessible, participants were less likely to choose shortcuts and instead reverted to familiar routes, underscoring the impact of acute stress on spatial decision-making (Varshney et al., 2024).

Furthermore, participants reporting higher trait spatial anxiety experienced greater stress and demonstrated reduced efficiency under high-pressure conditions, suggesting an interaction between individual differences and stress-induced navigation impairments (Varshney et al., 2024).

CONCLUSION

As researchers working daily with spatial navigation and memory paradigms, we have witnessed firsthand that VR is not merely a technological innovation but a transformative experimental platform. It allows us to study cognitive processes in conditions that are both controlled and ecologically valid, bridging the gap between laboratory paradigms and real-world behavior. By systematically manipulating spatial cues, cognitive load, and environmental stressors, VR provides an unprecedented opportunity to investigate how memory systems operate in dynamic and naturalistic contexts.

From an applied perspective, VR offers tangible benefits across multiple domains. In clinical practice, VR-based paradigms enhance the detection of subtle spatial memory deficits and support the design of personalized cognitive interventions, improving patient engagement and adherence to treatment. In educational and professional contexts, immersive simulations foster situated learning by promoting active exploration, decision-making, and problem-solving in complex environments. Moreover, the automated collection of behavioral and physiological metrics, such as trajectories, response times, and navigation strategies, provides objective, high-resolution indicators that complement and surpass traditional assessment tools. However, methodological challenges remain. Standardizing experimental protocols, minimizing simulator sickness, and ensuring cross-platform comparability are essential next steps for consolidating VR as a robust research tool.

REFERENCES

Ben-Zeev, T., Weiss, I., Ashri, S., Heled, Y., Ketko, I., Yanovich, R., & Okun, E. (2020). Mild Physical Activity Does Not Improve Spatial Learning in a Virtual Environment. *Frontiers in Behavioral Neuroscience*, *14*, 584052. DOI: 10.3389/fnbeh.2020.584052

Chirico, A., Lucidi, F., De Laurentiis, M., Milanese, C., Napoli, A., & Giordano, A. (2016). Virtual Reality in Health System: Beyond Entertainment. A Mini-Review on the Efficacy of VR During Cancer Treatment. *Journal of Cellular Physiology*, *231*(2), 275–287. DOI: 10.1002/jcp.25117

Chirico, A., Maiorano, P., Indovina, P., Milanese, C., Giordano, G. G., Alivernini, F., Iodice, G., Gallo, L., De Pietro, G., Lucidi, F., Botti, G., De Laurentiis, M., & Giordano, A. (2020). Virtual reality and music therapy as distraction interventions to alleviate anxiety and improve mood states in breast cancer patients during chemotherapy. *Journal of Cellular Physiology*, *235*(6), 5353–5362. DOI: 10.1002/jcp.29422

Chitale, V., Baghaei, N., Playne, D., Liang, H.-N., Zhao, Y., Erensoy, A., & Ahmad, Y. (2022). The Use of Videogames and Virtual Reality for the Assessment of Anxiety and Depression: A Scoping Review. *Games for Health Journal*, *11*(6), 341–354. Advance online publication. DOI: 10.1089/g4h.2021.0227

Cimadevilla, J. M., Nori, R., & Piccardi, L. (2023). Application of Virtual Reality in Spatial Memory. *Brain Sciences*, *13*(12), 1621. DOI: 10.3390/brainsci13121621

Cipresso, P., Giglioli, I. A. C., Raya, M. A., & Riva, G. (2018). The Past, Present, and Future of Virtual and Augmented Reality Research: A Network and Cluster Analysis of the Literature. *Frontiers in Psychology*, *9*, 2086. DOI: 10.3389/fpsyg.2018.02086

Cogné, M., Taillade, M., N'Kaoua, B., Tarruella, A., Klinger, E., Larrue, F., Sauzéon, H., Joseph, P.-A., & Sorita, E. (2017). The contribution of virtual reality to the diagnosis of spatial navigation disorders and to the study of the role of navigational aids: A systematic literature review. *Annals of Physical and Rehabilitation Medicine*, *60*(3), 164–176. DOI: 10.1016/j.rehab.2015.12.004

D'Cunha, N. M., Nguyen, D., Naumovski, N., McKune, A. J., Kellett, J., Georgousopoulou, E. N., Frost, J., & Isbel, S. (2019). A Mini-Review of Virtual Reality-Based Interventions to Promote Well-Being for People Living with Dementia and Mild Cognitive Impairment. *Gerontology*, *65*(4), 430–440. DOI: 10.1159/000500040

Dale, R. H. (1986). Spatial and temporal response patterns on the eight-arm radial maze. *Physiology & Behavior*, *36*(4), 787–790. DOI: 10.1016/0031-9384(86)90370-7

Eichenbaum, H. (1999). The hippocampus and mechanisms of declarative memory. *Behavioural Brain Research, 103*(2), 123–133. DOI: 10.1016/S0166-4328(99)00044-3

Fernández-Batanero, J. M., Montenegro-Rueda, M., & Fernández-Cerero, J. (2022). Use of Augmented Reality for Students with Educational Needs: A Systematic Review (2016–2021). *Societies (Basel, Switzerland), 12*(2), 36. DOI: 10.3390/soc12020036

Flexner, J. B., Flexner, L. B., & Stellar, E. (1963). Memory in Mice as Affected by Intracerebral Puromycin. *Science, 141*(3575), 57–59. DOI: 10.1126/science.141.3575.57

Hofmann, M., Rösler, A., Schwarz, W., Müller-Spahn, F., Kräuchi, K., Hock, C., & Seifritz, E. (2003). Interactive computer-training as a therapeutic tool in Alzheimer's disease. *Comprehensive Psychiatry, 44*(3), 213–219. DOI: 10.1016/S0010-440X(03)00006-3

Hořejší, P., Lochmannová, A., Jezl, V., & Dvořák, M. (2025). Virtual reality locomotion methods differentially affect spatial orientation and cybersickness during maze navigation. *Scientific Reports, 15*(1), 26255. DOI: 10.1038/s41598-025-12143-y

Jonson, M., Avramescu, S., Chen, D., & Alam, F. (2021). The Role of Virtual Reality in Screening, Diagnosing, and Rehabilitating Spatial Memory Deficits. *Frontiers in Human Neuroscience, 15*, 628818. DOI: 10.3389/fnhum.2021.628818

Josselyn, S. A., Köhler, S., & Frankland, P. W. (2017). Heroes of the Engram. *The Journal of Neuroscience : The Official Journal of the Society for Neuroscience, 37*(18), 4647–4657. DOI: 10.1523/JNEUROSCI.0056-17.2017

Kandel, E. R. (2012). The molecular biology of memory: cAMP, PKA, CRE, CREB-1, CREB-2, and CPEB. *Molecular Brain, 5*(1), 14. DOI: 10.1186/1756-6606-5-14

Kellems, R. O., Eichelberger, C., Cacciatore, G., Jensen, M., Frazier, B., Simons, K., & Zaru, M. (2020). Using Video-Based Instruction via Augmented Reality to Teach Mathematics to Middle School Students With Learning Disabilities. *Journal of Learning Disabilities, 53*(4), 277–291. DOI: 10.1177/0022219420906452

Kim, H., Park, J. Y., & Kim, K. K. (2018). Spatial Learning and Memory Using a Radial Arm Maze with a Head-Mounted Display. *Psychiatry Investigation, 15*(10), 935–944. DOI: 10.30773/pi.2018.06.28.3

Krajčovič, M., Matys, M., Gabajová, G., & Komačka, D. (2024). Utilization of Immersive Virtual Reality as an Interactive Method of Assignment Presentation. *Electronics (Basel), 13*(8), 1430. DOI: 10.3390/electronics13081430

Ma, C.-W., Cheng, P.-S., Chan, Y.-S., & Tipoe, G. L. (2023). Virtual reality: A technology to promote active learning of physiology for students across multiple disciplines. *Advances in Physiology Education*, *47*(3), 594–603. DOI: 10.1152/advan.00172.2022

Martelli, D., Prado, A., Xia, B., Verghese, J., & Agrawal, S. K. (2019). Development of a Virtual Floor Maze Test—Effects of Distal Visual Cues and Correlations With Executive Function in Healthy Adults. *IEEE Transactions on Neural Systems and Rehabilitation Engineering: A Publication of the IEEE Engineering in Medicine and Biology Society*, *27*(10), 2229–2236. DOI: 10.1109/TNSRE.2019.2938103

McGaugh, J. L. (2000). Memory—A Century of Consolidation. *Science*, *287*(5451), 248–251. DOI: 10.1126/science.287.5451.248

Mei, J., Kohler, J., Winter, Y., Spies, C., Endres, M., Banneke, S., & Emmrich, J. V. (2020). Automated radial 8-arm maze: A voluntary and stress-free behavior test to assess spatial learning and memory in mice. *Behavioural Brain Research*, *381*, 112352. DOI: 10.1016/j.bbr.2019.112352

Merlo, S. A., Belluscio, M. A., Pedreira, M. E., & Merlo, E. (2024). Memory persistence: From fundamental mechanisms to translational opportunities. *Translational Psychiatry*, *14*(1), 98. DOI: 10.1038/s41398-024-02808-z

Minderer, M., Harvey, C. D., Donato, F., & Moser, E. I. (2016). Neuroscience: Virtual reality explored. *Nature*, *533*(7603), 324–325. DOI: 10.1038/nature17899

Montana, J. I., Tuena, C., Serino, S., Cipresso, P., & Riva, G. (2019). Neurorehabilitation of Spatial Memory Using Virtual Environments: A Systematic Review. *Journal of Clinical Medicine*, *8*(10), 1516. DOI: 10.3390/jcm8101516

Pacheco, D., Sánchez-Fibla, M., Duff, A., & Verschure, P. F. M. J. (2017). A Spatial-Context Effect in Recognition Memory. *Frontiers in Behavioral Neuroscience*, *11*, 143. DOI: 10.3389/fnbeh.2017.00143

Parmar, D., Lin, L., DSouza, N., Jörg, S., Leonard, A. E., Daily, S. B., & Babu, S. V. (2023). How Immersion and Self-Avatars in VR Affect Learning Programming and Computational Thinking in Middle School Education. *IEEE Transactions on Visualization and Computer Graphics*, *29*(8), 3698–3713. DOI: 10.1109/TVCG.2022.3169426

Reijmers, L. G., Perkins, B. L., Matsuo, N., & Mayford, M. (2007). Localization of a Stable Neural Correlate of Associative Memory. *Science*, *317*(5842), 1230–1233. DOI: 10.1126/science.1143839

Rolls, E. T. (2022). The hippocampus, ventromedial prefrontal cortex, and episodic and semantic memory. *Progress in Neurobiology, 217*, 102334. DOI: 10.1016/j.pneurobio.2022.102334

Sagaspe, P., Amieva, H., Dartigues, J.-F., Olive, J., de la Rivière, J.-B., Chartier, C., Taillard, J., & Philip, P. (2023). Validity and diagnostic performance of a virtual reality-based supermarket application "MEMOSHOP" for assessing episodic memory in normal and pathological aging. *Digital Health, 9*, 20552076231218808. DOI: 10.1177/20552076231218808

Tischmeyer, W., & Grimm, R. (1999). Activation of immediate early genes and memory formation. *Cellular and Molecular Life Sciences : CMLS, 55*(4), 564–574. DOI: 10.1007/s000180050315

van der Ham, I. J. M., Faber, A. M. E., Venselaar, M., van Kreveld, M. J., & Löffler, M. (2015). Ecological validity of virtual environments to assess human navigation ability. *Frontiers in Psychology, 6*, 637. DOI: 10.3389/fpsyg.2015.00637

Varela-Aldás, J., Palacios-Navarro, G., Amariglio, R., & García-Magariño, I. (2020). Head-Mounted Display-Based Application for Cognitive Training. *Sensors (Basel), 20*(22), 6552. DOI: 10.3390/s20226552

Varshney, A., Munns, M. E., Kasowski, J., Zhou, M., He, C., Grafton, S. T., Giesbrecht, B., Hegarty, M., & Beyeler, M. (2024). Stress affects navigation strategies in immersive virtual reality. *Scientific Reports, 14*(1), 5949. DOI: 10.1038/s41598-024-56048-8

Wang, E. H. J., Lai, F. H. Y., Leung, W. M., Shiu, T. Y., Wong, H., Tao, Y., Zhao, X., Zhang, T. Y. T., & Yee, B. K. (2025). Assessing rapid spatial working memory in community-living older adults in a virtual adaptation of the rodent water maze paradigm. *Behavioural Brain Research, 476*, 115266. DOI: 10.1016/j.bbr.2024.115266

Weiss, P. L. T., Bialik, P., & Kizony, R. (2003). Virtual reality provides leisure time opportunities for young adults with physical and intellectual disabilities. *Cyberpsychology & Behavior, 6*(3), 335–342. DOI: 10.1089/109493103322011650

Wiebe, A., Kannen, K., Selaskowski, B., Mehren, A., Thöne, A.-K., Pramme, L., Blumenthal, N., Li, M., Asché, L., Jonas, S., Bey, K., Schulze, M., Steffens, M., Pensel, M. C., Guth, M., Rohlfsen, F., Ekhlas, M., Lügering, H., Fileccia, H., & Braun, N. (2022). Virtual reality in the diagnostic and therapy for mental disorders: A systematic review. *Clinical Psychology Review, 98*, 102213. DOI: 10.1016/j.cpr.2022.102213

Xu, D., Hao, X., Wang, Z., Duan, Y., Liu, F., Marsh, R., Yu, S., & Peterson, B. S. (2012). A Virtual Radial Arm Maze for the Study of Multiple Memory Systems in a Functional Magnetic Resonance Imaging Environment. *The International Journal of Virtual Reality : a Multimedia Publication for Professionals*, *11*(2), 63–76. DOI: 10.20870/IJVR.2012.11.2.2844

Chapter 13
Integrating Generative AI for Personalized Learning in Cryptography Education:
A Case Study With LLM-Driven Learning Activities

César Alejandro García
https://orcid.org/0000-0002-8781-575X
Universidad de Guadalajara, Mexico

Carolina Livier Recio-Colmenares
Universidad de Guadalajara, Mexico

Roxana B. Recio-Colmenares
Universidad de Guadalajara, Mexico

Eduardo F. Mejia-Lucatero
https://orcid.org/0009-0006-4437-978X
Universidad de Guadalajara, Mexico

José Luis Fernández-Robles
https://orcid.org/0000-0002-2273-529X
Universidad de Guadalajara, Mexico

ABSTRACT

This chapter presents a longitudinal case study on the integration of generative artificial intelligence (AI), specifically Large Language Models (LLMs), into the

DOI: 10.4018/979-8-3373-4657-1.ch013

teaching of cryptography at the undergraduate level. Conducted over eight academic terms at the Universidad de Guadalajara, the study analyzes how LLM-driven activities—such as personalized explanations, automated problem generation, and cryptanalysis simulations—impacted student learning. The implementation of a standardized final examination beginning in 2024B enabled consistent cross-cohort comparisons. Results show an initial performance dip during the transition phase, followed by stabilization and improved consistency. The findings suggest that LLMs can serve as adaptive scaffolding tools, supporting diverse learners in mastering abstract technical content. The chapter also explores the ethical, legal, and pedagogical considerations of using AI in education, offering a replicable model for integrating generative AI into STEM curricula.

1. INTRODUCTION

Cryptography is a core component of digital security and is essential to protocols governing confidentiality, authentication, and data integrity in information systems. In university-level computing curricula, cryptography is situated at the intersection of discrete mathematics, algorithm design, and cybersecurity—a combination that makes it both conceptually rich and pedagogically demanding. Undergraduate students often encounter difficulty connecting theoretical models underpinning encryption systems with their algorithmic implementations, particularly when instruction relies on lectures and static exercises with limited interactivity.

Recent advances in generative artificial intelligence—especially the emergence of Large Language Models (LLMs)—have introduced new possibilities for enhancing instruction in complex technical fields. These tools are capable of producing tailored explanations, generating domain-specific exercises, simulating cryptographic operations, and assisting students with real-time feedback. Despite growing interest in their educational applications, there is limited empirical research on how such tools affect learning outcomes in algorithm-intensive domains like cryptography.

This chapter presents a longitudinal case study documenting the staged integration of LLM-supported learning activities in the IH063 Cryptography course at the Universidad de Guadalajara. Spanning eight academic terms from 2022A to 2025A, the study tracks evolving instructional practices and student performance across traditional, transitional, and standardized assessment phases. Rather than testing a single hypothesis, the chapter adopts an exploratory design to identify instructional patterns, challenges, and opportunities associated with the adoption of generative AI in a real-world STEM learning environment.

The chapter is organized into eight sections. Section 2 reviews the literature on cryptography education, gamification, and the emerging role of generative AI in learning. Section 3 situates cryptography within legal, ethical, and human rights frameworks relevant to data protection. Section 4 describes the design and implementation of AI-supported instructional activities. Section 5 presents observational results from eight academic terms, highlighting performance trends. Section 6 discusses pedagogical implications and the role of LLMs as cognitive scaffolds. Section 7 outlines future research priorities, and Section 8 offers concluding reflections on the use of generative AI in technical STEM education.

2. BACKGROUND AND RELATED WORK

Cryptography is a core subfield of computer science concerned with securing information through mathematical and algorithmic techniques. In the context of undergraduate education, standard learning objectives typically include understanding classical and modern cipher systems, implementing symmetric and asymmetric encryption schemes, analyzing cryptographic protocols, and applying number theory concepts such as modular arithmetic and probability. Traditional teaching approaches rely heavily on lectures, static problem sets, and pen-and-paper exercises. However, these strategies often fail to bridge the gap between abstract theory and real-world application, particularly for students with limited mathematical background or experience in formal systems. This pedagogical challenge has prompted increasing interest in interactive, gamified, and AI-supported methods to enhance conceptual understanding and learner engagement.

2.1. Pedagogical Challenges in Cryptography Education

Cryptography occupies a foundational role in computer science curricula, preparing students to design and secure digital systems in an increasingly interconnected world. However, teaching cryptography poses notable challenges. Students must master abstract mathematical constructs, algorithmic thinking, and information theory while applying this knowledge to implement secure protocols and analyze vulnerabilities. Traditional lecture-based methods and static exercises often fail to promote deep understanding or real-world application (Adamovic et al., 2018; Koblitz, 1997).

2.2. Active Learning and Gamification in Technical Domains

Active learning methodologies have emerged as effective strategies for improving student engagement and learning outcomes in technical fields such as cryptography. These approaches shift the learning experience from passive absorption of information to active student participation, problem-solving, and application of knowledge in realistic contexts (Sakalli et al., 2004).

Gamification and simulation-based learning environments have received growing attention due to their potential to increase motivation and support experiential learning. Tools such as **Crypto Go**—a card game designed to teach cryptographic algorithms—and **3D escape-room simulations** have demonstrated positive effects on student engagement and self-reported understanding (Deeb & Hickey, 2019; González-Tablas et al., 2020). However, these interventions are often implemented in small-scale pilot settings or extracurricular workshops, typically with students at the introductory or high school level. Their results, while promising, are not directly generalizable to university-level STEM instruction without further validation.

Moreover, most published studies of these tools emphasize qualitative feedback or short-term motivation gains, with limited evidence of effect sizes or long-term retention. For instance, Crypto Go has been praised for promoting peer discussion and concept exposure, but lacks formal evaluation through standardized assessments or comparative control designs. Similarly, the escape-room models create immersive contexts but are often time- and resource-intensive, reducing scalability in standard curricular environments.

Project-based learning approaches (Alhamdani, 2016) have also proven effective in technical fields, promoting collaboration and critical thinking. Yet these interventions often require extensive faculty training and do not scale easily in large undergraduate courses.

In this context, our study contributes a complementary perspective by exploring how generative AI—specifically Large Language Models—can support scalable, personalized, and adaptive learning activities within the formal structure of an undergraduate cryptography course. Rather than focusing solely on engagement, we examine longitudinal academic performance across multiple cohorts and assess how AI-driven instructional strategies can influence outcome consistency in high-complexity learning domains.

2.3. Generative AI and Large Language Models in Education

The rapid advancement of artificial intelligence, particularly in the domain of Large Language Models (LLMs), introduces a new dimension to technology-enhanced learning. Generative AI systems such as GPT-4, Gemini, and other LLM-based tools possess the ability to process natural language queries, generate customized content, and simulate interactive dialogue. These capabilities enable them to offer students real-time support in solving complex problems, understanding abstract concepts, and navigating technical procedures.

In our instructional design, LLMs are not treated as standalone instructional agents but as tools embedded within a broader theory of change rooted in cognitive apprenticeship and scaffolded learning. Specifically, we hypothesize that:

- Cognitive Load Reduction: By offloading procedural tasks—such as modular arithmetic or syntactic debugging—LLMs allow students to allocate more cognitive resources to conceptual reasoning.
- Immediate Feedback: LLMs simulate responsive tutoring, providing context-aware clarification and explanations that reduce frustration and improve learning efficiency.
- Personalized Exploration: The interactive nature of LLMs allows students to explore content at their own pace and revisit topics as needed, accommodating diverse learning styles and prior preparation levels.
- Situated Learning: Through simulation scenarios and cryptographic challenges, students apply theory in near-authentic contexts, reinforcing transfer of knowledge to practical tasks.

Rather than assuming impact, our study observes how these mechanisms correlate with changes in student performance and engagement over time. While causal inference is limited by the study design, the alignment between theory, practice, and observed stabilization in performance suggests that LLM integration supports conceptual learning in a high-complexity technical domain.

2.4. Need for Longitudinal, Contextualized Evidence

Despite promising developments, the literature reveals a gap in long-term, contextualized evaluations of generative AI in technical courses. Most studies examine short-term interventions or pilot implementations without rigorous tracking of academic performance. Few address the interplay between active learning, AI support, and gamified tasks in abstract disciplines like cryptography.

This chapter contributes to closing that gap by presenting a longitudinal case study of LLM-supported instruction across eight academic terms in a university-level cryptography course. By focusing on practical outcomes and instructional design evolution, it provides empirical grounding for future, more controlled investigations.

3. THEORETICAL AND LEGAL FOUNDATIONS OF CRYPTOGRAPHY AND DATA PROTECTION

3.1. Cryptography and Fundamental Rights

In the Mexican legal framework, the right to privacy and the protection of personal data are principally enshrined in Article 16 of the Political Constitution of the United Mexican States. This article explicitly recognizes individuals' rights to data protection and regulates access to personal information held by both public and private entities. Complementing this constitutional provision, the Federal Law on Protection of Personal Data Held by Private Parties (Ley Federal de Protección de Datos Personales en Posesión de los Particulares) and the General Law on Protection of Personal Data Held by Obligated Subjects (Ley General de Protección de Datos Personales en Posesión de Sujetos Obligados) establish comprehensive mechanisms for the lawful collection, storage, processing, and safeguarding of personal data.

In this context, cryptographic systems serve as essential technical enablers for the exercise of these rights. Encryption protocols allow individuals and institutions to enforce confidentiality, ensure secure communication, and control access to sensitive information in compliance with legal obligations. By framing cryptography within this legal foundation, particularly Article 16 and its associated regulatory instruments, this chapter situates technical instruction not only within a scientific and pedagogical framework but also within a normative one that highlights the civic relevance of secure information practices.

3.2. Legal Framework for Data Protection and Transparency in Mexico

Mexico's legal architecture concerning transparency and data protection has evolved significantly over the past two decades. While earlier discussions focused on the Federal Law on Transparency and Access to Public Government Information (2002), this framework has since been replaced and expanded by the General Law of Transparency and Access to Public Information (Ley General de Transparencia y Acceso a la Información Pública), enacted in 2015. This law establishes standardized mechanisms and principles for transparency across all levels of government and reaffirms the protection of classified and personal data as an essential counterbalance to public access.

In parallel, the General Law on Protection of Personal Data Held by Obligated Subjects (Ley General de Protección de Datos Personales en Posesión de Sujetos Obligados) governs how public institutions handle personal data, while the Federal Law on Protection of Personal Data Held by Private Parties applies to the private sector. These instruments collectively implement Article 16 of the Constitution, which enshrines the right to privacy and data protection.

Cryptographic systems are essential to ensuring compliance with these legal mandates. Encryption safeguards the confidentiality and integrity of sensitive digital records, supports data minimization and security by design, and enables institutions to meet their legal obligations regarding secure data handling, especially in digital government and academic environments.

3.3. Institutional Guidelines and Governance

In response to the ethical and legal complexities associated with the integration of artificial intelligence into educational environments, the Universidad de Guadalajara published the *Guía para el uso responsable de inteligencia artificial en contextos académicos* (2023), which establishes institutional principles for the responsible and pedagogically sound use of generative AI in higher education. The document outlines core ethical and academic principles, including: (a) transparency in the acknowledgment of AI-assisted work, (b) the cultivation of critical thinking and preservation of student authorship, (c) the avoidance of overreliance or passive dependence on AI systems, and (d) the protection of academic integrity through human-centered evaluation processes (Universidad de Guadalajara, 2023).

Although the guidelines are advisory rather than prescriptive, they reflect a growing institutional commitment to ethical AI governance that aligns with national legal frameworks and international human rights standards. Within the scope of this study, all uses of generative AI were governed by these institutional principles. Students were required to disclose when AI tools were used in the completion of academic tasks and were trained to critically evaluate AI-generated outputs for accuracy and bias. Faculty members retained full oversight of activity design, implementation, and evaluation, ensuring that AI served as a pedagogical aid rather than a substitute for authentic learning. As generative AI technologies continue to evolve, ongoing revisions to institutional policies will be essential to ensure continued compliance with ethical, legal, and educational standards.

4. METHODOLOGY

4.1. Course Context and Participants

This study was conducted in the IH063 Cryptography course, part of the undergraduate Computer Science Engineering program at the Universidad de Guadalajara. The course is mandatory for students pursuing specializations in cybersecurity and information systems and introduces both theoretical and practical components of classical and modern cryptographic systems. Topics include encryption and decryption algorithms, key exchange protocols, hash functions, basic cryptanalysis, and information security principles.

While the study was conducted within a single academic program, student cohorts varied naturally over time, and no random assignment or experimental manipulation was employed. The analysis therefore reflects **observational insights**, not controlled evaluation.

The study spans eight academic terms (2022A to 2025A), with a total of 282 students distributed across different schedules (morning, afternoon, and evening). The instructional approach evolved over time: early cohorts (2022A–2023B) received conventional instruction, while later cohorts (2024A–2025A) experienced progressive integration of LLM-enhanced activities. Starting in 2024B, a standardized final examination was implemented to allow for consistent cross-cohort performance comparisons.

A sample version of the exam, shown in Figure 1, includes both conceptual and applied questions to evaluate students' theoretical understanding and problem-solving ability in real-world cryptographic contexts. These standardized items ensure alignment with course learning objectives and support objective measurement of knowledge transfer.

Figure 1. Extract from the standardized departmental exam introduced in term 2024B, assessing core cryptography concepts and real-world application scenarios.

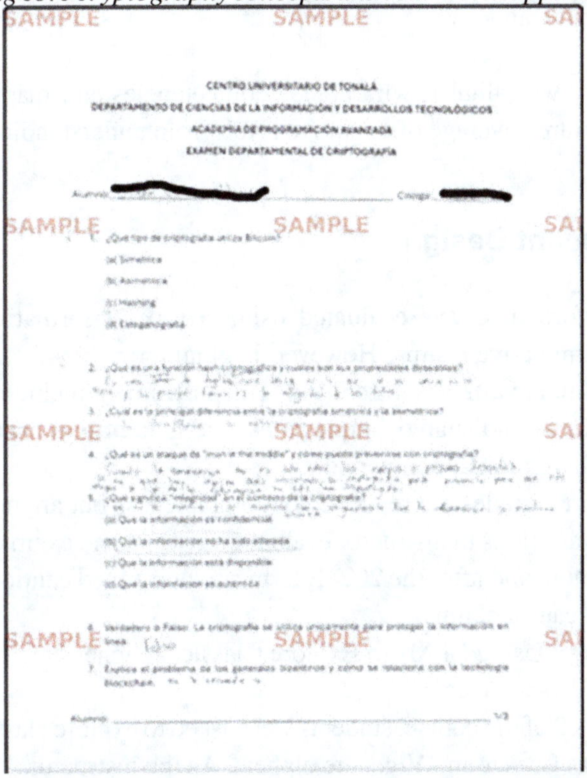

CENTRO UNIVERSITARIO DE TONALÁ

DEPARTAMENTO DE CIENCIAS DE LA INFORMACIÓN Y DESARROLLOS TECNOLÓGICOS

ACADEMIA DE PROGRAMACIÓN AVANZADA

EXAMEN DEPARTAMENTAL DE CRIPTOGRAFÍA

Alumno: ______ Código: ______

1. ¿Qué tipo de criptografía utiliza Bitcoin?

(a) Simétrica

(b) Asimétrica

(c) Hashing

(d) Esteganografía

2. ¿Qué es una función hash criptográfica y cuáles son sus propiedades deseables?

3. ¿Cuál es la principal diferencia entre la criptografía simétrica y la asimétrica?

4. ¿Qué es un ataque de "man in the middle" y cómo puede prevenirse con criptografía?

5. ¿Qué significa "integridad" en el contexto de la criptografía?

(a) Que la información es confidencial

(b) Que la información no ha sido alterada

(c) Que la información está disponible

(d) Que la información es auténtica

6. Verdadero o Falso: La criptografía se utiliza únicamente para proteger la información en línea.

7. Explica el problema de los generales bizantinos y cómo se relaciona con la tecnología blockchain.

Alumno: ______ 1/2

This is a descriptive longitudinal case study, not an experimental design. As such, no control group was established, and no random assignment was performed. Instead, the analysis focuses on naturalistic observation of performance trends and instructional evolution under real-world constraints.

4.2. Instructional Design and Phased Integration of LLM Activities

The LLM-based interventions were introduced progressively to ensure curricular alignment and instructor readiness. The implementation followed three main phases:

- Phase 1 (2023A–2023B): Pilot use of LLMs as voluntary, student-driven support tools.
- Phase 2 (2024A): Structured integration of LLM-generated content in class activities, including interactive problem sets and algorithm simulations.

- Phase 3 (2024B–2025A): Full curricular incorporation, with LLMs used to scaffold active learning tasks, generate personalized feedback, and simulate cryptographic attacks.

Each activity was aligned with course competencies and mapped to Bloom's taxonomy to ensure coverage of cognitive levels from understanding to application and analysis.

4.3. Assessment Design

Student performance was evaluated using a mix of formative assessments, projects, and summative exams. However, beginning in **2024B**, a **departmental standardized final exam** was introduced. This instrument includes a mix of algorithmic, procedural, and analytical questions, and is **identical across all cohorts**, allowing valid longitudinal comparisons.

Earlier cohorts' grades are reported for completeness but are not directly comparable due to variations in instructor evaluation criteria and exam difficulty. Thus, comparisons before and after the 2024B term are interpreted cautiously and are not used to support causal claims.

Case Scenario: Using LLMs to Explore Classical Ciphers

Instructor's Perspective:

During Week 3 of the course, students were asked to explore classical encryption methods, such as Caesar and Vigenère ciphers. As the instructor, I provided initial guidance and shared a curated prompt for students to use with an LLM:

"Simulate a Vigenère cipher encryption and decryption using the key 'CRYPTO' for the plaintext 'SECURITYMATTERS'. Show each step."

Students were encouraged to modify the prompt and reflect on the output. I reminded them that any AI-generated explanation should be critically evaluated and verified with course notes or manual calculations.

Student's Perspective (6th semester):

"At first, I copied the prompt and got the correct answer. But then I tried changing the key and realized the model made a mistake and it repeated a character where it shouldn't. That made me go back to the algorithm and figure out why. It was like having a lab partner who knows a lot but still needs checking."

This scenario exemplifies how generative AI was positioned as a **tool for sense-making** rather than answer retrieval, prompting students to reflect, verify, and ultimately deepen their understanding of cryptographic mechanisms.

4.4. Data collection and analysis

Final course grades were collected for each term. For standardized-exam cohorts, item-level data were also reviewed to evaluate the distribution of competencies. Data was anonymized and aggregated.

To identify trends, descriptive statistics (mean, range, standard deviation) were computed. We also examined grade dispersion to explore whether the LLM-based interventions helped reduce performance inequality. No inferential statistical tests (e.g., ANOVA, regression) were used due to the absence of randomization and small cohort sizes.

Additionally, informal qualitative feedback was collected through in-class reflections and unstructured comments. These were not coded systematically but were used to contextualize the quantitative findings.

4.5. Limitations and Design Considerations

This study relies on longitudinal comparisons of naturally occurring cohorts, with instructional design progressively evolving to integrate LLM-supported activities. However, no formal control groups were established, and variations in student populations across terms—such as differences in prior academic preparation, instructor styles, or contextual factors—introduce confounding elements that limit internal validity. As such, the trends observed should be interpreted as suggestive patterns, not causal claims.

This chapter is intended to be hypothesis-generating rather than hypothesis-testing. The aim is to document real-world instructional shifts, identify emerging patterns, and surface practical challenges that can inform future research. Subsequent studies will pursue more rigorous research designs, including matched cohort comparisons, mixed-method assessments of learning gains, and formal evaluations of LLM contributions to cognitive load reduction and conceptual mastery.

The results presented here serve as a practical foundation for controlled investigations, grounded in the realities of large-scale implementation within higher education contexts.

4.6. Ethical Safeguards and Data Governance

Although this study did not require formal approval from an Institutional Review Board (IRB) due to its instructional and non-invasive nature, all procedures were conducted in accordance with the ethical standards outlined in the *Guía para el uso responsable de inteligencia artificial en contextos académicos* (Universidad de Guadalajara, 2023).

All student data were anonymized prior to analysis, and only aggregate metrics were reported to preserve individual confidentiality. Activities involving LLMs were designed to avoid the inclusion of personally identifiable information. No sensitive student data were transmitted to external servers without prior sanitization. Interactions with generative AI were limited to publicly available platforms under educational licenses, and faculty maintained oversight of all AI-assisted exercises.

Additionally, plagiarism detection software (Turnitin) was employed to check all student submissions for originality, and any suspected misuse of AI tools was subject to manual review and follow-up by instructors. While this study does not test alternative hypotheses or causal explanations formally, these ethical safeguards support the integrity and transparency of the instructional intervention.

5. EXPERIMENTAL RESULTS

5.1. Data Collection

To evaluate the impact of LLM-driven learning activities on student performance, longitudinal data were collected from eight consecutive academic terms spanning from 2022A to 2025A. Each cohort's final grades were recorded, anonymized, and aggregated for analysis. The dataset captures both pre-intervention and post-intervention periods, offering a natural experiment to observe the transition from traditional instruction to LLM-enhanced pedagogy.

For cohorts prior to 2024B, final course grades were used as the primary performance metric. Beginning in 2024B, a standardized assessment instrument was introduced, allowing for direct cross-cohort comparisons and increased validity of performance measures in evaluating the impact of LLM-based learning activities.

It is important to note that final course grades in earlier cohorts were determined by instructors using diverse evaluation criteria, while a **standardized final exam** was introduced beginning in 2024B. As a result, direct comparison of average grades across all terms must be interpreted with caution. The results reflect a total of 282 students analyzed throughout the study period.

5.2. Verification of AI Output

To assess the reliability of LLM-generated outputs used in instructional activities, selected results were systematically compared against deterministic tools. For tasks such as modular arithmetic, frequency distribution analysis, and index of coincidence calculations, benchmark outputs were generated using independently verified Python scripts and established online cryptographic calculators.

The comparison revealed that LLMs such as ChatGPT and Gemini were able to produce correct results in most typical cases, particularly when prompts were well-structured and the mathematical context clearly specified. However, occasional errors were observed when the prompts were vague, or when multi-step reasoning was required. For example, in the calculation of modular inverses, LLMs sometimes failed to apply the extended Euclidean algorithm correctly when not explicitly prompted to do so.

These observations reinforce the importance of positioning LLMs as cognitive scaffolds rather than authoritative solvers. Students were trained to validate AI-generated results against known methods and to reflect on discrepancies as learning opportunities. In this sense, the integration of generative AI was framed not as automation of solution procedures but as a means to foster critical mathematical thinking within applied cryptography.

5.3. Observed Trends

The data reveal distinct performance patterns that correlate with the introduction and progressive integration of LLM-based instructional activities:

- Pre-Intervention Performance (2022A - 2022B): Students in these cohorts, who experienced fully traditional instruction, exhibited high average grades ranging from 91% to 96%, suggesting solid baseline performance under conventional teaching methods.
- Transitional Phase (2023A - 2023B): During the early experimental phases of AI integration, a temporary decline in average grades was observed, with averages dropping to 83%–85%. This period likely reflects the pedagogical and cognitive adjustment required as both instructors and students adapted to the new learning model.
- Stabilization and Recovery (2024A - 2025A): As the LLM-driven activities matured and instructional design stabilized, performance averages began to recover. A steady upward trend emerged, with average grades reaching 88% by 2025A. This suggests that, once fully integrated, LLM-based activities may contribute to improved comprehension, engagement, and outcome consistency.

The temporary decline and subsequent recovery in average grades reflect not only instructional design changes but also **shifts in assessment standardization**.

Performance data from 2024B and 2025A cohorts provide a more consistent basis for comparison due to the use of a common evaluation instrument.

To provide more transparency about performance variability, Table 1 summarizes the mean and standard deviation of final grades per cohort.

Table 1. Summary of Final Grade Statistics by Cohort

Period	Mean Grade (%)	Std. Deviation	Assessment Type
2022A	95.86	4.91	Instructor-based
2022B AM	93.54	6.02	Instructor-based
2022B PM	91.64	8.11	Instructor-based
2023A	85.00	10.23	Instructor-based
2023B	83.00	9.78	Instructor-based
2024A	86.00	7.62	Instructor-based
2024B	84.00	5.94	Standardized exam
2025A	88.00	4.87	Standardized exam

Figure 2 visualizes these distributions, illustrating the observed narrowing of grade dispersion in later terms. While these patterns are suggestive, we refrain from asserting statistical significance and instead present them as exploratory insights pending further controlled validation.

Figure 2. Average Grades and Standard Deviation by Cohort

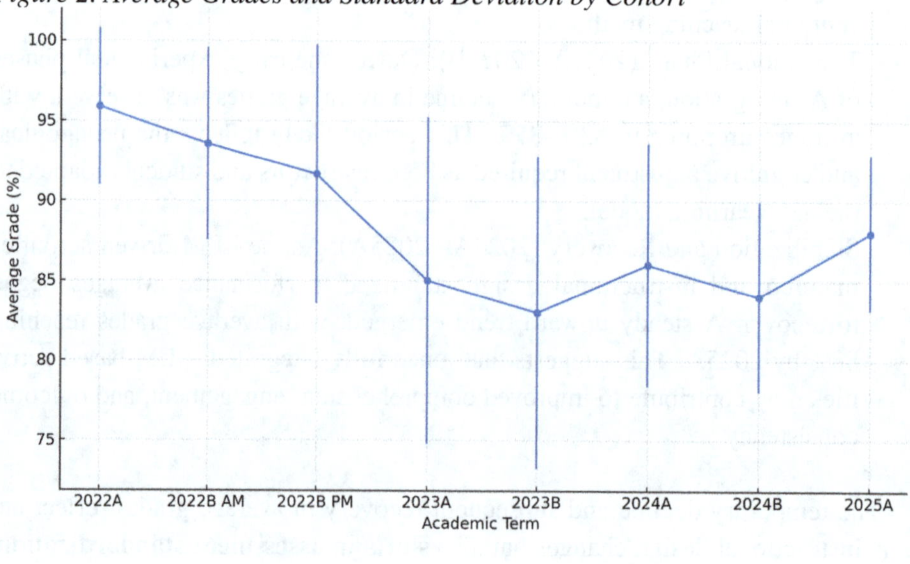

5.4. Statistical Interpretation

While formal statistical significance testing (ANOVA, Kruskal-Wallis, Mann-Whitney U tests) conducted during earlier phases of this research did not reveal conclusive differences between individual terms, the longitudinal aggregation of eight cohorts demonstrates meaningful trends in the broader evolution of student performance.

The temporary dip followed by recovery may reflect a natural adjustment curve common in the adoption of novel instructional technologies. Importantly, the narrowing of the performance range in later cohorts indicates a reduction in grade dispersion, suggesting that LLM-based scaffolding may help stabilize learning outcomes across diverse student populations.

To further illustrate individual learning trajectories within a single term, Figure 3 presents the progression of scores for 15 representative students from cohort 2024B. Each line tracks a student's performance across three sequential activities and the final standardized exam. While some variance in baseline performance is evident, the majority of students exhibit upward or stable trends, particularly between Activity 1 and the final assessment. This pattern suggests that sustained engagement with LLM-supported tasks may contribute to improved consolidation of concepts and problem-solving skills over time. The data also reflect that students with lower initial performance show the most pronounced gains, aligning with the scaffolding intentions of the AI-based instructional design.

Figure 3. Individual performance trajectories for 15 students in cohort 2024B across three activities and a standardized final exam. Most students exhibit upward trends, particularly those with lower initial performance.

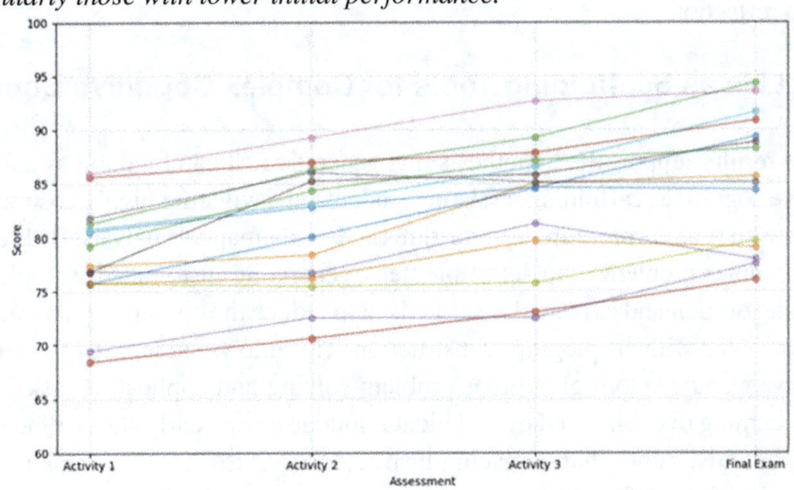

Additionally, informal student feedback collected throughout the intervention indicated positive perceptions of the LLM-driven activities. Students consistently reported greater confidence in tackling complex problems, increased engagement with cryptographic algorithms, and appreciation for the personalized explanations provided by the AI tools.

6. DISCUSSION AND IMPLICATIONS FOR EDUCATIONAL PRACTICE

The longitudinal findings from this study offer important insights into both the opportunities and challenges associated with integrating generative AI into cryptography education. While initial adoption produced temporary fluctuations in student performance, the subsequent stabilization and recovery observed in later cohorts suggest that LLM-driven learning activities can, over time, contribute meaningfully to student success in complex technical domains.

"At first I thought ChatGPT was just for solving problems, but then I used it to check if I truly understood what the question was asking. It helped me realize when I was memorizing versus when I actually knew the topic." — Student, 2024B

"The AI gave me good examples, but I had to ask the right question. That made me think more carefully about what I wanted to learn." — Student, 2025A

"Using the model for modular arithmetic helped me see the steps, but sometimes it made mistakes. That's when I learned to verify and not just copy." — Student, 2024A

These student voices reinforce the chapter's argument that LLMs can act as cognitive scaffolds—provided that their use is mediated by pedagogical intent and critical reflection.

6.1. LLMs as Scaffolding Tools for Complex Cognitive Domains

The results support the hypothesis that generative AI can function as a form of adaptive cognitive scaffolding, assisting students in navigating highly abstract content areas such as cryptographic algorithms and mathematical analysis. By breaking down complex problems into digestible steps, generating customized examples, and providing on-demand explanations, LLMs help reduce the cognitive load traditionally associated with cryptography instruction. This allows students to devote more cognitive resources to higher-order problem-solving and application tasks, rather than becoming overwhelmed by technical minutiae during early stages of learning.

Importantly, rather than replacing instructor expertise, LLMs complement the educator's role by offering individualized support at scale. Instructors can focus more intensively on areas requiring human judgment, ethical reasoning, collaborative learning, and deeper conceptual discussions, while the AI assists with mechanical computations, repetitive practice, and real-time content generation.

6.2. Mitigating Learning Gaps and Performance Dispersion

A notable trend observed in the stabilized cohorts (2024A onward) was a **reduction in performance dispersion**. The narrowing of grade ranges suggests that LLM-supported activities may be particularly effective in assisting lower-performing students to achieve baseline competencies, thereby reducing failure rates and improving overall classroom consistency. This supports the broader equity goals often associated with educational technology, whereby students with differing prior knowledge, learning styles, and academic preparation can receive tailored support to achieve success.

Such stabilization is especially relevant in cryptography, where students often enter the course with widely varying levels of mathematical fluency. LLMs offer flexible, patient, and nonjudgmental instructional support that can adapt to these individual needs in real time.

6.3. Limitations and Ethical Considerations

Despite these promising trends, the implementation of LLM-driven instruction raises several ethical and pedagogical challenges that warrant ongoing attention. Key issues include:

- Academic Integrity: The ease with which students can generate complete solutions using AI requires careful instructional design to ensure authentic engagement with the material.
- Overreliance Risk: Students may become dependent on AI assistance, potentially limiting their independent problem-solving skills if not properly guided.
- Bias and Accuracy: LLM-generated content may occasionally contain inaccuracies, requiring students and instructors to critically evaluate AI outputs.
- Privacy and Data Security: Institutional guidelines must address responsible data handling, especially when integrating third-party AI platforms.

The University of Guadalajara's institutional guidelines have served as an important framework for mitigating these risks, emphasizing transparency, responsible use, and critical reflection in the application of AI tools.

6.4. Implications for Broader STEM Education

The positive trends observed in cryptography education may generalize to other STEM disciplines characterized by high cognitive complexity, including mathematics, physics, engineering, and computer science more broadly. Generative AI tools have the potential to transform instructional design across technical fields by:

- Enabling personalized pacing for students.
- Offering scalable tutoring for large class sizes.
- Allowing instructors to focus on conceptual reasoning while automating routine exercises.
- Facilitating simulation-based learning scenarios that mirror professional problem-solving contexts.

As educational institutions worldwide grapple with how best to incorporate AI into pedagogy, this study contributes empirical evidence to inform best practices, identify risks, and demonstrate the transformative potential of generative AI when integrated thoughtfully into curriculum design.

7. FUTURE RESEARCH DIRECTIONS

The integration of generative AI into cryptography education represents only the initial phase of a broader research agenda that explores how emerging technologies can reshape complex technical learning environments. Based on the findings of this longitudinal study, several promising avenues for future research emerge.

7.1. Longitudinal Standardized Assessment

While the present analysis utilized final course grades as primary performance indicators, future studies should incorporate standardized assessment instruments that isolate specific learning objectives and conceptual competencies within cryptography. Developing validated assessment tools would allow for more precise measurement of student understanding, particularly in areas such as:

- Algorithm design and implementation
- Statistical cryptanalysis
- Key management protocols
- Mathematical foundations of encryption

Implementing department-wide or multi-institutional standardized assessments would enable more robust longitudinal comparisons across cohorts, instructional formats, and institutional contexts.

7.2. Expanded Use of Qualitative Data

Quantitative performance data, while valuable, capture only one dimension of learning outcomes. Future research should incorporate qualitative data sources, such as:

- Structured student interviews
- Focus groups
- Reflective journals
- Faculty observations

These data can provide richer insights into how students perceive LLM-based activities, how they experience learning autonomy, and how AI tools influence their confidence, engagement, and metacognitive skills.

7.3. Development of LLM-Powered Interactive Simulators

Building on the promising effects of dynamic problem generation and simulation exercises, future instructional designs could incorporate fully interactive AI-powered cryptography simulators. These environments would allow students to:

- Experiment with encryption algorithms in real time
- Simulate complex attacks on custom datasets
- Receive adaptive feedback based on their actions
- Explore real-world cryptographic applications in fields such as cybersecurity, blockchain, and data protection

Such simulators could further enhance engagement and bridge the gap between theoretical knowledge and applied technical proficiency.

7.4. Cross-Disciplinary Applications in STEM Education

The principles developed in this study may be transferable to other STEM domains characterized by abstract reasoning and complex algorithmic content. Future collaborative research could explore LLM-driven active learning designs for:

- Mathematical proofs and problem solving
- Algorithmic complexity and data structures
- Signal processing and encryption in engineering contexts
- Secure software development practices

Cross-disciplinary studies may reveal common instructional design principles for effectively integrating generative AI into highly technical STEM curricula.

7.5. Ethical AI Literacy and Faculty Development

As generative AI becomes more deeply embedded in educational contexts, research must also focus on developing AI literacy frameworks for both students and faculty. Faculty development programs should prepare instructors to:

- Design ethically sound AI-integrated activities
- Interpret AI-generated outputs critically
- Guide students in responsible AI use
- Monitor and evaluate the evolving capabilities and risks of emerging AI models

Establishing ethical AI literacy as a core competency in STEM education will be essential to ensure responsible, effective, and equitable adoption of generative AI technologies.

8. CONCLUSIONS

This chapter has presented an exploratory account of how generative AI, specifically Large Language Models, was progressively integrated into an undergraduate cryptography course over eight academic terms. The study aimed to observe trends rather than test causal hypotheses, and the data reflect both the challenges and opportunities that emerged during implementation.

While the introduction of a standardized final exam in the later academic terms improved internal consistency in assessment, it should be regarded as procedural refinement rather than a methodological innovation. This chapter does not claim causal inference but instead contributes a descriptive and practice-based account of the challenges and opportunities involved in integrating generative AI into technical education. Future work should build on this foundation using pre-registered protocols, controlled group comparisons, and mixed-method evaluation strategies to assess learning outcomes more rigorously.

REFERENCES

Adamovic, S., Sarac, M., Stamenkovic, U., & Radovanovic, D. (2018). The importance of the using software tools for learning modern cryptography. *International Journal of Engineering Education, 34*(1), 256–262.

Alhamdani, W. A. (2016). Teaching Cryptography Using Design Thinking Approach. *Journal of Applied Security Research, 11*(1), 78–89. DOI: 10.1080/19361610.2015.1069646

Deeb, F. A., & Hickey, T. J. (2019). Teaching Introductory Cryptography using a 3D Escape-the-Room Game. *2019 IEEE Frontiers in Education Conference (FIE)*, 1–6. DOI: 10.1109/FIE43999.2019.9028549

González-Tablas, A. I., González Vasco, M. I., Cascos, I., & Planet Palomino, Á. (2020). Shuffle, Cut, and Learn: Crypto Go, a Card Game for Teaching Cryptography. *Mathematics, 8*(11), 1993. DOI: 10.3390/math8111993

Koblitz, N. (1997). Cryptography as a teaching tool. *Cryptologia, 21*(4), 317–326. DOI: 10.1080/0161-119791885959

Sakalli, M. T., Bulus, E., & Buyuksaracoglu, F. (2004). Cryptography education for students. *Information Technology Based Proceedings of the FIfth International Conference OnHigher Education and Training, 2004. ITHET 2004.*, 621–626. DOI: 10.1109/ITHET.2004.1358246

Universidad de Guadalajara. (2023). *Orientaciones y definiciones sobre el uso de la inteligencia artificial generativa en los procesos académicos: Guía práctica.* Universidad de Guadalajara.

REFERENCES

Chapter 14
Molecules and Missions: A Game-Based Platform for Collaborative Pharmaceutical Innovation

Guillermo Jiménez-Hernández
https://orcid.org/0009-0008-6172-7269
Biodigital Innovation Lab, Translational Bioengineering Department, CUCEI, Universidad de Guadalajara, Mexico

Yajaira Zepeda-García
https://orcid.org/0000-0001-7529-9877
Biodigital Innovation Lab, Translational Bioengineering Department, CUCEI, Universidad de Guadalajara, Mexico

ABSTRACT

Molecules and Missions is a point-and-click strategy game that makes nanoscale science accessible through gamified learning. Set in a steampunk lab, players use virtual tools to explore cells, conduct experiments, and progress through campaigns. The chapter presents a citizen science proposal in which researchers can design downloadable content used so that players' results can be indicative of real experimentation. The project lowers barriers to molecular education, fosters critical thinking, and enables broader participation in pharmaceutical research.

1. INTRODUCTION: WHY MOLECULAR SCIENCES NEED A NEW LEARNING MODEL

Designing a drug to treat a specific disease is far from simply combining chemical compounds and hoping for the best. It represents one of the most fascinating and

DOI: 10.4018/979-8-3373-4657-1.ch014

complex challenges in modern molecular science, where researchers must navigate an invisible universe of atoms, molecules, and proteins arranged in intricate three-dimensional conformations.

Molecular sciences and chemistry naturally require working with highly abstract concepts, particularly when addressing cutting edge topics such as drug design. In this field, students and researchers become scientific polyglots, weaving together knowledge from multiple disciplines. Drug design involves the comprehension of fundamental concepts in chemistry, such as atomic and molecular structures, chemical bonding, and reactivity. It also requires a deep understanding of proteins, enzymes, and their interactions with small molecules. All of this knowledge must then be translated into the language of three-dimensional models, since biological interactions unfold in a spatial world where form determines function. This multidimensional character makes drug design not only one of the most intellectually demanding areas of molecular science, but also one of the most promising, holding the potential to redefine the boundaries of medicine.

One of the greatest challenges in teaching and learning molecular sciences is that many fundamental phenomena occur at the nanometric scale, completely invisible to the human eye. Processes such as molecular recognition, enzymatic catalysis, or receptor-ligand binding unfold in a hidden world, making them abstract and difficult for students to grasp. Understanding these three-dimensional conformations is often challenging for students but these conformations describe how atoms occupy space and adopt precise orientations. This is part of what gives molecular science its multidimensional nature, a concept that encompasses the structural, spatial, and dynamic levels at which molecular processes occur.

Consider the challenge: How do we help learners understand the way molecules adopt precise three-dimensional structures? How do we make their interactions tangible through subtle forces like hydrogen bonds and van der Waals interactions? More importantly, how do we bridge these microscopic events with the macroscopic effects we can actually observe? This persistent difficulty in explaining, visualizing, and reasoning about complex molecular concepts and their dynamic interactions represents a core pedagogical challenge, and it is precisely this problem that motivates the development of the proposed gamified learning strategy.

For many students, this invisible realm becomes a significant barrier. It demands innovative educational approaches that can transform the abstract into something tangible and make the complex understandable.

These environments not only reproduce the visual appearance of laboratory spaces but also emulate the functionality of instruments and the logic of experimental procedures. By engaging with virtual labs, students can manipulate simulated devices, observe experimental outcomes, and explore the behavior of reactants and substances under controlled digital conditions. In this way, they provide a close approximation to real laboratory practice while ensuring a safe, flexible, and scalable environment that expands opportunities for experimentation and learning.

Since the early 21st century, virtual labs have gained remarkable traction as tools for democratizing scientific knowledge and teaching. In many regions, especially those with limited financial or infrastructural resources; access to fully equipped physical laboratories simply isn't feasible. Virtual labs offer a practical solution, breaking down barriers of space, cost, and time (Byukusenge et al., 2022).

The rapid evolution of communication and information technologies has accelerated their global adoption. Today, these platforms serve multiple roles: preliminary training grounds before students enter physical labs, safe substitutes for dangerous or expensive experiments, and standalone alternatives where physical facilities are unavailable.

Beyond these practical benefits, digital platforms address a fundamental shift in educational philosophy, the move from passive to active learning methodologies. Traditional chemistry education often trapped students in cycles of rote memorization, where they learned reactions and structural models without truly engaging with the underlying processes.

Virtual labs flip this dynamic. They invite learners to actively participate in simulated experiments, test their own hypotheses, and directly observe results. This hands-on engagement deepens understanding, reduces errors in subsequent physical lab work, and builds genuine confidence in laboratory skills (Hawkins & Phelps, 2013).

An important question continues to spark discussion in educational circles: Can virtual labs fully replicate the knowledge and skills gained in traditional laboratories? While no absolute consensus exists, mounting evidence suggests that virtual labs significantly boost learning outcomes, improve exam performance, and enhance students' grasp of complex scientific concepts (Hawkins & Phelps, 2013).

However, most educators agree on one crucial point: virtual and physical laboratories work best as partners, not competitors. Together, they create a balanced educational experience that strengthens both conceptual understanding and hands-on practical skills.

Meanwhile, molecular science continues its explosive growth as one of today's most dynamic research areas. Its applications span drug development, medical diagnostics, and therapeutic innovation, making it increasingly relevant to solving humanity's most pressing health challenges (Tibell & Rundgren, 2010).

Drug design perfectly exemplifies the complexity of translating molecular science into real world solutions. Developing a new medication involves far more than identifying molecules that bind to a target; it's an intricate, multi-step journey. Researchers must evaluate manufacturability, safety, stability, solubility, selectivity, and long-term effectiveness.

Each candidate compound faces rigorous testing: Is it non-mutagenic? Non-toxic? Can it target biological systems with precision? These requirements reveal not only the intellectual demands of drug design but also the technical and ethical challenges of moving from theoretical models to life-saving treatments.

Given these complexities, interactive tools become even more crucial for molecular science education, particularly in drug design. While current evidence strongly supports their effectiveness, exciting opportunities lie ahead.

The integration of gamification strategies could transform abstract molecular problems into engaging, interactive challenges. Imagine students competing to design the most effective drug molecule or collaborating to solve complex binding puzzles.

Immersive technologies promise even greater breakthroughs. Virtual reality could allow learners to literally step inside molecular environments, visualize nanoscale interactions, and manipulate digital molecules with their hands, possibilities that seemed like pure science fiction just decades ago.

Virtual labs have already proven their worth in expanding access to scientific education. But their true potential lies in the next evolutionary step: creating deeply interactive, immersive learning experiences.

Few fields stand to benefit more than molecular sciences, where complexity and abstraction often challenge both learners and educators. By combining proven virtual lab strategies with innovative interactive tools, we can ignite curiosity, deepen understanding, and prepare the next generation of scientists for the demanding yet rewarding challenges of drug design and molecular research.

We present the concept of a platform designed for students with foundational knowledge in general chemistry and basic molecular biology. The primary target audience comprises undergraduate students in health sciences related fields (pharmacy, chemistry, medicine, biology, biomedicine, and related disciplines), although the progressive pedagogical design allows high school students with chemistry foundations to begin their approach to drug design. Because these learners often find highly abstract topics, such as three-dimensional molecular structures, protein–ligand interactions, and ion-channel dynamics, difficult to visualize through traditional instruction, the platform integrates gamified strategies precisely in those areas where interactive visualization improves understanding.

The stage-based learning system enables users with different educational backgrounds to advance at their own pace, from fundamental concepts to the application of molecular dynamics for rational drug design. This methodological flexibility also facilitates its use by professionals pursuing continuing education or early-career researchers seeking to strengthen specific competencies in computational medicinal chemistry.

At its core, drug design is the process of discovering and creating molecules capable of treating diseases by interacting with specific biological targets, typically proteins (Sulea et al., 2024). Proteins are the molecular machines of our cells: they catalyze reactions, transmit signals, and regulate virtually every biological process. Among these proteins, ion channels play a particularly critical role, acting as gateways that control the flow of ions across cell membranes. These channels are essential for nerve impulses, muscle contractions, heart rhythm, and countless other physiological processes (Zhang et al., 2024). When proteins malfunction, including ion channels that become overactive, underactive, or dysfunctional, disease often follows. These diseases can result in conditions ranging from epilepsy and cardiac arrhythmias to cystic fibrosis and certain types of pain disorders (Hernandez et al., 2024; Imbrici et al., 2016). Modern drug design seeks to create small molecules, drugs, that can bind to these proteins and either activate, inhibit, or modulate their function. This binding is highly specific; a drug molecule must fit into a protein's binding site like a key into a lock, forming stable interactions through chemical forces. To predict and optimize these interactions, researchers increasingly rely on molecular dynamics simulations: computational techniques that model how molecules move and interact over time at the atomic level (Ahmed et al., 2023; Gu et al., 2023). These simulations allow scientists to virtually test thousands of potential drug candidates before ever synthesizing them in a laboratory, dramatically accelerating the drug discovery process while reducing costs. Understanding this molecular recognition process, where form, function, and dynamics converge, is fundamental to modern pharmaceutical science (Weber et al., 2021).

These challenges in molecular science education point toward a promising solution: the strategic application of gamification principles to transform how students learn drug design.

2. EDUCATIONAL GAMES: FROM GAMIFICATION TO IMMERSION

Gamification refers to the incorporation of game design principles into educational settings, where elements such as dynamics, mechanics, and components are deliberately structured to influence motivation and learning outcomes (Figure 1). Rather than being a form of entertainment, it provides a conceptual framework that explains how game-like strategies can transform the learning process into a more engaging and goal-oriented experience.

Figure 1. **Framework of gamification in education**. *Dynamics represent motivational drivers and long-term engagement; mechanics define system behavior and progression; and components act as the basic building blocks that provide feedback and rewards. Created by the authors using ChatGPT, 2025.*

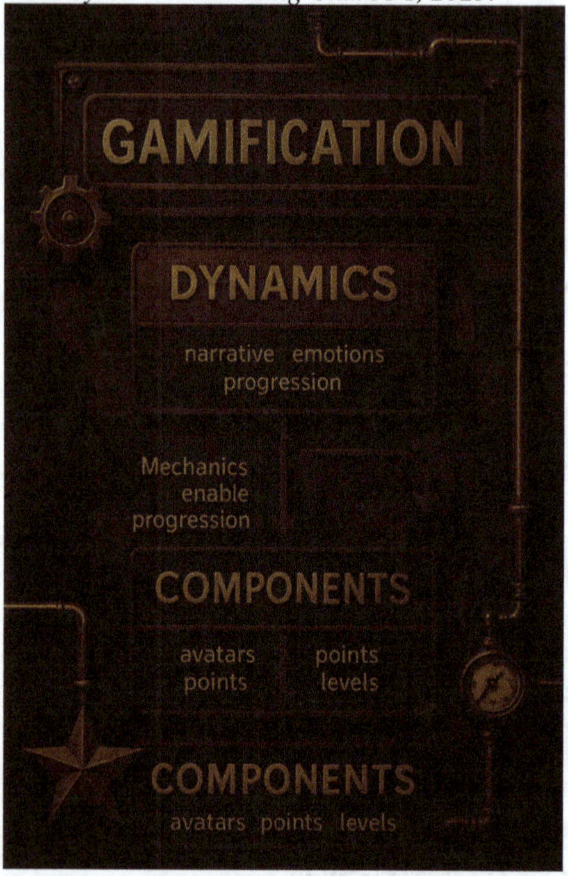

Educational games have emerged as a powerful perspective for learning, capable of attracting and maintaining student attention, something that has been consistently confirmed by several studies since 2014 (Ibarra-Herrera et al., 2019). Unlike traditional didactic methods, which often rely on passive reception of information, educational games promote active engagement, challenge-based progression, and meaningful interaction.

Currently, interactive video games have become innovative didactic tools that combine entertainment with learning. Their interactive nature allows users to actively engage in the experience, responding in real time to visual stimuli and in-game decisions. As educational resources, these games can facilitate the comprehension of complex content in a playful and meaningful way (Squire, 2003). A video game is defined as an electronic application that, through a visual interface, enables players to interact with virtual worlds and diverse narratives. When developed in networked formats, they become online video games, expanding their collaborative and social possibilities (Rollings & Adams, 2003). Within this framework, the proposed interactive video game seeks to integrate these elements to create a formative experience that is accessible and engaging for diverse audiences.

At the core of this approach lies gamification, defined as the application of game elements in non-game contexts. According to Werbach and Hunter (2012), gamification elements can be grouped into three main categories: dynamics, mechanics, and components.

Dynamics encompass elements such as narrative, emotions, and progression, providing a broad framework in which players become immersed in a storyline. Mechanics establish the rules that govern how the system operates, shaping user interaction and determining possible outcomes. At the most concrete level, components include avatars, badges, collections, points, and levels, which serve as tangible markers of achievement and progression.

An illustrative example of dynamic elements is storytelling, which offers learners a narrative structure that frames and guides their learning experience. Narratives foster imagination, help players contextualize abstract concepts, and generate emotional engagement with the educational content (Ibarra-Herrera et al., 2019).

These narrative and motivational strategies prove especially critical when addressing the technical challenges inherent in molecular sciences. Despite the transformative potential of molecular dynamics simulations in drug design (allow researchers to observe the movement of molecules, and predict their interactions and bonding), a significant barrier persists: the steep learning curve associated with research-grade simulation software. Even for computationally experienced users, mastering molecular dynamics implementation presents persistent challenges that extend beyond technical skills into areas of molecular biophysics, chemistry, and physical chemistry (Vieira et al., 2023). While highly effective for experts, their complexity poses a barrier for students or non-specialists.

This creates a paradox: the very tools needed to understand drug-protein interactions remain largely inaccessible to the students who would benefit most from hands-on experience with these technologies. The lengthy learning process often discourages students before they can appreciate the profound insights molecular dynamics can offer into drug design, limiting their ability to develop intuition about molecular recognition, binding dynamics, and structure-activity relationships.

Gamification emerges as a promising solution to democratize access to computational drug design while simultaneously enhancing student engagement and learning outcomes. The implementation of gamification in science education has attracted considerable research attention for its capacity to increase engagement and achieve learning more effectively, particularly as technology integration in science curricula has seen massive growth to combat declining student motivation toward science learning (Kalogiannakis et al. 2021). Studies demonstrate that gamification strategies significantly increase student motivation and engagement in chemistry education, improve attitudes toward the subject, and enhance academic performance (Chans et al. 2021). Perhaps most compellingly, the citizen science game Foldit has proven that non-experts can make genuine contributions to protein research: Foldit designs crafted by players with little or no biochemical training have proven as successful as those generated by experts or computers, with equivalent success rates in laboratory validation and similar folding stabilities (Koepnick et al. 2019). By transforming the abstract challenges of drug design into interactive, game-based experiences, students can develop genuine computational skills and chemical intuition while contributing to real scientific discovery, bridging the gap between educational gaming and authentic research participation.

Here lies the opportunity: gamification strategies could reduce this barrier by transforming the use of such sophisticated tools into interactive, engaging experiences that build understanding step by step, making advanced molecular science accessible to broader audiences. Bridging this gap requires approaches that not only lower the technical barriers of advanced tools but also invite broader participation in scientific practice. By framing complex processes through interactive and accessible formats, gamification can serve as a gateway for non-specialists to engage with scientific concepts. This aligns with a growing movement toward more open and participatory models of research, in which learning and discovery are no longer confined to experts alone.

This vision of democratizing scientific tools through gamification connects to a broader transformation happening across science itself. Science has long been perceived as the exclusive domain of experts, carried out in specialized laboratories and communicated primarily within academic circles. Yet, this perspective is beginning to shift as new approaches seek to make research more inclusive and participatory. The concept of citizen science captures this change: it invites individuals outside of academia to take part in the process of discovery, breaking down traditional barriers between professional researchers and the public (Giardullo et al., 2023). Through initiatives that range from large-scale data collection projects to collaborative platforms for analysis and interpretation, citizens can meaningfully contribute to advancing knowledge. In doing so, citizen science not only strengthens the connection between science and society, but also demonstrates that the generation of knowledge can be a collective endeavor, enriching both the scientific process and its societal impact (Johnson, 2023).

This approach not only democratizes science but also motivates learners by allowing them to contribute to real research challenges. To understand why these gamified approaches are so effective, it's worth examining the psychological mechanisms that make video games compelling.

As these participatory practices expand across different scientific fields, the question arises of how they might be applied within domains traditionally considered highly technical, such as drug discovery. Through gamified platforms, citizen science can extend participation in drug discovery by making processes accessible, understandable, and rewarding for broader audiences. This approach not only democratizes science but also motivates learners by allowing them to contribute to real research challenges.

The cultural phenomenon of video games helps explain why gamification is effective. From classics such as *Tetris* to globally recognized titles like *Mario Bros.*, video games engage players by assigning them a role as an avatar through which they confront obstacles, overcome challenges, and ultimately achieve victory. Although these experiences unfold in virtual environments, they hold significant meaning for players. Research from the University of Central Florida has shown that video games, by presenting progressive challenges, strengthen confidence and resilience in addressing real world problems (Shute, 2011). This finding is supported by additional research demonstrating that video games can enhance cognitive skills such as perception, attentional control, and decision-making, while also improving motivation and educational success through their interactive nature (Reynaldo et al., 2021). Unlike passive activities such as scrolling through social media, gaming is inherently active since it requires strategy, decision making, and problem solving.

This active nature explains why gaming transcends mere entertainment to become a training ground for real-world skills. Every mistake becomes a learning opportunity, while successes are immediately rewarded with points, levels, or victory music. This constant feedback creates a powerful psychological loop that reinforces competence and self-efficacy, something largely absent from daily adult life, where accomplishments often pass unrecognized despite their significance (Ryan et al., 2006).

The enduring appeal of video games stems from their unique ability to cast players as protagonists of their own journeys. Unlike passive entertainment such as social media or streaming, gaming demands focus, strategy, and decision making. Players don't simply observe; they actively shape outcomes through their choices and skills. With each attempt, they refine approaches and learn from setbacks while their brains register these virtual achievements as genuine accomplishments.

This psychological reinforcement proves particularly powerful because it fundamentally reshapes how players perceive their capacity to overcome challenges. Games provide what everyday life often lacks: consistent recognition for effort and progress. Through constant positive feedback loops, players develop stronger beliefs in their ability to reach goals and surmount obstacles, confidence that extends well beyond the virtual environment (Li et al., 2024).

The lessons learned transcend the screen itself. Games cultivate self-trust, resilience, and recognition of personal capability. By blurring the boundary between entertainment and empowerment, video games demonstrate how virtual victories can translate into real-world confidence and motivation, creating lasting psychological benefits that influence how players approach challenges in their daily lives.

3. CONCEPTUALIZING THE GAME: MOLECULES AND MISSIONS

Molecules and Missions is an immersive point-and-click science strategy video game that transforms players into molecular detectives working within a cutting edge research laboratory. Players embark on a scientific journey, progressing from basic cellular observation to sophisticated drug design, with the ultimate goal of developing therapeutic molecules that interact with cellular channels to treat human diseases.

The game adopts a first-person perspective, allowing players to assume the role of a laboratory apprentice who gradually evolves into an expert molecular scientist. The core gameplay revolves around strategic exploration of authentic laboratory equipment, microscopes, reagents, simulators, and advanced analytical instruments, while solving increasingly complex scientific puzzles. Each campaign presents unique challenges that blend scientific problem-solving with detailed observation and knowledge application, creating an educational atmosphere that mirrors real-world research environments that are summarized in Table 1.

Table 1. Structure of the gamified campaign for drug discovery education. Each campaign includes a defined entry point, prerequisite conditions, and a core learning objective, progressing from cellular exploration to real world medical applications.

Campaign	Entry Point	Prerequisites	Core Learning Objective
1: Foundations of Life	Advanced Research Microscope	*None*	Understanding cellular structures and protein channels
2: Molecular Highways	Patch-Clamp Station	*Complete Campaign 1*	Exploring ion channel function and metabolic pathways
3: Genes and the Web of Life	DNA Sequencer	*Complete Campaign 2*	Gene expression and molecular regulation
4: The Arsenal	Laboratory Storage System	*Complete Campaign 3*	Collecting and organizing therapeutic components

continued on following page

Table 1. Continued

Campaign	Entry Point	Prerequisites	Core Learning Objective
5: Molecular Architecture	Bioreactor Platform	*Complete Campaign 4*	Drug assembly and molecular design principles
6: Digital Validation	Computing Interface	*Complete Campaign 5*	Computational drug testing and optimization
7: Biological Reality	Microfluidic Organoid System	*Complete Campaign 6*	Cellular testing and side effect analysis
8: Global Impact	Golden Capsule Network	*Complete Campaign 7*	Addressing real-world medical challenges

The laboratory itself is designed in a distinctive steampunk style. Although the laboratory spans only a single room, every corner is filled with interactive devices and visual cues that immerse the player in the scientific world. This compact, yet richly detailed space allows for focused exploration while maintaining the aesthetic coherence of the steampunk theme, as illustrated in Figure 2.

Figure 2. **View of the laboratory**. *Laboratory highlighting its distinctive steampunk style. The room is packed with interactive devices, creating an immersive scientific environment. Created by the authors using Runaway, 2025.*

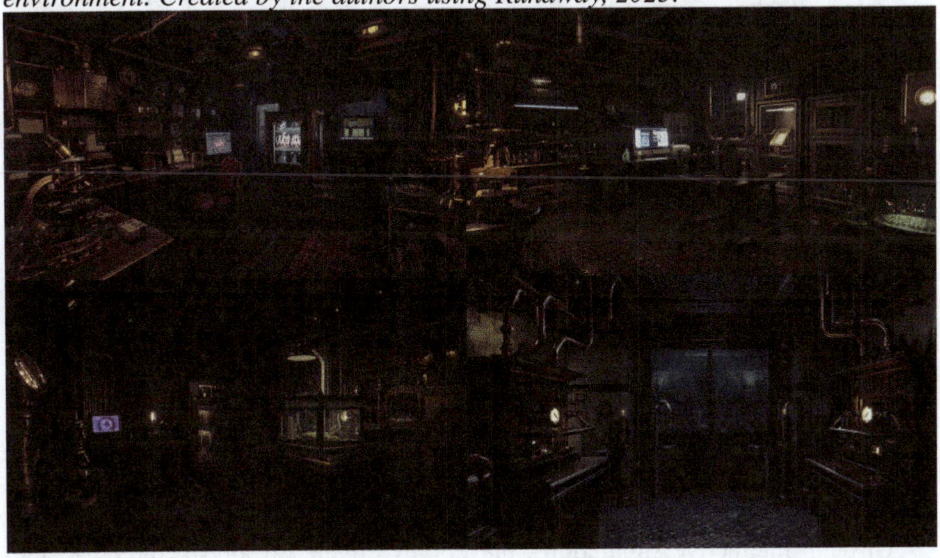

3.1 Campaign 1: Foundations of Life - Exploring the Microscopic World

The inaugural campaign introduces players to their primary research tool: a state-of-the-art microscope that serves as both educational instrument and gateway to discovery. Drawing inspiration from strategy games like Age of Empires II, the microscope functions as an interactive portal, launching players into the cellular universe.

Upon entering this microscopic realm, players begin a guided exploration of cellular diversity. They learn to navigate the microscope's controls while observing various cell types, systematically identifying fundamental structures: cell membranes, nuclei, organelles, and cytoplasm. Interactive tutorials teach players to distinguish between animal, plant, and bacterial cells, comparing their unique morphological features and functional adaptations.

The learning progression follows a carefully structured path. Players start with basic cell identification exercises, gradually advancing to more sophisticated observations that require recognizing subtle structural differences. Interactive prompts guide their attention to specific cellular components, while built-in assessment tools verify understanding before allowing progression.

The campaign culminates in a dramatic zooming sequence revealing the intricate architecture of cell membranes. Here, players encounter their first glimpse of protein channels, complex molecular structures that become the central focus of their entire research journey. This revelation serves as both the conclusion of basic cellular education and the foundation for subsequent campaigns.

3.2 Campaign 2: Molecular Highways - Understanding Metabolic Pathways and Ionic Channels

The second campaign expands the laboratory environment, shifting focus from passive observation to active experimentation. Players learn to manipulate experimental conditions, observing how different stimuli affect channel behavior and ionic flux across cellular membranes. The campaign introduces the interconnected world of cellular metabolism, where players explore major biochemical pathways that sustain cellular life.

Through interactive simulations, players investigate glycolysis, the citric acid cycle, and oxidative phosphorylation, learning how these processes generate cellular energy and maintain metabolic homeostasis. Advanced pathway visualization tools allow players to trace molecular interactions in real-time, unlocking components of a comprehensive metabolic map that serves as a reference guide for future campaigns.

The campaign's challenges require players to predict how changes in ion channel activity might affect metabolic flux, introducing concepts of cellular regulation and preparing them for the genetic control mechanisms explored in subsequent stages. Players learn to recognize the dynamic relationships between ion channels and metabolic processes, establishing crucial connections essential for drug design applications.

3.3 Campaign 3: Genes and the Web of Life - Genetics and Molecular Regulation

This campaign introduces players to the molecular mechanisms that control cellular behavior at the most fundamental level. Players delve into the central dogma of molecular biology, exploring how genetic information stored in DNA directs the synthesis of proteins that form ion channels and metabolic enzymes.

Interactive challenges guide players through gene expression, from transcription in the nucleus to translation at ribosomes. Players learn to identify regulatory sequences controlling when and where specific genes are expressed, understanding how cells coordinate the production of ion channels and metabolic enzymes in response to physiological demands.

Advanced simulation modules allow players to observe how mutations in ion channel genes can lead to altered protein function, introducing the concept of genetic diseases and their molecular basis. These exercises prepare players for therapeutic applications by establishing connections between genetic defects and disease states.

The campaign's culminating challenge requires players to map relationships between specific genes, their protein products, and the cellular processes these proteins control. Success unlocks access to the "genetic master code", a comprehensive database that becomes an essential reference tool for understanding molecular drug action.

3.4 Campaign 4: The Arsenal - Strategic Collection and Organization of Therapeutic Components

Drawing upon knowledge gained from previous campaigns, players now face the challenge of resource management and strategic selection. They must identify which proteins, metabolites, and genetic factors discovered in earlier stages have therapeutic potential and organize them systematically for future drug development efforts.

The campaign introduces players to the concept of druggability, the likelihood that a particular biological target can be modulated by therapeutic compounds. Through analysis exercises, players learn to evaluate potential drug targets based on their accessibility, selectivity, and therapeutic relevance. They explore how ion channels, metabolic enzymes, and regulatory proteins can serve as intervention points for treating disease.

Interactive molecular databases allow players to search for existing compounds with known biological activity, introducing them to the vast chemical space available for drug development. Players learn to classify molecules based on their structural features, biological targets, and therapeutic applications, building a comprehensive inventory of potential drug development resources.

Collection challenges become increasingly sophisticated as players advance, requiring them to identify subtle relationships between molecular structure and biological activity. The campaign concludes with players having assembled a comprehensive toolkit of biological targets and chemical starting points for molecular design.

3.5 Campaign 5: Molecular Architecture - The Art and Science of Drug Assembly

Within this campaign, players encounter the fundamental principles of medicinal chemistry and molecular design. They learn to analyze the three-dimensional structures of their target proteins, identifying binding sites where therapeutic molecules might interact effectively. Advanced visualization tools allow players to explore molecular surfaces, electrostatic properties, and dynamic behavior of their biological targets.

The core gameplay revolves around molecular assembly puzzles that simulate rational drug design logic. Players must consider multiple factors simultaneously: molecular complementarity with target binding sites, chemical stability, synthetic accessibility, and predicted biological selectivity. Each assembly challenge requires players to balance competing demands while creating molecules with optimal therapeutic properties.

Interactive chemistry modules teach players about chemical bonding, molecular geometry, and structure-activity relationships. They learn to predict how changes in molecular structure might affect biological activity, introducing concepts of pharmacophore mapping and molecular optimization. Advanced challenges introduce players to drug-like properties, teaching them to evaluate designs based on established criteria for oral bioavailability, metabolic stability, and toxicity potential.

The campaign concludes with players having designed several prototype molecules for each chosen target. These molecular designs serve as starting points for rigorous testing and optimization procedures explored in subsequent campaigns.

3.6 Campaign 6: Digital Validation - Computational Drug Testing and Optimization

Players gain access to an interactive "Molecular Simulation Library", a comprehensive digital resource guiding them through computational drug evaluation processes. This platform introduces players to quantitative methods used to predict drug efficacy, selectivity, and safety before expensive experimental testing begins.

The campaign's core mechanics center around molecular dynamics simulations, where players observe how their designed molecules interact with target proteins over time. These simulations reveal the dynamic nature of molecular recognition, showing players how binding affinities change with molecular flexibility, conformational changes, and environmental conditions.

Advanced docking studies allow players to explore how their designed molecules fit within target binding sites, teaching them to recognize favorable and unfavorable binding modes. Interactive scoring functions help players understand the energetics of molecular recognition, while comparative analysis tools enable ranking different molecular designs based on predicted binding affinity and selectivity.

3.7 Campaign 7: Biological Reality - Cellular Testing and Side Effect Analysis

Players transition from computational simulations to biological experimentation, introducing their most promising molecular designs to miniaturized cellular systems that model human tissue function. These organoid cultures represent significant advancement in complexity, exhibiting many characteristics of real human organs while remaining suitable for controlled experimentation.

The core challenge involves comprehensive drug evaluation across multiple biological parameters. Players must monitor whether their designed molecules produce intended therapeutic effects while identifying unexpected side effects or interference with normal cellular processes. Interactive monitoring systems allow players to track drug distribution within organoid cultures, observing how molecules traverse cellular barriers and accumulate in different tissue compartments.

The campaign introduces therapeutic windows—the dosage range where drugs provide beneficial effects without causing harmful side effects. Through dose-response experiments, players learn to identify optimal drug concentrations and recognize signs of toxicity that might limit therapeutic applications.

Players encounter realistic scenarios where designed molecules produce unexpected effects, requiring them to modify therapeutic strategies or return to earlier stages for molecular redesign. The campaign introduces ADMET properties (Absorption, Distribution, Metabolism, Excretion, and Toxicity), teaching players to use computational tools to predict how designed molecules might behave in biological systems. When simulations reveal problems with molecular designs, players can return to the assembly platform to modify chemical structures and retest their hypotheses, mirroring real-world drug discovery workflows.

3.8 Campaign 8: Global Impact - Addressing Real-World Medical Challenges

The final campaign connects players to real-world medical challenges through an innovative delivery system that periodically provides containers with detailed information about specific diseases and medical conditions. Each represents a new therapeutic challenge requiring players to integrate and apply all previously acquired skills.

Unlike previous campaigns focusing on individual competencies, this stage presents complex, multifaceted problems mirroring challenges faced by contemporary pharmaceutical researchers. Each disease capsule contains comprehensive information about the pathophysiology of specific medical conditions, including molecular mechanisms underlying disease development and progression.

Players must approach each medical challenge by systematically applying the complete drug discovery pipeline mastered through previous campaigns. This begins with detailed disease mechanism analysis, identification of potential therapeutic targets, and evaluation of existing treatment options to identify unmet medical needs.

The campaign design allows continuous expansion through downloadable content modules, each focusing on different disease areas or emerging health challenges. Advanced challenges introduce personalized medicine concepts, where genetic variations between patients affect drug response and optimal treatment strategies.

The campaign emphasizes the global nature of medical challenges, introducing diseases that disproportionately affect different geographic regions and socioeconomic populations. Success requires players to demonstrate mastery of the complete drug discovery process while adapting approaches to address unique requirements of each medical challenge, transforming the game from educational simulation into a platform for exploring contemporary medical challenges where scientific knowledge, strategic thinking, and social responsibility converge.

4. A FIRST-PERSON TOUR THROUGH THE LAB

To truly understand how Molecules and Missions transforms abstract molecular concepts into engaging learning experiences, we present this guided walkthrough that follows a player's journey through all eight campaigns. This immersive narrative demonstrates how the game's steampunk aesthetic, progressive challenges, and scientific authenticity work together to create meaningful educational outcomes.

The following walkthrough (table 2) captures the player experience from initial cellular exploration through complex drug design challenges, illustrating how each campaign builds upon previous knowledge while introducing new concepts and skills. Through this detailed exploration, readers can envision how gamified learning environments bridge the gap between theoretical understanding and practical application in molecular sciences.

Table 2. Guided walkthrough of mini-games, activities, and targeted learning outcomes across the eight Molecules and Missions campaigns, from initial cellular exploration to advanced drug-design challenges.

Campaign	Mini-game / Activity (Brief Description)	Skills / Concepts Learned
1	Microscope: Explore the cell and identify specific organelles by clicking on them	Organelle identification, cellular functions, attention to detail
2	Patch-clamp: Detect a blocking molecule and repair disrupted metabolic pathways	Membrane and ion channel function, metabolism, problem-solving
3	DNA Sequencer: Find start codons by tracing DNA sequences	Basic genetics, protein coding
	DNA Sequencer: Repair mutations to restore protein function	Gene-metabolism connections, precision, attention
4	Flask Collection: Select useful chemical fragments for future molecules	Chemical fragment recognition, chemical properties
	Temperature Balance: Maintain proper temperature and stability of flasks	Attention, precision, managing multiple variables
	Atom Collection: Collect individual atoms without disturbing assembled fragments	Coordination, observation, strategic planning
5	Bioreactor: Assemble simple molecules like water	Basic structure-function understanding, problem-solving
	Advanced Bioreactor: Assemble complex molecules from fragments with proper 3D orientation	3D skills, planning, applied chemistry
6	Molecular Docking: Align and place drugs into ion channels	3D orientation, molecular interactions, precision
	Bioreactor Production: Scale up production of functional molecules by adjusting parameters	Production scaling, observation, variable control
7	Drug Introduction: Introduce drugs into virtual cells	Efficacy evaluation, toxicity assessment, cause-effect reasoning
	Dose & Variant Analysis: Compare doses and genetic variants	Result analysis, critical thinking
8	Disease Scenario Application: Apply previous knowledge to various diseases	Knowledge integration, critical thinking, solution design

4.1 Campaign 1

You step into Molecules and Missions, you find yourself in a steampunk laboratory. You can see eight stations arranged around the room, each one marked by a unique machine or device that hints at the challenges and learning objectives it holds. The player begins with Campaign 1, and only by completing its objectives and mini-games will Campaign 2 be unlocked. The sequential progression ensures that players acquire the foundational knowledge before moving to the more complex challenges.

As a first time player, you approach the only available device: the microscope. The moment you select it, the world around you fades and you are transported inside an atlas style representation of a eukaryotic cell. A calm narrator begins to explain the basics: the cell, its membrane, and its bustling interior. Slowly, the organelles start to move around, each carrying out their mysterious functions.

Your first challenge appears: "Find three mitochondria." You don't know exactly which ones they are, so you begin to explore, clicking and tapping organelles to test your guesses. Each correct choice reveals a short description of its function and adds it to your experience log, while earning Experience points (XP). Mistakes cost some XP, but encourage careful observation and learning by trial and error.

As you advance, new tasks appear: select two organelles involved in transport, then another set involved in energy conversion. Each round gradually teaches you to recognize organelles by shape, behavior, and role within the cell, all while keeping the experience playful and rewarding. Successfully completing these challenges fills your experience log and unlocks the next campaign, readying you for the next adventure.

4.2 Campaign 2

Having completed enough mini-games, you unlock the second campaign. Back in the steampunk laboratory, you now select the second station, represented by a set of patch-clamp systems. As you click on it, the laboratory fades away and once again you are transported inside a cell. This time, the focus is on the cell membrane. You see several components held in place by delicate pipettes, and the narrator explains how these structures regulate what enters and leaves the cell. With each movement of molecules across the membrane, the pipettes project dynamic graphs, revealing the electrical potential of a neuron.

The narrator explains how these ion channels orchestrate cellular balance. Suddenly, an alarm echoes through the environment. One of the ion channels has malfunctioned, its gate is blocked by an unexpected molecule. The ion flow halts, and the projection shifts into a glowing map of metabolic pathways. What was once seamless now begins to fragment: proteins appear as simple shapes (circles, hexagons, and chains) that no longer connect to their substrates. Some look like a circle with a missing slice, others like puzzle pieces that no longer fit. As the pathways break apart, organelles slow down and the cell shows clear signs of stress. The challenge is no longer just to observe; you must identify the faulty molecule and complete the missing shapes, restoring connections before the system collapses.

Even after you manage to repair the pathways, the cell does not fully recover. The narrator's voice returns, calm but firm, explaining that the fix is only temporary. On the projection, you watch as the foreign molecule creeps back into the channel, blocking the gate once more. The graphs flicker, organelles hesitate, and the balance you worked so hard to restore begins to waver again. A new entry flashes in your logbook: 'The cell cannot stabilize on its own. A lasting solution must be found. A drug will be needed to prevent this malfunction.' The message lingers like a challenge, your next mission is no longer just to play, but to discover a cure.

4.3 Campaign 3

You enter Campaign 3: Genes and the Web of Life as the steampunk lab vibrates with new energy. The patch-clamp console stays activated after completing missions, while a nearby monitor glows, the DNA sequencer activating Campaign 3. This marks a deeper journey beyond proteins and pathways into life's fundamental blueprints.

Selecting the DNA sequencer dissolves the room, placing you inside an immense illuminated DNA scroll stretching infinitely. The double helix spins like a colossal track. The narrator explains: genes provide instructions determining protein construction and cellular organization.

Your first challenge: "Find the start codon." Letters unfold (A, T, C, G) requiring sequence tracing to identify correct signals. Success reveals ribosome visualization building protein strands. Errors pause machinery, emphasizing precision needed to decipher life's script.

Progressive mini-challenges arise: linking genes to metabolic pathways, repairing mutations to restore protein function, observing how genetic instructions become ion channels or active pathways. Each success adds entries to your genetic notebook, connecting DNA code to Campaign 2's proteins and systems.

The concept clarifies: genes aren't abstract code but architects of every encountered cellular structure and process. Overcoming genetic challenges unlocks Campaign 4, preparing the transition from theory to applied biotechnology.

4.4 Campaign 4

Back in the laboratory, the refrigerator unlocks. Clicking transports you to a chilled room filled with glowing flasks and tubes containing colored liquids and powders of various sizes and textures. The narrator explains these are chemical building blocks, potential ingredients for new molecules and drugs. However, not everything is usable, and you can unlock only limited components. Wise choices determine future drug design possibilities.

The narrator guides: "Each contains chemical fragments: building blocks for future molecules. Observation, collection, and recording are important, but not all prove useful."

Moving carefully along aisles, you select flasks. Holographic labels appear: "Hydroxyl group: forms hydrogen bonds," "Aromatic ring: provides structural stability," "Halogen atom: enhances binding affinity." Discoveries log automatically in your experience book, recording growing chemical knowledge. You feel the hunt's thrill, scanning for unusual items that might matter later.

A unique flask catches your eye, its glow different, almost pulsating. The narrator emphasizes: "This molecule is special. It helps defective ion channels open, key to restoring cellular balance." Upon collection, the Temperature Balance minigame begins.

This transcends simple collection. Each flask has hidden, precise temperature ranges. You adjust environments, moving sliders, controlling airflow, balancing temperatures, keeping flasks within safe ranges. Missteps shatter flasks, spilling contents and costing XP. The special ion-channel flask demands utmost attention; its glow intensifies as controls guide you toward perfect balance.

Other flasks respond: one reveals low-toxicity fragments, another cost-effective pieces, a third shows alkyl side chains, useful for membrane anchoring but imperfectly positioned, reducing effectiveness in some configurations. Stakes rise with every adjustment. When finally holding all flasks steady, cascading light fills the room, signaling success. Every preserved flask records in your logbook, each entry glowing with promise.

Finishing flask security reveals subtle shimmers around each. The narrator explains: "Every collected fragment contains individual atoms (carbon, hydrogen, oxygen, nitrogen, and more). These are molecular building blocks, awaiting assembly." Small atomic icons float above flasks, shimmering and moving as if alive.

A new challenge appears: collecting atoms without disturbing assembled fragments. You guide cursors or tap floating symbols, gathering individual elements into inventory. Each successful collection adds knowledge and earns XP. Fragments remain intact while providing individual components for future assembly. Some atoms move faster or shift positions, adding challenge testing attention and reflexes while maintaining engagement.

The narrator concludes: "You've collected several fragments, but the cell remains vulnerable. These are starting points. The solution is incomplete, and inventory capacity is limited. Whether you'll return for additional fragments remains uncertain." You leave with collected blocks, aware that future work builds on these discoveries.

4.5 Campaign 5

You enter Campaign 5: Molecular Architecture. The previously dormant bioreactor awakens; amber lights blinking among gears and copper pipes as if something awaits formation. This campaign unlocks only after completing Campaign 4's collection lessons. Now, the challenge involves giving pieces meaning and structure.

Activating the bioreactor enters virtual space where atoms and bonds float like luminous mechanical puzzle pieces. The narrator guides: each molecule exceeds its parts' sum—a symphony of atoms bound in precise patterns defining function.

Your first challenge: "Build a water molecule." Simple-sounding, but the system requires correct order and exact angles for bond stability. Misplaced connections cause collapse, forcing strategic rethinking.

Tasks grow complex as the narrator explains molecular formation. Brief tutorials precede challenges assembling increasingly complex structures. Each successful construction includes logs explaining biological relevance and drug creation potential.

Challenges evolve: manipulating individual atoms plus entire flasks containing pre-assembled Campaign 4 fragments. Flasks float in air, glowing softly, grabbable with cursors or hand controls. Each rotates, tilts, and positions in three-dimensional space. Orientation proves crucial that internal bonds connected only with proper fragment alignment. Wrong approaches or misaligned tilts cause connection failures.

Experimentation provides immediate feedback: successful bonds brighten fragments, emit light pulses, and trigger chimes. Incorrect placements flicker and bounce away. Achieving correct fragment angles prompts narrator commentary: "Notice perfect bond alignment, this angle enables optimal atomic interaction, ensuring molecular stability and function." XP rewards successful connections, with bonuses for perfect angles or sequential completions. Goals involve stabilizing bonds and correct assembly; sufficient XP unlocks advanced challenges and complex molecular structures, creating dynamic, strategic experiences rewarding precision and planning.

The experience teaches how molecular structure determines function beyond skill gaming. Each completed assembly triggers bioreactor valve steam expulsion, celebrating progress with mechanical light and energy spectacles.

Campaign completion teaches shaping life's fundamental materials, establishing groundwork for transforming assemblies into actual drugs, Campaign 6's awaiting challenge.

4.6 Campaign 6

The bioreactor-connected monitor flashes blue, inviting dimensional crossing. Valves hiss softly, gears turn steadily, announcing the lab's next revelation.

Activating the Campaign illuminates the bioreactor screen, entering three-dimensional environments where molecules, cell channels, and metabolic pathways animate. All previous campaign knowledge finds new expression stages.

The Molecular Docking Challenge begins with your assembled drug floating above cell membranes, glowing against digital ion channel models. You guide it toward binding sites, navigating repelling charges and moving gates. Approaching requires rotation and tilting for precise alignment, following subtle visual cues like channel light gradients. The narrator explains: "Notice molecular fit orientation enables interactions potentially triggering channel opening." Proper alignment allows binding; channel gates open slowly, ions flow, and energy ripples spread through simulations. Interactions prove functional, not merely visual: incorrect angles or misaligned conditions cause molecular bouncing and closed gates. XP rewards successful binding, perfect orientation, and efficiency, with bonuses for stable interaction maintenance.

Progressive challenges increase complexity. You simulate reactions across scenarios: temperature changes, pH alterations, genetic variant introductions. Successful simulations unlock dynamic reports displaying graphs, models, and patterns explaining results in accessible yet profound language.

After successfully guiding molecules into channels and achieving stable interactions, the narrator gestures toward the bioreactor: "Now that your drug works, production scaling begins." The bioreactor hums alive: gears spinning, amber lights blinking faster. Controls appear for flow rate, temperature, and reagent supply.

Fine-tuning parameters fills flasks with glowing molecular copies. Successful batches provide immediate feedback: light pulses, chimes, and XP for precise control. Misadjustments slow production or create imperfect molecules, encouraging careful observation and iterative improvement. This stage demonstrates scaling from single successful molecules to multiple functional copies requiring detailed attention, mirroring real-world drug manufacturing.

Campaign completion provides both molecular-level interaction and macro-level production experience. You've guided drugs into ion channels, adjusted angles and environmental factors precisely, and overseen bioreactor production. The campaign closes with narrator words: "You've brought molecules to life, from design to production. Every choice matters, and cells may now benefit from your work. Remember, new challenges await, every adjustment counts."

4.7 Campaign 7

The steampunk laboratory assumes a serious air as if machines recognize approaching responsibility. Lights flicker with reddish and golden hues while valve systems release slow, solemn steam. The organoid microfluidics station illuminates—your new learning portal.

Activation transports you inside detailed virtual cells where experiments become critical evaluations of previously designed drugs. The narrator warns: "Every compound has purpose but also cost. Today you learn to measure both."

Your first challenge: introduce drugs into cells and observe pathways. Environments respond immediately, you see molecular interactions with ion channels, metabolic pathway activation or blockage, beneficial or dangerous process triggers.

Some simulations show expected results: restored energy, optimized cellular functions. Others reveal unexpected side effects: channel saturation, metabolic pathway interruptions, toxic accumulation. Each reaction projects light and shadow choreography through cells, spectacles both beautiful and disturbing.

Tasks grow complex. You compare different doses, analyze genetic variants, introduce mutations, and evaluate how cellular responses change. Mistakes subtract points while opening new learning opportunities: understanding science lacks absolute certainties but involves delicate action-consequence balances.

Overcoming challenges displays results dashboards with dynamic graphs, interactive reports, and repeatable simulations reinforcing learned concepts. The narrator concludes: "Creating drugs isn't enough. You must understand how they live inside organisms, what helps and harms, what saves and risks."

Ending slowly shuts down organoid stations. In the steampunk lab, you hear a golden capsule transport tube hissing. A container emerges with disease names: notice that Campaign 8 downloadable content (DLC) awaits, elevating learning to more challenging levels.

4.8 Campaign 8

Iterative Global Impact reveals the steampunk laboratory's most ambitious purpose. Copper and bronze lights flicker rhythmically while hidden gear humming echoes like heartbeats heralding new beginnings. The golden capsule transport tube vibrates gently, releasing contents: sealed containers with disease names inscribed in glowing letters.

The AI-voiced narrator explains solemnly: "You've learned observing cells, deciphering channels, assembling molecules, and testing drugs. But science doesn't exist in vacuums, disease always challenges it. Today, you must revisit learned concepts and demonstrate knowledge transformation into solutions."

Opening capsules transform simulation screens into scenarios representing selected disease physiology. These may be nervous systems with defective channels, uncontrolled tumor cell growth, or altered metabolisms requiring delicate adjustments. Each mission dynamically adapts to presented challenges.

Your task involves iterating through previous campaigns: returning to microscopes, analyzing pathways, adjusting genes, assembling and testing molecules. Now everything connects to real contexts, every decision measures in terms of efficacy, safety, and potential side effects within disease settings.

Progress releases new capsules from transport systems, each representing different diseases. Each container presents separate challenges like new worlds requiring rethinking and applying learned concepts with unique strategies. Some prove simpler, others more complex, but all require creativity, precision, and patience.

The lab responds to your progress: machines glow brighter with completed challenges as if celebrating breakthroughs. The narrator concludes inspiringly: "Science doesn't end with discovery but renews with each new question. This laboratory is infinite, like diseases challenging humanity. Your role involves iterating, learning, and creating, again and again."

As the iterative disease campaign unfolds, new capsules are periodically released by the transport system, each representing a distinct challenge. Upon opening these new packages or DLCs, the player is invited to participate in additional research-driven campaigns offered by scientists as part of a citizen science initiative. Participation is entirely voluntary, and players are presented with clear terms and conditions along with an informed consent form. This ensures that any simulations, decisions, and results generated during these extended campaigns can be ethically and securely used by researchers for academic and scientific purposes, allowing players to contribute directly to ongoing studies while continuing their immersive experience.

5. EDUCATIONAL OUTCOMES AND RESEARCH INTEGRATION

Imagine stepping into a virtual world where you can design a new drug, exploring every stage of the process from cellular architecture to final protein interaction. Molecules and Missions is designed to guide players through this comprehensive journey, blending fundamental scientific principles with cutting-edge advances in molecular science. Learning progresses systematically, with each stage building upon previous knowledge while challenging players to think both critically and creatively about complex biological systems.

5.1 Progressive Learning Through Authentic Scientific Resources

Once cellular architecture is understood, attention naturally shifts to proteins and their functional roles. At this crucial stage, UniProt (The UniProt Consortium, 2023) provides essential information about protein sequences and gene encoding, enabling learners to understand how molecular structures directly relate to biological function. The game transforms this complex database information into interactive experiences, converting abstract sequence data into tangible insights about protein behavior. Players can experiment with protein variants virtually, observing how subtle amino acid changes influence three-dimensional structure and enzymatic activity, a process that closely mirrors actual scientific investigation methodologies used in contemporary research laboratories.

The journey then advances into the chemical domain, where comprehensive databases such as PubChem (Kim et al., 2021), ChEMBL (Zdrazil et al., 2024), and DrugBank (n.d) provide access to vast collections of small molecules and their documented properties. Through these resources, players explore molecular diversity, visualize complex chemical structures, and develop foundational understanding of how therapeutic compounds are systematically designed and optimized. This stage proves critical because it translates abstract chemical data into meaningful visual representations that guide the drug discovery process, helping players understand structure-activity relationships that form the backbone of medicinal chemistry.

From these chemical foundations, the learning path leads to three-dimensional molecular simulations, where theoretical concepts take spatial form and dynamic behavior becomes observable. In this immersive stage, learners manipulate molecular structures within virtual environments, directly observing how conformational changes influence binding interactions and biological functions. This hands-on approach underscores the fundamental importance of molecular geometry in determining drug efficacy while providing intuitive understanding of drug-target relationships. Beyond their scientific fidelity, these interactive simulations strengthen conceptual understanding and sustain motivation, particularly benefiting learners with limited prior expertise in molecular sciences.

The simulation experience culminates when players evaluate drug-protein interactions using structural data from the Protein Data Bank (PDB) (Burley et al., 2021). The detailed three-dimensional structures of proteins and ligands enable learners to manipulate molecular models, predict optimal binding sites, and assess the therapeutic potential of their designed compounds. This immersive experience provides tangible understanding of how molecules behave within biological systems, successfully translating abstract theoretical concepts into interactive, engaging educational environments that feel authentic and scientifically relevant.

5.2 From Individual Learning to Collective Discovery

The integration of educational gaming with authentic scientific databases creates opportunities that extend beyond traditional classroom learning. Through carefully designed gamified platforms, citizen science initiatives can meaningfully extend participation in drug discovery by making complex processes accessible, understandable, and rewarding for diverse audiences regardless of their formal scientific training background.

This democratization approach transforms the traditional paradigm of exclusive expert-driven research into more collaborative models where educated participants can contribute substantively to pharmaceutical research challenges. Players develop not only theoretical understanding but also practical skills that enable them to generate hypotheses, test molecular designs, and contribute data that may inform actual drug development efforts.

The educational framework creates a bidirectional relationship between learning and discovery. Students gain knowledge while simultaneously contributing to databases of potential therapeutic compounds, creating a virtuous cycle where educational engagement generates scientific value. This approach transforms drug discovery from an exclusive scientific endeavor into a collective experience where participants gain both knowledge and genuine sense of contribution to meaningful research outcomes.

Furthermore, the collaborative nature of these platforms models the increasingly interdisciplinary character of contemporary pharmaceutical research, where biologists, chemists, computer scientists, and data analysts work together to address complex medical challenges. By experiencing this collaborative process firsthand, learners develop appreciation for scientific teamwork while building confidence in their ability to contribute to cutting-edge research initiatives.

Through this comprehensive integration of education and research, Molecules and Missions demonstrates how gamified learning environments can simultaneously achieve pedagogical goals while advancing scientific knowledge, creating sustainable models for broader public engagement in pharmaceutical innovation.

6. IMPLEMENTATION CHALLENGES

Implementing gamified platforms and virtual labs in drug discovery education presents significant opportunities alongside substantial obstacles. While these tools have demonstrated potential to democratize access, foster motivation, and engage learners in authentic scientific processes, their successful deployment requires addressing challenges that span technical infrastructure, pedagogical integration, accessibility, scientific rigor, and resource sustainability. Understanding these implementation barriers is essential for transforming innovative concepts into viable, lasting educational practices.

6.1 Technical Barriers

The foundation of effective gamified learning platforms rests on robust technical infrastructure, which remains unevenly distributed across educational contexts. Although valuable databases such as UniProt, PubChem, ChEMBL (Zdrazil et al., 2024), DrugBank (n.d.), and the PDB are freely accessible, the computational demands of interactive molecular simulations can be substantial. High-speed internet connectivity, adequate memory capacity, and updated graphics capabilities represent prerequisites that many educational institutions and individual learners cannot readily access.

This technological gap risks creating a paradox where tools designed to democratize scientific education inadvertently reinforce existing inequalities. Students in resource-constrained environments may find themselves excluded from three-dimensional molecular visualizations and real-time simulations, while institutions lacking technical infrastructure struggle to provide necessary support. The digital divide extends beyond hardware limitations to include variations in technical literacy among both students and educators.

Addressing these disparities requires strategic approaches that acknowledge resource limitations. Solutions might include developing platforms with scalable complexity, implementing offline functionality for essential components, creating local caching systems for large datasets, or establishing shared computational resources through institutional partnerships. The goal is ensuring that technological requirements enhance rather than limit educational accessibility.

6.2 Pedagogical and Curricular Integration

Integrating gamified approaches into established educational frameworks presents complex pedagogical challenges that extend beyond technical implementation. Traditional academic structures often emphasize standardized assessment methods and content delivery models that may not align naturally with exploratory, game-based learning approaches. The shift from passive information reception to active problem-solving through gameplay requires fundamental reconsideration of how learning is structured, assessed, and validated.

Effective integration demands alignment between gamified activities and intended learning outcomes, ensuring that playful exploration translates into disciplinary understanding. Assessment strategies must evolve to recognize skills such as creative problem-solving, collaborative inquiry, and systems thinking, rather than focusing exclusively on factual recall. This pedagogical shift requires educators to reconceptualize their roles from information providers to learning facilitators and mentors.

Professional development emerges as a critical factor in successful implementation. Many educators lack experience with game-based learning environments, which can lead to underutilization or inappropriate application of these tools. Comprehensive training programs must address both technical proficiency and pedagogical rationale, helping instructors design meaningful activities that connect gameplay experiences to disciplinary knowledge while maintaining academic rigor.

6.3 Accessibility and Inclusion

Ensuring equitable access represents both an ethical imperative and a practical challenge in developing gamified educational platforms. While these tools may reduce certain learning barriers by making science more engaging, they can inadvertently create new obstacles if accessibility considerations are not integrated from the initial design phase rather than added as afterthoughts.

Students with visual impairments require alternative approaches to molecular visualization, such as haptic feedback systems or detailed audio descriptions of molecular structures and interactions. Learners with motor impairments need adaptive interfaces that accommodate different interaction capabilities when manipulating three-dimensional molecular models. Cognitive accessibility considerations include providing multiple ways to process information, adjustable complexity levels, and clear navigation structures.

Implementing universal design principles benefits all learners, not just those with identified disabilities. Features such as customizable interfaces, multiple representation formats, and flexible interaction methods create more inclusive learning environments while modeling the collaborative and diverse nature of contemporary scientific practice. This inclusivity is particularly relevant in drug discovery education, where diverse perspectives and approaches strengthen both learning outcomes and scientific progress.

6.4 Scientific Validity and Data Integrity

Balancing engagement with scientific accuracy presents ongoing challenges in gamified educational design. The simplification necessary to make complex molecular processes accessible to learners carries risks of creating misconceptions or oversimplified understanding that may hinder rather than enhance scientific comprehension. The challenge lies in identifying which aspects of scientific complexity are essential to preserve and which can be appropriately simplified without compromising educational integrity.

Effective gamification requires maintaining what might be termed "authentic complexity", preserving the essential logic and relationships of scientific processes while making them approachable for learners at different levels. This involves careful consideration of how molecular interactions, protein dynamics, and drug mechanisms are represented, ensuring that simplifications enhance understanding rather than distort scientific reality.

Quality assurance mechanisms become particularly important when gamified platforms incorporate citizen science elements. While non-specialist contributions can provide valuable learning experiences and potentially useful data, robust validation systems are essential to maintain scientific credibility. These systems might include automated error detection, expert oversight protocols, and cross-validation procedures that ensure meaningful scientific engagement without compromising data integrity.

6.5 Institutional and Policy Constraints

Long-term viability of gamified educational platforms depends on sustainable funding models and institutional commitment beyond initial implementation. While scientific databases remain freely accessible, interactive platforms require ongoing investment in server infrastructure, technical support, content updates, and educator training programs.

Educational institutions face competing demands for limited resources, making it challenging to justify investments in innovative educational approaches. Costs extend beyond initial development to include maintenance, compatibility updates, and professional development. Policy frameworks often lag behind educational innovation, potentially undervaluing learning outcomes achieved through non-traditional methods, which limits institutional support and recognition.

Alternative approaches merit consideration, including collaborative development where institutions share costs, partnerships with technology companies, or integration with research initiatives that benefit from citizen science contributions. The goal is creating sustainable ecosystems that support ongoing innovation without placing unsustainable burdens on individual institutions.

6.6 Moving Forward

Addressing implementation challenges requires coordinated approaches that recognize the interconnected nature of technical, pedagogical, and institutional obstacles. Successful deployment depends on strategic planning that addresses multiple barriers simultaneously.

Key strategies include developing flexible, scalable platforms that function across diverse technological contexts; implementing gradual deployment with pilot programs to build institutional confidence; integrating accessibility from the design phase rather than as afterthoughts; and creating professional development programs that provide ongoing support as educators develop competence with new approaches.

The promise of gamified virtual labs lies in transforming abstract molecular concepts into engaging, accessible learning experiences. Realizing this potential requires acknowledging challenges while working systematically to address them through thoughtful planning, collaborative approaches, and sustained commitment to educational innovation that serves all learners effectively.

7. CONCLUSION: TOWARD A NEW PARADIGM IN SCIENCE EDUCATION

The journey through molecular science education stands at a transformative crossroads where the traditional boundaries between learning and discovery, between student and researcher, between virtual simulation and real-world application are dissolving. This proposal considers the merging of education, scientific research, and interactive design into a unified framework that reimagines how we can democratize access to one of science's most complex fields.

The Molecules and Missions framework demonstrates how carefully designed interactive experiences can transform abstract molecular concepts into tangible learning adventures. By progressing through eight interconnected campaigns, from basic cellular observation to addressing global medical challenges, learners develop not just knowledge, but the scientific intuition and problem-solving skills essential for real drug discovery. In this context, gamification is not merely a pedagogical tool, but a pathway for pharmaceutical innovation where the game serves as a collaborative space where students, researchers, and developers tackle real-world problems together.

Interactive video games are increasingly recognized as innovative educational tools that blend entertainment with learning (Prensky, 2008). Their interactive nature engages users in real-time responses to visual stimuli and decision-making (Gee, 2008). Educational games have been shown to enhance the understanding of complex topics in an enjoyable and meaningful way (Squire, 2003). Within this framework, the integration of gamification principles with authentic scientific processes creates unprecedented opportunities for broader participation in drug discovery research.

By incorporating real scientific challenges, the platform fosters a transdisciplinary approach, bringing together experts in video game design, artificial intelligence, bioinformatics, and educational theory. Students become active contributors rather than passive recipients; solving problems, generating molecules, and populating a growing database of potential solutions. Beyond learning, gameplay generates actionable knowledge for drug discovery and development, transforming learners into contributors to actual pharmaceutical research.

The implementation challenges examined (technical infrastructure, pedagogical integration, accessibility, and sustainability) are significant but not insurmountable. They require coordinated responses that acknowledge the interconnected nature of these obstacles while building solutions that serve diverse learners and contexts. The key lies in developing flexible, scalable platforms that maintain scientific rigor across varied technological environments.

This approach addresses a critical need in science education: making the invisible world of molecular interactions visible and comprehensible. The nanoscale realm where drug molecules bind to protein channels has traditionally been accessible only through abstract representations. Virtual labs with immersive visualization capabilities transform these abstractions into manipulable, observable phenomena that learners can explore directly.

The potential impact extends beyond individual learning outcomes to encompass broader societal benefits. As students progress through gamified drug discovery experiences, they develop deeper appreciation for pharmaceutical research complexity, fostering more informed public discourse about health policies and scientific investment. The collaborative nature of these platforms models the interdisciplinary character of contemporary research, where diverse expertise converges to address complex challenges.

While virtual labs have already demonstrated their importance in expanding access to scientific education, the future lies in enhancing their interactivity and immersion. Molecular sciences, with their inherent complexity and abstraction, stand to benefit the most from these innovations. Looking forward, advances in virtual reality, artificial intelligence, and collaborative platforms will continue to expand educational possibilities, creating increasingly sophisticated personalized learning experiences.

By combining evidence-based virtual lab practices with new interactive tools, educators and researchers can foster deeper understanding, spark curiosity, and better prepare future scientists for the demanding challenges of drug design and molecular research. The proposed game offers an interactive, accessible, and compelling learning experience for a wide range of audiences, transforming how we approach molecular science education.

The journey is just beginning, and the possibilities are as exciting as the molecules we study. The molecular world awaits exploration, and the tools to make that exploration accessible to all are within our reach.

8. REFERENCES

Ahmed, M., Maldonado, A. M., & Durrant, J. D. (2023). From byte to bench to bedside: Molecular dynamics simulations and drug discovery. *BMC Biology*, *21*(1), 299. DOI: 10.1186/s12915-023-01791-z PMID: 38155355

Burley, S. K., Bhikadiya, C., Bi, C., Bittrich, S., Chen, L., Crichlow, G. V., Christie, C. H., Dalenberg, K., Di Costanzo, L., Duarte, J. M., Dutta, S., Feng, Z., Ganesan, S., Goodsell, D. S., Ghosh, S., Green, R. K., Guranović, V., Guzenko, D., Hudson, B. P., & Zhuravleva, M. (2021). RCSB Protein Data Bank: Powerful new tools for exploring 3D structures of biological macromolecules for basic and applied research and education in fundamental biology, biomedicine, biotechnology, bioengineering and energy sciences. *Nucleic Acids Research*, *49*(D1), D437–D451. DOI: 10.1093/nar/gkaa1038 PMID: 33211854

Byukusenge, C., Nsanganwimana, F., & Tarmo, A. P. (2022). Effectiveness of virtual laboratories in teaching and learning biology: A review of literature. *International Journal of Learning Teaching and Educational Research*, *21*(6), 1–17. DOI: 10.26803/ijlter.21.6.1

Chans, G. M., & Portuguez Castro, M. (2021). Gamification as a Strategy to Increase Motivation and Engagement in Higher Education Chemistry Students. *Computers*, *10*(10), 132. DOI: 10.3390/computers10100132

DrugBank. (n.d.). Retrieved June 13, 2025, from https://go.drugbank.com/

Gee, J. P. (2008). *What video games have to teach us about learning and literacy* (2nd ed.). Palgrave Macmillan.

Giardullo, P., Neresini, F., Marín-González, E., Luís, C., Magalhães, J., & Arias, R. (2023). Citizen science and participatory science communication: An empirically informed discussion connecting research and theory. *JCOM, Journal of Science Communication*, *22*(2). Advance online publication. DOI: 10.22323/2.22020201

Gu, S., Shen, C., Yu, J., Zhao, H., Liu, H., Liu, L., Sheng, R., Xu, L., Wang, Z., Hou, T., & Kang, Y. (2023). Can molecular dynamics simulations improve predictions of protein-ligand binding affinity with machine learning? *Briefings in Bioinformatics*, *24*(2), bbad008. Advance online publication. DOI: 10.1093/bib/bbad008 PMID: 36681903

Hawkins, I., & Phelps, A. J. (2013). Virtual laboratory vs. traditional laboratory: Which is more effective for teaching electrochemistry? *Chemistry Education Research and Practice*, *14*(4), 516–523. DOI: 10.1039/C3RP00070B

Hernandez, C. C., Gimenez, L. E., Strassmaier, T., Rogers, M., & Taymans, J.-M. (2024). Editorial: Targeting ion channels for drug discovery: emerging challenges for high throughput screening technologies. *Frontiers in Molecular Neuroscience*, *17*, 1414816. Advance online publication. DOI: 10.3389/fnmol.2024.1414816 PMID: 38883981

Ibarra-Herrera, C. C., Carrizosa, A., Yunes-Rojas, J. A., & Mata-Gómez, M. A. (2019). Design of an app based on gamification and storytelling as a tool for biology courses. [IJIDeM]. *International Journal on Interactive Design and Manufacturing*, *13*(4), 1271–1282. DOI: 10.1007/s12008-019-00600-8

Imbrici, P., Liantonio, A., Camerino, G. M., de Bellis, M., Camerino, C., Mele, A., Giustino, A., Pierno, S., de Luca, A., Tricarico, D., Desaphy, J.-F., & Conte, D. (2016). Therapeutic Approaches to Genetic Ion Channelopathies and Perspectives in Drug Discovery. *Frontiers in Pharmacology*, *7*. Advance online publication. DOI: 10.3389/fphar.2016.00121 PMID: 27242528

Johnson, B. A. (2023). *A molecular construction game based on principles from game-based learning sciences* (Master's thesis, University of California, Merced). eScholarship.

Kalogiannakis, M., Papadakis, S., & Zourmpakis, A.-I. (2021). Gamification in Science Education. A Systematic Review of the Literature. *Education Sciences*, *11*(1), 22. DOI: 10.3390/educsci11010022

Kim, S., Chen, J., Cheng, T., Gindulyte, A., He, J., He, S., Li, Q., Shoemaker, B. A., Thiessen, P. A., Yu, B., Zaslavsky, L., Zhang, J., & Bolton, E. E. (2021). PubChem in 2021: New data content and improved web interfaces. *Nucleic Acids Research*, *49*(D1), D1388–D1395. DOI: 10.1093/nar/gkaa971 PMID: 33151290

Koepnick, B., Flatten, J., Husain, T., Ford, A., Silva, D.-A., Bick, M. J., Bauer, A., Liu, G., Ishida, Y., Boykov, A., Estep, R. D., Kleinfelter, S., Nørgård-Solano, T., Wei, L., Players, F., Montelione, G. T., DiMaio, F., Popović, Z., Khatib, F., & Baker, D. (2019). De novo protein design by citizen scientists. *Nature*, *570*(7761), 390–394. DOI: 10.1038/s41586-019-1274-4 PMID: 31168091

Li, L., Hew, K. F., & Du, J. (2024). Gamification enhances student intrinsic motivation, perceptions of autonomy and relatedness, but minimal impact on competency: A meta-analysis and systematic review. *Educational Technology Research and Development*, *72*(2), 765–796. DOI: 10.1007/s11423-023-10337-7

Prensky, M. (2008). *Digital game-based learning*. Paragon House.

Reynaldo, C., Christian, R., Hosea, H., & Gunawan, A. A. S. (2021). Using Video Games to Improve Capabilities in Decision Making and Cognitive Skill: A Literature Review. *Procedia Computer Science*, *179*, 211–221. DOI: 10.1016/j.procs.2020.12.027

Rollings, A., & Adams, E. (2003). *Andrew rollings and Ernest Adams on game design*. New Riders Publishing.

Ryan, R. M., Rigby, C. S., & Przybylski, A. (2006). The Motivational Pull of Video Games: A Self-Determination Theory Approach. *Motivation and Emotion*, *30*(4), 344–360. DOI: 10.1007/s11031-006-9051-8

Shute, V. J. (2011). Stealth assessment in computer-based games to support learning. In Tobias, S., & Fletcher, J. D. (Eds.), *Computer games and instruction* (pp. 503–524). IAP Information Age Publishing. DOI: 10.1108/978-1-61735-410-620251025

Squire, K. (2003). Video games in education. *Int. J. Intell. Games & Simulation*, *2*(1), 49–62.

Sulea, T., Kumar, S., & Kuroda, D. (2024). Editorial: Progress and challenges in computational structure-based design and development of biologic drugs. *Frontiers in Molecular Biosciences*, *11*, 1360267. Advance online publication. DOI: 10.3389/fmolb.2024.1360267 PMID: 38389897

Tibell, L. A. E., & Rundgren, C.-J. (2010). Educational challenges of molecular life science: Characteristics and implications for education and research. *CBE Life Sciences Education*, *9*(1), 25–33. DOI: 10.1187/cbe.08-09-0055 PMID: 20194805

The UniProt Consortium. (2023). UniProt: The universal protein knowledgebase in 2023. *Nucleic Acids Research*, *51*(D1), D523–D531. DOI: 10.1093/nar/gkac1052

Vieira, I. H. P., Botelho, E. B., de Souza Gomes, T. J., Kist, R., Caceres, R. A., & Zanchi, F. B. (2023). Visual dynamics: A WEB application for molecular dynamics simulation using GROMACS. *BMC Bioinformatics*, *24*(1), 107. DOI: 10.1186/s12859-023-05234-y PMID: 36949402

Weber, C., Sipos, M., Paczal, A., Balint, B., Kun, V., Foloppe, N., Dokurno, P., Massey, A. J., Walmsley, D. L., Hubbard, R. E., Murray, J., Benwell, K., Edmonds, T., Demarles, D., Bruno, A., Burbridge, M., Cruzalegui, F., & Kotschy, A. (2021). Structure-Guided Discovery of Potent and Selective DYRK1A Inhibitors. *Journal of Medicinal Chemistry*, *64*(10), 6745–6764. DOI: 10.1021/acs.jmedchem.1c00023 PMID: 33975430

Werbach, K., & Hunter, D. (2012). *For the win*. Wharton Digital Press.

Zdrazil, B., Felix, E., Hunter, F., Manners, E. J., Blackshaw, J., Corbett, S., de Veij, M., Ioannidis, H., Lopez, D. M., Mosquera, J. F., Magarinos, M. P., Bosc, N., Arcila, R., Kizilören, T., Gaulton, A., Bento, A. P., Adasme, M. F., Monecke, P., Landrum, G. A., & Leach, A. R. (2024). The ChEMBL Database in 2023: A drug discovery platform spanning multiple bioactivity data types and time periods. *Nucleic Acids Research*, *52*(D1), D1180–D1192. DOI: 10.1093/nar/gkad1004 PMID: 37933841

Zhang, J., Sabatier, J.-M., Chahine, M., & Tricarico, D. (2024). Editorial: Reviews in pharmacology of ion channels and channelopathies. *Frontiers in Pharmacology, 15*, 1449967. Advance online publication. DOI: 10.3389/fphar.2024.1449967 PMID: 39228529

Compilation of References

Abdulhussain, Y., Ghelani, H., Henderson, H., Sudhir, M., Mascarenhas, S., Radhakrishnan, R., & Jan, R. K. (2022). The use and effectiveness of high-fidelity simulation in health professions education: Current update. *Simulation*, *98*(12), 1085–1095. Advance online publication. DOI: 10.1177/00375497221101066

Abidin, S. R. Z., Noor, S. F. M., Ashaari, N. S., & Yadegaridehkordi, E. (2024). Improving literacy skills using the serious game model compatible with brain-based learning. *Multimedia Tools and Applications*, *84*(1), 95–129. DOI: 10.1007/s11042-024-20305-9

Acevedo-Osorio, G. O., Cortes-Benítez, P. L., Blanco-Vanegas, A. M., & Montero-Caicedo, L. L. (2025). Impact of virtual reality on the strengthening of psychomotor skills in Surgical Instrumentation students in Pereira, Colombia. *Medical Education*, *26*(5), 101083. DOI: 10.1016/j.edumed.2025.101083

Adamovic, S., Sarac, M., Stamenkovic, U., & Radovanovic, D. (2018). The importance of the using software tools for learning modern cryptography. *International Journal of Engineering Education*, *34*(1), 256–262.

Aguilera, D., & Vílchez-González, J. M. (2024). ¿De qué hablamos cuando hablamos de educación STEAM? Una revisión de experiencias educativas. *Revista Fuentes*, *2*(26), 211–224. DOI: 10.12795/revistafuentes.2024.15412

Ahmed, M., Maldonado, A. M., & Durrant, J. D. (2023). From byte to bench to bedside: Molecular dynamics simulations and drug discovery. *BMC Biology*, *21*(1), 299. DOI: 10.1186/s12915-023-01791-z PMID: 38155355

Al Shamsi, H., Al Mashrafi, S., Al Kalbani, T., & Almutairi, A. G. (2020). Implications of Language Barriers for Healthcare: A Systematic Review. *Oman Medical Journal*, *35*(2), 1–7. DOI: 10.5001/omj.2020.40

Alcántara Pineda, A. (2017). *Métodos estadísticos para comparar perfiles de disolución requeridos por la NOM-177.* https://farmazine.mx/articulos/metodos-estadisticos-para-comparar-perfiles-de-disolucion-requeridos-por-la-nom-177

Alhamdani, W. A. (2016). Teaching Cryptography Using Design Thinking Approach. *Journal of Applied Security Research, 11*(1), 78–89. DOI: 10.1080/19361610.2015.1069646

Aliyu, H. (2025). A review of instructional strategies for maximizing the effectiveness of PhET interactive simulations in chemistry education. *Rima International Journal of Education, 4*(1), 479–487.

Almelhi, A. M. (2021). Effectiveness of the ADDIE Model within an E-Learning Environment in Developing Creative Writing in EFL Students. *English Language Teaching, 14*(2), 20. DOI: 10.5539/elt.v14n2p20

Álvarez Magallán, B. A., Acosta-Díaz, R., & Morales-Vanegas, E. A. (2024). Privacy-Aware Artificial Intelligence: A Review of Design Principles and Applications. *Avances En Interacción Humano-Computadora, 9*(1), 209–213. DOI: 10.47756/aihc.y9i1.169

Ammar, M., Amjad, I., Nisar, M., & Ghoneim, O. S. (2024). Effects of board games on balance in association with cognition in community-dwelling older adults. *Journal of Musculoskeletal Surgery and Research : Official Publication of Saudi Orthopaedic Association, 8*(3), 256–263. DOI: 10.25259/JMSR_122_2024

Amorim, A. N., Jeon, L., Abel, Y., Albuquerque, E. X. S., Soares, M., Silva, V. C., & Oliveira Neto, J. R. (2022). Escribo play learning games can foster early reading and writing for low-income kindergarten children. *Computers & Education, 177*, 104364. DOI: 10.1016/j.compedu.2021.104364

Angulo, B. P., Gaxiola, A. A., Peñuelas, E. G., & Lagarda, A. C. (2018). Incidence and degree of anxiety in higher level students in the area of health sciences. *Salud en Tabasco, 24*(1), 21-26. Retrieved from https://tabasco.gob.mx/sites/default/files/users/ssaludtabasco/21.pdf

Aparicio Gómez, W. O. (2023). Artificial Intelligence and its Impact on Education: Transforming Learning for the 21st Century. *International Journal of Pedagogy and Educational Innovation, 3*(2), 217–230. DOI: 10.51660/ripie.v3i2.133

Armendáriz Espadas, P. (2018). *Los videojuegos educativos en México* (Universidad de las Américas Puebla). Retrieved from http://catarina.udlap.mx/u_dl_a/tales/documentos/lnd/armendariz_espadas_p/etd_3021084549481.pdf

Arnold, B. J. (2014). Gamification in education. *Proceedings of the American Society of Business and Behavioral Sciences*, *21*(1), 32–39.

Asad, M., Naz, A., Churi, P., & Tahanzadeh, M. (2021). Virtual reality as a pedagogical tool to improve experiential learning: a systematic review of the literature. *International Research in Education*, 1–17. https://doi.org/DOI: 10.1155/2021/7061623

Asemani Barekat, N. (2023). The Effect of Board Games on the Academic Achievement and Learning Motivation of Fourth-Grade Elementary Student. *International Journal of Elementary Education*, *12*(3), 68–75. DOI: 10.11648/j.ijeedu.20231203.13

Asociación Interamericana de Contabilidad. (2024). *Desventajas y Riesgos de la Inteligencia Artificial en la Educación Universitaria - AIC*. AIC. https://contadores-aic.org/desventajas-y-riesgos-de-la-inteligencia-artificial-en-la-educacion-universitaria-originalidad-de-ensayos-y-plagios/

Aster, A., Laupichler, M. C., Zimmer, S., & Raupach, T. (2024). Game design elements of serious games in the education of medical and healthcare professions: A mixed-methods systematic review of underlying theories and teaching effectiveness. *Advances in Health Sciences Education : Theory and Practice*, *29*(5), 1825–1848. DOI: 10.1007/s10459-024-10327-1 PMID: 38563873

Aulia, P. F. (2025). The effectiveness of gamification in enhancing English language learning outcomes. *Jurnal Pendidikan Dan Sastra Inggris*, *5*(2), 304–320. https://journalshub.org/index.php/JUPENSI/article/view/5238/5082

Baek, Y., Xu, Y., Han, S., & Cho, J. (2015). Exploring effects of intrinsic motivation and prior knowledge on student achievements in game-based learning. *Smart Computing Review*, *5*(4), 368–377. DOI: 10.6029/smartcr.2015.10.001

Balart-Sánchez, S. A., Vélez-Pérez, H., Rivera-Tello, S., Gómez Velázquez, F. R., González-Garrido, A. A., & Romo-Vázquez, R. (2019). A step forward in the quest for a mobile EEG-designed epoch for psychophysiological studies. *Biomedizinische Technik*, *64*(6), 655–667. DOI: 10.1515/bmt-2017-0189 PMID: 31322998

Bao, S., Chan, V. T., & Merzenich, M. M. (2001). Cortical remodelling induced by activity of ventral tegmental dopamine neurons. *Nature*, *412*(6842), 79–83. DOI: 10.1038/35083586 PMID: 11452310

Baranowski, T., Buday, R., Thompson, D. I., & Baranowski, J. (2008). Playing for real: Video games and stories for health-related behavior change. *American Journal of Preventive Medicine*, *34*(1), 74–82. DOI: 10.1016/j.amepre.2007.09.027 PMID: 18083454

Barrows, H. S. (1986). A taxonomy of problem-based learning methods. *Medical Education, 20*(6), 481–486. DOI: 10.1111/j.1365-2923.1986.tb01386.x

Bavelier, D., & Green, C. S. (2019). Enhancing attentional control: Lessons from action video games. *Neuron, 104*(1), 147–163. DOI: 10.1016/j.neuron.2019.09.031 PMID: 31600511

Beck, A. T., Epstein, N., Brown, G., & Steer, R. A. (1988). An inventory for measuring clinical anxiety: Psychometric properties. *Journal of Consulting and Clinical Psychology, 56*(6), 893–897. DOI: 10.1037/0022-006X.56.6.893 PMID: 3204199

Beck, A. T., Steer, R. A., & Brown, G. K. (1996). *Manual for the Beck Depression Inventory-II*. Psychological Corporation.

Bediou, B., Adams, D. M., Mayer, R. E., Tipton, E., Green, C. S., & Bavelier, D. (2018). Meta-analysis of action video game impact on perceptual, attentional, and cognitive skills. *Psychological Bulletin, 144*(1), 77–110. DOI: 10.1037/bul0000130 PMID: 29172564

Belli, S., & López Raventós, C. (2008). Breve historia de los videojuegos. *Athenea Digital, 179*(14), 159–179. DOI: 10.5565/rev/athenead/v0n14.570

Beltrán Fuentes, A. F. (2024). El impacto del uso de la inteligencia artificial en los estudiantes de Administración de Empresas de la Pontificia Universidad Javeriana (Tesis de licenciatura, Pontificia Universidad Javeriana, Bogotá, Colombia). Repositorio Institucional PUJ. https://apidspace.javeriana.edu.co/server/api/core/bitstreams/8f23fe21-53ad-4ea1-8f62-ff250d48cf05/content

Ben-Zeev, T., Weiss, I., Ashri, S., Heled, Y., Ketko, I., Yanovich, R., & Okun, E. (2020). Mild Physical Activity Does Not Improve Spatial Learning in a Virtual Environment. *Frontiers in Behavioral Neuroscience, 14*, 584052. DOI: 10.3389/fnbeh.2020.584052

Berson, I. R., & Berson, M. J. (2019). Digital citizenship and emotional literacy: Building empathy in online environments. *Journal of Social Studies Education Research, 10*(2), 1–20.

Biggs, J. B., & Collis, K. F. (1982). *Evaluating the Quality of Learning: The SOLO Taxonomy (structure of the Observed Learning Outcome)*. Academic Press. https://books.google.com.mx/books?id=x4qcAAAAMAAJ

Birk, M. V., Mandryk, R. L., & Krolczyk, Z. (2020). The effects of avatar customization on player engagement in educational games [Conference session]. 2020 IEEE International Conference on Teaching, Assessment, and Learning for Engineering (TALE), Takamatsu, Japan (virtual). https://doi.org/DOI: 10.1109/TALE48869.2020.9368315

Borleffs, E., Glatz, T. K., Daulay, D. A., Richardson, U., Zwarts, F., & Maassen, B. A. M. (2018). GraphoGame SI: The development of a technology-enhanced literacy learning tool for Standard Indonesian. *European Journal of Psychology of Education, 33*(4), 595–613. DOI: 10.1007/s10212-017-0354-9

Boudadi, N., & Gutiérrez-Colón, M. (2020). Effect of Gamification on students' motivation and learning achievement in Second Language Acquisition within higher education: A literature review 2011-2019. *The EUROCALL Review, 28*(1), 40–69. DOI: 10.4995/eurocall.2020.12974

Boyle, E. A., Hainey, T., Connolly, T. M., Gray, G., Earp, J., Ott, M., Lim, T., Ninaus, M., Ribeiro, C., & Pereira, J. (2016). An update to the systematic literature review of empirical evidence of the impacts and outcomes of computer games and serious games. *Computers & Education, 94*, 178–192. DOI: 10.1016/j.compedu.2015.11.003

Brooke, J. (1996). SUS: A quick and dirty usability scale. In Jordan, P. W., Thomas, B., Weerdmeester, B. A., & McClelland, A. L. (Eds.), *Usability Evaluation in Industry* (pp. 189–194). Taylor & Francis.

Brophy, S. B., & Lowe, T. A. (2017). *A Learning Trajectory for Developing Computational Thinking and Programming*. Purdue e-Pubs. https://docs.lib.purdue.edu/enepubs/14/

Brown-Jeffy, S., & Cooper, J. E. (2011). Toward a Conceptual Framework of Culturally Relevant Pedagogy: An Overview of the Conceptual and Theoretical Literature. *Teacher Education Quarterly (Claremont, Calif.), 38*(1), 65–84.

Buheji, M. (2019). Gamification techniques to re-invent public healthcare services: A case study. *International Journal of Human Resource Studies, 9*(2), 339. DOI: 10.5296/ijhrs.v9i2.14888

Burley, S. K., Bhikadiya, C., Bi, C., Bittrich, S., Chen, L., Crichlow, G. V., Christie, C. H., Dalenberg, K., Di Costanzo, L., Duarte, J. M., Dutta, S., Feng, Z., Ganesan, S., Goodsell, D. S., Ghosh, S., Green, R. K., Guranović, V., Guzenko, D., Hudson, B. P., & Zhuravleva, M. (2021). RCSB Protein Data Bank: Powerful new tools for exploring 3D structures of biological macromolecules for basic and applied research and education in fundamental biology, biomedicine, biotechnology, bioengineering and energy sciences. *Nucleic Acids Research, 49*(D1), D437–D451. DOI: 10.1093/nar/gkaa1038 PMID: 33211854

Burns, M. S., Griffin, J., & Snows, C. E. (1999). *Starting out right. A guide promoting children s reading success*. National Academic Press.

Byukusenge, C., Nsanganwimana, F., & Tarmo, A. P. (2022). Effectiveness of virtual laboratories in teaching and learning biology: A review of literature. *International Journal of Learning Teaching and Educational Research, 21*(6), 1–17. DOI: 10.26803/ijlter.21.6.1

Byusa, E., Kampire, E., & Mwesigye, A. R. (2022). Game-based learning approach on students' motivation and understanding of chemistry concepts: A systematic review of literature. *Heliyon, 8*(5), e09541. DOI: 10.1016/j.heliyon.2022.e09541

Cabero-Almenara, J., & Costas, J. (2016). La utilización de simuladores para la formación de los alumnos. *Revista Prisma Social, 17*, 343–372.

Camacho-Quiroz, R. (2013). La lectura en México, un problema multifactorial. *Contribuciones Desde Coatepec*, (25), 153–156.

Cámara de Diputados. (2010). *Ley Federal de Protección de Datos Personales en Posesión de los Particulares*. Diario Oficial de la Federación. https://www.diputados.gob.mx/LeyesBiblio/pdf/LFPDPPP.pdf

Cárdenas Rodríguez, H. Lilia., Cortés Arroyo, A. Rosa., & Universidad Autónoma Metropolitana (México). Unidad Xochimilco. (1996). *Aspectos biofarmacéuticos de la evaluación de medicamentos / Hilda Lilia Cárdenas Rodríguez, Alma Rosa Cortés Arroyo.* Casa abierta al tiempo, Universidad Autónoma Metropolitana.

Cárdenas, A., Castro, C., Chacón, M. J., Cabrera, Z., & Hernández, V. (2023). Health habits in university students and perceptions about weight and diet during the SARS-CoV2 pandemic. Science and Humanism in Health 2023, Vol. 10, No 3, pp85-91 Retrieved from. http://revista.medicina.uady.mx

Casallas-Hernández, N., Castillo-Daza, C. A., & González-Guzmán, V. A. (2025). Acceptance and effectiveness of high-fidelity simulation in nursing education: Application of the Technology Acceptance Model (TAM). *Clinical Simulation in Nursing, 105*, 101765. DOI: 10.1016/j.ecns.2025.101765

Castells, M. (2000). *La era de la información: Economía, sociedad y cultura* (2. ed). Alianza.

CEMTRO Clinic. (2019). *Da Vinci robotic surgery.* Robotic Surgery. Retrieved September 6, 2025, from http://www.icirugiarobotica.com/cirugia-robotica-da-vinci/

Cès, P., Duflos, M., Tricard, E., Jhean-Larose, S., & Giraudeau, C. (2024). Playing board games to increase emotional competencies in school-age children and older people: A systematic review. *Leisure Sciences*, •••, 1–24. DOI: 10.1080/01490400.2024.2373415

Chamorro, E., Cárdenas, J., Melo, L., Vallejo, O., Arcos, J., Bolaños, A., Poveda, J., Pinchao, L., Vianey, A., & Rodríguez, J. (2022). Competent human formation: Project-based learning experiences. https://doi.org/DOI: 10.31948/editorialunimar.164

Changoluisa Jaya, L. G. (2024). Effects of Artificial Intelligence on the Socioemotional Development of Adolescents. *Ciencia Latina Multidisciplinary Journal*, *8*(3), 3423–3440. DOI: 10.37811/cl_rcm.v8i3.11565

Chans, G. M., & Portuguez Castro, M. (2021). Gamification as a Strategy to Increase Motivation and Engagement in Higher Education Chemistry Students. *Computers*, *10*(10), 132. DOI: 10.3390/computers10100132

Checa-Romero, M., & Gimenez-Lozano, J. M. (2024). Video games and metacognition in the classroom for the development of 21st century skills: A systematic review. *Frontiers in Education*, *9*, 1485098. Advance online publication. DOI: 10.3389/feduc.2024.1485098

Chen, L., & Xia, M. (2025). Adolescent psychological adaptation: The impact of daily levels and instability in psychological need satisfaction and frustration. Journal of Adolescence, Advance online publication. https://www.researchgate.net/publication/390355467_Adolescent_Psychological_Adaptation_The_Impact_of_Daily_Levels_and_Instability_in_Psychological_Need_Satisfaction_and_Frustration. DOI: 10.1002/jad.12495

Chirico, A., Lucidi, F., De Laurentiis, M., Milanese, C., Napoli, A., & Giordano, A. (2016). Virtual Reality in Health System: Beyond Entertainment. A Mini-Review on the Efficacy of VR During Cancer Treatment. *Journal of Cellular Physiology*, *231*(2), 275–287. DOI: 10.1002/jcp.25117

Chirico, A., Maiorano, P., Indovina, P., Milanese, C., Giordano, G. G., Alivernini, F., Iodice, G., Gallo, L., De Pietro, G., Lucidi, F., Botti, G., De Laurentiis, M., & Giordano, A. (2020). Virtual reality and music therapy as distraction interventions to alleviate anxiety and improve mood states in breast cancer patients during chemotherapy. *Journal of Cellular Physiology*, *235*(6), 5353–5362. DOI: 10.1002/jcp.29422

Chitale, V., Baghaei, N., Playne, D., Liang, H.-N., Zhao, Y., Erensoy, A., & Ahmad, Y. (2022). The Use of Videogames and Virtual Reality for the Assessment of Anxiety and Depression: A Scoping Review. *Games for Health Journal*, *11*(6), 341–354. Advance online publication. DOI: 10.1089/g4h.2021.0227

Choi, E., Shin, S. H., Ryu, J. K., Jung, K. I., Kim, S. Y., & Park, M. H. (2020). Commercial video games and cognitive functions: Video game genres and modulating factors of cognitive enhancement. *Behavioral and Brain Functions : BBF*, *16*(1), 2. DOI: 10.1186/s12993-020-0165-z PMID: 32014027

Cimadevilla, J. M., Nori, R., & Piccardi, L. (2023). Application of Virtual Reality in Spatial Memory. *Brain Sciences*, *13*(12), 1621. DOI: 10.3390/brainsci13121621

Cipresso, P., Giglioli, I. A. C., Raya, M. A., & Riva, G. (2018). The Past, Present, and Future of Virtual and Augmented Reality Research: A Network and Cluster Analysis of the Literature. *Frontiers in Psychology*, *9*, 2086. DOI: 10.3389/fpsyg.2018.02086

Clapson, M. L., Gilbert, B. C. T., & Musgrove, A. (2020). Race to the reactor and other chemistry games: Game-based and experiential learning experiences in materials and polymer chemistry. *Journal of Chemical Education*, *97*(12), 4391–4399. DOI: 10.1021/acs.jchemed.0c01135

Clark, D. B., Tanner-Smith, E. E., & Killingsworth, S. S. (2016). Digital games, design, and learning: A systematic review and meta-analysis. *Review of Educational Research*, *86*(1), 79–122. DOI: 10.3102/0034654315582065 PMID: 26937054

Clark, T. M. (2024). Using multiple PhET sims to investigate greenhouse gases within a real-world context. *Journal of Chemical Education*, *101*(10), 4242–4250. DOI: 10.1021/acs.jchemed.4c00551

CodeCombat. (s.f.). *CodeCombat*. Recuperado el 15 de noviembre de 2025, de https://codecombat.com/

CodinGame. (s.f.). *CodinGame – Start Coding*. Recuperado el 15 de noviembre de 2025, de https://www.codingame.com/start/

Cogné, M., Taillade, M., N'Kaoua, B., Tarruella, A., Klinger, E., Larrue, F., Sauzéon, H., Joseph, P.-A., & Sorita, E. (2017). The contribution of virtual reality to the diagnosis of spatial navigation disorders and to the study of the role of navigational aids: A systematic literature review. *Annals of Physical and Rehabilitation Medicine*, *60*(3), 164–176. DOI: 10.1016/j.rehab.2015.12.004

Connolly, T. M., Boyle, E. A., MacArthur, E., Hainey, T., & Boyle, J. M. (2012). A systematic literature review of empirical evidence on computer games and serious games. *Computers & Education*, *59*(2), 661–686. DOI: 10.1016/j.compedu.2012.03.004

Costa, P., & Sousa Lobo, J. M. (2001). Modeling and comparison of dissolution profiles. *European Journal of Pharmaceutical Sciences*, *13*(2), 123–133. DOI: 10.1016/S0928-0987(01)00095-1

Craig, D. (2024). *PELIGRO IA – Los riesgos de la Inteligencia Artificial en la Educación | Diego F. Craig*. https://craig.ar/peligro-ia/?utm_source=chatgpt.com

Cristofori, I., Shalom, D., & Grafman, J. (2019). Executive functions. In D'Esposito, M., & Byrne, J. H. (Eds.), *Encyclopedia of the cognitive neurosciences* (2nd ed.). Elsevier., DOI: 10.1016/B978-0-12-804281-6.00011-2

Cruz Pérez, M. A., Pozo Vinueza, M. A., Andino Jaramillo, A. F., & Arias Parra, A. D. (2018). Las Tecnologías de la Información y la Comunicación (TIC) como forma investigativa interdisciplinaria con un enfoque intercultural para el proceso de formación de los estudiantes. *E-Ciencias De La Información*, *9*(1). Advance online publication. DOI: 10.15517/eci.v1i1.33052

Csikszentmihalyi, M., Abuhamdeh, S., & Nakamura, J. (2014). Flow. In M. Csikszentmihalyi, *Flow and the Foundations of Positive Psychology* (pp. 227–238). Springer Netherlands. DOI: 10.1007/978-94-017-9088-8_15

D'Astous, A., & Gagnon, K. (2007). An inquiry into the factors that impact on consumer appreciation of a board game. *Journal of Consumer Marketing*, *24*(2), 80–89. DOI: 10.1108/07363760710737085

D'Cunha, N. M., Nguyen, D., Naumovski, N., McKune, A. J., Kellett, J., Georgousopoulou, E. N., Frost, J., & Isbel, S. (2019). A Mini-Review of Virtual Reality-Based Interventions to Promote Well-Being for People Living with Dementia and Mild Cognitive Impairment. *Gerontology*, *65*(4), 430–440. DOI: 10.1159/000500040

Dale, R. H. (1986). Spatial and temporal response patterns on the eight-arm radial maze. *Physiology & Behavior*, *36*(4), 787–790. DOI: 10.1016/0031-9384(86)90370-7

Dana. (2023). *The immersive simulation application allows physicians to practice robotic surgery with virtual reality transmission.* Health Simulation Network. Retrieved September 6, 2025, from https://reddesimulacionensalud.com/tecnologia/la-aplicacion-de-simulacion-inmersiva-permite-a-los-medicos-practicar-cirugia-robotica-con-transmision-de-realidad-virtual/

Darlami, J., & Sharma, S. (2024). The role of physicochemical and topological parameters in drug design. *Frontiers in Drug Discovery, Volume 4-2024*. DOI: 10.3389/fddsv.2024.1424402

Data México. (2025). *Distribución de estudiantes Instituto Tecnológico Superior de Xalapa* https://www.economia.gob.mx/datamexico/es/profile/institution/instituto-tecnologico-superior-de-xalapa de Diego-Cordero, R., Fernández-García, E., & Badanta Romero, B. (2017). Use of ICT to promote healthy lifestyles in children and adolescents: The case of overweight. *Spanish Journal of Health Communication*, *8*(1), 79–91. DOI: 10.20318/recs.2017.3607

De la Riva, B. (2024). *Beyond screens: An approach to the responsible use of AI through ICTs.* Edetania. *Estudios y Propuestas Sicoeducativos*, (65), 97–115. DOI: 10.46583/edetania_2024.65.1139

Deeb, F. A., & Hickey, T. J. (2019). Teaching Introductory Cryptography using a 3D Escape-the-Room Game. *2019 IEEE Frontiers in Education Conference (FIE)*, 1–6. DOI: 10.1109/FIE43999.2019.9028549

Dehghanzadeh, H., Fardanesh, H., Hatami, J., Talaee, E., & Noroozi, O. (2021). Using gamification to support learning English as a second language: A systematic review. *Computer Assisted Language Learning*, *34*(7), 934–957. DOI: 10.1080/09588221.2019.1648298

Dehghanzadeh, H., Farrokhnia, M., Dehghanzadeh, H., Taghipour, K., & Noroozi, O. (2024). Using gamification to support learning in K-12 education: A systematic literature review. *British Journal of Educational Technology*, *55*(1), 34–70. DOI: 10.1111/bjet.13335

Demuyakor, J. (2021). Battling Underaged Online Video Gamers: Probing the Negative Effects of Online Video Gaming Addictions on Young Adolescents. *Asian Journal of Media and Communication*, *5*(2). Advance online publication. DOI: 10.20885/asjmc.vol5.iss2.art3

Desfilis, E. S., Martínez, I., & Serna, C. (2020). Chapter 3. Adolescents of postmodernity. Growing up in the digital age. *New Perspectives on Life Cycle Psychology*, 63-88.

Deterding, S., Dixon, D., Khaled, R., & Nacke, L. (2011). From game design elements to gamefulness: Defining "gamification". En *Proceedings of the 15th International Academic MindTrek Conference: Envisioning Future Media Environments* (pp. 9–15). ACM. https://doi.org/DOI: 10.1145/2181037.2181040

Diamond, A. (2012). Activities and programs that improve children's executive functions. *Current Directions in Psychological Science*, *21*(5), 335–341. DOI: 10.1177/0963721412453722 PMID: 25328287

Diamond, L. C., & Jacobs, E. A. (2024). Language barriers and health inequity. *AMA Journal of Ethics*, *26*(1), E1–E8. https://journalofethics.ama-assn.org/article/how-should-clinicians-respond-language-barriers-exacerbate-health-inequity/2021-02

Diario Oficial de la Federación. (2017). *Ley General de Protección de Datos Personales en Posesión de Sujetos Obligados*. https://www.dof.gob.mx/nota_detalle.php?codigo=5478205&fecha=26/01/2017

Dietrich, N. (2018). Escape classroom: The Leblanc process—An educational "escape game.". *Journal of Chemical Education, 95*(6), 996–999. DOI: 10.1021/acs.jchemed.7b00690

Do, T. T. N., Lin, C. T., & Gramann, K. (2021). Human brain dynamics in active spatial navigation. *Scientific Reports, 11*(1), 13036. Advance online publication. DOI: 10.1038/s41598-021-92246-4 PMID: 34158525

Douglas, D. (2000). *Assessing languages for specific purposes*. Cambridge University Press.

Douglas, D. (2001). Language for Specific Purposes assessment criteria: Where do they come from? *Language Testing, 18*(2), 171–185. DOI: 10.1177/026553220101800204

DrugBank. (n.d.). Retrieved June 13, 2025, from https://go.drugbank.com/

Dunwell, I., de Freitas, S., Petridis, P., Hendrix, M., Arnab, S., Lameras, P., & Stewart, C. (2014). *A game-based learning approach to road safety: The code of everand*. 3389–3398. DOI: 10.1145/2556288.2557281

Duque, P., & Cervantes-Cervantes, L.-S. (2019). Responsabilidad Social Universitaria: Una revisión sistemática y análisis bibliométrico. *Estudios Gerenciales*, 451–464. DOI: 10.18046/j.estger.2019.153.3389

Ebnesajjad, S. (2013). Fluoroplastics, Volume 1: Non-melt processible fluoropolymers. William Andrew Publishing.

Educar, E. (25 de mayo de 2018). *Diez cosas que un educador puede hacer para lograr una enseñanza eficaz*. Recuperado de https://eligeeducar.cl/noticias/10-cosas-que-puede-hacer-un-educador-para-lograr-una-ensenanza-efectiva/

Eichenbaum, H. (1999). The hippocampus and mechanisms of declarative memory. *Behavioural Brain Research, 103*(2), 123–133. DOI: 10.1016/S0166-4328(99)00044-3

Elashmawi, W. H., Ayman, A., Antoun, M., Mohamed, H., Mohamed, S. E., Amr, H., Talaat, Y., & Ali, A. (2024). A Comprehensive Review on Brain–Computer Interface (BCI)-Based Machine and Deep Learning Algorithms for Stroke Rehabilitation. *Applied Sciences (Basel, Switzerland), 14*(14), 6347. DOI: 10.3390/app14146347

Eliosa, V. (2022). 6 types of learning that can be reinforced through simulation. https://blog.pearsonlatam.com/columna-de-opinion/6-tipos-de-aprendizaje-que-pueden-reforzarse-mediante-la-simulacion

Endeavor & Santander. (2025). Game On: El auge del Gaming en México. Retrieved from https://mexico.endeavor.org/gaming/

Entertainment Software Association. (2023). *Essential facts about the computer and video game industry*. Entertainment Software Association. Retrieved from https://www.theesa.com/resources/essential-facts-about-the-us-video-game-industry/

Erickson, F. (1977). Some Approaches to Inquiry in School-Community Ethnography. *Anthropology & Education Quarterly*, *8*(2), 58–69. https://www.jstor.org/stable/3216407. DOI: 10.1525/aeq.1977.8.2.05x1396r

Eriksson, M., Kenward, B., Poom, L., & Stenberg, G. (2021). The behavioral effects of cooperative and competitive board games in preschoolers. *Scandinavian Journal of Psychology*, *62*(3), 355–364. DOI: 10.1111/sjop.12708 PMID: 33543787

Esparza Meza, E. M., Campillo Labrandero, M., Stincer Gómez, D., Sánchez Xicotencatl, C. O., Téllez Rojo, A. L., & Aveleyra Ojeda, E. (2022). Experiences of Mexican youth facing the COVID-19 pandemic and lockdown. *Psicumex*, *13*(1), 1–27. DOI: 10.36793/psicumex.v13i1.526

Espinoza, M., Baños, R. M., García-Palacios, A., & Botella, C. (2013). Virtual reality in psychological interventions with cancer patients. *Psycho-Oncology*, *10*(2-3), 247–261. DOI: 10.5209/rev_PSIC.2013.v10.n2-3.43447

Estrada-Plana, V., Martínez-Escribano, A., Ros-Morente, A., Mayoral, M., Castro-Quintas, Á., Vita-Barrull, N., Terés-Lleida, N., March-Llanes, J., Badia-Bafalluy, A., & Moya-Higueras, J. (2024). Benefits of playing at school: Filler board games improve visuospatial memory and mathematical skills. *Brain Sciences*, *14*(7), 642. DOI: 10.3390/brainsci14070642 PMID: 39061383

Evans, F., Spinelli, A., Zapirain, E., Soriano, F., & Massa, S. M. (2016). Proceso de desarrollo de serious games. Diseño centrado en el usuario, jugabilidad e inmersión. *III Congreso Argentino De Ingeniería (Cadi) - IX Congreso Argentino De Enseñanza de la Ingeniería (Caedi)*.

Federal Telecommunications Institute. (IFT) (2024). *National Survey on the Availability and Use of Information Technologies in Households (ENDUTIH) 2023*. Retrieved from https://www.ift.org.mx/comunicacion-y-medios/comunicados-ift/es/el-inegi-el-ift-y-la-sct-presentan-los-resultados-de-la-endutih-2023

Fernández Castrillo, C., & González-González, A. (2025). Youth magazines from the millennial generation to the Alpha: Analysis of the evolution in the consumption habits of Spanish adolescents. *Studies on the Journalistic Message*, *31*(2), 527–540. DOI: 10.5209/emp.98143

Fernández-Abascal, E. G. (2018). *Human Emotion and Motivation: Fundamentals psychological aspects of well-being*. Pirámide.

Fernández-Batanero, J. M., Montenegro-Rueda, M., & Fernández-Cerero, J. (2022). Use of Augmented Reality for Students with Educational Needs: A Systematic Review (2016–2021). *Societies (Basel, Switzerland)*, *12*(2), 36. DOI: 10.3390/soc12020036

Fernández-Sánchez, M. R., González-Fernández, A., & Acevedo-Borrega, J. (2023). Conceptual Approach to the Pedagogy of Serious Games. *Information (Basel)*, *14*(2), 132. Advance online publication. DOI: 10.3390/info14020132

Figueroa Flores, J. F. (2015). Using Gamification to Enhance Second Language Learning. *Digital Education Review*, *27*, 32–54. DOI: 10.1344/der.2015.27.32-54

Fisher, N., & Kulshreshth, A. K. (2024). Exploring Dynamic Difficulty Adjustment Methods for Video Games. *Virtual Worlds*, *3*(2), 230–255. DOI: 10.3390/virtualworlds3020012

Flexner, J. B., Flexner, L. B., & Stellar, E. (1963). Memory in Mice as Affected by Intracerebral Puromycin. *Science*, *141*(3575), 57–59. DOI: 10.1126/science.141.3575.57

Flores, G. (2006). Language Barriers to Health Care in the United States. *The New England Journal of Medicine*, *355*(3), 229–231. DOI: 10.1056/NEJMp058316

Fogg, B. J. (2003). *Persuasive technology: Using computers to change what we think and do*. Morgan Kaufmann. DOI: 10.1016/B978-155860643-2/50011-1

Fortune Business Insights. (n.d.). *Board games market size, share & trends analysis [2032]*. Retrieved September 3, 2025, from https://www.fortunebusinessinsights.com/board-games-market-104972

Franceschini, S., & Bertoni, S. (2019). Improving action video games abilities increases the phonological decoding speed and phonological short-term memory in children with developmental dyslexia. *Neuropsychologia*, *130*, 100–106. DOI: 10.1016/j.neuropsychologia.2018.10.023 PMID: 30395809

Franceschini, S., Gori, S., Ruffino, M., Viola, S., Molteni, M., & Facoetti, A. (2013). Action video games make dyslexic children read better. *Current Biology*, *23*(6), 462–466. DOI: 10.1016/j.cub.2013.01.044 PMID: 23453956

Franceschini, S., Trevisan, P., Ronconi, L., Bertoni, S., Colmar, S., Double, K., Facoetti, A., & Gori, S. (2017). Action video games improve reading abilities and visual-to-auditory attentional shifting in English-speaking children with dyslexia. *Scientific Reports*, *7*(1), 5863. Advance online publication. DOI: 10.1038/s41598-017-05826-8 PMID: 28725022

Fundamental, X. R. (n.d.). FUNDAMENTAL SURGERY. The flight simulator for surgeons [Video]. YouTube. https://www.youtube.com/watch?v=0NtCRXOuLto

GameMaker. (2025). *Características y herramientas del motor*. https://gamemaker.io/es/features

Gao, Z., Yan, H., Liu, J., ... Tracing distinct learning trajectories in introductory programming course: a sequence analysis of score, engagement, and code metrics for novice computer science vs. math cohorts. *IJ STEM Ed* **12**, 27 (2025). https://doi.org/DOI: 10.1186/s40594-025-00546-2

García, L., Pernett, A., & Cano, J. (2017). Estudio exploratorio de usabilidad para niños de Colombia. *Zona Próxima, 9444*(26), 12–30. Retrieved from https://www.redalyc.org/pdf/853/85352029002.pdf

Garcia, C., & Garcia, R. (2021). Developing cultural competence in an occupational therapy program in a border institution in South Texas. In Sellers, M. D. S., & Johnson, M. E. (Eds.), *Cultural Competence in Applied Psychology* (pp. 138–157). IGI Global., https://scholarworks.utrgv.edu/context/tl_fac/article/1086/viewcontent/145841.pdf

García-Peñalvo, F. J. (2018). Interaction in technological learning ecosystems. [EKS]. *Education in the Knowledge Society, 19*(3), 7–13. DOI: 10.14201/eks.19341

Garfield, J. B., Ben-Zvi, D., Chance, B., Medina, E., Roseth, C., & Zieffler, A. (2008). *Developing students' statistical reasoning* (SCOPUS:84891388863). Springer Netherlands. DOI: 10.1007/978-1-4020-8383-9

Gaviria, D. (2021) Pedagogy de la Gamification. Colombia: Creative Commons. www.gamifiquemos.com

Gay, G. (2018). *Culturally responsive teaching: theory, research, and practice*. Teachers College Press.

Gaytan-Lugo, L., Hernandez, S., Santana-Mancilla, P. C., & Garcia-Ruiz, M. (2014). *A contextual study and usability testing of videogames to inform the design of a serious game to improve reading comprehension. Memorias ENC 2014. Encuentro Nacional de Ciencias de la Computación (ENC 2014)*. Ocotlán.

Gee, J. P. (2007). What video games have to teach us about learning and literacy. Palgrave Macmillan. Recuperado de https://dl.acm.org/doi/abs/10.1145/950566.950595

Gee, J. P. (2003). What video games have to teach us about learning and literacy. *Computers in Entertainment, 1*(1), 20. DOI: 10.1145/950566.950595

Gee, J. P. (2008). *What video games have to teach us about learning and literacy* (2nd ed.). Palgrave Macmillan.

Gené, O. B. (n.d.). *Gamificación en educación* [Unpublished manuscript]. Universidad Politécnica de Madrid.

Ghazali, N., Ab Rahim, I. S., & Syed Idrus, S. Z. (2024). Challenges and Opportunities of Cybersecurity Education for Non-technical Majors. [JCSI]. *Journal of Communication in Scientific Inquiry*, *6*(1), 47–55. DOI: 10.58915/jcsi.v6i1.873

Giardullo, P., Neresini, F., Marín-González, E., Luís, C., Magalhães, J., & Arias, R. (2023). Citizen science and participatory science communication: An empirically informed discussion connecting research and theory. *JCOM, Journal of Science Communication*, *22*(2). Advance online publication. DOI: 10.22323/2.22020201

GOB. (2023, June 27). *The National Survey on Mental Health and Addictions begins.* Government of Mexico. https://www.gob.mx/salud/prensa/inicia-levantamiento-de-la-encuesta-nacional-de-salud-mental-y-adicciones

Gómez Fuentes, M. (2011). *Notas del Curso: Análisis de Requerimientos*. Retrieved from https://www.cua.uam.mx/pdfs/conoce/libroselec/Notas_Analisis_Requerimiento.pdf

Gómez-Urquiza, J. L., Velando-Soriano, A., Membrive-Jiménez, M. J., Ramírez-Baena, L., Aguayo-Estremera, R., Ortega-Campos, E., & Cañadas-De la Fuente, G. A. (2023). Prevalence and levels of burnout in nursing students: A systematic review with meta-analysis. *Nurse Education in Practice*, *72*, 103753. Advance online publication. DOI: 10.1016/j.nepr.2023.103753 PMID: 37651959

González González, C. S., & Blanco Izquierdo, F. (2011). Videojuegos educativos sociales en el aula. *Revista ICONO14. Revista Científica de Comunicación y Tecnologías Emergentes*, *9*(2), 59. DOI: 10.7195/ri14.v9i2.46

González, V. A., & Gewerc, B. (2021). Public and private spaces for adolescents on social networks: State of the art. *IX International Multidisciplinary Congress of Educational Research, July 1–2.* Universitat de Lleida. https://dialnet.unirioja.es/servlet/libro?codigo=976466

González-González, C. S. (2023). El impacto de la inteligencia artificial en la educación: Transformando la forma en que enseñamos y aprendemos. *Revista Qurriculum*, (36), 51–60. DOI: 10.25145/j.qurricul.2023.36.03

González, M. J., & Delgado, M. (2009). Rendimiento académico y enseñanza-aprendizaje de la lectoescritura en Educación Infantil y Primaria: Un estudio longitudinal. *Infancia y Aprendizaje*, *32*(3), 265–276. DOI: 10.1174/021037009788964114

Gonzalez, R. A J., & De La Rosa, M. I. (2025). Self-perception of the personal image in social networks of university women: A comparative study between generations Z and Y. Social Trends. *Journal of Sociology (Melbourne, Vic.)*, *14*, 75–90.

González-Tablas, A. I., González Vasco, M. I., Cascos, I., & Planet Palomino, Á. (2020). Shuffle, Cut, and Learn: Crypto Go, a Card Game for Teaching Cryptography. *Mathematics*, *8*(11), 1993. DOI: 10.3390/math8111993

Government of the State of Jalisco. (2021). *Jalisco State Governance and Development Plan 2018-2024, vision 2030. Update 2021* (2nd ed.). Secretariat of Planning and Citizen Participation. https://plan.jalisco.gob.mx/

Gozzo, L., Caraci, F., & Drago, F. (2022). Bioequivalence, Drugs with Narrow Therapeutic Index and The Phenomenon of Biocreep: A Critical Analysis of the System for Generic Substitution. *Healthcare (Basel)*, *10*(8), 1392. Advance online publication. DOI: 10.3390/healthcare10081392

Granić, A. (2023). Technology Acceptance and Adoption in Education. In *Handbook of Open, Distance and Digital Education* (pp. 183–197). Springer., DOI: 10.1007/978-981-19-2080-6_11

Green, C. S., & Bavelier, D. (2012). Learning, attentional control, and action video games. *Current Biology*, *22*(6), R197–R206. DOI: 10.1016/j.cub.2012.02.012 PMID: 22440805

Green, C. S., & Bavelier, D. (2015). Action video game training for cognitive enhancement. *Current Opinion in Behavioral Sciences*, *4*, 103–108. DOI: 10.1016/j.cobeha.2015.04.012

Gros Salvat, B. (2009). Certezas e interrogantes acerca del uso de los videojuegos para el aprendizaje. *Comunicación: Revista Internacional de Comunicación Audiovisual. Publicidad y Estudios Culturales*, *1*(7), 251–264.

Güemes-Hidalgo, M., Ceñal, M. J., & Hidalgo, M. I. (2017). Puberty and adolescence. *Adolescere. Journal of Continuing Education of the Spanish Society of Adolescent Medicine*, *5*(1), 7–22. https://www.adolescere.es/revista/pdf/volumen-V-n1-2017/Adolescere-2017-1.pdf

Guerrero-Martínez, S. F. & Martínez-Castillo, M. F. (2022). YouTube, Instagram, emerging educational environments in times of remote teaching and collaborative learning. INNOVA Research Journal, 7(3.1), 1-12. DOI: 10.33890/innova.v7.n3.1.2022.2146

Guillén-Parra, L. S., & Moscoso-Bernal, S. A. (2024). Artificial intelligence and education: Proposal for use with 16-year-old youth. *MQRInvestigar*, *8*(3), 2631–2653. DOI: 10.56048/MQR20225.8.3.2024.2631-2653

Gunia, A., Moraresku, S., & Vlček, K. (2021). Brain mechanisms of visuospatial perspective-taking in relation to object mental rotation and the theory of mind. *Behavioural Brain Research*, *407*, 113247. DOI: 10.1016/j.bbr.2021.113247 PMID: 33745982

Gu, S., Shen, C., Yu, J., Zhao, H., Liu, H., Liu, L., Sheng, R., Xu, L., Wang, Z., Hou, T., & Kang, Y. (2023). Can molecular dynamics simulations improve predictions of protein-ligand binding affinity with machine learning? *Briefings in Bioinformatics*, *24*(2), bbad008. Advance online publication. DOI: 10.1093/bib/bbad008 PMID: 36681903

Gutierrez, A., Sanchez, E., & Rios, C. (2024). Proposal for psychoeducational intervention in adolescents in the first year of secondary school. *Contemporary Dilemmas Journal: Education, Politics and Values.*, *X I*(3). https://dilemascontemporaneoseducacionpoliticayvalores.com/index.php/dilemas/article/view/4160

Gutiérrez-Ochoa, S. M., Díaz-Torres, C. H., & Belandria-Vivas, L. M. (2024). Influence of new technologies on adolescence: Risks and benefits. *Gestión y Desarrollo Libre*, *9*(18), 1–24. DOI: 10.18041/2539-3669/gestionlibre.18.2024.12104

Guzhñay Vélez, K. J. (2021). Aprendizaje de lengua y literatura mediante rúbricas de evaluación. *Sociedad & Tecnología*, *4*(2), 174–190. DOI: 10.51247/st.v4i2.103

Guzmán Acosta, C. (2025). Private higher education in Mexico. *Journal of Psychology of the Autonomous University of the State of Mexico*, *14*(41), 68–92. https://revistapsicologia.uaemex.mx/article/view/26051

Haber, S. N., & Knutson, B. (2010). The reward circuit: Linking primate anatomy and human imaging. *Neuropsychopharmacology : Official Publication of the American College of Neuropsychopharmacology*, *35*(1), 4–26. DOI: 10.1038/npp.2009.129 PMID: 19812543

Hakim, A. R., Ramli, K., Gunawan, T. S., & Windarta, S. (2023). A Novel Digital Forensic Framework for Data Breach Investigation. *IEEE Access : Practical Innovations, Open Solutions*, *11*, 42644–42659. DOI: 10.1109/ACCESS.2023.3270619

Hamari, J., Koivisto, J., & Sarsa, H. (2014). Does gamification work? — A literature review of empirical studies on gamification. In *Proceedings of the 47th Hawaii International Conference on System Sciences* (pp. 3025–3034). IEEE. https://doi.org/DOI: 10.1109/HICSS.2014.377

Hamari, J., Shernoff, D. J., Rowe, E., Coller, B., Asbell-Clarke, J., & Edwards, T. (2016). Challenging games help students learn: An empirical study on engagement, flow and immersion in game-based learning. *Computers in Human Behavior, 54*, 170–179. DOI: 10.1016/j.chb.2015.07.045

Hamp-Lyons, L., & Lumley, T. (2001). Assessing language for specific purposes. *Language Testing, 18*(2), 127–132. DOI: 10.1177/026553220101800201

Happify, Inc. (s.f.). *The Science Behind Happify*. Recuperado de https://www.happify.com/public/science-behind-happify/

HashStudioz Technologies. (s.f.). *Mental Health Meets Gamification: Designing Emotionally Intelligent Apps*. Recuperado de https://www.hashstudioz.com/blog/mental-health-meets-gamification-designing-emotionally-intelligent-apps/

Hastuti, D., & Malihah, N. (2024). Systematic Literature Review (SLR): Implementation of The Project-Based Learning (PJBL) Approach to Improve Students' Speaking Skills. *Proceeding of International Interdiciplinary Conference And Research Expo, 1*(1), 88-107. https://doi.org/https://doi.org/10.18326/iicare.v1i1.634

Hawkins, I., & Phelps, A. J. (2013). Virtual laboratory vs. traditional laboratory: Which is more effective for teaching electrochemistry? *Chemistry Education Research and Practice, 14*(4), 516–523. DOI: 10.1039/C3RP00070B

Henrich, S., & Worthington, R. (2023). Let your clients fight dragons: A rapid evidence assessment regarding the therapeutic utility of 'Dungeons & Dragons.'. *Journal of Creativity in Mental Health, 18*(3), 383–401. DOI: 10.1080/15401383.2021.1987367

Hernandez, C. C., Gimenez, L. E., Strassmaier, T., Rogers, M., & Taymans, J.-M. (2024). Editorial: Targeting ion channels for drug discovery: emerging challenges for high throughput screening technologies. *Frontiers in Molecular Neuroscience, 17*, 1414816. Advance online publication. DOI: 10.3389/fnmol.2024.1414816 PMID: 38883981

Hernández-Sampieri, R., & Mendoza-Torres, C. (2018). Metodología de la investigación: las rutas cuantitativa, cualitativa y mixta 2ed. Cd. de México: McGraw-Hill.

Hidalgo Cajo, B. G., Mayacela Alulema, Á. G., & Hidalgo Cajo, I. M. (2017). Estrategias didácticas para potenciar el aprendizaje de Farmacología clínica. *Revista Habanera de Ciencias Médicas, 16*(3), 439–453.

Hofmann, M., Rösler, A., Schwarz, W., Müller-Spahn, F., Kräuchi, K., Hock, C., & Seifritz, E. (2003). Interactive computer-training as a therapeutic tool in Alzheimer's disease. *Comprehensive Psychiatry, 44*(3), 213–219. DOI: 10.1016/S0010-440X(03)00006-3

Ho-Minh, T., & Suppasetseree, S. (2025). Enhancing Vietnamese EFL Students' Speaking Skills Through Augmented Reality: A Mixed-Method Study in English for Tourism and Hospitality. *Education Process: International Journal, 15*(1). Advance online publication. DOI: 10.22521/edupij.2025.15.139

Hořejší, P., Lochmannová, A., Jezl, V., & Dvořák, M. (2025). Virtual reality locomotion methods differentially affect spatial orientation and cybersickness during maze navigation. *Scientific Reports, 15*(1), 26255. DOI: 10.1038/s41598-025-12143-y

Hourcade, J. P. (2015). *Child-Computer Interaction. University of Iowa's Department of Computer Science*. Editorial Board of Interacting with Computers.

Howard-Jones, P. A. (2014). Neuroscience and education: Myths and messages. *Nature Reviews. Neuroscience, 15*(12), 817–824. DOI: 10.1038/nrn3817 PMID: 25315391

Huang, B., Hew, K. F., & Lo, C. K. (2019). Investigating the effects of gamification-enhanced flipped learning on undergraduate students' behavioral and cognitive engagement. *Interactive Learning Environments, 27*(8), 1106–1126. DOI: 10.1080/10494820.2018.1495653

Huon, J.-F., Nizet, P., Tollec, S., Vene, E., Fronteau, C., Leichnam, A., Tching-Sin, M., Michelet-Barbotin, V., Foucault-Fruchard, L., & Nativel, F. (2024). A systematic review of the impact of simulation on students' confidence in performing clinical pharmacy activities. *International Journal of Clinical Pharmacy, 46*(4), 795–810. DOI: 10.1007/s11096-024-01715-z

Hwang, J., & Lu, A. S. (2018). Narrative and active video game in separate and additive effects of physical activity and cognitive function among young adults. *Scientific Reports, 8*(1), 11020. Advance online publication. DOI: 10.1038/s41598-018-29274-0 PMID: 30030456

Ibarra-Herrera, C. C., Carrizosa, A., Yunes-Rojas, J. A., & Mata-Gómez, M. A. (2019). Design of an app based on gamification and storytelling as a tool for biology courses. [IJIDeM]. *International Journal on Interactive Design and Manufacturing, 13*(4), 1271–1282. DOI: 10.1007/s12008-019-00600-8

Ibarra, M., Ataucusi, P., Barzola, B., & Huaman, J. (2017). Mejorando la disponibilidad de recursos educativos digitales para enseñar en escuelas rurales sin acceso a internet. *Revista Brasileira de Informática Na Educação, 25*(03), 80. DOI: 10.5753/rbie.2017.25.03.80

Iftikhar, S., Guerrero-Roldán, A., & Mor, E. (2022). Practice Promotes Learning: Analyzing Students' Acceptance of a Learning-by-Doing Online Programming Learning Tool. *Applied Sciences (Basel, Switzerland)*, *12*(24), 12613. DOI: 10.3390/app122412613

Imbrici, P., Liantonio, A., Camerino, G. M., de Bellis, M., Camerino, C., Mele, A., Giustino, A., Pierno, S., de Luca, A., Tricarico, D., Desaphy, J.-F., & Conte, D. (2016). Therapeutic Approaches to Genetic Ion Channelopathies and Perspectives in Drug Discovery. *Frontiers in Pharmacology*, *7*. Advance online publication. DOI: 10.3389/fphar.2016.00121 PMID: 27242528

INEGI. (2018). Disminuye la Población Lectoraern México: Módulo de Lectura (MOLEC) 2018. Instituto Nacional de Estadística y Geografía. Retrieved from https://www.inegi.org.mx/contenidos/saladeprensa/boletines/2018/EstSociodemo/MOLEC2018_04.pdf

Inter-institutional Commission for the Training of Human Resources for Health (CIFRHS). (2023). National Exam for Medical Residency Applicants. https://cifrhs.salud.gob.mx/site1/enarm/2023/index.html

Ishaq, K., Mat Zin, N. A., Rosdi, F., Jehanghir, M., Ishaq, S., & Abid, A. (2021). Mobile-assisted and gamification-based language learning: A systematic literature review. *PeerJ. Computer Science*, *7*, e496. Advance online publication. DOI: 10.7717/peerj-cs.496

Issleib, M., Geiger, A., Pinnschmidt, H. O., Hilz, P., Zöllner, C., & Moll-Khosrawi, P. (2025). Virtual reality as a training method for basic life support of the medical staff on general wards: A randomized controlled non-inferiority trial. *Virtual Reality (Waltham Cross)*, *29*(3), 141. Advance online publication. DOI: 10.1007/s10055-025-01216-y

Jackson, G. T., & McNamara, D. S. (2013). Motivation and Performance in a Game-Based Intelligent Tutoring System. *Journal of Educational Psychology*, *105*(4), 1036–1049. DOI: 10.1037/a0032580

Jackson, J. (2009). Game-based teaching: What educators can learn from videogames. *Teaching Education*, *20*(3), 291–304. DOI: 10.1080/10476210902912533

Jacobs, E., Chen, A. H., Karliner, L. S., Agger-Gupta, N. I. E. L. S., & Mutha, S. (2006). The need for more research on language barriers in health care: A proposed research agenda. *The Milbank Quarterly*, *84*(1), 111–133. DOI: 10.1111/j.1468-0009.2006.00440.x

Jaramillo, J. A. (1996). Tu and usted: Address etiquette in the Mexican American family. *Hispanic Journal of Behavioral Sciences, 18*(4), 522–532. DOI: 10.1177/07399863960184006

Jaramillo-Mediavilla, L., Basantes-Andrade, A., Cabezas-González, M., & Casillas-Martín, S. (2024). Impact of gamification on motivation and academic performance: A systematic review. *Education Sciences, 14*(6), 639. DOI: 10.3390/educsci14060639

Jartelius, M. (2020). The 2020 Data Breach Investigations Report – a CSO's perspective. *Network Security, 2020*(7), 9–12. DOI: 10.1016/S1353-4858(20)30079-9

Jiménez, D. (2018). Niños ya no juegan en la calle, nuevos entretenimientos causan obesidad. Retrieved from https://www.excelsior.com.mx/comunidad/2018/01/08/1211772

Jiménez, A. S. A., Ramírez, N. A. B., Santana-Mancilla, P. C., Romero, J. C. M., & Acosta-Díaz, R. (2018).. . *Heuristic Evaluation of a Gamified Application for Education in Patients with Diabetes, 1–4*, 1–4. Advance online publication. DOI: 10.1145/3293578.3293593

Johnson, B. A. (2023). *A molecular construction game based on principles from game-based learning sciences* (Master's thesis, University of California, Merced). eScholarship.

Jonassen, D. H. (1999). Designing constructivist learning environments. In Reigeluth, C. M. (Ed.), *Instructional-design theories and models: A new paradigm of instructional theory* (Vol. II, pp. 215–239). Lawrence Erlbaum Associates.

Jonson, M., Avramescu, S., Chen, D., & Alam, F. (2021). The Role of Virtual Reality in Screening, Diagnosing, and Rehabilitating Spatial Memory Deficits. *Frontiers in Human Neuroscience, 15*, 628818. DOI: 10.3389/fnhum.2021.628818

Josselyn, S. A., Köhler, S., & Frankland, P. W. (2017). Heroes of the Engram. *The Journal of Neuroscience : The Official Journal of the Society for Neuroscience, 37*(18), 4647–4657. DOI: 10.1523/JNEUROSCI.0056-17.2017

Juul, J. (2005). *Half-real: Video games between real rules and fictional worlds.* MIT Press.

Kaddoura, R., Faraji, H., Otaki, F., Radhakrishnan, R., Stanley, A., Paulus, A., Jackson, L., Jayyousi, R. A., Mascarenhas, S., Sudhir, M., Alfroukh, J., Ghelani, H., Azar, A. J., Khamis, A. H., & Jan, R. K. (2024). High-fidelity simulation versus case-based tutorial sessions for teaching pharmacology: Convergent mixed methods research investigating undergraduate medical students' performance and perception. *PLoS One, 19*(8), e0302609. DOI: 10.1371/journal.pone.0302609

Kalogiannakis, M., Papadakis, S., & Zourmpakis, A.-I. (2021). Gamification in science education: A systematic review of the literature. *Education Sciences*, *11*(1), 22. DOI: 10.3390/educsci11010022

Kandel, E. R. (2012). The molecular biology of memory: cAMP, PKA, CRE, CREB-1, CREB-2, and CPEB. *Molecular Brain*, *5*(1), 14. DOI: 10.1186/1756-6606-5-14

Kapp, K. M. (2012). The gamification of learning and instruction: Game-based methods and strategies for training and education. Pfeiffer. Recuperado de https://scholar.google.com/citations?view_op=view_citation&hl=es&user=UEujZfUAAAAJ&citation_for_view=UEujZfUAAAAJ:u5HHmVD_uO8C

Kapp, K. M. (2012). *The gamification of learning and instruction: Game-based methods and strategies for training and education*. Pfeiffer.

Katz, D., Horváth, Z., Pontes, H. M., Koncz, P., Demetrovics, Z., & Király, O. (2024). How much gaming is too much? An analysis based on psychological distress. *Journal of Behavioral Addictions*, *13*(3), 716–728. DOI: 10.1556/2006.2024.00036 PMID: 39024045

Kellems, R. O., Eichelberger, C., Cacciatore, G., Jensen, M., Frazier, B., Simons, K., & Zaru, M. (2020). Using Video-Based Instruction via Augmented Reality to Teach Mathematics to Middle School Students With Learning Disabilities. *Journal of Learning Disabilities*, *53*(4), 277–291. DOI: 10.1177/0022219420906452

Khaldi, A., Bouzidi, R., & Nader, F. (2023). Gamification of e-learning in higher education: A systematic literature review. *Smart Learning Environments*, *10*(1), 10. DOI: 10.1186/s40561-023-00227-z PMID: 40478066

Kim, H., Park, J. Y., & Kim, K. K. (2018). Spatial Learning and Memory Using a Radial Arm Maze with a Head-Mounted Display. *Psychiatry Investigation*, *15*(10), 935–944. DOI: 10.30773/pi.2018.06.28.3

Kim, K. W. (2025). Go and the brain: Cognitive and neural impacts of training. *Psychiatry Investigation*, *22*(4), 357–364. DOI: 10.30773/pi.2024.0387 PMID: 40262784

Kim, S., Chen, J., Cheng, T., Gindulyte, A., He, J., He, S., Li, Q., Shoemaker, B. A., Thiessen, P. A., Yu, B., Zaslavsky, L., Zhang, J., & Bolton, E. E. (2021). PubChem in 2021: New data content and improved web interfaces. *Nucleic Acids Research*, *49*(D1), D1388–D1395. DOI: 10.1093/nar/gkaa971 PMID: 33151290

Klein, J. D. (1992). Effect of instructional gaming and reentry status on performance and motivation. *Contemporary Educational Psychology*, *17*(4), 364–370. DOI: 10.1016/0361-476X(92)90074-9

Koblitz, N. (1997). Cryptography as a teaching tool. *Cryptologia, 21*(4), 317–326. DOI: 10.1080/0161-119791885959

Koepnick, B., Flatten, J., Husain, T., Ford, A., Silva, D.-A., Bick, M. J., Bauer, A., Liu, G., Ishida, Y., Boykov, A., Estep, R. D., Kleinfelter, S., Nørgård-Solano, T., Wei, L., Players, F., Montelione, G. T., DiMaio, F., Popović, Z., Khatib, F., & Baker, D. (2019). De novo protein design by citizen scientists. *Nature, 570*(7761), 390–394. DOI: 10.1038/s41586-019-1274-4 PMID: 31168091

Koepp, M. J., Gunn, R. N., Lawrence, A. D., Cunningham, V. J., Dagher, A., Jones, T., Brooks, D. J., Bench, C. J., & Grasby, P. M. (1998). Evidence for striatal dopamine release during a video game. *Nature, 393*(6682), 266–268. DOI: 10.1038/30498 PMID: 9607763

Koivisto, J., & Hamari, J. (2019). The rise of motivational information systems: A review of gamification research. *International Journal of Information Management, 45*, 191–210. DOI: 10.1016/j.ijinfomgt.2018.10.013

Kowal, M., Conroy, E., Ramsbottom, N., Smithies, T., Toth, A., & Campbell, M. (2021). Gaming Your Mental Health: A Narrative Review on Mitigating Symptoms of Depression and Anxiety Using Commercial Video Games. *JMIR Serious Games, 9*(2), e26575. DOI: 10.2196/26575 PMID: 34132648

Krajčovič, M., Matys, M., Gabajová, G., & Komačka, D. (2024). Utilization of Immersive Virtual Reality as an Interactive Method of Assignment Presentation. *Electronics (Basel), 13*(8), 1430. DOI: 10.3390/electronics13081430

Krath, J., Schürmann, L., & Von Korflesch, H. F. O. (2021). Revealing the theoretical basis of gamification: A systematic review and analysis of theory in research on gamification, serious games and game-based learning. *Computers in Human Behavior, 125*, 106963. DOI: 10.1016/j.chb.2021.106963

Kühn, S., Romanowski, A., Schilling, C., Lorenz, R., Mörsen, C., Seiferth, N., Banaschewski, T., Barbot, A., Barker, G. J., Büchel, C., Conrod, P. J., Dalley, J. W., Flor, H., Garavan, H., Ittermann, B., Mann, K., Martinot, J.-L., Paus, T., Rietschel, M., & Gallinat, J. (2011). The neural basis of video gaming. *Translational Psychiatry, 1*(11), e53–e53. DOI: 10.1038/tp.2011.53 PMID: 22833208

Laamarti, F., Eid, M., & El Saddik, A. (2014). An overview of serious games. *International Journal of Computer Games Technology, 2014*(1), 358152. DOI: 10.1155/2014/358152

Ladson-Billings, G. (2021). Three decades of culturally relevant, responsive, & sustaining pedagogy: What lies ahead? In *The educational forum* (Vol. 85, No. 4, pp. 351-354). Routledge. https://doi.org/DOI: 10.1080/00131725.2021.1957632

Ladson-Billings, G. (1995). Toward a theory of culturally relevant pedagogy. *American Educational Research Journal, 32*(3), 465–491. DOI: 10.3102/00028312032003465

Ladson-Billings, G. (2014). Culturally relevant pedagogy 2.0: Aka the remix. *Harvard Educational Review, 84*(1), 74–84. DOI: 10.17763/haer.84.1.p2rj131485484751

Lampropoulos, G., & Sidiropoulos, A. (2024). Impact of Gamification on Students' Learning Outcomes and Academic Performance: A Longitudinal Study Comparing Online, Traditional, and Gamified Learning. *Education Sciences, 14*(4), 367. DOI: 10.3390/educsci14040367

Latorre, A. (2003). *La investigación-Acción: Conocer y cambiar la práctica educativa.* Editorial Graó.

Ledbetter, E., Lau, S., Enterline, A., Sibbitt, B., & Chen, A. M. H. (2020). A Simulation Activity to Assess Student Pharmacists' Knowledge and Perceptions of Oncology Pharmacy. *American Journal of Pharmaceutical Education, 84*(5), 7474. DOI: 10.5688/ajpe7474

Lee, T., Jo, H. J., Kim, M., & Kwon, J. S. (2025). The neural basis of intuitive approximate number system in board game Go (Baduk) experts. *Scientific Reports, 15*(1), 16400. DOI: 10.1038/s41598-025-98605-9 PMID: 40355626

Lei, Y.-Y., Zhu, L., Sa, Y. T. R., & Cui, X.-S. (2022). Effects of high-fidelity simulation teaching on nursing students' knowledge, professional skills and clinical ability: A meta-analysis and systematic review. *Nurse Education in Practice, 60,* 103306. DOI: 10.1016/j.nepr.2022.103306

Lemus, M. (2017). Young people in front of the world: Digital technologies as a support for everyday life. *Latin American Journal of Social Sciences. Childhood and Youth, 15*(1), 161–172. DOI: 10.11600/1692715x.1510902022016

Lightbot. (s.f.). *Lightbot.* Recuperado el 15 de noviembre de 2025, de https://lightbot.lu/

Li, L., Hew, K. F., & Du, J. (2024). Gamification enhances student intrinsic motivation, perceptions of autonomy and relatedness, but minimal impact on competency: A meta-analysis and systematic review. *Educational Technology Research and Development, 72*(2), 765–796. DOI: 10.1007/s11423-023-10337-7

Li, M., Ma, S., & Shi, Y. (2023). Examining the effectiveness of gamification as a tool promoting teaching and learning in educational settings: A meta-analysis. *Frontiers in Psychology, 14*, 1253549. DOI: 10.3389/fpsyg.2023.1253549 PMID: 37876838

Limberger, J. B. (2013). Metodologias ativas de ensino-aprendizagem para educação farmacêutica: Um relato de experiência. *Interface: Comunicacao, Saude, Educacao, 17*(47), 969–975. DOI: 10.1590/1807-57622013.3683

Liu, Y. C., Wang, W. T., & Lee, T. L. (2021). An Integrated View of Information Feedback, Game Quality, and Autonomous Motivation for Evaluating Game-Based Learning Effectiveness. *Journal of Educational Computing Research, 59*(1), 3–40. DOI: 10.1177/0735633120952044

Llamas-Alonso, J. C., & Llamas-Alonso, L. A. (2025). Videojuegos y aprendizaje: Impacto cognitivo, neurobiológico y aplicaciones educativas. Video Games and Learning: Cognitive, Neurobiological Impact, and Educational Applications. *Humanus Nexus, 9*(16), nueva época. ISSN 3061-7235.

Llamas-Alonso, J., Guevara, M. A., Hernández-González, M., Hevia-Orozco, J. C., & Almanza-Sepúlveda, M. L. (2019). Action video game players require greater EEG coupling between prefrontal cortices to adequately perform a dual task. *Entertainment Computing, 30*, 100302. Advance online publication. DOI: 10.1016/j.entcom.2019.100302

Long, M. K. & International Symposium on Languages for Specific Purposes. (2017). *Language for specific purposes : trends in curriculum development* (M. K. Long, Ed.). Georgetown University Press.

Looyestyn, J., Kernot, J., Boshoff, K., Ryan, J., Edney, S., & Maher, C. (2017). Does gamification increase engagement with online programs? A systematic review. *PLoS One, 12*(3), e0173403. Advance online publication. DOI: 10.1371/journal.pone.0173403 PMID: 28362821

Lopez De Ramos, A. L., Casado Robles, E., Atagua-Díaz, Z., Prado, J. F., Álvarez Franco, A. M., Cáceres, A., & Ramos Fortuna, V. (2024). Análisis de la alfabetización digital: Explorando la brecha de género en estudiantes universitarios panameños. *Latitude, 1*(19), 22–46. DOI: 10.55946/latitude.v1i19.242

López Raventós, C. (2016). El videojuego como herramienta educativa. Posibilidades y problemáticas acerca de los serious games. *Apertura, Revista de Innovación Educativa, 8*(1), 1–51. Retreived from http://www.udgvirtual.udg.mx/apertura//index.php/apertura/article/view/825

López, J. Y. A., Nuñoncca Huaycho, R. N., Yallercco Santos, F. I., Talavera-Mendoza, F., & Rucano Paucar, F. H. (2023). The impact of serious games on learning in primary education: A systematic literature review. *International Journal of Learning. Teaching and Educational Research*, *22*(3), 379–395. DOI: 10.26803/ijlter.22.3.23

Lorenz, R. C., Gleich, T., Gallinat, J., & Kühn, S. (2015). Video game training and the reward system. *Frontiers in Human Neuroscience*, *9*, 40. DOI: 10.3389/fnhum.2015.00040 PMID: 25698962

Ma, C.-W., Cheng, P.-S., Chan, Y.-S., & Tipoe, G. L. (2023). Virtual reality: A technology to promote active learning of physiology for students across multiple disciplines. *Advances in Physiology Education*, *47*(3), 594–603. DOI: 10.1152/advan.00172.2022

Magazine, U. X. (2017). Participatory Design in Practice. Retrieved from https://uxmag.com/articles/participatory-design-in-practice

Maqbool, M., Farooq, M., Imran, M., Alghafli, M., & Fatima, N. (2025). Mental health and academic performance of students at tertiary level: The role of housing. *Frontiers in Education*, *10*, 1627192. Advance online publication. DOI: 10.3389/feduc.2025.1627192

Marcano, B. (2008). Juegos Serios Y Entrenamiento En La Sociedad Digital. *Teoría de La Educación Educación y Cultura En La Sociedad de La Información, 9*, 5. Retrieved from https://dialnet.unirioja.es/servlet/articulo?codigo=2778746&info=resumen

Marfisi-Schottman, I., George, S., & Tarpin-Bernard, F. (2010, October). Tools and methods for efficiently designing serious games. In *Proceedings of the 4th Europeen Conference on Games Based Learning ECGBL* (pp. 226-234).

Marinelli, C. V., Nardacchione, G., Trotta, E., Di Fuccio, R., Palladino, P., Traetta, L., & Limone, P. (2023). The Effectiveness of Serious Games for Enhancing Literacy Skills in Children with Learning Disabilities or Difficulties: A Systematic Review. *Applied Sciences (Basel, Switzerland)*, *13*(7), 4512. DOI: 10.3390/app13074512

Marín-Marín, J., Moreno-Guerrero, A., Dúo-Terrón, P., & López-Belmonte, J. (2021). STEAM in education: A bibliometric analysis of performance and co-words in Web of Science. *International Journal of STEM Education*, *8*(1), 41. DOI: 10.1186/s40594-021-00296-x PMID: 34189015

Mark, H. F. (Ed.). (2020). *Encyclopedia of polymer science and technology* (4th ed.). Wiley., DOI: 10.1002/0471440264

Martelli, D., Prado, A., Xia, B., Verghese, J., & Agrawal, S. K. (2019). Development of a Virtual Floor Maze Test—Effects of Distal Visual Cues and Correlations With Executive Function in Healthy Adults. *IEEE Transactions on Neural Systems and Rehabilitation Engineering: A Publication of the IEEE Engineering in Medicine and Biology Society, 27*(10), 2229–2236. DOI: 10.1109/TNSRE.2019.2938103

Martinez, S. (2024). 21 Hispanics: Richness in Diversity. *Cultural Sensitivity and Responsiveness in Neurorehabilitation: A Personalized Approach for Speech-Language Pathologists, 1*, 419.

Martínez-García, M., González-Caminal, G., & Gomar-Sancho, C. (2025). Quantitative analysis of communication and patient safety competencies included in a clinical simulation program for the degree in Medicine. *Medical Education, 26*(4), 101041. DOI: 10.1016/j.edumed.2025.101041

Martinez, L., Gimenes, M., & Lambert, E. (2023). Video games and board games: Effects of playing practice on cognition. *PLoS One, 18*(3), e0283654. Advance online publication. DOI: 10.1371/journal.pone.0283654 PMID: 36972271

Mavroeidi, A.-G., Kitsiou, A., Kalloniatis, C., & Gritzalis, S. (2019). Gamification vs. Privacy: Identifying and Analysing the Major Concerns. *Future Internet, 11*(3), 67. DOI: 10.3390/fi11030067

McGaugh, J. L. (2000). Memory—A Century of Consolidation. *Science, 287*(5451), 248–251. DOI: 10.1126/science.287.5451.248

McGonigal, J. (2011). *Reality is broken: Why games make us better and how they can change the world*. Penguin Press.

McNaughton, B. L., Battaglia, F. P., Jensen, O., Moser, E. I., & Moser, M. B. (2006). Path integration and the neural basis of the "cognitive map.". *Nature Reviews. Neuroscience, 7*(8), 663–678. DOI: 10.1038/nrn1932 PMID: 16858394

MedicalExpo. (2024). Osso VR surgical training simulator. https://www.medicalexpo.com/prod/osso-vr/product-301294-1007883.html

Medtronic Digital Surgery. (2021, September 28). Tactile surgery. Medtronic Enterprise [Video]. YouTube. Retrieved September 4, 2025, https://www.youtube.com/watch?v=_Fhqd070FBw [REMOVED HYPERLINK FIELD]

Meier, S. K., Ray, K. L., Mastan, J. C., Salvage, S. R., & Robin, D. A. (2021). Meta-analytic connectivity modelling of deception-related brain regions. *PLoS One, 16*(8), e0248909. Advance online publication. DOI: 10.1371/journal.pone.0248909 PMID: 34432808

Mei, J., Kohler, J., Winter, Y., Spies, C., Endres, M., Banneke, S., & Emmrich, J. V. (2020). Automated radial 8-arm maze: A voluntary and stress-free behavior test to assess spatial learning and memory in mice. *Behavioural Brain Research, 381*, 112352. DOI: 10.1016/j.bbr.2019.112352

Mejillones Picazo, R. N. (2024). Impact of social media use with artificial intelligence on adolescents' self-esteem and identity. *Innovarium International Journal, 2*(2), 1–13. https://revinde.org/index.php/innovarium/article/view/21

Méndez, R. M. S., Ocampo, R. D. L. S., Rebilla, E. E. R., & Azuero, D. P. S. (2024). El impacto del mal uso de la inteligencia artificial en la realización del trabajo autónomo en el entorno de educación superior. *South Florida Journal of Development*, *5*(2), 681–687. DOI: 10.46932/sfjdv5n2-020

Mendoza, L. (2023, August 11). *Unraveling the MIMO method and its importance in feedback.* Health Simulation Network. https://reddesimulacionensalud.com/desarrollo-profesional/desentranando-el-metodo-mimo-y-su-importancia-en-el-feedback/

Menon, D., Romero, M., & Viéville, T. (2019). Computational thinking development and assessment through tabletop escape games. *International Journal of Serious Games*, *6*(4), 3–18. DOI: 10.17083/ijsg.v6i4.319

Merlo, S. A., Belluscio, M. A., Pedreira, M. E., & Merlo, E. (2024). Memory persistence: From fundamental mechanisms to translational opportunities. *Translational Psychiatry*, *14*(1), 98. DOI: 10.1038/s41398-024-02808-z

Merry, S. N., Stasiak, K., Shepherd, M., Frampton, C., Fleming, T., & Lucassen, M. F. (2012). The effectiveness of SPARX, a computerised self help intervention for adolescents seeking help for depression: Randomised controlled non-inferiority trial. *BMJ (Clinical Research Ed.)*, *344*(apr18 3), e2598. https://www.bmj.com/content/344/bmj.e2598. DOI: 10.1136/bmj.e2598 PMID: 22517917

Meuter, R. F., Gallois, C., Segalowitz, N. S., Ryder, A. G., & Hocking, J. (2015). Overcoming language barriers in healthcare: A protocol for investigating safe and effective communication when patients or clinicians use a second language. *BMC Health Services Research*, *15*(1), 371. DOI: 10.1186/s12913-015-1024-8

Miller, G. E. (1990). The assessment of clinical skills/competence/performance. *Academic Medicine*, *65*(9), S63–S67. DOI: 10.1097/00001888-199009000-00045

Minderer, M., Harvey, C. D., Donato, F., & Moser, E. I. (2016). Neuroscience: Virtual reality explored. *Nature*, *533*(7603), 324–325. DOI: 10.1038/nature17899

Ministry of Health & National Institute of Public Health. (2024). Report on the Results of the National Health and Nutrition Survey - Continuous 2023. In *ENSANUT.* National Institute of Public Health. Retrieved August 15, 2025, from https://ensanut.insp.mx/encuestas/ensanutcontinua2023/doctos/informes/ensanut_23_112024.pdf

Ministry of Public Education. (2025, August 26). *Bulletin 113: SEP starts the start of the 2024-2025 school year* [Press release]. Government of Mexico. https://www.gob.mx/sep/articulos/boletin-113-arranca-sep-inicio-del-ciclo-escolar-2024-2025?idiom=es

Mitra, A., & Wu, Y. (2012). Challenges and Opportunities in Achieving Bioequivalence for Fixed-Dose Combination Products. *The AAPS Journal, 14*(3), 646–655. DOI: 10.1208/s12248-012-9378-x

Molina-Carmona, R., & Llorens-Largo, F. (2020). Gamification and Advanced Technology to Enhance Motivation in Education. *Informatics (MDPI), 7*(2), 20. DOI: 10.3390/informatics7020020

Monné Bellmunt, A. (2025). Impact of technologies and AI on human development: From childhood to old age. *DIM: Didactics, Innovation, and Multimedia, (43).* https://www.raco.cat/index.php/DIM/article/view/10000003804

Montana, J. I., Tuena, C., Serino, S., Cipresso, P., & Riva, G. (2019). Neurorehabilitation of Spatial Memory Using Virtual Environments: A Systematic Review. *Journal of Clinical Medicine, 8*(10), 1516. DOI: 10.3390/jcm8101516

Morais, Y. de J., dos Santos, V. R. C., & Soler, O. (2021). Simulação realística como mediadora do processo ensino-aprendizagem na graduação em Farmácia: Revisão sistemática. *Research. Social Development, 10*(10), e241101018783–e241101018783. DOI: 10.33448/rsd-v10i10.18783

Moral Álvarez, J., & Almazán Ruíz, E. (2017). El uso de los videojuegos como recurso didáctico para el aprendizaje de inglés (Tesis para licenciatura). Universidad de Jaén, Andalucía, España. Retrieved from http://tauja.ujaen.es/bitstream/10953.1/5745/1/Moral_lvarez_Jess_TFG_Educacin_Primaria.pdf

Moreno Arellano, C. (2025). Towards universal coverage in higher education? Perspectives on the increase in enrollment in Mexico. *The Journal of Higher Education, 54*(214), 19–42. DOI: 10.36857/resu.2025.214.3268

Moreno Infante, C. R., Cuenca Peláez, K. F., Cool Cedeño, D., Murillo León, M. E., & Quintana Monar, A. M. (2025). El impacto de la tecnología en la vida social de los adolescentes: The Impact of Technology on Adolescents' Social Life. *Multidisciplinary Journal of General Studies, 4*(2), 1370–1390. DOI: 10.70577/reg.v4i2.148

Moya-Higueras, J., Solé-Puiggené, M., Vita-Barrull, N., Estrada-Plana, V., Guzmán, N., Arias, S., Garcia, X., Ayesa-Arriola, R., & March-Llanes, J. (2023). Just Play Cognitive Modern Board and Card Games, It's Going to Be Good for Your Executive Functions: A Randomized Controlled Trial with Children at Risk of Social Exclusion. *Children (Basel, Switzerland), 10*(9), 1492. Advance online publication. DOI: 10.3390/children10091492 PMID: 37761453

Mukherjee, M., Le, N. T., Chow, Y.-W., & Susilo, W. (2024). Strategic Approaches to Cybersecurity Learning: A Study of Educational Models and Outcomes. *Information (Basel), 15*(2), 117. DOI: 10.3390/info15020117

Multimedia, C. I. B. A. L. (2004). Ven a jugar con Pipo. CIBAL Multimedia S.L. Retrieved from http://www.pipoclub.com/webonline/guia/catalogo.pdf

Murch, W. S., & Clark, L. (2016). Games in the brain: Neural substrates of gambling addiction. *The Neuroscientist, 22*(5), 534–545. DOI: 10.1177/1073858415591474 PMID: 26116634

Navarro-Mateos, C. (s/f). *Análisis del rol docente en una propuesta de gamificación en el máster de profesorado Analysis of the teaching role in a gamification proposal in the teacher's master's degree*. https://doi.org/DOI: 10.4438/1988-592X-RE-2024-405-635

Neves, C., Oliveira, T., Cruz-Jesus, F., & Venkatesh, V. (2025). Extending the unified theory of acceptance and use of technology for sustainable technologies context. *International Journal of Information Management, 80*, 102838. DOI: 10.1016/j.ijinfomgt.2024.102838

Nguyen, V. T. T., Darville, N., & Vermeulen, A. (2023). Pharmacokinetics of Long-Acting Aqueous Nano-/Microsuspensions After Intramuscular Administration in Different Animal Species and Humans—A Review. *The AAPS Journal, 25*(4), 4. Advance online publication. DOI: 10.1208/s12248-022-00771-5

Nielsen, J. (2012). Usability 101: Introduction to Usability. Nielsen Norman Group. Retrieved from https://www.nngroup.com/articles/usability-101-introduction-to-usability/

Norman, D. A. (2004). *Emotional design: Why we love (or hate) everyday things*. Basic Books. DOI: 10.1145/985600.966013

Nyberg, L., & Eriksson, J. (2016). Working memory: Maintenance, updating, and the realization of intentions. *Cold Spring Harbor Perspectives in Biology, 8*(2), a021816. Advance online publication. DOI: 10.1101/cshperspect.a021816 PMID: 26637287

O'Reilly, J. X., Mesulam, M. M., & Nobre, A. C. (2008). The cerebellum predicts the timing of perceptual events. *The Journal of Neuroscience : The Official Journal of the Society for Neuroscience*, *28*(9), 2252–2260. DOI: 10.1523/JNEUROSCI.2742-07.2008 PMID: 18305258

O'Sullivan, B. (2012). Assessment issues in languages for specific purposes. *Modern Language Journal*, *96*(s1), 71–88. DOI: 10.1111/j.1540-4781.2012.01298.x

Ojanen, E., Ronimus, M., Ahonen, T., Chansa-Kabali, T., February, P., Jere-Folotiya, J., Kauppinen, K.-P., Ketonen, R., Ngorosho, D., & Pitk, Ã¤nen, M., Puhakka, S., Sampa, F., Walubita, G., Yalukanda, C., Pugh, K., Richardson, U., Serpell, R., & Lyytinen, H. (. (2015). GraphoGame â€" a catalyst for multi-level promotion of literacy in diverse contexts. *Frontiers in Psychology*, *6*. Advance online publication. DOI: 10.3389/fpsyg.2015.00671

Orozco-Rodriguez, C., Palafox González, A., & Valenzuela García, C. (2023). A realistic situation, proposed from data generated within the GeOrder Simulator to elicit the statistical reasoning. *Heliyon*, *9*(9), e19330. DOI: 10.1016/j.heliyon.2023.e19330

Orta, J., & Sánchez Sánchez, E. (2018). Niveles de razonamiento sobre variación estadística de estudiantes de nivel medio superior al resolver problemas en un contexto de riesgo. *Educación Matemática*, *30*(1), 47–71. DOI: 10.24844/EM3001.02

Ortiz, R. (2017). Educación globalizada: Tendencias y retos de la educación superior en México y el mundo. *RIESED - Revista Internacional De Estudios Sobre Sistemas Educativos, 2*(6), 24–39.

Osso, V. R. (2017, August 23). Osso VR virtual surgery. Real results [Video]. YouTube. https://www.youtube.com/watch?v=bqra7wslwCM

Osso, V. R. (2023). Guide to using virtual reality in medical education programs. Osso's virtual reality blog. https://www.ossovr.com/post/guide-to-using-vr-in-medical-education-programs

Pacheco, D., Sánchez-Fibla, M., Duff, A., & Verschure, P. F. M. J. (2017). A Spatial-Context Effect in Recognition Memory. *Frontiers in Behavioral Neuroscience*, *11*, 143. DOI: 10.3389/fnbeh.2017.00143

Palaus, M., Marron, E. M., Viejo-Sobera, R., & Redolar-Ripoll, D. (2017). Neural basis of video gaming: A systematic review. *Frontiers in Human Neuroscience*, *11*, 248. DOI: 10.3389/fnhum.2017.00248 PMID: 28588464

Papert, S. (1993). The children's machine. Perseus Book Group. Retrieved from https://pdfs.semanticscholar.org/e744/f03a3586f8e79dee595a3dbdef2e327b28cd.pdf

Papert, S. (1998). Does Easy Do It? Children, Games, and Learning. Retrieved from http://www.papert.org/articles/Doeseasydoit.html

Parmar, D., Lin, L., DSouza, N., Jörg, S., Leonard, A. E., Daily, S. B., & Babu, S. V. (2023). How Immersion and Self-Avatars in VR Affect Learning Programming and Computational Thinking in Middle School Education. *IEEE Transactions on Visualization and Computer Graphics*, *29*(8), 3698–3713. DOI: 10.1109/TVCG.2022.3169426

Parody, L., Santos, J., Trujillo-Cayado, L. A., & Ceballos, M. (2022). Gamification in Engineering Education: The Use of Classcraft Platform to Improve Motivation and Academic Performance. *Applied Sciences (Basel, Switzerland)*, *12*(22), 11832. DOI: 10.3390/app122211832

Parra-Taboada, M. E., Trujillo-Arteaga, J. C., Álvarez-Abad, D. R., Arias-Domínguez, A. S., & Santillán-Gordón, E. (2024). El impacto de la inteligencia artificial en la educación. *Revista Científica Retos de la Ciencia*, *1*(4), 169–181. DOI: 10.53877/rc.8.19e.202409.14

Participate in Design. (2019). Our Design Philosophy. Retrieved from https://participateindesign.org/approach/what

Partovi, T., & Razavi, M. R. (2019). The effect of game-based learning on academic achievement motivation of elementary school students. *Learning and Motivation*, *68*, 101592. DOI: 10.1016/j.lmot.2019.101592

Parvate, S., Dixit, P., & Chattopadhyay, S. (2020). Superhydrophobic surfaces: Insights from theory and experiment. *The Journal of Physical Chemistry B*, *124*(8), 1323–1360. DOI: 10.1021/acs.jpcb.9b08567

Pasqualotto, A., Altarelli, I., de Angeli, A., Menestrina, Z., Bavelier, D., & Venuti, P. (2022). Enhancing reading skills through a video game mixing action mechanics and cognitive training. *Nature Human Behaviour*, *6*(4), 545–554. DOI: 10.1038/s41562-021-01254-x

Piaget, J. (1952). *The origins of intelligence in children* (Cook, M., Trans.). International Universities Press., DOI: 10.1037/11494-000

Piazza, A., Vasudevan, S., & Carr, M. (2023). Cybersecurity in UK Universities: Mapping (or managing) threat intelligence sharing within the higher education sector. *Journal of Cybersecurity*, *9*(1), tyad019. Advance online publication. DOI: 10.1093/cybsec/tyad019

Piquette, N. A., Savage, R. S., & Abrami, P. C. (2014). A cluster randomized control field trial of the ABRACADABRA web-based reading technology: Replication and extension of basic findings. *Frontiers in Psychology, 5*, 1413. DOI: 10.3389/fpsyg.2014.01413

Polli, J. E. (2008). In Vitro Studies are Sometimes Better than Conventional Human Pharmacokinetic In Vivo Studies in Assessing Bioequivalence of Immediate-Release Solid Oral Dosage Forms. *The AAPS Journal, 10*(2), 289–299. DOI: 10.1208/s12248-008-9027-6

Pozzi, F. E., Appollonio, I., Ferrarese, C., & Tremolizzo, L. (2023). Can traditional board games prevent or slow down cognitive impairment? A systematic review and meta-analysis. *Journal of Alzheimer's Disease, 95*(3), 829–845. DOI: 10.3233/JAD-230473 PMID: 37638443

Pramod, D. (2025). Gamification in cybersecurity education; a state of the art review and research agenda. *Journal of Applied Research in Higher Education, 17*(4), 1162–1180. DOI: 10.1108/JARHE-02-2024-0072

Prathyusha, N. (2020). Role of gamification in language learning. [IJRAR]. *International Journal of Research and Analytical Reviews, 7*(2), 577–583.

Prensky, M. (2008). *Digital game-based learning*. Paragon House.

Prieto, Y. S., Garzón, A. D., & Martínez, A. P. (2024). *Life skills for adolescents in the strengthening of the life project from rural identity*. [Applied project]. UNAD Institutional Repository. https://repository.unad.edu.co/handle/10596/63858

Psicosmart. (2024, September 21). *The influence of gamification on students' mental health: benefits and risks*. Retrieved from https://psicosmart.pro/articulos/articulo-la-influencia-de-la-gamificacion-en-la-salud-mental-de-los-estudiantes-beneficios-y-riesgos-200608

Quinde-Moncerrate, H. G., Quinde-Zambrano, L. F., & Franco-Arroyo, P. P. (2025). Impact of artificial intelligence on contemporary education: Systematic review. *Sociedad & Tecnología, 8*(2), 358–368. DOI: 10.51247/st.v8i2.505

Rabek, J. F. (2012). *Polymer photodegradation: Mechanisms and experimental methods*. Springer Science & Business Media.

Ramgobin, A., Fontaine, G., & Bourbigot, S. (2020). A Case Study of Polyether Ether Ketone (I): Investigating the Thermal and Fire Behavior of a High-Performance Material. *Polymers, 12*(8), 1789. DOI: 10.3390/polym12081789

Ramírez-Sánchez, N. A., Vega-Peña, N. V., Domínguez-Torres, L. C., & Sanabria-Quiroga, Á. E. (2018). Mental training and surgeons: A strategy for improvement. *Iatreia, 31*(2), 180–190. DOI: 10.17533/udea.iatreia.v31n2a06

Raos, G., & Zappone, B. (2021). Polymer adhesion: Seeking new solutions for an old problem. *Macromolecules, 54*(23), 10617–10644. DOI: 10.1021/acs.macromol.1c01182

Ratinho, E., & Martins, C. (2023). The role of gamified learning strategies in student's motivation in high school and higher education: A systematic review. *Heliyon, 9*(8), e19033. DOI: 10.1016/j.heliyon.2023.e19033 PMID: 37636393

Reijmers, L. G., Perkins, B. L., Matsuo, N., & Mayford, M. (2007). Localization of a Stable Neural Correlate of Associative Memory. *Science, 317*(5842), 1230–1233. DOI: 10.1126/science.1143839

Revelo-Sánchez, O., Collazos-Ordoñez, C. A., & Jiménez-Toledo, J. A. (2018). La Gamificación como estrategia didáctica para la enseñanza/aprendizaje de la programación: Un mapeo sistemático de literatura. [revista Descontinuada]. *Lámpsakos, 1*(19), 31–46. DOI: 10.21501/21454086.2347

Reynaldo, C., Christian, R., Hosea, H., & Gunawan, A. A. S. (2021). Using Video Games to Improve Capabilities in Decision Making and Cognitive Skill: A Literature Review. *Procedia Computer Science, 179*, 211–221. DOI: 10.1016/j.procs.2020.12.027

Rivas, K. A., Lemus García, C. R., Montelong, M. V., Cortez Álvarez, C. R., Barajas Menzoza, M. A., Avalos, A. V., & Garduño, A. C. (2023). Estudio Comparativo de Perfiles de Disolución de Tabletas de 500 mg de Paracetamol para Determinar su Intercambiabilidad. *Artículos del Congreso Internacional de Investigación Academia Journals Chetumal, 15*(5), 2.1-2.6.

Robinson, L., Cotten, S. R., Ono, H., Quan-Haase, A., Mesch, G., Chen, W., Schulz, J., Hale, T. M., & Stern, M. J. (2015). Digital inequalities and why they matter. *Information Communication and Society, 18*(5), 569–582. DOI: 10.1080/1369118X.2015.1012532

Rodríguez, A. N. S., Romero, M. E. M., Agreda, C. J. R., Saldarriaga, J. G. R., & Saldarriaga, M. A. R. (2024). Impacto de la inteligencia artificial en las prácticas educativas: Percepciones y actitudes del profesorado. *LATAM Revista Latinoamericana de Ciencias Sociales y Humanidades, 5*(2). Advance online publication. DOI: 10.56712/latam.v5i2.1933

Rodríguez-Abitia, G., Ramírez-Montoya, M. S., López-Caudana, E. O., & Romero-Rodríguez, J. M. (2021, 31 julio). *Factores para el desarrollo del pensamiento computacional en estudiantes de pregrado*. Campus Virtuales, Virtuales, 10(2), 153-164. http://uajournals.com/ojs/index.php/campusvirtuales/article/view/893

Rodríguez-Fernández, A., Ruíz-De la Fuente, M., Maury-Sintjago, E., Petersen, S., Paredes, V., & Montero, B. (2024). Sociodemographic Factors Associated with Video Game Addiction in Schoolchildren from the South-Central Region of Chile. *Children (Basel, Switzerland)*, *11*(10), 1156. DOI: 10.3390/children11101156 PMID: 39457120

Rollings, A., & Adams, E. (2003). *Andrew rollings and Ernest Adams on game design*. New Riders Publishing.

Rolls, E. T. (2022). The hippocampus, ventromedial prefrontal cortex, and episodic and semantic memory. *Progress in Neurobiology*, *217*, 102334. DOI: 10.1016/j.pneurobio.2022.102334

Romero Agudelo, L. N., Salinas Urbina, V., & Mortera Gutiérrez, F. J. (2010). Learning styles based on Kolb's model in virtual education. *Apertura (Guadalajara, Jal.)*, *2*(1).

Romero Castillo, J. S. (2025). Educational Innovations in Laparoscopy: A Comparative Meta-Analysis Between Mechanical Simulation and Traditional Training [Undergraduate Thesis, Universidad Veracruzana. "Dr. Rafael Lucio" High Specialty Center]. Veracruz. https://cdigital.uv.mx/handle/1944/53563

Romero López, E. (2024, October 4). Chapala has recorded three suicides so far this year. *Laguna Weekly*. Retrieved from http://semanariolaguna.com/82002/

Romero, M., Usart, M., & Ott, M. (2015). Can serious games contribute to developing and sustaining 21st century skills? *Games and Culture*, *10*(2), 148–177. DOI: 10.1177/1555412014548919

Romero-Mendez, E. A., Santana-Mancilla, P. C., Garcia-Ruiz, M., Montesinos-López, O. A., & Anido-Rifón, L. E. (2023). The Use of Deep Learning to Improve Player Engagement in a Video Game through a Dynamic Difficulty Adjustment Based on Skills Classification. *Applied Sciences (Basel, Switzerland)*, *13*(14), 8249. DOI: 10.3390/app13148249

Roussin, C. J., & Weinstock, P. (2017). SimZones: An organizational innovation for simulation programs and centers. *Academic Medicine*, *92*(8), 1114–1120. DOI: 10.1097/ACM.0000000000001746 PMID: 28562455

Russo, M., Kosman, G., Ginsburg, A., Thompson-Hoffman, S., & Pederson, J. (1998). *A compact for reading and School-home Links*. Department of Education.

Ryan, R. M., & Deci, E. L. (2000). Self-determination theory and the facilitation of intrinsic motivation, social development, and well-being. *The American Psychologist*, *55*(1), 68–78. https://psycnet.apa.org/doiLanding?doi=10.1037%2F0003-066X.55.1.68. DOI: 10.1037/0003-066X.55.1.68 PMID: 11392867

Ryan, R. M., & Deci, E. L. (2020). Intrinsic and extrinsic motivation: Classic definitions and new directions. *Contemporary Educational Psychology*, *61*, 101863. DOI: 10.1016/j.cedpsych.2020.101863

Ryan, R. M., Rigby, C. S., & Przybylski, A. (2006). The Motivational Pull of Video Games: A Self-Determination Theory Approach. *Motivation and Emotion*, *30*(4), 344–360. DOI: 10.1007/s11031-006-9051-8

Sagaspe, P., Amieva, H., Dartigues, J.-F., Olive, J., de la Rivière, J.-B., Chartier, C., Taillard, J., & Philip, P. (2023). Validity and diagnostic performance of a virtual reality-based supermarket application "MEMOSHOP" for assessing episodic memory in normal and pathological aging. *Digital Health*, *9*, 20552076231218808. DOI: 10.1177/20552076231218808

Sakalli, M. T., Bulus, E., & Buyuksaracoglu, F. (2004). Cryptography education for students. *Information Technology Based Proceedings of the FIfth International Conference OnHigher Education and Training, 2004. ITHET 2004.*, 621–626. DOI: 10.1109/ITHET.2004.1358246

Sala, G., Tatlidil, K. S., & Gobet, F. (2018). Video game training does not enhance cognitive ability: A comprehensive meta-analytic investigation. *Psychological Bulletin*, *144*(2), 111–139. DOI: 10.1037/bul0000139 PMID: 29239631

Salas, M. A. (2017). The use of simulation in medical education. Mini physiological checks, 4 (1), 3-10. http://sedici.unlp.edu.ar/handle/10915/126449

Salas-Flores, L. O., Rojas Espinoza, B. I., Pinedo Paz, M. A., & Vega Vilca, C. S. (2024). ICT and collaborative learning in higher education: A systematic review. Court. *Journal of Education Sciences and Legal Sciences*, *4*(9), 579–591. DOI: 10.59659/revistatribunal.v4i9.94

Samba, D. (n.d.). *The 10 Best Apps for Virtual Support in Mental Health*. Digital Samba Blog. Retrieved from https://www.digitalsamba.com/es/blog/the-top-10-apps-for-virtual-mental-health-support

Sánchez Sánchez, E., Silvestre Castro, E., & García Ríos, V. N. (2019). Patrones de razonamiento sobre pruebas de significación de estudiantes de bachillerato. *Patterns of reasoning on signification tests of high school students.* http://hdl.handle.net/10481/55045

Santana-Mancilla, P. C., Gaytán-Lugo, L. S., & Rodríguez-Ortiz, M. A. (2016). Usability Testing of Serious Games: The Experience of the IHCLab. In *Games User Research: A Case Study Approach* (pp. 271–283). CRC Press.

Santana-Mancilla, P. C., Rodríguez-Ortiz, M., Gaytán-Lugo, L., & Garcia-Ruiz, M. (2015). User Experience Evaluation to El Encanto: A Serious Game for Learning Community Intervention. *Research in Computing Science*, *108*(1), 81–88. DOI: 10.13053/rcs-108-1-9

Schenk, S., Lech, R. K., & Suchan, B. (2017). Games people play: How video games improve probabilistic learning. *Behavioural Brain Research*, *335*, 208–214. DOI: 10.1016/j.bbr.2017.08.027 PMID: 28842270

Schleicher, A. (2019). PISA 2018: Insights and Interpretations. Retrieved from https://www.oecd.org/pisa/PISA%202018%20Insights%20and%20Interpretations%20FINAL%20PDF.pdf

Schouten, B. C., Cox, A., Duran, G., Kerremans, K., Banning, L. K., Lahdidioui, A., van den Muijsenbergh, M., Schinkel, S., Sungur, H., Suurmond, J., Zendedel, R., & Krystallidou, D. (2020). Mitigating language and cultural barriers in healthcare communication: Toward a holistic approach. *Patient Education and Counseling*, *103*(12), 2604–2608. DOI: 10.1016/j.pec.2020.05.001

Schultz, C., & Bryant, R. (2011). *Game Testing All in One*. Mercury Learning & Information, Herndon.

Schultz, W. (2016). Dopamine reward prediction error coding. *Dialogues in Clinical Neuroscience*, *18*(1), 23–32. DOI: 10.31887/DCNS.2016.18.1/wschultz PMID: 27069377

Scratch. (s.f.). *Scratch – Imagine, Program, Share*. Recuperado el 15 de noviembre de 2025, de https://scratch.mit.edu/

Seaborn, K., & Fels, D. I. (2015). Gamification in theory and action: A survey. *International Journal of Human-Computer Studies*, *74*, 14–31. DOI: 10.1016/j.ijhcs.2014.09.006

Secretaría de Salud. (2013). *NORMA Oficial Mexicana NOM-177-SSA1-2013, Que establece las pruebas y procedimientos para demostrar que un medicamento es intercambiable. Requisitos a que deben sujetarse los Terceros Autorizados que realicen las pruebas de intercambiabilidad. Requisitos para realizar los estudios de biocomparabilidad. Requisitos a que deben sujetarse los Terceros Autorizados, Centros de Investigación o Instituciones Hospitalarias que realicen las pruebas de biocomparabilidad.* https://www.dof.gob.mx/

Serag-Bolos, E. S., Chudow, M., Perkins, J., & Patel, R. V. (2018). Enhancing Student Knowledge Through a Comprehensive Oncology Simulation. *American Journal of Pharmaceutical Education*, *82*(3), 6245. DOI: 10.5688/ajpe6245

Serrano Herrera, R. A. (2021). *Sistema de tutoría afectiva para apoyar el proceso de enseñanza y aprendizaje de estructuras de datos* [Tesis de licenciatura, Tecnológico Nacional de México]. Repositorio Institucional TecNM. https://rinacional.tecnm.mx/handle/TecNM/2700

Serrate-González, S., Sánchez-Rojo, A., Andrade-Silva, L. E., & Muñoz-Rodríguez, J. M. (2023). Onlife Identity: The Question of Gender and Age in Teenagers' Online Behaviour. *Comunicar: Media Education Research Journal*, *31*(75), 9–19.

Shandley, K., Austin, D., Klein, B., & Kyrios, M. (2010). An evaluation of 'Reach Out Central': an online gaming program for supporting the mental health of young people. . Recuperado de https://academic.oup.com/her/article-abstract/25/4/563/573881?redirectedFrom=fulltext&login=falseDOI: 10.1093/her/cyq002

Showstack, R. (2019). Patients don't have language barriers; the healthcare system does. *Emergency Medicine Journal : EMJ*, *36*(10), 580–581. DOI: 10.1136/emermed-2019-208929

Shute, V. J. (2011). Stealth assessment in computer-based games to support learning. In Tobias, S., & Fletcher, J. D. (Eds.), *Computer games and instruction* (pp. 503–524). IAP Information Age Publishing. DOI: 10.1108/978-1-61735-410-620251025

Sierra-Daza, M. C., Martín-del Pozo, M., & Sánchez, M. R. F. (2023). Videojuegos para el desarrollo de competencias en Educación Superior. *Revista Fuentes*, *25*(2), 228–241. DOI: 10.12795/revistafuentes.2023.22687

Signori, G. G., Guimaraes, J. C. F. D., Severo, E. A., & Rotta, C. (2018). Gamification as an innovative method in the processes of learning in higher education institutions. *International Journal of Innovation and Learning*, *24*(2), 115. DOI: 10.1504/IJIL.2018.094066

Silva, G. M., Souto, J. J. de S., Fernandes, T. P., Bolis, I., & Santos, N. A. (2021). Interventions with serious games and entertainment games in autism spectrum disorder: A systematic review. *Developmental Neuropsychology*, *46*(7), 463–485. DOI: 10.1080/87565641.2021.1981905 PMID: 34595981

Simonsen, J., & Robertson, T. (Eds.). (2013). *Routledge international handbook of participatory design* (Vol. 711). Routledge.

Simulation Center for Clinical and Surgical Excellence. Jalisco (CeSiECQ Jalisco). https://sites.google.com/view/cesiecq/p%C3%A1gina-principal

Singun, A. (2025). Unveiling the barriers to digital transformation in higher education institutions: A systematic literature review. *Discover Education*, *4*(1), 37. DOI: 10.1007/s44217-025-00430-9

Skinner, B. F. (1953). *Science and human behavior*. Macmillan.

Slavin, R. E., Madden, N. A., Dolan, L., & Wasik, B. A. (1996). *Every child, every school: Success for all*. Corwin Press, Inc.

Sleeter, C. E. (2011). An agenda to strengthen culturally responsive pedagogy. *English Teaching*, *10*(2), 7–23.

Smartico Help Center. (2024, March). *March 2024*. Smartico.ai. Retrieved from https://help.smartico.ai/welcome/more/release-notes/march-2024

Smidt, A., Balandin, S., Sigafoos, J., & Reed, V. A. (2009). Kirkpatrick's model: A useful tool for evaluating training outcomes. *Journal of Intellectual & Developmental Disability*, *34*(3), 266–274. DOI: 10.1080/13668250903093125 PMID: 19681007

Sosa de la Cruz, G. A. (2020). *Aplicación web para apoyar la toma de decisiones en el proceso de enseñanza de la programación* [Tesis de licenciatura, Tecnológico Nacional de México]. Repositorio Institucional TecNM. https://rinacional.tecnm.mx/handle/TecNM/2681

Sousa Lima, M. A., Monteiro, Á. C., Melo Leite Junior, A. J., de Andrade Matos, I. S., Alexandre, F. S. O., Nobre, D. J., ... & da Silva Júnior, J. N. (2019). Game-based application for helping students review chemical nomenclature in a fun way. DOI: 10.1021/acs.jchemed.8b00540

Spahl, W., Carter, M., Guillemin, M., & Young, D. (2024). *Gamified Digital Mental Health Interventions for Young People: Scoping Review of Ethical Aspects During Development and Implementation*.

Speer, N. K., Reynolds, J. R., Swallow, K. M., & Zacks, J. M. (2009). Reading stories activates neural representations of visual and motor experiences. *Psychological Science, 20*(8), 989–999. DOI: 10.1111/j.1467-9280.2009.02397.x PMID: 19572969

Squire, K. (2003). Video games in education. *Int. J. Intell. Games & Simulation, 2*(1), 49–62. https://www.biblioteken.fi/sites/default/files/content/10.1.1.100.8500.pdf

Starosta, J., Kiszka, P., Szyszka, P. D., Starzec, S., & Strojny, P. (2024). The tangled ways to classify games: A systematic review of how games are classified in psychological research. *PLoS One, 19*(6), e0299819. Advance online publication. DOI: 10.1371/journal.pone.0299819 PMID: 38913664

Statista. (2018). Number of active video gamers worldwide from 2014 to 2021. Retrieved from https://www.statista.com/statistics/748072/number-pc-gamers-world-platform

Statista. (2023, January 10). *Video game industry - Statistics & Facts*. Video Gaming & ESports. https://www.statista.com/topics/868/video-game-industry/

Statista. (2025, July 4). *Industria del videojuego: valor de mercado global*. https://es.statista.com/estadisticas/598622/valor-de-mercado-del-videojuego-en-el-mundo/

Stockdale, L., Morrison, R. G., Palumbo, R., Garbarino, J., & Silton, R. L. (2017). Cool, callous and in control: Superior inhibitory control in frequent players of video games with violent content. *Social Cognitive and Affective Neuroscience, 12*(12), 1869–1880. DOI: 10.1093/scan/nsx115 PMID: 29040750

Suárez López, D., Colón López, C., Cohen Jiménez, J., & Colpas, E. (2016). Appropriation of social networks for applying the Socratic method in critical thinking. *Zona Próxima, (25)*, 118–128. https://www.redalyc.org/journal/853/85350504009/html/

Subhash, S., & Cudney, E. A. (2018). Gamified learning in higher education: A systematic review of the literature. *Computers in Human Behavior, 87*, 192–206. DOI: 10.1016/j.chb.2018.05.028

Sulea, T., Kumar, S., & Kuroda, D. (2024). Editorial: Progress and challenges in computational structure-based design and development of biologic drugs. *Frontiers in Molecular Biosciences, 11*, 1360267. Advance online publication. DOI: 10.3389/fmolb.2024.1360267 PMID: 38389897

Sun, D., Looi, C., Li, Y., Zhu, C., Zhu, C., & Cheng, M. (2024). Block-based versus text-based programming: A comparison of learners' programming behaviors, computational thinking skills and attitudes toward programming. *Educational Technology Research and Development, 72*(2), 1067–1089. DOI: 10.1007/s11423-023-10328-8

Sung, H., Kim, M., Park, J., Shin, N., & Han, Y. (2024). Effectiveness of Virtual Reality in Healthcare Education: Systematic Review and Meta-Analysis. *Sustainability (Basel), 16*(19), 8520. DOI: 10.3390/su16198520

Swartz, S. L., Shook, R. E., & Klein, A. F. (2000). California Early Literacy Learning. Redlaus, CA: Foundation for California early literacy learning.

Taddeo, G. (2023). Life Long/Insta-Learning: The Use of Influencers as Informal Educators. *Italian Journal of Sociology of Education, 15*(2), 147–167. DOI: 10.14658/PUPJ-IJSE-2023-2-8

Tafur-Méndez, F., Almao-Malvacias, V., & Zambrano-Chamba, M. (2023). Conocimiento sobre la gamificación como técnica para reforzar el aprendizaje en la educación superior. *593 Digital Publisher CEIT, 8*(3), 209–218. DOI: 10.33386/593dp.2023.3.1628

Taylor, M. E., Liu, M., Abelson, S., Eisenberg, D., Lipson, S. K., & Schueller, S. M. (2024). Scope, effectiveness, adoption, implementation, and maintenance of digital mental health interventions for college students: A systematic review. *Current Psychiatry Reports, 26*(12), 683–693. DOI: 10.1007/s11920-024-01545-w PMID: 39392547

Team, S., & Team, S. (2021, 29 julio). *Headspace vs Calm Meditation App Comparison | Sleepopolis*. Sleepopolis. https://sleepopolis.com/headspace-vs-calm-meditation-app-comparison/

Technologies, U. (2020). Unity as a Library. Unity Documentation. Retrieved from https://docs.unity3d.com/Manual/UnityasaLibrary.html

Tejera-Martínez, F., Aguilera, D., & Vílchez-González, J. M. (2020). Lenguajes de programación y desarrollo de competencias clave. Revisión sistemática. *Revista Electrónica de Investigación Educativa, 22*, 1–16. DOI: 10.24320/redie.2020.22.e27.2869

Tene, T., Vique López, D. F., Valverde Aguirre, P. E., Cabezas Oviedo, N. I., Vacacela Gomez, C., & Bellucci, S. (2025). A systematic review of serious games as tools for STEM education. *Frontiers in Education, 10*, 1432982. DOI: 10.3389/feduc.2025.1432982

The Stanford Daily. (2025, January 12). *Stanford students release Sharotonin, a new app to gamify mental health* [Satirical article]. Retrieved from https://stanforddaily.com/2025/01/12/mental-health-gamified/

The UniProt Consortium. (2023). UniProt: The universal protein knowledgebase in 2023. *Nucleic Acids Research, 51*(D1), D523–D531. DOI: 10.1093/nar/gkac1052

Tibell, L. A. E., & Rundgren, C.-J. (2010). Educational challenges of molecular life science: Characteristics and implications for education and research. *CBE Life Sciences Education, 9*(1), 25–33. DOI: 10.1187/cbe.08-09-0055 PMID: 20194805

Ting, T. T., Han, K. M., Feng, S. Y., Tan, B. Z., Kit, C. J., Husin, W. N. A.-A. W., Aitizaz, A., Shabbir, M., Khattak, U. F., & Sunday, A. (2024). Afolalu. Exploring Video Games Impact on Mental Health among University (2024). *Pakistan Journal of Life and Social Sciences, 22*(2), 23912–23939. DOI: 10.57239/PJLSS-2024-22.2.001706

Tirocchi, S. (2024). Generation Z, values, and media: From influencers to BeReal, between visibility and authenticity. *Frontiers in Sociology, 8*, 1304093. Advance online publication. DOI: 10.3389/fsoc.2023.1304093 PMID: 38274837

Tischmeyer, W., & Grimm, R. (1999). Activation of immediate early genes and memory formation. *Cellular and Molecular Life Sciences : CMLS, 55*(4), 564–574. DOI: 10.1007/s000180050315

Tobias, S., Fletcher, J. D., & Wind, A. P. (2014). Game-Based Learning. In Spector, J. M., Merrill, M. D., Elen, J., & Bishop, M. J. (Eds.), *Handbook of Research on Educational Communications and Technology* (pp. 485–503). Springer New York., DOI: 10.1007/978-1-4614-3185-5_38

Toda, A. M., Valle, P. H. D., Isotani, S., Cristea, A. I., Bittencourt, I. I., & Lima, F. (2018). The dark side of gamification: An overview of negative effects of gamification in education. In *Higher Education for All: From challenges to novel technology-enhanced solutions* (p. 14). Springer. DOI: 10.1007/978-3-319-97934-2_9

Tokuno, J., Knobovitch, R. M., Botelho, F., Fried, H. B., Carver, T. E., & Fried, G. M. (2025). Immersive Virtual Reality Simulation for Medical Student Procedural Training: Assessment of Cognitive Load and Usability. *Surgical Innovation, 32*(4), 378–384. DOI: 10.1177/15533506251339920 PMID: 40298260

Toral Aguilar, L. (2022). *Notas: «Programación básica»* [Tesis de licenciatura, Tecnológico Nacional de México]. Repositorio Institucional TecNM. https://rinacional.tecnm.mx/handle/TecNM/8191

Torres-Hernández, N., Pessoa, T., & Gallego-Arrufat, M. J. (2019). Intervención y evaluación con tecnologías de la competencia en seguridad digital. *Digital Education Review*, 111–129. DOI: 10.1344/der.2019.35.111-129

Treloar, L. R. G. (2013). *The physics of rubber elasticity* (3rd ed.). Oxford University Press.

Triplett, W. J. (2023). Addressing Cybersecurity Challenges in Education. *International Journal of STEM Education for Sustainability*, *3*(1), 47–67. DOI: 10.53889/ijses.v3i1.132

Türkoğlu, B. (2019). The effect of educational board games training programme on the social skill development of the fourth graders. *Elementary Education Online*, *18*(3), 1326–1344. DOI: 10.17051/ilkonline.2019.612180

U.S. Department of Health and Human Services, Food and Drug Administration, Center for Drug Evaluation and Research. (1997, agosto). *Guía para la industria: Pruebas de disolución de formas de dosificación oral sólidas de liberación inmediata*. https://www.fda.gov/

Ubitus. (2022). *Empowering Surgeons! HuiShu Technology's AI-assisted system and virtual reality platform boost hands-on training for medical students*. Retrieved September 6, 2025 from https://smartsurgerytek.com/empowering-surgeons-huishu-technologys-ai-assisted-system-and-vr-platform-boost-practical-training-for-medical-students/ [REMOVED HYPERLINK FIELD]

Ullah, M., Amin, S. U., Munsif, M., Yamin, M. M., Safaev, U., Khan, H., Khan, S., & Ullah, H. (2022). Serious games in science education: A systematic literature review. *Virtual Reality & Intelligent Hardware*, *4*(3), 189–209. DOI: 10.1016/j.vrih.2022.02.001

UNESCO IESALC. (2024, November 11). *New report: Supporting the mental health of higher education students*. Retrieved from https://www.iesalc.unesco.org/es/articles/nuevo-informe-apoyando-la-salud-mental-de-los-estudiantes-de-educacion-superior

UNESCO. (2020a). *Education for sustainable development: A roadmap*. UNESCO., DOI: 10.54675/YFRE1448

UNESCO. (2020b). Learning through radio and television in the time of COVID-19 [Global Education Coalition]. *Global Education Coalition*. https://en.unesco.org/news/learning-through-radio-and-television-time-covid-19

UNESCO. (2021). *AI and education: Guidance for policy-makers*.

Ungau, S., Nasip, F., Linyaw, K., & Yusop, Y.Tang Tien Mee. (2023). Gamification in Improving Reading Skills of Preschool Children: Blending Through Puzzle Game. *Journal of Cognitive Sciences and Human Development*, *9*(1), 193–220. DOI: 10.33736/jcshd.5479.2023

United Nations. (n.d.). *The Universal Declaration of Human Rights*. United Nations. https://www.un.org/es/about-us/universal-declaration-of-human-rights

UNIVERSAE. (21 de marzo de 2022). La *Gamificación en la educación: concepto y ejemplos*. Recuperado de https://universae.com/en/blog/gamification-in-education/

Universidad de Guadalajara. (2023). *Orientaciones y definiciones sobre el uso de la inteligencia artificial generativa en los procesos académicos: Guía práctica*. Universidad de Guadalajara.

Universidad de Guadalajara. Centro Universitario de Ciencias Exactas e Ingenierías (CUCEI) & Coordinación Licenciatura en Químico Farmacéutico Biólogo. (2025). *Perfil de Ingreso y Egreso*. https://www.cucei.udg.mx/carreras/farmaceutica/es/perfil-de-ingreso-y-egreso

University of Guadalajara. (2023, June 27). *60 percent of CUCS students suffer academic stress*. https://www.udg.mx/es/noticia/sufre-estres-academico-60-por-ciento-de-estudiantes-del-cucs

UN-UNICEF-Uruguay. (2020). *Social networks and adolescents, what you need to know*. Retrieved from https://www.unicef.org/uruguay/crianza/digital/redes-sociales-y-adolescentes-lo-que-tenes-que-saber

Usán Supervía, P., & Salavera Bordás, C. (Eds.). (2020). *Gamificación educativa: Innovación en el aula para potenciar el proceso de enseñanza-aprendizaje*. Pregunta Ediciones. https://dialnet.unirioja.es/servlet/libro?codigo=972682

Valdés Montecinos, M. (2019). Internacionalización del currículo universitario virtual en el contexto de la globalización. *Telos: Revista de Estudios Interdisciplinarios En Ciencias Sociales*, *21*(3), 754–775. DOI: 10.36390/telos213.13

van der Ham, I. J. M., Faber, A. M. E., Venselaar, M., van Kreveld, M. J., & Löffler, M. (2015). Ecological validity of virtual environments to assess human navigation ability. *Frontiers in Psychology*, *6*, 637. DOI: 10.3389/fpsyg.2015.00637

Varela-Aldás, J., Palacios-Navarro, G., Amariglio, R., & García-Magariño, I. (2020). Head-Mounted Display-Based Application for Cognitive Training. *Sensors (Basel)*, *20*(22), 6552. DOI: 10.3390/s20226552

Vargas, F., Restrepo, S., & Tapia, M. (2023). Fomento al hábito por la lectura en estudiantes de educación básica primaria en el Estado de México. (2023). *Revista de Ciencias Sociales*, *3*(3), 282–291. https://www.cienciaysociedaduatf.com/index.php/ciesocieuatf/article/view/97

Varshney, A., Munns, M. E., Kasowski, J., Zhou, M., He, C., Grafton, S. T., Giesbrecht, B., Hegarty, M., & Beyeler, M. (2024). Stress affects navigation strategies in immersive virtual reality. *Scientific Reports*, *14*(1), 5949. DOI: 10.1038/s41598-024-56048-8

Venkatesh, V., Thong, J. Y. L., & Xu, X. (2012). Consumer Acceptance and Use of Information Technology: Extending the Unified Theory of Acceptance and Use of Technology. *Management Information Systems Quarterly*, *36*(1), 157–178. DOI: 10.2307/41410412

Vera Velázquez, R., Maldonado Zúñiga, K., Castro Piguave, C., & Batista Garcet, Y. (2021). Metodología del aprendizaje basado en problemas como una herramienta para el logro del proceso de enseñanza- aprendizaje: Metodología del aprendizaje basado en problemas. *Sinapsis: La revista científica del ITSUP, 1*(19), 15. DOI: 10.37117/s.v19i1.465

Vera-Monroy, S. P., Mejía-Camacho, A., & Gamboa Mora, M. C. (2020). C=OCAR-BOHIDRATOS: Efecto del juego sobre el aprendizaje. *Educación en la Química*, *31*(1), 23–35. DOI: 10.22201/fq.18708404e.2020.1.68522

Vieira, I. H. P., Botelho, E. B., de Souza Gomes, T. J., Kist, R., Caceres, R. A., & Zanchi, F. B. (2023). Visual dynamics: A WEB application for molecular dynamics simulation using GROMACS. *BMC Bioinformatics*, *24*(1), 107. DOI: 10.1186/s12859-023-05234-y PMID: 36949402

Villamil, J. (2013). Entre 108 países, México es penúltimo lugar en lectura. Revista Proceso. Retrieved from_https://www.proceso.com.mx/339874/entre-108-paises-mexico-es-penultimo-lugar-en-lectura

VirtaMed. (n.d.). ArthroSTM. Retrieved September 6, 2025, from https://www.virtamed.com/en/products-and-solutions/simulators/arthros

VirtaMed. (s.f.). VirtaMed ArthroSTM Tobillo [Video]. YouTube. https://www.youtube.com/watch?v=psXNC2XrLS0

Vita-Barrull, N., Estrada-Plana, V., March-Llanes, J., Sotoca-Orgaz, P., Guzmán, N., Ayesa, R., & Moya-Higueras, J. (2024). Do you play in class? Board games to promote cognitive and educational development in primary school: A cluster randomized controlled trial. *Learning and Instruction*, *93*, 101946. DOI: 10.1016/j.learninstruc.2024.101946

Vygotsky, L. S. (1978). *Mind in society: The development of higher psychological processes* (Cole, M., John-Steiner, V., Scribner, S., & Souberman, E., Eds.). Harvard University Press., DOI: 10.2307/j.ctvjf9vz4

Wang, E. H. J., Lai, F. H. Y., Leung, W. M., Shiu, T. Y., Wong, H., Tao, Y., Zhao, X., Zhang, T. Y. T., & Yee, B. K. (2025). Assessing rapid spatial working memory in community-living older adults in a virtual adaptation of the rodent water maze paradigm. *Behavioural Brain Research*, *476*, 115266. DOI: 10.1016/j.bbr.2024.115266

Wanniarachchi, V. U., Greenhalgh, C., Choi, A., & Warren, J. R. (2025). Personalization variables in digital mental health interventions for depression and anxiety in adolescents and youth: A scoping review. *Frontiers in Digital Health*, *7*, 1500220. DOI: 10.3389/fdgth.2025.1500220 PMID: 40444184

Weber, C., Sipos, M., Paczal, A., Balint, B., Kun, V., Foloppe, N., Dokurno, P., Massey, A. J., Walmsley, D. L., Hubbard, R. E., Murray, J., Benwell, K., Edmonds, T., Demarles, D., Bruno, A., Burbridge, M., Cruzalegui, F., & Kotschy, A. (2021). Structure-Guided Discovery of Potent and Selective DYRK1A Inhibitors. *Journal of Medicinal Chemistry*, *64*(10), 6745–6764. DOI: 10.1021/acs.jmedchem.1c00023 PMID: 33975430

Wehmeyer, M. L., Palmer, S. B., Smith, S. J., Davies, D. K., & Stock, S. (2008). The efficacy of technology use by people with intellectual disability: A single-subject design meta-analysis. *Journal of Special Education Technology*, *23*(3), 21–30. DOI: 10.1177/016264340802300303

Weinstein, A., & Lejoyeux, M. (2020). Neurobiological mechanisms underlying internet gaming disorder. *Dialogues in Clinical Neuroscience*, *22*(2), 113–126. DOI: 10.31887/DCNS.2020.22.2/aweinstein PMID: 32699511

Weiss, P. L. T., Bialik, P., & Kizony, R. (2003). Virtual reality provides leisure time opportunities for young adults with physical and intellectual disabilities. *Cyberpsychology & Behavior*, *6*(3), 335–342. DOI: 10.1089/109493103322011650

Werbach, K., & Hunter, D. (2012). *For the win*. Wharton Digital Press.

Werbach, K., & Hunter, D. (2015). *The Gamification Toolkit: Dynamics, Mechanics, and Components for the Win*. Wharton Digital Press.

Wiebe, A., Kannen, K., Selaskowski, B., Mehren, A., Thöne, A.-K., Pramme, L., Blumenthal, N., Li, M., Asché, L., Jonas, S., Bey, K., Schulze, M., Steffens, M., Pensel, M. C., Guth, M., Rohlfsen, F., Ekhlas, M., Lügering, H., Fileccia, H., & Braun, N. (2022). Virtual reality in the diagnostic and therapy for mental disorders: A systematic review. *Clinical Psychology Review*, *98*, 102213. DOI: 10.1016/j.cpr.2022.102213

Wiggins, B. E. (2016). An Overview and Study on the Use of Games, Simulations, and Gamification in Higher Education. *International Journal of Game-Based Learning*, *6*(1), 18–29. DOI: 10.4018/IJGBL.2016010102

World Health Organization. (2021). *International statistical classification of diseases and related health problems* (5th ed.). https://icd.who.int

Wu, K., Kwon, S. H., Zhou, X., Fuller, C., Wang, X., Vadgama, J., & Wu, Y. (2024). Overcoming Challenges in Small-Molecule Drug Bioavailability: A Review of Key Factors and Approaches. *International Journal of Molecular Sciences, 25*(23), 13121. Advance online publication. DOI: 10.3390/ijms252313121

Xu, D., Hao, X., Wang, Z., Duan, Y., Liu, F., Marsh, R., Yu, S., & Peterson, B. S. (2012). A Virtual Radial Arm Maze for the Study of Multiple Memory Systems in a Functional Magnetic Resonance Imaging Environment. *The International Journal of Virtual Reality : a Multimedia Publication for Professionals, 11*(2), 63–76. DOI: 10.20870/IJVR.2012.11.2.2844

Yacoub, M. S. W., & Holton, A. J. (2023). Development and implementation of an online narrative game to aid studying and review in an online general chemistry course. *Journal of Chemical Education, 100*(9), 3688–3693. DOI: 10.1021/acs.jchemed.3c00266

Zamani, S., Rostami, A., Nguyen, M., Sinha, R., & Madanian, S. (2025). A Gamified AI-Driven Systemfor Depression Monitoringand Management. *Applied Sciences (Basel, Switzerland), 15*(13), 7088. DOI: 10.3390/app15137088

Zdrazil, B., Felix, E., Hunter, F., Manners, E. J., Blackshaw, J., Corbett, S., de Veij, M., Ioannidis, H., Lopez, D. M., Mosquera, J. F., Magarinos, M. P., Bosc, N., Arcila, R., Kizilören, T., Gaulton, A., Bento, A. P., Adasme, M. F., Monecke, P., Landrum, G. A., & Leach, A. R. (2024). The ChEMBL Database in 2023: A drug discovery platform spanning multiple bioactivity data types and time periods. *Nucleic Acids Research, 52*(D1), D1180–D1192. DOI: 10.1093/nar/gkad1004 PMID: 37933841

Zembylas, M. (2023). The decolonisation of humanising pedagogies in higher education: Implications for culturally responsive pedagogies. In *Global Perspectives and New Challenges in Culturally Responsive Pedagogies* (pp. 36–49). Routledge., DOI: 10.4324/9781003335719-5

Zendle, D., & Cairns, P. (2019). Loot boxes are again linked to problem gambling: Results of a replication study. *PLoS One, 14*(3), e0213194. DOI: 10.1371/journal.pone.0213194 PMID: 30845155

Zepeda Hurtado, M. E., Cardoso Espinoso, E. O., & Cortés Ruiz, J. A. (2019). El aprendizaje orientado en proyectos para el desarrollo de habilidades blandas en el nivel medio superior del IPN. *RIDE Revista Iberoamericana para la Investigación y el Desarrollo Educativo, 10*(19). Advance online publication. DOI: 10.23913/ride.v10i19.530

Zhang, J., Sabatier, J.-M., Chahine, M., & Tricarico, D. (2024). Editorial: Reviews in pharmacology of ion channels and channelopathies. *Frontiers in Pharmacology, 15*, 1449967. Advance online publication. DOI: 10.3389/fphar.2024.1449967 PMID: 39228529

About the Contributors

José Luis David Bonilla Carranza holds a Doctorate in Electronic and Computer Sciences from the University of Guadalajara's Center for Exact Sciences and Engineering (CUCEI-UDG), Mexico. He currently serves as a Professor in the Department of Innovation Based on Information and Knowledge at CUCEI-UDG, where he teaches courses on programming, video game development, and emerging technologies. His academic and professional endeavors are deeply rooted in his affiliation with the University of Guadalajara, an institution where he actively contributes to research projects and technological initiatives aimed at bridging academia with industry. A visionary scholar at the intersection of technology and education, Dr. Bonilla Carranza has dedicated his career to advancing innovative pedagogical tools. His research focuses on integrating artificial intelligence (AI), serious games, and virtual reality (VR) to enhance STEM (Science, Technology, Engineering, and Mathematics) education. Notably, he pioneered frameworks for leveraging AI platforms like ChatGPT as dynamic aids in cultivating critical STEM skills, emphasizing their role in fostering interactive and adaptive learning environments. His work on serious games has redefined competency assessments for Industry 4.0, offering novel methodologies to evaluate professional skills through immersive game-based simulations. Additionally, he has explored the pedagogical potential of open-source software and VR, publishing influential studies on their application in designing educational video games. Beyond his core focus, Dr. Bonilla Carranza has collaborated on interdisciplinary projects, including the use of nanoparticles and hydrogels to optimize agricultural processes, showcasing his commitment to addressing real-world challenges through technology. Professionally, he is a founding member of the College of Information Systems Professionals of Jalisco (COPSIJAL) and COPSIAL, organizations dedicated to advancing professional standards in information technology. His industry experience includes leadership roles at Mexico's Federal Electricity Commission (CFE), where he spearheaded system development projects and technological process improvements.

Recognized for his dynamic teaching style, Dr. Bonilla Carranza consistently receives outstanding evaluations from students, who praise his clarity, enthusiasm, and dedication to mentoring the next generation of technologists. Looking ahead, he is exploring the synergy between computational logic and interactive learning, designing video games that cultivate software engineering skills—a testament to his unwavering commitment to adaptive education and applied technology. Dr. Bonilla Carranza's legacy lies in his ability to merge academic rigor with practical innovation, shaping both the minds of future professionals and the tools that will drive tomorrow's technological advancements.

Adriana Peña Pérez Negrón holds a Ph.D. in Computer Science from the Technical University of Madrid (2009) and currently serves as a Research Professor in the Department of Electronics and Computing at the University of Guadalajara's Center for Exact Sciences and Engineering (CUCEI-UDG) in Mexico. At CUCEI-UDG, she teaches courses such as Experimental and Statistical Design and leads interdisciplinary research at the crossroads of virtual environments, artificial intelligence (AI), and education. A founding member of the College of Information Systems Professionals of Jalisco (COPSIJAL), she also contributes to the academic community as the Editor-in-Chief of ReCIBE, a peer-reviewed journal focused on computing, biomedicine, and electronics. Dr. Peña Pérez Negrón is a pioneering scholar in collaborative virtual environments, virtual reality (VR), and AI-driven educational tools. Her research bridges theoretical innovation and practical applications, with notable contributions including the development of frameworks for analyzing nonverbal communication in avatars—advancements that enhance human collaboration in digital spaces. Her work, published in leading journals such as Virtual Reality and Journal on Multimodal User Interfaces, has redefined how virtual interactions are designed and understood. A strong advocate for technology's role in education, she has spearheaded projects integrating VR and open-source software to create educational video games, including methodologies for training professionals in Industry 4.0 competencies. Her interdisciplinary approach extends to gamifying international software engineering standards (e.g., ISO/IEC 29110) for academic settings in Mexico, fostering best practices in software development teams. Beyond education, she has contributed to smart city frameworks using big data algorithms and sentiment analysis in Spanish, offering scalable solutions for urban decision-making. Committed to diversity in STEM, Dr. Peña Pérez Negrón co-edited Latin American Women and Research Contributions to the IT Field (2020), a groundbreaking anthology highlighting women's leadership in technology across Latin America. Her editorial leadership also includes Virtual Reality Designs (2020), a seminal text exploring VR applications in behavioral analysis and education. With over 50 publications in indexed journals and international conferences, she has collaborated on projects ranging from synthetic perception in autonomous characters to nanoparticle applications in agriculture, underscoring her dedication to solving societal challenges through technology. Recognized for her visionary scholarship, she continues to explore the synergies between VR, gamification, and collaborative learning, aiming to cultivate high-performing teams in software engineering. Her work not only advances academic discourse but also empowers industries and communities, cementing her legacy as a researcher who transcends disciplinary boundaries to drive innovation in education, equity, and technology.

Marco Antonio Pérez-Cisneros holds a Ph.D. in Science from the University of Manchester's Institute of Science and Technology (UMIST), United Kingdom, awarded in 2004. He currently serves as a Professor and Dean of the Electronics and Computer Science Division at the University of Guadalajara's Center for Exact Sciences and Engineering (CUCEI-UDG), Mexico. A distinguished member of Mexico's National Research System (SNI) and the Mexican Academy of Sciences, he is also affiliated with prominent international organizations such as the Institute of Electrical and Electronics Engineers (IEEE) and the Institution of Engineering and Technology (IET). Dr. Pérez-Cisneros is a leading scholar in computational intelligence and evolutionary algorithms, with a prolific career spanning robotics, computer vision, automated control, and medical technology. His research has yielded over 130 indexed publications and seven authoritative textbooks, establishing him as a pivotal figure in applied computational methodologies. Among his groundbreaking contributions are the development of the Whale Optimization Algorithm and the Water Strider Algorithm, innovative metaheuristic frameworks designed to tackle complex multi-objective engineering challenges. His work in medical image analysis, particularly his metaheuristic approaches to COVID-19 detection and machine learning models for diagnosing conditions like flatfoot disease, underscores his commitment to merging technology with healthcare solutions. A pioneer in image processing, Dr. Pérez-Cisneros has advanced techniques for contrast enhancement, multi-level segmentation, and thermal analysis using nature-inspired algorithms. His interdisciplinary collaborations extend to smart city initiatives, where he applies agent-based modeling and big data analytics to optimize urban safety and energy efficiency. Beyond research, he is a dedicated educator and advocate for technological literacy. As co-editor of Virtual Reality Designs (2020), he explores virtual reality's potential in behavioral studies and education, while his textbooks on computational intelligence serve as foundational resources for students and professionals alike. Currently, Dr. Pérez-Cisneros focuses on AI-driven systems for emergency evacuation planning and gamified educational tools, reflecting his vision of technology as a force for societal advancement. Recognized for his rigorous scholarship and leadership, he continues to mentor emerging engineers and shape the future of computational intelligence, leaving an indelible mark on both academia and industry.

***

Pablo A. Alcaraz Valencia is a professor of the Universidad de Colima, who specializes in technologies for supporting second language learning. He has more than 5 years of experience as a developer.

Daisy Alvarado is an occupational therapist and occupational scientist in El Paso, Texas. Her research focuses on understanding occupational identity and the biopsychosocial mechanisms of occupation that impact health and well-being. Her teaching emphasizes the importance of blending research and practice skills. She currently serves as a faculty member in the University of Texas at El Paso's Department of Occupational Therapy. Dr. Alvarado was recently recognized as a 2025 Change Maker: Borderland Woman in Health for her contributions to research and practice in occupational therapy at UTEP and in the borderland. Her scholarly contributions include national and international conference presentations and publications in journals, such as Psychosomatic Medicine and the Scandinavian Journal of Occupational Therapy. She serves as a special volunteer researcher for the National Institutes of Health Clinical Center and secretary of the Society for the Study of Occupation: USA.

Jesús Cabral-Araiza, Graduate in psychology. Mr. in Education from ITESM Guadalajara campus, PhD in Sciences for Sustainable Development from CUCOSTA-UdeG. Member of the Academic Body CA: 1130 Biolaw, Bioethics, Education and Human Rights. His academic work is related to the use of technologies for learning and various aspects of applied bioethics. Likewise, he maintains research on ethical aspects and clinical psychology in areas of social psychology, including gentrification, thanatology, and artificial intelligence. He serves as director of the Bachelor's Degree in Psychology at the Puerto Vallarta campus of the University of Guadalajara.

Madeleine Contreras holds a PhD in Systems and Educational Environments from the University of Guadalajara (Mexico). She is a professor in virtual programs at CUCEA-UDG and CUGDL-UDG, participating in educational and organizational development projects and teaching emotional intelligence. She also collaborates in the Master's program in Family Relational Therapy at the University of Valle de Atemajac. Her research focuses on learning in virtual environments, communicative and psychological processes from an ecosystem approach, and the use of serious games in education, mental health, and non-profit contexts. She has published on interdisciplinary collaborative work and collaborates as a clinical psychologist with the Ministry of Health. She practices psychotherapy in public and private settings, with research interests in group work, gender perspective, violence, and vulnerable populations.

Karla Cruz Vera In 2022, she joined as a professor at the University of Guadalajara. She is a full member of the College of Psychology Professionals of the State of Jalisco, a founding and full member of the Mexican Association of Psychologists A.C., where she is responsible for the children's area at the state and national levels. She holds a Bachelor's degree in Psychology from the University of Guadalajara. In 2023, she was awarded the Professional Merit Award in Psychology in the Golden Psyche category in the field of Educational Psychology by the Alumni Society of the Bachelor's Degree in Psychology of the University of Guadalajara, A.C. She has given lectures at CPPEJAC, UNIVA, and INAESA, holds the title of Peace Manager, and is a member of the Peace Managers Network. She is currently pursuing a Master's degree in Health Sciences Education, collaborates with the Academic Body CA-990 called Applied Data Science, and teaches at CUCEI in the Department of Innovation Based on Information and Knowledge.

Nelson Bruno Cunha, Ph.D. in Behavioral Sciences with a specialization in Behavior Analysis from the University of Guadalajara, Mexico. Master's degree in Cognitive Neuroscience and Behavior from the Federal University of Paraíba, Brazil. Bachelor's degree in Pharmacy from the State University of Paraíba, Brazil. Main line of research focuses on addictions. I have produced scientific publications and disseminated knowledge at national and international conferences. My research emphasizes the pharmacological, neurobiological, and behavioral aspects of addictions, as well as the use of natural substances for the treatment of smoking.

Jose Juan Espinosa holds a degree in Communications and Electronics Engineering from the Faculty of Engineering of the University of Guadalajara. He also holds a Bachelor's degree in Mathematics from the Universidad Abierta y a Distancia de México (UNADM), a Master's degree in Electrical Engineering from the Center for Research and Advanced Studies of the National Polytechnic Institute (CINVESTAV), and a Doctorate in Educational Competencies Development from IPESUJ. He is currently a researcher and professor in the Department of Computer Science and is a member of the Academic Body CA-990 called Applied Data Science.

José Luis Fernández, Professor affiliated with the Department of Information Systems at the University Center for Economic and Administrative Sciences of the University of Guadalajara. He holds a Ph.D. in Information Technologies (2018) and a Master's degree in Learning Technologies (2012) from the University of Guadalajara. His teaching areas include IT Project Management, IT Service Management, Graphic Design, and Video Editing. He also collaborates with university professors in seminars on instructional design and the development of educational materials. His research interests focus on the planning and development of educational materials for teaching children in primary education, particularly the use of video games (serious games) for teaching mathematics.

David Fernández Quezada is a Professor and Researcher at the University of Guadalajara (CUCS) with a Ph.D. in Biomedical Sciences specializing in Neurosciences. He has authored multiple peer-reviewed articles and book chapters. His research focuses on developing virtual reality environments for studying cognition and behavior and implementing machine learning models based on digital biomarkers for applications in biomedical sciences.

Abraham Figueroa is a Digital Animation and Visual Effects Engineer with a Master's degree in 3D Organic Modeling. His passion for animation and 3D modeling has led him to explore different areas, from character and environment creation to product and space visualization. His goal is to continue innovating and refining his skills to deliver high-quality results and meet the needs of both his clients and students.

Jorge Jesus Galvez Rodriguez obtained his Ph.D. degree from the University of Guadalajara, Mexico. He currently is an associate professor at the University of Guadalajara. His research interests include evolutionary computation, computer vision, computer graphic, virtual reality and robotics.

Miguel A. Garcia-Ruiz graduated in Computer Systems engineering and obtained his MSc in Computer Science from the University of Colima, Mexico. Miguel received his PhD in Computer Science and Artificial Intelligence from the Centre for Research in Cognitive Science (COGS), University of Sussex, UK. Dr. Miguel Garcia-Ruiz took a virtual reality workshop at Salford University, England, and a computer graphics techniques internship at the Madrid Polytechnic University, Spain. Dr. Miguel Garcia-Ruiz has published various books and many scientific papers in academic journals, and has directed a video documentary about an introduction to virtual reality. Dr. Miguel was a Visiting Professor at the Faculty of Business and IT of the University of Ontario, Canada, where he participated in a research project on combating social deviations with technology, He was an Assistant Professor with the School of Telematics, University of Colima, Mexico. Currently, Miguel is a Full Professor with the Faculty of Computer Science and

Technology from Algoma University, Canada. Dr. Garcia-Ruiz was a member of Mexico's National System of Researchers (SNI) of the National Council of Science and Technology (CONACYT), and was awarded the Innovation Educator of the Year, given by the Sault Ste. Marie Innovation Centre (SSMIC) in 2015.

Francisco Gonzalez holds a degree in Computer Systems Engineering from the Instituto Tecnológico Superior de Chapala and a Master's in Computer Graphics Processing. With more than twenty years of professional experience, he has specialized in the development of interactive, three-dimensional, and immersive environments, as well as in the application of advanced visualization and graphics processing techniques. His career combines both research and applied practice, focused on the design and optimization of computer systems that drive innovative digital experiences.

Armando Ariel Gutierrez Lopez, Graduated in Psychology from the University Center of the Coast of the University of Guadalajara, currently a professor at the Valles del Tintoque Educational Group at the High School and University levels, as well as a collaborator of CA: 1130 Biolaw, Bioethics, Education and Human Rights, participating in various research projects for the publication of Magazine Articles, Book Chapters, giving conferences and workshops, as well as the organization of academic and cultural events

Jacqueline Gutiérrez, Graduate in psychology. Master in systemic family therapy. University of the Atejamac Valley. Mexico. Doctorate in Educational Systems and Environments. Professor at UNIVA in Postgraduate Studies and at the University of Guadalajara in Undergraduate Studies. Clinical psychologist for the Secretary of Health in mental health promotion, different programs, bullying, suicide prevention, gender violence, among others. Individual, family and couples psychotherapy.

Humberto Gutiérrez Pulido, Professor of Mathematics at CUCEI, University of Guadalajara (UdG). He earned his Master's and PhD in Probability and Statistics from CIMAT (Mexico), and his Bachelor's degree in Mathematics from UdG. He holds Level I distinction of the Mexican National System of Researchers (SNI), a recognition first awarded in 2004. He is the author of more than 10 books, several of them published by McGraw-Hill, which are used as textbooks across Latin America and Spain. He has published over 70 research articles and has received more than 11,000 citations on Google Scholar. He has provided training and consulting services to various companies and institutions in Mexico and Latin America, and has held leadership positions within the Government of Jalisco and the University of Guadalajara.

Rosaura Hernández Montelongo is a tenured professor and researcher at the Department of Translational Bioengineering, CUCEI (University of Guadalajara). Her academic work focuses on the development and application of new materials and biomaterials, with particular emphasis on polymers, composites, and hydrogels aimed at both aqueous contaminant removal and biomedical applications. Her scientific production covers topics such as polymer synthesis and modification, the use of smart materials for heavy metal capture, mathematical modeling of diffusion and transport processes, and the application of image analysis techniques in biology and agriculture. She also participates in interdisciplinary projects related to materials engineering and applied bioengineering.

Salvador H.-V. earned his B.Sc. in Physics and Artificial Intelligence from the Universidad Veracruzana, his M.Sc. in Electrical Engineering from the Universidad Autónoma de San Luis Potosí, and his Ph.D. in Physics from the Universidad de Guanajuato, where he specialized in the computational simulation of soft condensed matter. He has been a full-time faculty member at the Instituto Tecnológico Superior de Xalapa for more than eleven years, with research interests spanning soft condensed matter simulation, biomolecular systems, and computer programming education.

Miguel Hidalgo-Reyes, PhD in Computer Science with experience in research and technological development. His research interests are data mining, usability in software development and information visualization. He has participated in national and international forums and has published in scientific journals and digital media. He is currently a SECIHTI researcher at the Institute of Ecology, participating in the data governance, data repositories and data science projects.

María Isabel Mendoza-Rodríguez holds a Master degree degree in Psychology, with a Master's degree in Sexuality and Gender Equity from UMEP, a PhD student in Inclusion, Public Policy and Research from UMEP. Teacher for 11 years at the Preparatory level of the University of Guadalajara, currently with a management position as Secretary of the Regional High School of Ixtlahuacán de los Membrillos.

Guillermo Jiménez-Hernández holds a B.A. in Arts and an M.Sc. in Bioengineering and Intelligent Computing. He is currently pursuing a Ph.D. in Electronics and Computer Science. His research focuses on digital creativity for science communication, exploring innovative methodologies that merge generative algorithms, interactive media, and educational design to make complex scientific concepts more accessible to diverse audiences.

Julio César Llamas Alonso is a cognitive neuroscientist and experimental psychologist. His research focuses on the neurophysiological and cognitive bases of video game practice, as well as involuntary cognitive processes. He is passionate about video games, particularly those with rich narratives and role-playing elements.

Luis A. Llamas-Alonso is a psychologist with a Ph.D. in Behavioral Neuroscience and a professor specializing in psychophysiology, with expertise in EEG and eye-tracking techniques. His research focuses on the effects of video gaming on cognition, emotion and brain dynamics. He is deeply passionate about video games.

Sonia Elizabeth Martínez Solís is a Computer Systems Engineer, trained at the Higher Technological Institute of Chapala, with a specialization in the Development of Teaching Skills from the Technological Institute of Advanced Education. She also holds a Diploma in Teaching Competencies at the high school level from the Western Institute of Technology and Higher Studies. She has participated in state-level educational science conferences and is an active member of experimental clubs in the institutions where she collaborates. Her professional work in education has provided her with tools to understand technological advances and to foster collaborative learning with her students. She is deeply committed to teaching and is passionate about promoting learning, exploration, and curiosity in the classroom.

José Martínez Chávez. Surgeon Midwife. University of Guadalajara. Medical Specialist in General Surgery. University of Guadalajara. Medical Specialist in Abdominal Organ Transplantation. Mexican Social Security Institute. Nanotechnology Engineer. University of Guadalajara. Teacher of the Didactics in Health Sciences program. Anahuac University Mexico. Master in Health Sciences Education. University of Guadalajara. Master degree in Health Services Administration program. Institute Veracruzano of the Health Services Administration program. Veracruzano University Institute. Physician assigned to the abdominal organ transplant program of the Centro Médico de Occidente.

Diana Emilia Martínez, PhD, has developed a distinguished scientific career at the intersection of immunogenetics, neuroimmunology, bioinformatics, and analytical sciences, with a transdisciplinary vision that bridges molecular research and applied innovation. Her research contributions span across immunology, chronic degenerative diseases.

Luis Medellín has been a professor at the University of Guadalajara since 2001 and is a founding member of the College of Information Systems Professionals of Jalisco. He holds a bachelor's degree in Computer Science and a master's degree in Information Systems from the University of Guadalajara. As part of a team with other professors, he won the Jalisco State Award for Innovation, Science, and

Technology in the Outreach category. He has given lectures at ANIEI (National Institute of Information Technology), published popular books, and co-authored articles in academic journals in Mexico. He has collaborated with the Center for Data Analysis and Supercomputing (CADS) to provide support and collaboration, and is the Coordinator of Artificial Intelligence. He is currently a full-time professor at the CUCEI and CUCEA universities. He belongs to the CA-990 academic body called Applied Data Science.

Laura E. Mendoza is an Assistant Professor of Instruction in the Department of Chicano Studies, Languages, and Linguistics at the University of Texas at El Paso. She holds a Ph.D. in Literacy and Biliteracy, and her research and teaching focus on inclusive pedagogies that foster belonging and success for emergent bilinguals and transnational students. With over a decade of experience as a language educator, Dr. Mendoza integrates culturally responsive teaching, open educational resources, and innovative practices—such as learning communities and gamification—into her classroom and scholarship.

Elba Abigail Morales Vanegas is a professor at the School of Telematics at the Universidad de Colima, Mexico. She holds a Ph.D. in Economic and Administrative Sciences, two master's degrees in Transparency and Personal Data Protection and in Engineering, as well as degrees in Law and Telematics Engineering. Her multidisciplinary background bridges legal, technological, and ethical perspectives, with research focused on the societal impact of Artificial Intelligence and Industry 4.0, transparency, and personal data protection. She has participated as a speaker in local and national forums and has published in peer-reviewed journals and books on privacy-aware design of intelligent applications and privacy-centered artificial intelligence. Her work reflects a strong commitment to responsible, human-centered technological solutions that respect fundamental rights.

Carmen Leticia Salcedo-Quevedo is a university professor with more than 17 years of teaching experience. She has completed her doctoral training in Pedagogy and Research and is a full-time professor at the Instituto Tecnológico de Jalisco, Chapala campus. Her professional background is in Computer Systems Engineering at both undergraduate and master's levels. Throughout her career, she has worked in the field of Business Intelligence, enabling her to integrate technology with strategic decision-making. She also engages in continuous training in data science to strengthen her academic and professional profile at the intersection of education and technology. She is the leader of the academic body Applied Technology, Animation, and Robotics.

María Ramirez Jimenez, University professor, researcher, and technologist with more than 18 years of experience at the University of Guadalajara. Specialist in cybersecurity, databases, and programming, she has developed innovative projects such as the Mi Protector Digital platform. Her work combines teaching, research, and educational innovation aimed at digital transformation and the responsible training of new generations.

Carolina Livier Recio Colmenares is a distinguished researcher and member of the National System of Researchers in Mexico, recognized as a Candidate for National Researcher for the period 2022-2025. Her expertise lies in the field of Design and Optimization of Advanced Materials, contributing to the Lines of Generation and Application of Knowledge at the University of Guadalajara, specifically within the Department of Water and Energy Studies. In addition to her research endeavors, Dr. Recio Colmenares is the Program Coordinator for the bachelor's degree in Energy Engineering at the University of Guadalajara. Dr. Recio Colmenares holds a bachelor's degree in chemical engineering, a master's degree in water and energy engineering, and a Doctorate in Water and Energy, all from the University of Guadalajara. Her current research interests are ecological remediation using advanced materials and energy efficiency. Dr. Recio-Colmenares is a Member of IEEE.

Roxana Berenice Recio-Colmenares was born in Guadalajara, Mexico, in 1988. She received the B.S. degree in industrial engineering, in 2012, and the M.S. degree in water and energy engineering and the Ph.D. degree in water and energy from the Centro Universitario de Tonalá, Universidad de Guadalajara, in 2015 and 2021, respectively. She also completed a postdoctoral fellowship with the Environmental Technology Unit, CIATEJ. Since 2018, she has been a Professor with the Centro Universitario de Tonalá, Universidad de Guadalajara, in the Division of Engineering and Technological Innovation. She has excelled in her involvement in technological and environmental development projects, including as the Project Manager for the FORDECYT 190603 Project with UNAM, focused on solar drying plants. She has contributed with an international patent ("Modular Air Heater") and book chapters, such as Artificial Neural Networks for Engineering Applications and Thermal Applications of Solar Energy in Industrial Sectors. She is also a Candidate in the Mexican National System of Researchers (SNI) and actively participates in academic and technological initiatives to promote sustainability. Her research interests include applied neural networks, technology, and sustainability, emphasizing innovative solutions for agro-industrial and environmental processes.

Martín Rivera holds a Doctorate in Educational Competencies Development from IPESUJ, and earned her degree in Computer Engineering and a Master's in Strategic Quality Management from the University of Guadalajara. She is currently a researcher, professor, and CISCO instructor at the University of Guadalajara in the Department of Computer Science, and a professor in the Master's in Information Technologies program at CUCEA. Her areas of interest are computer networks, computer architecture, quality management, and educational research. Furthermore, she is a member of the Academic Body CA-990 called Applied Data Science.

Sergio Rivera-Tello is a biomedical engineer with a Ph.D. in Neurosciences and a current professor specializing in EEG and cognitive neuroscience. His research bridges engineering and brain science, focusing on the neural mechanisms of time perception, attention, and working memory. He is also an enthusiastic board game player.

María Teresa Romero Gutiérrez is a Professor at the University Center of Tlajomulco, University of Guadalajara. She holds a degree in Pharmaceutical Chemistry and Biology, a Master's in Medical Sciences, and a Ph.D. in Biomedical Sciences. She is a member of the National System of Researchers (Level I), with an academic record that includes 19 JCR-indexed articles, one book chapter, and an H-index of 9. Her research focuses on venom systems, the design of bioinspired artifacts, and the study of neurodevelopmental disorders through multi-omic approaches. Her objective is to advance scientific and medical knowledge in ways that generate a positive impact on society.

Pedro C. Santana Mancilla is a full professor at the School of Telematics at the Universidad de Colima in Mexico. He earned his Ph.D. in Information and Communications Technology from the University of Vigo (Spain), a Master's degree in Engineering from the Autonomous University of Baja California (Mexico), and a degree in Telematics Engineering from the Universidad de Colima (Mexico). His research focuses on Human-Computer Interaction, intelligent systems and environments, the Internet of Things, smart transportation, and the development of support technologies for older adults and learning. He is a level 2 member of the National System of Researchers (SNII) of the Ministry of Science, Humanities, Technology, and Innovation (SECIHTI). He is a member of the Mexican Academy of Computing, where he coordinates the Academic Section on Human-Computer Interaction. Additionally, he serves as the president of the Mexican Association of Human-Computer Interaction and leads the research group "UCOL-CA-118: Intelligent, Interactive, and Accessible Environments" at the School of Telematics.

His scientific work includes publications in books, journals, and conferences nationally and internationally.

Yajaira Zepeda-García is a PhD student at the University of Guadalajara. Her research focuses on computational chemistry, with emphasis on drug delivery systems. She is part of the Biodigital Innovation Lab, an interdisciplinary research group that integrates biology, computation and design to explore innovative solucions at the intersection of science and technology. She collaborates in science culture and outreach initiatives to promote public engagement with research.

Index

A

B

C

D

E

G

H

I

L

M

N

P

R

S

T

U

V

www.ingramcontent.com/pod-product-compliance
Lightning Source LLC
LaVergne TN
LVHW061530290926
849162LV00004B/742